DIALYSIS ACCESS

A MULTIDISCIPLINARY APPROACH

DIALYSIS ACCESS

A MULTIDISCIPLINARY APPROACH

Editor

RICHARD J. GRAY, M.D. F.S.C.V.I.R.

Clinical Director, Interventional Radiology
Washington Hospital Center
Washington, DC

Assistant Editor

JEFFREY J. SANDS, M.D.

Vice President
Vascular Access Programs
Fresenius Medical Care, NA
Winter Park, Florida

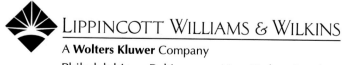

LIPPINCOTT WILLIAMS & WILKINS
A **Wolters Kluwer** Company
Philadelphia • Baltimore • New York • London
Buenos Aires • Hong Kong • Sydney • Tokyo

Acquisitions Editor: Beth Barry
Developmental Editor: Pamela Sutton
Production Editor: Jonathan Geffner
Manufacturing Manager: Colin Warnock
Cover Designer: Christine Jenney
Compositor: Maryland Composition
Printer: Maple Press

Library of Congress Cataloging-in-Publication Data
Dialysis access : a multidisciplinary approach / [edited by] Richard J. Gray, Jeffrey J. Sands.
   p.; cm.
  Includes bibliographical references and index.
  ISBN 0-7817-3100-3 (alk. paper)
   1. Hemodialysis. 2. Arteriovenous shunts, Surgical. I. Gray, Richard J. (Richard James) II. Sands, Jeffrey J.
  [DNLM: 1. Renal Dialysis—methods. 2. Dialysis—methods. WJ 378 D53408 2002]
  RC901.7.H45 D5223 2002
  617.4′61059—dc21
                                            2002018389

Care has been taken to confirm the accuracy of the information presented and to describe generally accepted practices. However, the authors, editors, and publisher are not responsible for errors or omissions or for any consequences from application of the information in this book and make no warranty, expressed or implied, with respect to the currency, completeness, or accuracy of the contents of the publication. Application of this information in a particular situation remains the professional responsibility of the practitioner.

The authors, editors, and publisher have exerted every effort to ensure that drug selection and dosage set forth in this text are in accordance with current recommendations and practice at the time of publication. However, in view of ongoing research, changes in government regulations, and the constant flow of information relating to drug therapy and drug reactions, the reader is urged to check the package insert for each drug for any change in indications and dosage and for added warnings and precautions. This is particularly important when the recommended agent is a new or infrequently employed drug.

Some drugs and medical devices presented in this publication have Food and Drug Administration (FDA) clearance for limited use in restricted research settings. It is the responsibility of the health care provider to ascertain the FDA status of each drug or device planned for use in their clinical practice.

10 9 8 7 6 5 4 3 2

To my wonderful children, Alexis and Austin, who light up my life;
and my loving wife, Denise, for her unlimited understanding
and support of the academic endeavors that awaken me
in the hours that precede the sunrise.

Richard Gray

To my wife Lynn, whose love and support makes everything possible;
my children, Michael, Laura, and Kevin, who bring freshness and joy to life;
my parents, Harry and Helene, who are a continued source of inspiration;
and to the patients whom I have had the privilege to serve.

Jeffrey Sands

CONTENTS

CONTRIBUTING AUTHORS

Michael Allon, M.D. Professor, Department of Medicine, University of Alabama at Birmingham; Nephrologist, Department of Nephrology, University Hospital, Birmingham, Alabama

Sanford D. Altman, M.D. Director, Open Access Vascular Access Center, North Miami, Florida

Barbara Alving, M.D. Deputy Director; National Heart, Lung, and Blood Institute; National Institutes of Health; Bethesda, Maryland

W. Perry Arnold, M.D. Medical Director, RMS Lifeline Inc., Timonium, Maryland

Enrico Ascher, M.D. Professor, Department of Surgery, State University of New York at Brooklyn, Health Sciences; Director, Division of Vascular Surgery, Maimonides Medical Center, Brooklyn, New York

Mohammad A. Aslam, M.D. Third Year Fellow, Department of Nephrology, Louisiana State University; Interventional Nephrology Fellow, Department of Nephrology, Louisiana State University Health Sciences Center, Shreveport, Louisiana

Gerald A. Beathard, M.D., Ph.D. Vice President, RMS Lifeline, Austin, Texas

Anatole Besarab, M.D. Senior Staff; Director of Clinical Research, Division of Nephrology and Hypertension, Henry Ford Hospital, Detroit, Michigan

Changyi Chen, M.D., Ph.D. Professor, Michael E. DeBakey Department of Surgery, Baylor College of Medicine, Houston, Texas

Martin R. Crain, M.D. Associate Professor, Department of Radiology and Vascular Surgery, Director of Vascular and Interventional Radiology, Medical College of Wisconsin, Milwaukee, Wisconsin

Jacob Cynamon, M.D. Professor of Clinical Radiology, Department of Radiology, Albert Einstein College of Medicine; Director, Division of Vascular and Interventional Radiology, Montefiore Medical Center, Bronx, New York

Thomas A. Depner, M.D. Professor, Department of Medicine, Division of Nephrology, University of California–Davis; University of California–Davis Medical Center, Sacramento, California

Paul W. Eggers, Ph.D Program Director, Kidney and Urology Epidemiology, National Institute of Diabetes and Digestive and Kidney Diseases, Bethesda, Maryland

Pamela A. Flick, M.D. Chief of Vascular Interventional Radiology, Associate Professor, Department of Radiology, Georgetown University Medical Center, Washington, DC

Stanley Frinak, M.S.E.E. Electrical Engineer, Section of Nephrology, Henry Ford Health Systems, Detroit, Michigan

Gary Gelbfish, M.D. Assistant Clinical Professor, Department of Surgery, Mount Sinai School of Medicine, Vascular Access Unit, North General Hospital, New York, New York

Richard J. Gray, M.D., F.S.C.V.I.R. Clinical Director, Interventional Radiology, Washington Hospital Center, Washington, DC

Mitchell L. Henry, M.D. Professor of Surgery, Director, Clinical Transplantation, Department of Surgery, Division of Transplantation, The Ohio State University Medical Center, Columbus, Ohio

Jonathan Himmelfarb, M.D. Clinical Professor, Department of Medicine, University of Vermont College of Medicine, Burlington, Vermont; Director, Division of Nephrology and Renal Transplantation, Department of Nephrology, Maine Medical Center, Portland, Maine

Anil P. Hingorani, M.D. Clinical Assistant Professor, Department of Surgery, State University of New York at Brooklyn, Health Sciences; Vascular Attending Surgeon, Division of Vascular Surgery, Maimonides Medical Center, Brooklyn, New York

Przemyslaw Hirszel, M.D. Professor, Department of Medicine, Director, Division of Nephrology, Uniformed Services University of the Health Sciences; Attending Physician, Nephrology Service, National Naval Medical Center, Bethesda, Maryland

Michael R. Jaff, D.O., R.V.T. Director, Department of Vascular Medicine, The Heart and Vascular Institute, Morristown, New Jersey

Hyun S. Kim, M.D.   Assistant Professor, Department of Radiology and Surgery, The Russell H. Morgan Department of Radiology and Radiological Sciences, Cardiovascular and Interventional Radiology, The Johns Hopkins University School of Medicine and Medical Institutions, Baltimore, Maryland

Michael A. Kraus, M.D.   Associate Professor, Department of Clinical Medicine, Indiana University; Clinical Director of Nephrology, Department of Internal Medicine, University Hospital, Indianapolis, Indiana

Dorene Kuhn, M.S., C.R.N.P., C.C.R.N.   Nurse Practitioner, Department of Medicine, Division of Nephrology, Johns Hopkins University Medical Center, Baltimore, Maryland

Peter H. Lin, M.D.   Assistant Professor, Department of Surgery, Baylor College of Medicine; Chief, Department of Vascular Surgery, Houston VA Medical Center, Houston, Texas

Susan P. Loughlin, B.S.N., R.N., C.C.R.C.   Clinical Research Coordinator, Department of Medicine, Section of Nephrology, Washington Hospital Center, Washington, DC

Alan B. Lumsden, Mb.Chb.   Professor and Chief, Division of Vascular Surgery and Endovascular Therapy, Michael E. DeBakey Department of Surgery, Baylor College of Medicine; Chief, Vascular Surgery, The Methodist Hospital, Houston, Texas

Gunnar B. Lund, M. D.   Professor, Department of Radiology, University of Maryland Medical School, Baltimore, Maryland

Patrick C. Malloy, M.D.   Chairman, Department of Radiology, Danbury Hospital, Danbury, Connecticut

William A. Marston, M.D.   Associate Professor, Department of Surgery, Division of Vascular Surgery, University of North Carolina, Chapel Hill, North Carolina

Roger Milam, B.S.   Baltimore, Maryland

Jack Moore, Jr., M.D.   Associate Professor, Department of Medicine, Uniformed Services University of the Health Sciences, Bethesda, Maryland; Director, Department of Medicine, Section of Nephrology, Washington Hospital Center, Washington, DC

Christopher E. Pierpont, M.D.   Albert Einstein College of Medicine; Chief Resident, Department of Radiology, Montefoire Medical Center, Bronx, New York

Amer Rajab, M.D., Ph.D.   Assistant Professor, Department of Surgery, Division of Transplantation, The Ohio State University Medical Center, Columbus, Ohio

Alain C. Raynaud, M.D.   Vascular Radiologist, Department of Vascular Radiology, Hôpital Européen Georges Pompidou; Chief, Department of Vascular Radiology, Alleray Labrouste Clinic, Paris, France

John H. Rundback, M.D.   Associate Professor, Department of Interventional Radiology, College of Physicians & Surgeons of Columbia University; Director of Clinical Reserach, Department of Vascular and Interventional Radiology, New York Presbyterian Hospital, New York, New York

Jeffrey J. Sands, M.D.   Vice President, Vascular Access Programs, Fresenius Medical Care NA, Winter Park, Florida

Scott Savader, M.D.   Department of Radiology, Methodist Hospital, Indianapolis, Indiana

Harry Schanzer, M.D.   Clinical Professor, Department of Surgery, Mount Sinai School of Medicine, New York, New York

Paul J. Scheel, Jr., M.D.   Associate Professor, Department of Medicine, The Johns Hopkins University; Vice Chairman, Department of Medicine, The Johns Hopkins Hospital, Baltimore, Maryland

Gerald Schulman, M.D.   Associate Professor, Department of Medicine, Division of Nephrology, Vanderbilt University; Physician, Department of Medicine, Vanderbilt Medical Center, Nashville, Tennessee

Steve J. Schwab, M.D.   Professor and Vice Chairman, Department of Medicine, Duke University Medical Center, Durham, North Carolina

Melhem J. Sharafuddin, M.D.   Assistant Professor, Department of Radiology, University of Iowa Hospitals and Clinics, Iowa City, Iowa

Surendra Shenoy, M.D., Ph.D.   Assistant Professor, Department of Surgery, Washington University School of Medicine; Barnes–Jewish Hospital, St. Louis, Missouri

Anton N. Sidawy, M.D., M.P.H.   Professor, Department of Surgery, George Washington and Georgetown Universities; Chief, Surgery Service, Veterans Administration Medical Center, Washington, DC

Michael B. Silva, Jr., M.D.   Professor of Surgery and Radiology, Departments of Vascular Surgery and Vascular Interventional Radiology, Texas Tech University Health Sciences Center; Chief, Vascular Surgery and Vascular Interventional Radiology, University Medical Center, Lubbock, Texas

Kurt B. Stevenson, M.D., M.P.H.   Associate Professor (Adjunct), Department of Medicine, Division of Clinical Epidemiology, University of Utah School of Medicine, Salt Lake City, Utah; Principal Clinical Coordinator, PRO-West, Boise, Idaho

Jan H. M. Tordoir, M.D., Ph.D. Associate Professor, Department of Surgery, University Hospital Maastricht, Maastricht, The Netherlands

Luc Turmel-Rodrigues, M.D. Department of Radiology, Clinque St.-Gatien, Tours, France

Karim Valji, M.D. Professor, Department of Radiology, University of California–San Diego, San Diego, California

Mark D. Vannorsdall, M.D. Division of Nephrology, Maine Medical Center, Portland, Maine

Judith H. Veis, M.D. Assistant Professor, Department of Medicine, Uniformed Services University of the Health Sciences, Bethesda, Maryland; Associate Director, Section of Nephrology, Washington Hospital Center, Washington, DC

Thomas M. Vesely, M.D. Associate Professor of Radiology and Surgery, Vascular and Interventional Radiology Section, Mallinckrodt Institute of Radiology, Washington University School of Medicine, St. Louis, Missouri

Dierk Vorwerk, M.D. Professor of Radiology, Chairman, Department of Diagnostic and Interventional Radiology, Ingolstadt Clinic, Ingolstadt, Germany

Ron Waksman, M.D. Clinical Professor of Medicine, Department of Cardiology, Georgetown University Medical Center; Associate Director, Division of Cardiology, Washington Hospital Center, Washington, DC

Joshua L. Weintraub, M.D. Assistant Professor, Department of Radiology, College of Physicians & Surgeons of Columbia University; Department of Radiology, New York Presbyterian Hospital, New York, New York

David W. Windus, M.D. Associate Professor, Department of Medicine, Renal Division, Washington University School of Medicine, St. Louis, Missouri

Jack Work, M.D. Professor, Department of Medicine, Director of Interventional Nephrology, Emory University, Atlanta, Georgia

Jane Y. Yeun, M.D. Assistant Professor, Department of Medicine, University of California–Davis, Sacramento, California; Section Chief, Nephrology Section, Sacramento Veterans Administration Medical Center, Mather, California

William R. Yorkovich, R.P.A. Physician Assistant, Division of Vascular Surgery, Maimonides Medical Center, Brooklyn, New York

PREFACE

Since the first reports of successful dialysis through separate arterial and venous cannulas in the early 1960's, the medical community has endeavored to create and maintain satisfactory life-sustaining accesses. The success of this effort is reflected in the estimated 300,000 Americans who are dialysis-dependent. Nevertheless, provision of functional accesses that are readily available, easy to place, easy to use, reliable, and acceptable to patients remains problematic. Access failure and complications are a leading cause of hospitalization for patients with end-stage renal disease, with annual expenditures of over one billion dollars in the United States alone. This combination of morbidity and cost has placed an increasing burden upon patients, providers, health care delivery systems, and payers alike. On a personal level, frequent failure of dialysis accesses is a frustrating and time-consuming problem for dialysis patients and their health care providers. The critical role of the dialysis access has resulted in a rapid proliferation of procedures to improve patient outcomes and generated intense multidisciplinary interest in all aspects of vascular access creation and management.

The central importance of vascular access led the National Kidney Foundation (NKF) to devote one of four sections in the Dialysis Outcomes Quality Initiative (DOQI) solely to vascular access. The central themes of these vascular access guidelines are increased creation of autogenous arteriovenous fistulas, surveillance with early intervention to prevent access failure, decreased dependence on catheters, and venous preservation. Although the original NKF-DOQI and updated K-DOQI (Kidney Disease Outcomes Quality Initiative) have provided explanations of the rationale for each guideline, a comprehensive central source of information on dialysis vascular access has heretofore been lacking. We intend for this text to fill that void. This book provides an in-depth review of the issues and data supporting current access management practices written by the specialists who pioneered them. All forms of dialysis access are presented, with basic science information contributed by authors, including some European colleagues, who performed the original research. We anticipate that this text will serve as a resource for the numerous health professionals involved in vascular access management at all levels of expertise. The broad scope of background information provided in each area will fulfill the need for a basic text that can be used by trainees from all medical disciplines. At the same time, the detailed depth of information presented will also be a valuable reference source for seasoned professionals and investigators.

Only an integrated multidisciplinary team that coordinates the efforts of nephrologists, interventional radiologists, surgeons, nurses, dietitians, social workers, and dialysis clinic personnel can consistently provide state-of-the-art access care. It is our intention for this text to remain a living document that will periodically be updated with the new and rapid advances in this emerging multidisciplinary field.

Richard J. Gray, M.D., F.S.C.V.I.R.
Jeffrey J. Sands, M.D.

ACKNOWLEDGMENT

We would like to thank the authors who contributed their time, effort, and expertise for this text. In addition, several individuals made invaluable contributions during the conception of this book. At the risk of excluding someone, specific thanks are due to Drs. W. Perry Arnold, Gary Gelbfish, Jack Moore, Jr., Scott J. Savader, Anton N. Sidawy, Scott O. Trerotola, and Thomas M. Vesely, who perused the proposed table of contents and suggested additional topics or authors that are included herein. Thanks also to Pamela Sutton, Beth Barry, Jonathan Geffner, and their staffs at Lippincott Williams & Wilkins for their tireless editorial guidance. Last but not least, we thank the remarkable patients whom we have the privilege to serve.

DIALYSIS ACCESS

A MULTIDISCIPLINARY APPROACH

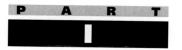

PART I

DIALYSIS OUTCOMES QUALITY INITIATIVE FOR VASCULAR ACCESS

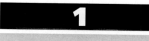

NATIONAL KIDNEY FOUNDATION'S DIALYSIS OUTCOMES QUALITY INITIATIVE: GOALS AND GENERAL PRINCIPLES

STEVE J. SCHWAB

The National Kidney Foundation's Dialysis Outcomes Quality Initiative (NKF-DOQI) was established in 1995. It was driven by the NKF's belief that patient outcomes and survivals could be improved by developing a series of evidence-based clinical practice guidelines. These clinical practice guidelines were envisioned as documenting and recommending clinical best practice. The NKF identified four areas where they believed variations in clinical practice in the care of patients with end-stage renal disease (ESRD) could be improved with evidence-based guidelines (Table 1.1).

Following a generous unrestricted educational grant from AMGEN, the NKF then convened multidisciplinary panels to select work group chairs and, ultimately, work group members. These work groups were selected to encompass established experts from each field involved in the guideline area. In addition, each specialty group of major clinical practitioners was to be involved in the formation of the guidelines. Thus, in the area of hemodialysis vascular access, representatives from not only nephrology but also from vascular and transplant surgery, nephrology nursing, and interventional nephrology/interventional vascular radiology were needed. These individuals usually served as representatives of their respective specialty and subspecialty organizations (Table 1.2).

Initially, these practice guidelines were published by the NKF in 1997, both in the *American Journal of Kidney Disease* and in stand-alone monograph form (1). These practice guide-lines subsequently were updated by additional review of the literature as the K-DOQI (Kidney Disease Outcomes Quality Initiative) and again published by the NKF in 2000–2001 (2). These guidelines are available not only from the published references but also from the NKF and at the NKF website.

GUIDELINE DEVELOPMENT

The initial efforts to develop the vascular access DOQI practice guidelines required a 2-year period during which the world literature on hemodialysis vascular access was critically reviewed. The Institute of Medicine has defined *practice guidelines* as "systematically developed statements to assist practitioner and patient decisions about appropriate health care for specific clinical circumstances." The NKF-DOQI had four guiding principles in these guideline developments:

1. The practice guideline would be developed using scientific rigorous processes, and the rationale and evidentiary basis for each guideline would be clearly explained.
2. Multidisciplinary work groups with expertise in the area of interest would develop the guidelines.

TABLE 1.1. NKF-DOQI WORK GROUPS 1995

Hemodialysis vascular access
Adequacy of hemodialysis
Adequacy of peritoneal dialysis
Management of anemia in patients with uremia

NFK-DOQI, National Kidney Foundation's Dialysis Outcomes Quality Initiative.

TABLE 1.2. VASCULAR ACCESS WORK GROUP MEMBERS 1995

S.J. Schwab, M.D., Chair	Nephrologist
A. Besarab, M.D., Co-Chair	Nephrologist
G. Beathard, M.D. Ph.D.	Interventional nephrologist
D. Brouwer, R.N. C.N.N.	Nephrology nurse
E. Etheredge, M.D.	Transplant surgeon
M. Hartigan, R.N., M.S.N., C.N.N.	Nephrology nurse
M. Levine, M.D.	Nephrologist
R. McCann, M.D.	Vascular surgeon
R. Sherman, M.D.	Nephrologist
S. Trerotola, M.D.	Vascular interventional radiologist

3. The work groups would work independently of any organizational affiliation and would have unfettered responsibility for determining the guideline content.
4. The guidelines would undergo widespread systematic review by multiple organizations before being finalized.

The NKF used two separate groups of facilitators to assist the working group's development of the practice guidelines. These groups (Covance Health Economics and Outcomes Services, Inc., and Medical Education Institute) not only performed computer review and recall of the world's published literature on vascular access but also provided a mechanism of structured review so that multiple on-point articles could be evaluated rigorously for validity and be assigned a priority score. These specialists then assisted in providing internal consistency for guideline development process.

LITERATURE REVIEW PROCESS

The NKF principle that guidelines ideally should be evidence based required a massive and systematic review of the world literature on vascular access. Initially, this was accomplished by the identification of topics and key words. Subsequently, using computerized bibliographic databases, the world literature was reviewed (Table 3). On the topic of hemodialysis vascular access, more than 3,577 articles were identified at the time of the initial screening. Abstracts from these articles were reviewed by at least three members of the committee, and articles considered to have significant value were retrieved in full. These full-text articles were read by at least three members of the work group committee. Then 941 full-text articles were retrieved and reviewed. Of these 941 articles, 221 were determined to be key articles that dealt with substantial critical areas in the area of vascular access. These 221 articles then underwent structured review by an outside process to determine the validity and analysis of the way the observations were obtained. This structured review allowed comparisons of multiple observations across time in areas of interest to individual practice guidelines. Subsequently, 207 articles were cited in the final practice guideline body. Preliminary practice guidelines were formulated.

The guidelines underwent a series of peer reviews. At each step in the peer review, the guidelines and critical comments were returned to members of the working group to evaluate conclusions and to evaluate for internal consis-

TABLE 1.3. LITERATURE REVIEW PROCESS NKF/DOQI

Total articles identified	3,577
Full-text retrieval and review	941
Structured review	221
Articles cited	207

NFK-DOQI, National Kidney Foundation's Dialysis Outcomes Quality Initiative.

tency. The initial review was by the NKF Advisory Council. All the professional and patient organizations involved in the practice guideline development performed secondary review. These included the American Society of Nephrology, the American Society of Vascular Surgeons, the American Society of Transplant Surgeons, the American Association of Kidney Patients, the Council of the ESRD networks, the American Nephrology Nurses Association, and the American Society of Vascular Interventional Radiology. Additional reviews were done by managed care organizations and by representatives from the large dialysis chains as well as the dialysis industry in general. Following each review, the guidelines were modified based on evidence-based clinical commentary. After these revisions, the guidelines were made available to the general public for comments. On receipt of comments from the public and appropriate revisions, the initial practice guidelines were published by the NKF in October 1997 (1). It is important to note that each of the involved specialty societies and their representatives reviewed and accepted the final clinical practice guidelines.

WHY VASCULAR ACCESS CLINICAL GUIDELINES

Complications of hemodialysis vascular access are not only a major cause of morbidity in hemodialysis patients but are also a major cost to ESRD system. The U.S. Renal Data System (USRDS) estimated that the cost of access morbidity approaches $8,000 per patient yearly (3). Others have estimated that hemodialysis vascular access may account for 17% of the total spending for hemodialysis patients (3). This estimate may be conservative because access-related morbidity has been reported to account for almost 25% of all hospital stays for ESRD patients and in various ways may contribute to as much as 50% of total hospitalization costs. Managed care organizations, when planning for a capitated environment, estimate that as much as a third of the total cost of ESRD is spent on the creation and maintenance of hemodialysis vascular access. Thus, maintenance of vascular access not only reflects an enormous problem for patients struck with ESRD but also represents an enormous financial drain on the ESRD program.

KEY MESSAGES FROM THE DIALYSIS OUTCOMES QUALITY INITIATIVE

The hemodialysis vascular access guidelines in its final rendition represented 38 practice guidelines. Each individual practice guideline is clearly defined as to whether it is evidence or opinion based. Accompanying the guideline are the rationale and the references that define it as either an opinion- or an evidence-based guideline. Interestingly, to be an opinion-based guideline, it was necessary to achieve consensus among all members of the working committee, which in many cases was no small feat. When present, it represented a major consensus statement. Nonetheless, despite 38 practice guidelines ranging from physical examination before placement of access, and ending with guidelines for cumulative patency rates for primary arteriovenous fistula (AVF), three major messages emerged.

1. Native AVFs have a dramatically lower complication rate and longer patency rate than any other form of permanent vascular access. Thus, the guidelines' focus on methods for increasing the prevalence of AVF in the North American hemodialysis population. Multiple strategies are proposed, but early referral to a nephrologist and ultimately to vascular access surgeons is the only sure way to increase the likelihood of native AVF formation. Early patient education about the importance of protecting vascular anatomy and significant attempts to form and maintain a native AVF before the onset of ESRD therapy are essential.

2. When arteriovenous (AV) accesses are placed, detecting access dysfunction before thrombosis is essential to maintaining long-term patency. Thus, the guidelines focus on both monitoring and surveillance techniques to identify problematic areas in vascular access prior to thrombosis or infection. It is the belief of the guideline committee, supported heavily by the literature, that prophylactic monitoring and surveillance combined with prophylactic intervention dramatically can improve AV fistula and AV graft patency.

3. It is absolutely essential to minimize the long-term dependence on tunneled hemodialysis access catheters because of the overall complication rate in terms of infection and dysfunction. The committee stressed that hemodialysis catheter access to the circulation is essential and that tunneled catheters have dramatically improved the welfare of our patients when used for short- or intermediate-term access to the circulation. Long-term or permanent access to the circulation accompanied by a catheter should be reserved as a final, or last, resort.

DIALYSIS OUTCOMES QUALITY INITIATIVE BECOMES KIDNEY DISEASE OUTCOMES QUALITY INITIATIVE

Evidence-based practice guidelines remain evidentiary in basis only if they are continually updated. Thus, the NKF committed itself to updating these practice guidelines continually to maintain their applicability. The publication of K-DOQI in 2001 represents a substantial review of the literature published since 1997 (2). Practice guidelines were updated and, where appropriate, additional changes in the practice guidelines were made. It is interesting to note that the practice guidelines were changed only modestly as a result of the literature. Nonetheless, significant new advances have occurred, mandating guideline changes. Finally, any group impaneled to maintain guidelines develops biases during the course of literature review. Acknowledging this, the NKF plans to impanel new practice guideline groups for subsequent practice guideline renditions and updates.

REFERENCES

1. National Kidney Foundation: Dialysis Outcomes Quality Initiative (NFK-DOQI). Clinical practice guidelines for hemodialysis vascular access. *Am J Kidney Dis* 1977;30:5154–5196.
2. National Kidney Foundation: Kidney Disease Outcomes Quality Initiative (NKF K/DOQI. Clinical practice guidelines for vascular access. *Am J Kidney Dis* 2001;37(Suppl 1):s137–s181.
3. Schwab SJ. Hemodialysis vascular access: the forum. *Kidney Int* 1999;55:2078–2090.

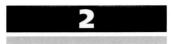

IMPLEMENTING A VASCULAR ACCESS PROGRAM: IMPROVED OUTCOMES WITH MULTIDISCIPLINARY APPROACHES

MICHAEL ALLON

The National Kidney Foundation's Dialysis Outcomes Quality Initiative (NKF-DOQI) guidelines spell out the goals of vascular access management in hemodialysis patients in broad strokes. These include (a) a concerted effort to increase the construction of arteriovenous (AV) fistulas, (b) ongoing monitoring for vascular access dysfunction with elective intervention to minimize access thrombosis, and (c) attempts to minimize the use of dialysis catheters. Whereas most physicians agree on the importance of following these clinical guidelines, there are substantial logistic obstacles to implementing these guidelines in practice:

1. Multiple disciplines are involved in ensuring optimal vascular access in dialysis patients, including nephrologists, access surgeons, interventional radiologists, and dialysis nurses. Optimal management of vascular access requires close communication among the disciplines involved.
2. Vascular access procedures are performed largely on an outpatient basis, thereby adding complexity to the scheduling of the appointments.
3. The access appointments and procedures need to be coordinated in a way that minimizes disruption of the outpatient dialysis schedule.
4. Improving outcomes requires prospective, complete, and accurate information on all vascular access events and procedures.

A number of clinical centers in the United States have developed a coordinated approach to improving vascular access outcomes (1–8). The key features common to all the successful centers include a multidisciplinary team approach, a dedicated vascular access coordinator, devising clinical care pathways, maintaining a computerized database, and continuously assessing outcomes resulting from the implemented changes. To address these issues at the University of Alabama at Birmingham (UAB), we created a full-time position for a dialysis access coordinator in 1996. The clinical re-

sponsibilities of this person include the following:

1. The coordinator acts as a liaison among the nephrologists, surgeons, radiologists, and dialysis nurses, thereby providing consistency of communication. In the absence of a coordinator, communication breaks down at multiple levels. For example, a patient may be referred for a fistulogram to be performed for a suspected graft stenosis. The radiologist observes a severe stenosis at the venous anastomosis that is refractory to angioplasty and pages the patient's nephrologist to recommend surgical revision of the graft. The nephrologist never answers the radiologist's page because he or she is out of town; so a surgical appointment is never made. Eventually, the graft thromboses because it has not been revised in a timely fashion. In contrast, under the multidisciplinary approach, the radiologist informs the access coordinator of the problem. The access coordinator immediately schedules the patient to see the surgeon regarding elective revision of the graft. The graft is revised in a timely fashion and remains patent. Most of the communication occurs by e-mail or fax, and copies are sent to all the involved persons. For example, notification of an appointment for a fistulogram in interventional radiology is copied to the patient's nephrologist, clinical secretary, and nurse manager of the patient's outpatient dialysis unit.
2. The coordinator schedules all vascular access procedures with the radiology and surgery departments and provides these services with the relevant clinical information. The access coordinator is familiar with the patient's dialysis schedule and makes every effort to schedule vascular access appointments so that they do not conflict with the dialysis schedule. The access coordinator automatically follows up on every appointment and ensures that the patient actually shows for the appointment. If not, the access coordinator reschedules the patient's appointment. In the absence of an access coordinator, the patient might miss a surgical appointment for placement of an AV fistula and is not rescheduled promptly. As a result, the patient may continue to un-

dergo dialysis with a catheter for several weeks or months before the surgery appointment is rescheduled. In the meantime, the patient is likely to receive inadequate dialysis or develop catheter-associated bacteremia.

3. The coordinator follows up on all vascular access procedures performed by surgery and radiology. It is critical to find out exactly what access procedure was performed and whether an additional procedure is indicated. If attempted thrombectomy of a graft by interventional radiology was unsuccessful, the patient needs to be referred promptly to the surgery department for revision of the graft or construction of a new vascular access if revision is not feasible. If the dialysis nurses are now using a new fistula, the access coordinator schedules prompt removal of the dialysis catheter. If the new fistula has not matured in a reasonable time frame (about 6–8 weeks), the access coordinator refers the patient for a diagnostic ultrasound or fistulogram. If this diagnostic study reveals large tributary vessels, the access coordinator refers the patient to the surgeon for ligation of the tributaries. The access coordinator follows up with the dialysis nurses to find out whether the fistula has matured.

4. The coordinator maintains a prospective computerized database to track all vascular access procedures. Meaningful analysis of outcomes or complications is critically dependent on having a complete and accurate record of all vascular access procedures performed. This database is useful in a variety of ways. First, a chronological list of all vascular access procedures in a single patient can be generated from these data. This information is valuable for the surgeon or radiologist in planning the next access procedure. Second, these data can facilitate the generation of a list of all procedures of a certain type and during a specified time period. For example, the nephrologist may be interested in knowing how many grafts clotted during the past 3 months, how many cases of catheter-associated bacteremia were encountered, or how many postoperative complications occurred following new graft construction. Such information can be sorted by dialysis unit and can assist the medical director and nurse manager of the unit in identifying problems or proposing solutions. Likewise, a detailed list of surgical complications can be provided to each surgeon to assist him or her in reducing future surgical complications.

5. The coordinator identifies specific problems related to vascular access that need to be addressed. The access coordinator is in a unique position to identify vascular access-related problems early. For example, one nephrologist may have two dialysis patients referred for catheter exchange for poor flow and not think much of it. On the other hand, the access coordinator might observe that during a 1-month period, ten catheters had to be exchanged within 2 weeks of being placed. The access coordinator alerts the interventional radiologist to this worrisome pattern. Prompt investigation reveals that the problem is with a specific brand of catheter, and a decision is made to switch to a different brand. Without an access coordinator, this problem might not have been recognized and remedied for many months.

From this description of the clinical responsibilities of the access coordinator, it should be apparent that careful selection of this person is critical to the success of the multidisciplinary approach to vascular access. Some of the important attributes of a successful access coordinator include the following:

1. The coordinator must be extremely knowledgeable about dialysis and vascular access. He or she must have had hands-on experience with dialysis patients and a thorough understanding of all the issues involved in optimizing vascular access. At UAB, we have had a physician assistant and two dialysis nurses fill this position successfully. It is doubtful that a clinical secretary would be able to fulfill the role as well.

2. The coordinator must be very organized, efficient, and detail oriented. Every referral for a procedure entails multiple steps to have a successful outcome. For example, if a patient comes to dialysis with a clotted graft, the access coordinator receives an initial referral from the dialysis unit. He or she needs to schedule the patient for a thrombectomy procedure in interventional radiology and inform the dialysis unit so that the patient can be instructed about the time and place. The access coordinator needs to provide interventional radiology with a detailed vascular access history for that patient. If the thrombectomy is successful, the patient needs to be scheduled for a "makeup" dialysis session. If the declotting attempt is unsuccessful, the interventional radiologist places a tunneled dialysis catheter in the patient for temporary dialysis. The access coordinator then needs to schedule a surgery appointment for the patient, inform the dialysis unit of the appointment, and then follow up to learn when a surgical procedure is intended. The patient's nephrologist needs to be notified of all these events. Finally, the access information needs to be entered promptly and accurately into the computer database.

3. The access coordinator must have excellent communication skills. In a busy dialysis practice, this job is extremely stressful. The access coordinator is constantly communicating with nephrologists, radiologists, surgeons, dialysis nurses, and dialysis patients. These communications may occur by phone, fax, e-mail, paging, or in person. At UAB, it is not unusual for the access coordinator to be simultaneously on the phone with one person, communicating by e-mail regarding another patient, receiving a faxed report on a third patient, being paged about a fourth patient, and having a nephrology fellow in the office wanting to discuss a fifth patient. The access coordinator needs to be able to meet these multiple demands without becoming flustered and without losing his or her temper.

The success of the team approach to vascular access is critically dependent on the maintenance of a prospective computerized database. Different programs have used a number of commercially available software programs successfully; however, certain features are common to these computerized record systems:

1. Keep it simple. Someone has to enter all these data. It is important to prioritize what information is really needed regarding each procedure. It is preferable to have less information about each procedure but have all the information available rather than having a huge amount of information collected on each procedure but have only partial information on many procedures.

2. Use consistent terminology. For the purpose of data analysis, it is critical that a given procedure is always referred to in a standard fashion. If the same procedure is labeled as a *thrombectomy* in some instances and as a *declot* in other instances, meaningful analysis will be extremely difficult.

3. Data must be entered promptly. The rule at UAB is that all the access procedures from that day must be entered in the computer database by the end of that day. Information that is not entered promptly is likely to be forgotten. Having multiple scraps of paper and Post-it notes all over the place is a prescription for disaster. When the details of a procedure are not available by the end of the day, the access coordinator enters a preliminary entry into the computer, which is subsequently revised when further information becomes available.

4. Only one or two people enter all the data. Minimizing the number of people entering access information into the database ensures a high level of consistency.

5. Use the database for scheduling, not just for record keeping.

6. Review entries periodically.

The basic continuous quality improvement (CQI) process involves several steps. First, a particular problem that requires improvement is identified. Second, a plan of action is developed to improve the desired outcome. Third, the plan of action is implemented. Finally, one evaluates the outcomes following the change to determine whether there has been an objective improvement in the outcomes. A critical aspect of the entire process is the ability to measure rapidly and accurately outcomes before and after a given change is introduced. The following is a description of how the CQI process was used at UAB to improve vascular access outcomes.

1. Approach to clotted grafts: Over a 6-month period, we were averaging 12.5 clotted grafts per month. At the time, management of clotted grafts consisted of inpatient surgical thrombectomies. Because of delays in scheduling surgical procedures, the patients often required one or two dialysis sessions with a femoral catheter. Moreover, only 48% of declotted grafts remained patent until the next scheduled dialysis treatment. In an attempt to improve the turnaround time and outcomes of clotted grafts, we began to refer all clotted grafts to interventional radiology for outpatient thrombectomy. Angioplasty of the stenotic lesion

was performed at the same time. If the declot was unsuccessful, a tunneled dialysis catheter was placed during the same visit, and the patient was referred to the surgery department for revision of the existing graft or placement of a new vascular access if revision was not feasible. As a result of this approach, the vast majority of thrombosed grafts underwent a thrombectomy within 24 hours of referral. Moreover, the success rate increased from 48% to 69% (1).

2. Decreasing graft thrombosis: Although the medical literature clearly documented that grafts clotted as a result of myointimal hyperplasia and progressive stenosis, there was minimal surveillance of grafts for evidence of stenosis. To remedy this problem, we began to educate aggressively the nephrologists and dialysis nurses about the importance of graft surveillance and prompt referral of patients with suspected graft stenosis for a fistulogram. Specifically, patients were referred to interventional radiology department if they had persistent elevation of dynamic dialysis venous pressures at a low blood flow, unexplained decline in Kt/V, prolonged bleeding from the needle sites, or abnormal inspection or auscultation of the graft. This program of aggressive clinical monitoring of grafts reduced the frequency of graft thrombosis by 60%, from 0.70 to 0.28 per graft-year (1). Similar improvements in the rate of graft thrombosis have been reported by other centers using a multidisciplinary team approach to vascular access. Glazer and associates (3), with the Kaiser Permanente Group in Southern California, reported a decrease in the rate of graft thrombosis from 0.97 to 0.41 per patient-year. Similarly, Duda and colleagues (4) applied this approach in the Gambro units in Southeast Georgia and observed a 44% decrease in the incidence of graft thrombosis, from 1.04 to 0.58 per patient-year (see also Chapter 22).

3. Decreasing complications of access surgery: Prospective tracking of surgical complications after new AV graft construction was performed. A *surgical complication* was defined as any complication occurring within 1 month of the surgery that resulted in the need for a second access procedure. This included an unsuccessful attempt at graft construction, graft thrombosis, graft infection, or severe steal syndrome. During the initial tracking period, we noted that 25% of new grafts had a postoperative complication. In an attempt to reduce the frequency of this complication, we provided each surgeon with a confidential, detailed list of graft procedures that he or she had performed, along with the associated complications. We then had a face-to-face meeting to discuss potential changes to reduce the frequency of postoperative complications. In the subsequent tracking period, the frequency of postoperative complications following new graft surgery decreased to 11%. Moreover, a decrease was observed for each of the three surgeons performing access surgery (1).

4. Increasing the rate and success of AV fistula placement: Although the medical literature clearly documents the superiority of fistulas over grafts, we found that the initial permanent vascular access placed in new dialysis patients was an autologous fistula in only 33% of patients. We had a face-

to-face meeting with the surgeons to discuss a strategy to improve the proportion of patients receiving a fistula. As a result of this concerted effort, we were able to increase the proportion of fistulas in new dialysis patients to 69% (1). The increase was particularly dramatic among female patients. Unfortunately, analysis of the outcomes of fistulas revealed that only 47% of new fistulas matured sufficiently to be usable for dialysis. The adequacy rate of new fistulas was substantially better for upper-arm fistulas compared with forearm fistulas. Moreover, the adequacy of forearm fistulas was particularly poor among female, diabetic, and elderly patients (9). A literature review showed that a multidisciplinary approach to increasing fistulas by Sands and Miranda (2), with preferential placement of upper arm fistulas, resulted in a dramatic increase in the proportion of dialysis patients using a fistula, from 28% to 44%. Glazer and colleagues (3) increased the placement of fistulas in new dialysis patients from 27% to 71%. Similarly, Duda and associates (4) used a multidisciplinary approach to increase the prevalence of fistulas in their dialysis population from 14.6% to 25.2%. Silva and colleagues (10) collaborated with radiologists to perform preoperative sonographic vascular mapping before the placement of fistulas. Using this approach, they achieved a dramatic increase in fistula placement and maturation. To improve the outcomes of the fistulas placed at UAB, we developed a collaborative program between nephrologists, radiologists, and surgeons to perform routine preoperative venous mapping to assist the surgeons in planning their vascular access procedures. The effect of this program on fistula adequacy is currently being assessed.

5. Shifting surgical access procedures to the outpatient setting: When we implemented our multidisciplinary approach to vascular access, the vast majority of vascular access procedures were being performed in the inpatient setting. Most of the nephrologists and surgeons believed that dialysis patients were too medically complicated to have outpatient surgery. Only 16% of access procedures were performed as same-day surgery procedures because those patients' insurance companies would not authorize an inpatient procedure. Review of the outcomes of patients whose access procedures were performed as same-day surgery revealed no difference in complications compared with patients whose procedures were performed on an inpatient basis. After a face-to-face meeting with the surgeons, we began to schedule elective access procedures routinely as same-day surgery procedures. As the surgeons and nephrologists became progressively more comfortable with this approach, more and more patients were being discharged from the recovery area without being admitted for overnight hospital observation. Finally, the surgeons began to schedule a substantial proportion of the elective access cases to be performed in the outpatient clinic. Overall, the proportion of elective access procedures performed in the inpatient setting decreased from 84% to 19%. This approach has resulted in a dramatic savings in costs for hospitalization of patients, without an adverse effect on patient outcomes. The cost for hospitalizations related to placement of new AV grafts decreased from $1,370 to $598 (1). Similarly, Duda and colleagues (4) were able to decrease vascular access admissions by 30% and to decrease by 45% the number of outpatient dialysis sessions missed because of vascular access procedures. Finally, Becker and colleagues (7) implemented a vascular access care pathway at Vanderbilt University Medical Center and observed substantial decreases in patient charges and major complications.

In an effort to improve the efficiency of vascular access procedures, a number of centers recently developed freestanding vascular access centers dedicated exclusively to the outpatient management of vascular access problems in dialysis patients (11–13) (see Chapter 40). These centers typically are staffed by interventional radiologists or nephrologists and provide rapid turnaround as well as prospective tracking of complications and outcomes of radiologic access interventions. These outpatient centers appear to provide faster turnaround than hospital-based programs and offer more consistent communication with referring nephrologists and dialysis units. It is likely that we will witness substantial growth in vascular access centers over the next decade.

REFERENCES

1. Allon M, Bailey R, Ballard R, et al. A multidisciplinary approach to hemodialysis access: prospective evaluation. *Kidney Int* 1998; 53:473–479.
2. Sands J, Miranda C. Optimizing hemodialysis access: a teaching tool. *Nephrology News & Issues* 1996;10:16–27.
3. Glazer S, Crooks P, Shapiro M, et al. Using CQI and the DOQI guidelines to improve vascular access outcomes: the Southern California Kaiser Permanente experience. *Nephrol News & Issues* 2000;14:21–26.
4. Duda C, Spergel LM, Holland J, et al. How a multidisciplinary vascular access care program enables implementation of the DOQI guidelines. *Nephrol News & Issues* 2000;14:13–17.
5. Spergel LM. DOQI guidelines and the vascular access puzzle: finding the pieces that fit. *Nephrol News & Issues* 1998;12:46–50.
6. Pflederer TA, Darras FS, Welch K, et al. How to organize hemodialysis vascular access quality assurance efforts into a cohesive whole for better patient outcomes. *Contemp Dial Nephrol* 2000;1:18–21.
7. Becker BN, Breiterman-White R, Nylander W, et al. Care pathway reduces hospitalizations and cost of hemodialysis vascular access surgery. *Am J Kidney Dis* 1977;30:525–531.
8. Welch KA, Pflederer TA, Knudsen J, et al. Establishing the vascular access coordinator: breaking ground for better outcomes. *Nephrology News & Issues* 1998;12:43–46.
9. Miller PE, Tolwani A, Luscy CP, et al. Predictors of adequacy of arteriovenous fistulas in hemodialysis patients. *Kidney Int* 1999;56:275–280.
10. Silva MB, Hobson RW, Pappas PJ, et al. A strategy for increasing use of autogenous hemodialysis access procedures: impact of preoperative noninvasive evaluation. *J Vasc Surg* 1998;27:302–308.
11. Rasmussen RL. The interventional nephrologist: initial experience in a 'dialysis access center'. *Contemp Dial Nephrol* 1998;19:16–19.
12. Guilarte JM. An innovative approach to restoring and preserving vascular access in hemodialysis patients. *Contemp Dial Transplant* 1999;20:21–22.
13. Beathard GA. Has the time come for a dedicated dialysis vascular access laboratory? *Contemp Dial Transplant* 1999;20:18–20.

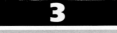

DIALYSIS OUTCOMES QUALITY INITIATIVE IMPLEMENTATION: THE WASHINGTON UNIVERSITY SCHOOL OF MEDICINE EXPERIENCE

SURENDRA SHENOY
DAVID W. WINDUS
THOMAS M.VESELY

The purpose of this chapter is to relate the lessons learned during a process of implementation of the Dialysis Outcomes Quality Initiative (DOQI) guidelines for vascular access management. Published in 1997, the DOQI clinical practice guidelines were based on the collective wisdom and information available at that time. Over the past 10 years, we have developed and practiced a multidisciplinary approach to vascular access management at our institution. Our multidisciplinary team already had been practicing many of the DOQI recommendations, and we have intensified our efforts since that time. This experience has often been challenging but also rewarding and educational.

This chapter describes the viewpoints and pertinent issues we faced using a multidisciplinary approach from the perspective of a nephrologist, surgeon, and interventional radiologist. We focused on the DOQI guidelines that required the most effort and organization to implement. These include the selection of vascular access, timing of access placement, an access monitoring program, and surgical and interventional approaches to the management of complications. At times, the differing viewpoints of the individual members of the vascular access team are emphasized. Several unresolved issues for implementation of the guidelines are addressed in the end.

OVERVIEW OF PROGRAM

The formation of a multidisciplinary hemodialysis vascular access team began informally in the early 1990s. At that time, there was the fortuitous combination of a nephrologist, surgeon, and interventional radiologist, all with similar interests in vascular access for hemodialysis. In addition, a registered nurse with extensive dialysis and access experience from the dialysis unit was integral. In our opinion, the ulti-

mate benefit of this combination was to develop a consensus approach to most of the commonly encountered vascular access problems.

For several years, the access team met on a weekly basis to discuss and develop management plans for each patient with a vascular access problem. At each meeting, the patient's clinical problem was discussed, the appropriate imaging studies reviewed, and a treatment plan devised. These meetings were also a forum for new issues, plans, and review of research proposals. A written summary of each patient's problem and future treatment plans then was distributed by electronic mail to all physicians involved with the patient's access care. This plan became part of the patient's record and was to be implemented by the dialysis nurse when a problem became manifest. The key benefit of this face-to-face discussion process was the gradual development of a consensus approach to vascular access problems. We do not believe this could have been achieved without the weekly team meeting. Because of the inevitable time constraints, our team meeting has devolved after several years into a weekly circulation of access notes via electronic mail and almost daily communication between the members of the vascular access team. The nurse coordinator is responsible for continually updating the vascular access records and circulating information. The access notes communicate current information between members of the team, are used to record past and future treatment plans, and are a means for requesting a treatment plan. It must be emphasized that these notes are not a substitute for timely action or direct communication. An example of this document is shown in Table 3.1.

From the perspective of the radiologist, one of the most important aspects of each meeting was a discussion of recent endovascular procedures. The angiographic images were reviewed, and the radiologist described the pertinent findings

TABLE 3.1. EXAMPLES OF VASCULAR ACCESS NOTES

Patient A: (Surgeon) Fistulogram for low flows 9/19. Small pseudoaneurysm arterial limb of graft. Mild stenosis venous limb, which did not appear flow limiting. No hemodynamic stenoses identified. Surgeon to review films. Flows continues to be low, 335. Kt/V 1.2, too low. Clotted 11/17. Interventional 11/17. Thrombolysis with angioplasty of severe venous anastomosis stenosis with approx. 20% residual. Angioplasty of moderate stenosis in arterial limb just proximal to pseudoaneurysm. Mild residual stenosis over a 4-cm area in venous limb. Office appt. with surgeon 11/29.

Patient B: (Surgeon) Fistulogram 10/31 for recurrent leg swelling. INR too high. Rescheduled for 11/15. Angioplasty of long stenotic segment of moderate to severe narrowing in right common femoral vein distal to confluence of superficial femoral veins and profunda. This is a recurrent stenosis and will persist. Suggest revision/jump graft for long-term improvement.

Patient C: (Surgeon) Pseudoaneurysm rupture 10/18. Fistula tied off. Ash catheter placed 10/23. Incisions healed. ?Plan.

Patient D: (Surgeon) Low flows and low KT/V. Review previous fistulogram. ?Needs new access. Kt/V is low (inadequate dialysis and flows are 460) ?Plan

and indications for the endovascular procedure. The radiologic outcome of the procedure was compared with clinical measures of success, such as improvement of access flow rate, arm swelling, or adequacy of dialysis. Awareness of the clinical response to treatment is critical for formulating future management plans. If the endovascular procedure was a success, the patient was returned to interventional radiology when future problems developed. Alternatively, if the endovascular procedure was unsuccessful and surgical revisions of the vascular access limited, plans were made for a new vascular access. The details of any future intervention, either radiologic or surgical, were formulated and documented in the access notes for future reference.

From the surgical point of view, the access meeting was an opportunity to discuss new referrals, share surgical opinions, and review the imaging studies. It was interesting to note differences in the interpretation of information and the formulation of treatment plans among the different physicians. This meeting became a platform for the initiation of institutional protocols and algorithms for vascular access management. For example, percutaneous thrombectomy was the standard treatment following the first episode of thrombosis. The radiologist usually would identify the underlying problem and repair it, if possible, during this thrombectomy procedure. If the results were suboptimal, the patient underwent a surgical procedure to correct the problem. This approach nearly eliminated the use of simple surgical thrombectomies at our institution. Prophylactic graft revisions or thrombectomy with revisions became the primary surgical procedures for maintaining the graft patency.

COMMENTS ON SELECTED GUIDELINES

Guideline 2: Diagnostic Evaluation Prior to Permanent Access Selection

Many nephrologists and vascular access surgeons are unaware of the importance of preoperative imaging before placement of a vascular access. This guideline describes and supports the use of preoperative venography, and other complementary imaging studies, in selected patients before placement of a permanent vascular access. It is particularly important to assess the patency of the central veins in patients who have had central venous catheters or implanted cardiac pacemakers. There has been nonuniformity in the implementation of this guideline, and preoperative venography is one of the more underutilized aspects of our vascular access program. Although some surgeons commonly refer appropriate patients for venography, other surgeons seem to be unaware of the importance of this preoperative assessment. Patients with renal failure often have other systemic disease that resulted in prior hospitalization and central venous catheterization. Failure to do central vein imaging to identify a central stenosis results in problems with venous hypertension and failure of access. It is not unusual for the interventional radiologist to see patients with arm swelling following creation of a new access; these patients are referred for outflow vein mapping. Even with appropriate use of preoperative vein imaging, however, we occasionally encounter central venous obstruction resulting from an enlarged aortic knob compressing the left brachiocephalic vein, which becomes symptomatic after creation of arteriovenous (AV) access.

From a surgical perspective, preoperative imaging studies should be used in appropriate patients. Our attempts to optimize the creation of primary fistulae have increased the utilization of preoperative imaging, specifically the use of ultrasound to map upper arm cephalic veins. Preoperative ultrasound is also useful for identifying forearm veins in obese patients.

Guideline 3: Selection of Permanent Vascular Access

Our center experience was similar to many others through the 1980s to mid-1990s in that we had resigned ourselves to the use of graft-based vascular access. We had a prevalence of graft accesses of about 85%. The reasons for this high prevalence included a perceived high failure rate of AV fistulas, a desire to avoid catheter access, and a desire to provide sufficient blood flow for efficient dialysis. In fact, our nephrology group actively discouraged placement of AV fistulas by the surgeons. This resulted from a poor experience of fistula maturation, lack of availability of reliable catheter access, and a wish to use high blood flows in an attempt to minimize treatment times for the then-accepted urea kinetics outcomes.

TABLE 3.2. INCIDENCE OF HEMODIALYSIS VASCULAR ACCESS PLACED FOR THE YEARS 1996–2000

Year	Fistulae	Grafts	Total New Access	Fistula %
1996	21	50	71	30
1997	41	53	94	44
1998	76	82	158	48
1999	77	77	154	50
2000	75	50	125	60

Over the past 5 years, attempted AV fistula as first access has increased. The reasons for this increase are earlier referral and an active effort by surgeons to place this type of access. In addition, patients with failed forearm grafts have had upper-arm AV fistulas placed. The prevalence of AV fistulas in the hospital-based dialysis facility has increased to about 25%. Although this prevalence remains below our goal, the trend is upward. Surgical records reflect a similar trend. Fistula placement rates have increased from 38% before 1997 to an average of 52% for the ensuing 3 years (Table 3.2).

Patients who are considered good candidates for fistula creation based on clinical and imaging criteria undergo fistula creation regardless of their time of referral and dialysis status. Patients who are marginal candidates for native vein fistulae receive a fistula if they are not on dialysis or have a long life expectancy. Upper-arm basilic vein transposition is not offered as a primary access.

From the radiologic perspective, the increasing prevalence of AV fistulae in our hemodialysis population was observed with apprehension. Although the radiologists are not responsible for the creation of fistulae, they frequently become involved with treating the problems that occur. Our concern was due in part to our unfamiliarity with fistulae and the substantial time commitment required when treating this type of vascular access, particularly for thrombectomy procedures. The evaluation and treatment of fistulae-related problems necessitate learning new techniques and often require a high level of experience. For these reasons, our participation in the treatment of fistulae-related problems evolved slowly. Unlike the management of dysfunctional grafts that is primarily provided by interventional radiologists, fistulae that develop problems of stenosis or thrombosis are treated primarily by surgeons.

Guideline 4: Type and Location of Dialysis Arteriovenous Graft Placement

Patients who are poor candidates for fistulae receive forearm loop grafts. The timing of surgery depends on dialysis status. We prefer to place a loop graft 4 to 6 weeks before initiation of dialysis. With this approach, however, many patients who are awaiting graft placement tend to get the grafts after initiation of dialysis. Once the forearm graft develops outflow vein problems necessitating surgical revision, veins in and around the cubital fossa region are used. All attempts are made to preserve upper arm basilic and brachial veins. This is a significant deviation from our previous practice of performing forearm to upper-arm jump grafts. For patients with good upper- arm brachial and basilic veins, the grafts are given up after attempts for revisions in and around the cubital fossa fail. These patients then get an upper-arm brachial/basilic vein transposition fistula as the next access. We perform an upper-arm loop graft for patients who do not have upper-arm veins suitable for upper-arm transposition fistula or when the transposition fails.

Guideline 6: Acute Hemodialysis Vascular Access

Our philosophy is to avoid the use of nontunneled (acute) catheters whenever possible. Our use of these catheters has dropped considerably in the past 5 years. Reasons for this decline are use of same- or next-day thrombectomies by interventional radiology, avoiding prolonged waiting times for surgical thrombectomies and increased use of tunneled catheters for long-term use. Although the nephrologists place most of these nontunneled catheters, interventional radiologists occasionally are needed to insert catheters into patients with occluded or otherwise problematic central veins. The internal or external jugular veins are used primarily for these nontunneled catheters. If these veins are occluded, the catheter is placed into a femoral vein. The subclavian veins are used only as a last resort. In addition, patients who need only one dialysis treatment usually will have a femoral catheter placed just before and removed immediately after dialysis.

Guideline 8: Timing of Access Placement

Timing of modality planning and initiation of dialysis has a major impact on access planning. It has been clearly shown that late referral (or diagnosis) of patients with advanced renal failure has been a major factor in late vascular access planning and placement (1). We support the goal of patient referral to the access surgeon when the creatinine clearance is around 25 mL per minute and dialysis is anticipated within the year. We analyzed initial access for the group of patients starting dialysis in our center over the past 2 years. About one fourth of patients initiated dialysis without prior evaluation by a nephrologist or within 3 months of the initial office visit. We also discovered that a significant number of patients who had been followed up by us in clinic for longer than 3 months initiated dialysis with a catheter. Common reasons for the necessity of a catheter included a precipitous decline in renal function, awaiting AV fistula development, and patient refusal for access placement.

Guideline 9: Access Maturation

Assessing access maturation has not been a problem with polytetrafluoroethylene (PTFE) graft material. Our preference is to wait 4 to 5 weeks before the first needle stick. In our experience, the incidence of tunnel hematoma and graft infections resulting from inadequate incorporation of the graft material is nearly eliminated by using such an approach. Autologous fistula maturation, however, has always been a matter of opinion. Even the DOQI guidelines do not provide an objective method of analysis of fistula maturation. We consider a fistula mature when there is a minimum of 8 cm of subcutaneous vein that is greater than 5 mm in diameter with a flow greater than 600 mL per minute. The fistula flow is measured by Doppler ultrasound in the feeding blood vessel to the limb bearing the fistula (e.g., brachial artery flow measurement for forearm radiocephalic fistula) (2). On occasion, we use superficial outflow veins that have adequate flow and diameter if they are deep and are not accessible for needle sticks (unpublished data). Through timely referral or tunneled-catheter use, most patients with the potential for an AV fistula should have that option available.

From the nephrology perspective, the surgical service has made an effort to place more AV fistulas, which has led to an emphasis on several issues. First, patients are starting dialysis with nonmature fistulas and catheters. Second, marginal AV fistulae have poor flow rates and frequent needle placement problems. Third, there are no quantitative criteria to predict which fistulae will ultimately mature. In our experience, AV fistulae that are not usable by 3 months ever mature beyond that time despite salvage attempts.

Guideline 10: Monitoring Dialysis Arteriovenous Grafts for Stenosis

Methods for monitoring AV grafts for stenosis have improved dramatically over the past several years. The main barriers to an access monitoring program, however, are financial and personnel issues. We continue to struggle with both these problems. The DOQI guidelines emphasize intra-access flow measurement, static intra-access pressure, and dynamic venous pressure measurements as the most evidenced-based options for access monitoring. Before the release of DOQI guidelines, we assessed access dysfunction indirectly using parameters to assess the adequacy of hemodialysis. Patients with an unexplained reduction in Kt/V would undergo a urea recirculation study. We reported that surgical or percutaneous repair of outflow stenoses detected by an elevated urea recirculation resulted in reduced recirculation and improved dialysis quality (3). In a separate study, we found that about 25% of declining urea kinetics could be explained by access related problems (4). Although urea kinetics are monitored on a monthly basis, our continued high rate of access complications seemed to be unaffected by this approach.

In 1997, we obtained a device that utilizes an ultrasonic dilution method to determine access flow rates (Transonic HD01, Transonic Systems, Inc., Ithaca, NY, U.S.A.) because promising data had become available demonstrating that these measurements are useful for the detection of outflow stenoses and a harbinger to thrombosis (5,6). Currently, we monitor access flow in all patients with PTFE grafts on an every 1- or 3-month basis, depending on the patient's prior history of graft problems. Although patients who have had prior access complications are targeted for monthly evaluation, we believe that monthly monitoring, as suggested by DOQI guidelines, is untenable given the constraints described subsequently. The technician is scheduled about 1 day a week and can realistically do about 15 blood-flow studies per day. The results of consecutive flow studies are kept on a computer spreadsheet that is available throughout the dialysis unit. Patients with blood flows of less than 600 mL per minute are referred to interventional radiology for a fistulogram.

We have encountered several significant barriers to implementation of our monitoring program. First, the initial cost of the equipment is substantial and no reimbursement was available for the testing when we initiated the program. Second, salary costs were incurred from use of the technician's time. Third, the dialysis technician trained to do the flow testing sometimes was rescheduled to do dialysis treatments because of recurring staff shortages and illness. On the positive side, an experienced dialysis technician can learn the procedure easily, and flow-rate measurements allow us to focus on elective interventions in grafts with impending failure. We remain uncertain about whether frequent flow testing reduces overall costs. The issue of reimbursement remains unclear at this time.

With an increase in the number of AV fistulae, monitoring native-vein fistulae could evolve into a potential problem. Unlike PTFE grafts, intra-access flow measurements in primary fistulae may not be as predictive of developing stenoses. Measurement of recirculation could be a more useful tool. We have noted fistula dysfunction in several of our patients who either have presented with thrombosis or have experienced the problems of inadequate dialysis that led to the diagnosis. Doppler blood-flow measurements could evolve as the primary tool for measuring fistula flows. Currently, we prefer the use of a clinical examination combined with measurement of flow in the feeding artery (easily reproducible) to monitor the AV fistulae. A fistulogram could be useful to identify the extent of the problem. It is also important to study the arterial inflow because arterial disease could be responsible for the decrease in fistula flows.

Guidelines 16–18: Management of Complications

Postoperative vascular and neurologic complications, seen primarily in diabetic patients, can be devastating. We currently evaluate these patients using pulse oximetry to monitor distal extremity perfusion in the postoperative period

(7). High-risk patients with poor pulse oximetric readings associated with a decrease in waveforms are closely monitored; if necessary, they are observed overnight in the hospital. Patients with ischemic limbs are treated by external banding or ligation of the vascular access.

Guideline 19: Treatment of Stenoses without Thromboses

From a radiologist's perspective, it was gratifying to discover that the DOQI guidelines supported nearly all of our clinical practices pertaining to the diagnosis and treatment of vascular access-related problems. Patients with patent but dysfunctional vascular accesses are referred to interventional radiology for a diagnostic fistulogram. The referral can be prompted by an abnormality discovered during a physical examination of the vascular access, an abnormality detected during hemodialysis treatment, or an abnormal value detected during routine monitoring studies performed in the hemodialysis unit.

The use of ultrasonic dilution flow measurements to monitor periodically the intragraft blood flow as our primary surveillance method led to an improvement in the detection of venous stenoses before graft thrombosis. Prevention of graft thrombosis is only one benefit of a surveillance program, however. A significant (>50%) stenosis also can decrease the hemodynamic performance of a vascular access and thereby decrease the efficiency of hemodialysis treatment. Thus, the early detection and treatment of significant stenoses will not only prevent thrombosis but also will improve the efficiency of hemodialysis.

The DOQI criteria for angioplasty are similar to those that were already in use at our institution. As stated in guideline 19, an intervention (i.e., angioplasty) should not be performed unless two criteria are fulfilled. First, the patient must have an abnormal clinical finding, such as arm swelling, or an abnormal physiologic parameter, such as decreased intragraft blood flow. Second, the patient must have a greater than 50% stenosis demonstrated by angiography. It is important that the stenosis is responsible for the clinical or physiologic abnormality. At our institution, patients who are referred to interventional radiology for a fistulogram already demonstrated a clinical or physiologic abnormality, most commonly a decrease in intragraft blood flow. If the fistulogram then reveals a greater than 50% stenosis, the angioplasty procedure is performed immediately.

As expected, using measurements of access flow as our primary surveillance method has decreased the number of thrombectomy procedures and, correspondingly, increased the number of elective angioplasty procedures. Furthermore, the measurement of access blood flow provided valuable insights into other factors that contribute to the performance of a vascular access. These factors include stenoses in the proximal native arteries and intragraft stenoses. By measuring the intragraft blood flow immediately following en-

dovascular interventions, we have learned that the successful repair of venous stenoses does not always improve blood flow (8). We also learned that arterial inflow disease is more prevalent than has been reported. About 20% of our patients have native arterial lesions, most commonly atherosclerotic disease in the proximal brachial artery. We now perform retrograde arteriography, via vascular access, in patients who are presenting with the first vascular access problem.

Guideline 20: Treatment of Central Venous Stenoses

The guidelines were particularly important in reference to the controversial issue of using vascular stents to treat stenoses at the venous anastomosis and in peripheral veins. Guidelines 19 and 20 state that vascular stents should be used only in "selected instances," such as elastic central vein stenoses, surgically inaccessible lesions, or in patients with contraindications to surgery. Although we have used vascular stents for the treatment of recurring stenoses in large central veins, we have remained conservative in our use of stents at the venous anastomosis and in the peripheral veins. We continue to believe that a conservative approach is supported by the published literature. It is our belief that the use of vascular stents does not provide superior patency rates compared with those achieved using standard angioplasty. In addition, our vascular access surgeons disapprove of using stents in the peripheral veins. They believe that vascular stents will interfere with future surgical revisions and provide minimal long-term benefit.

Guideline 21: Treatment of Thrombosis and Associated Stenosis in Dialysis Arteriovenous Grafts

Most patients with thrombosed PTFE grafts are referred to interventional radiology for evaluation and treatment. Commonly, the patient is sent to radiology on the same day that the access thrombosis is discovered. The radiologist evaluates the graft and native veins and determines whether an endovascular thrombectomy is appropriate. If so, the thrombectomy and subsequent endovascular repairs are performed at that time. If the endovascular thrombectomy was a success, the patient will continue to return to interventional radiology when future problems develop. Details of the diagnostic findings and endovascular procedures are documented in the radiology report, and a summary is provided in the access notes. Alternatively, if the radiologist evaluates the graft and determines that endovascular salvage is not appropriate, the patient's hemodialysis center is notified and a hemodialysis catheter is inserted. The surgeon responsible for the patient is informed of these events and the diagnostic findings, and plans for surgical management of the vascular access are formulated.

The disadvantage of such a system is that the interventional radiologist becomes the first stop. Any delay because of institutional problems in scheduling percutaneous thrombectomy invariably leads to catheter dialysis because scheduling surgery needs some lead time. Incorporating C-arm technology into operative suites is a potential solution that could obviate such a delay. With such a setup, percutaneous thrombectomy could be performed in the operating room, and surgical intervention could be provided at the same time.

Guideline 22: Treatment of Thrombosis in Primary Arteriovenous Fistulae

Surgeons typically manage and repair thrombosed primary fistulae. Although one radiologist may be willing to treat thrombosed primary fistulae, other radiologists may not be. Mature fistulae usually have an underlying outflow or inflow problem that precipitates the thrombosis. Along with a thrombectomy, surgeons typically perform patch venoplasty using a vein or PTFE patch. Fistulae that are not fully mature tend to fail thrombectomy attempts.

Guideline 23: Treatment of Tunneled Cuffed Catheter Dysfunction

The DOQI guidelines define a *dysfunctional* catheter as one that cannot sustain a blood flow of at least 300 mL per minute. In our opinion, this value is often difficult to achieve and sustain in our patient population. A significant number of our patients would have dysfunctional catheters if we used this definition. For clinical purposes, we define a dysfunctional catheter, one necessitating an intervention, as having a blood flow less than 250 mL per minute. These patients are referred to interventional radiology for evaluation and treatment. Initially, the course of the catheter is examined under fluoroscopy to identify catheter kinks or tip malposition. A contrast study then is performed to evaluate for the presence of a fibrin sheath or pericatheter thrombus. The multi-side-hole Ash Split catheter (Medcomp, Harleysville, PA, U.S.A.) is our primary tunneled hemodialysis catheter. In our experience, the most frequent cause of catheter dysfunction is thrombotic occlusion of the distal end hole or multiple side holes. We use a brushing technique to remove this thrombotic debris and restore catheter patency (9). If this technique is unsuccessful, or if catheter dysfunction is a frequent occurrence, the catheter is replaced over a guidewire through the original tract.

Guideline 26: Treatment of Infection of Tunneled Cuffed Catheters

Before publication of the DOQI guidelines, we had a somewhat disorganized approach to the treatment of catheter-related infections. The DOQI guidelines provided us with an educated opinion and direction for the management of these commonly encountered problems. The most useful suggestions within guideline 26 regarded the treatment of catheter exit-site infections. This supported our opinion that these types of minor wound infections could often be treated with local site care and parenteral antibiotics.

One of the most divisive issues continues to be the management of patients with tunneled catheters and bacteremia. Positive blood cultures usually prompt a discussion of catheter removal. The DOQI opinion-based guideline is removal of all catheters with a demonstrated bacteremia. From the radiology perspective, there is a desire be more protective of the patient's central veins because another catheter will have to be inserted when the bacteremia resolves. The radiologist often prefers to leave the catheter in place and treat the patient with intravenous antibiotics. Even with acceptance of the DOQI guidelines, this issue continues to be difficult. We have a reasonable consensus for some common scenarios: (a) immediate catheter removal for all unstable or persistently ill patients and (b) attempted catheter salvage with 4 weeks antibiotics in stable patients with exhausted alternative vascular access sites. We also virtually always remove catheters in patients with *Staphylococcus aureus* infections. We continue to struggle with a consensus approach to the stable patient with relatively nonvirulent infections.

Guideline 28: Aneurysm of Primary Arteriovenous Fistulae

This DOQI guideline outlines indications for intervention in primary fistula. Fistula monitoring still has many unresolved problems. Our opinion is that aneurysmal dilations in AV fistulae usually are associated with distal venous stenosis. These mandate a careful clinical examination. A pulsatile flow leads the examiner to the stenotic segment. In fistulae with high blood flow, weblike focal stenotic lesions in large-caliber veins can be difficult to demonstrate on routine fistulogram; such occult lesions can be fully appreciated only by observing a resistant waist on an inflated angioplasty balloon. Elective repair of the stenosis helps increase fistula flow, prevents further increase in size of the aneurysm, and prevents associated complications.

UNRESOLVED ISSUES

Guideline 1: Patient History and Physical Examination before Permanent Access Selection

The modality of dialysis (hemodialysis versus peritoneal dialysis) is most often decided before referral for access creation. The specific type of hemodialysis access decision is often left to the surgeon, however. DOQI guidelines clearly outline the importance of evaluating key elements of history, physical examination, and preoperative diagnostic evaluation to determine the timing, type, and location of access procedures. What is not emphasized is the need to understand comprehensively the overall ESRD plan in a given patient. For example, the guidelines emphasize the importance of early referral to the surgeon. Early referral often ends with placement of a permanent access. It is not unusual to see a patient with potential for living related transplantation being evaluated for dialysis access. Permanent access should be avoided in such a patient unless hemodialysis is needed for an indefinite period. This avoids the unnecessary use of peripheral vessels that may be required in the future if the transplant fails. In addition, we have observed that dialysis accesses clot more expeditiously with normalization of renal (and platelet) function following transplantation. Similarly, comprehensive understanding of end-stage renal disease (ESRD) is also necessary when access decisions are made in elderly patients, debilitated patients, or patients with incurable disease. In our opinion, life expectancy should be factored into treatment algorithms. Any patient with clinical findings conducive to native-vein fistula creation should be offered this procedure. A synthetic graft arteriovenous fistula that can be accessed within 2 to 3 weeks of placement, however, may be a suitable first procedure when clinical findings are ambiguous for a native-vein fistula creation. This access may be more suitable for patients with limited life expectancy.

Guideline 5: Type and Location of Tunneled Cuffed Catheter Placement

Unfortunately, one of our most common indications for placement of a tunneled hemodialysis catheter is following a failed percutaneous thrombectomy procedure. About 10% to 15% of our thrombectomy procedures are terminated because of untreatable lesions in the native venous outflow. If the thrombectomy procedure is abandoned immediately following the diagnostic venogram, the nephrologist is notified. Unfortunately, placement of a tunneled hemodialysis catheter frequently becomes necessary because scheduling surgery often needs some lead time. It is essential that surgical thrombectomy and revision be scheduled as soon as possible to avoid prolonged catheter use. As mentioned earlier, incorporating C-arm technology into operative suites could be a potential solution. With such a setup, percutaneous thrombectomy could be performed in the operating room, and surgical intervention could be provided at the same time.

Guideline 7: Preservation of Veins for Arteriovenous Access

Preservation of peripheral veins has been a difficult goal. We have had considerable success in placing medical alerts once chronic renal failure or ESRD has been established in the hospital. Although many nephrologists educate patients regarding the importance of vein preservation, most hospital personnel are ignorant of this issue. Venipuncture, peripheral intravenous catheters, placement of subclavian catheters, use of radial artery for coronary artery bypass surgery and autologous transplantation of parathyroid in the fore-

arm decrease the options available for creating dialysis access. Educating the medical community is an important aspect of access planning and management.

Guideline 8: Timing of Access Placement

We have attempted graft placement when the anticipated need for dialysis is 4 to 6 weeks away. This attempt has resulted in an unacceptably high number of patients initiating dialysis with tunneled dialysis catheters. Given the unpredictability of renal disease progression, one wonders whether the grafts should be placed sooner. If so, when they should be placed is still an unresolved problem. Vascular access blood flow monitoring shows decreasing flow in most grafts with time. It is unknown whether earlier placement (e.g., 8–12 weeks before anticipated dialysis) of graft access will lead to earlier stenosis formation.

SUMMARY

In summary, developing a multidisciplinary team for dialysis access planning and treatment has helped us to develop a consensus approach to managing dialysis access. Establishment of the DOQI guidelines reinforced this consensus approach and further improved outcome. Yet implementation of the DOQI guidelines has not been without problems. We are continuing to address these issues in an effort to achieve the DOQI goals of increasing efficiency of patient care and positively impacting the patient outcome.

REFERENCES

1. Arora P, Obrador GT, Ruthazer R, et al. Prevalence, predictors, and consequences of late nephrology referral at a tertiary care center. *J Am Soc Nephrol* 1999;10:1281–1286.
2. Shenoy S, Middleton W, Windus D. Brachial artery flow measurement as an indicator of forearm native vein fistula maturation—early experience. In: Henry M, Ferguson R, eds. *Vascular access for hemodialysis*. Chicago: Precept Press, 2001:233–237.
3. Windus DW, Audrain J, Vanderson R, et al. Optimization of high-efficiency hemodialysis by detection and correction of fistula dysfunction. *Kidney Int* 1990;38:337–341.
4. Coyne DW, Delmez J, Spence G, et al. Impaired delivery of hemodialysis prescriptions: an analysis of causes and an approach to evaluation. *J Am Soc Nephrol* 1997;8:1315–1318.
5. Strauch BS, O'Connell RS, Geoly KL, et al. Forecasting thrombosis of vascular access with Doppler color flow imaging. *Am J Kidney Dis* 1992;19:554–557.
6. Sands JJ, Miranda CL. Prolongation of hemodialysis access survival with elective revision. *Clin Nephrol* 1995;44:329–333.
7. Shenoy S, Lowell J, Ramachandran V, et al. Pulse oximetry to monitor distal extremity perfusion in the postoperative period. In: Henry M, Ferguson R, eds. *Vascular access for hemodialysis*. Chicago: Precept Press, 1999:61–67.
8. Ahya SA, Windus DW, Vesely TM. Utility of radiologic criteria for predicting access flow after percutaneous transluminal angioplasty. *Kidney Int* 2001;59:1974–1978.
9. Cox K, Vesely TM, Windus DW, et al. The utility of brushing dysfunctional hemodialysis catheters. *J Vasc Interv Radiol* 2000;11:979–983.

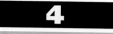

TRENDS IN VASCULAR ACCESS PROCEDURES AND EXPENDITURES IN MEDICARE'S END-STAGE RENAL DISEASE PROGRAM

PAUL W. EGGERS
ROGER MILAM

The creation and maintenance of vascular access sites for dialysis patients are not only a source of considerable morbidity within the dialysis population, but they also constitute a major cost to the Medicare end-stage renal disease (ESRD) program. This chapter examines recent trends in vascular access procedures and compares the costs to Medicare following placement of fistula, graft, and catheter access procedures.

The Dialysis Outcomes Quality Initiative (DOQI) clinical guidelines for vascular access have an autologous fistula placement goal of 40% in prevalent hemodialysis patients. As of 1998, only 27% of patients nationwide had a fistula, with 20% using a central venous catheter for access. Although fistula rates were higher in the Northeast, none of the ESRD networks met the DOQI guideline level. The Health Care Financing Association (HCFA) billing data, however, show that fistula placement has been increasing the past few years and that more vascular procedures are performed in the outpatient setting. As a result, expenditures for vascular access are decreasing in absolute terms and as a percent of all dialysis costs.

Total Medicare per capita expenditures following access placements are $77,600 in the first year after placement and $54,200 in the second year. Adjusted annual costs for fistulae are $4,500 less than for grafts and $9,000 less than for catheters. Unmeasured patient comorbidities, however, probably account for some of these differences.

BACKGROUND

The creation, maintenance, and replacement of vascular access in dialysis patients are recognized as major sources of morbidity and costs of Medicare's ESRD program (1–3). In addition, recent evidence suggests that costs may be increasing as a percent of program expenditures (4–7) and that fistulae are decreasing as a percent of vascular access procedures (6,8). The importance of vascular access in the care of dialysis patients was recognized in the development of the DOQI guidelines by the National Kidney Foundation (9). All these studies deal with trends preceding publication of DOQI. Post-DOQI trends have not yet been documented.

Barriers to autologous fistula placement include a large percentage of patients with inadequate sites for creation of artery-to-vein anastomoses and late referrals to dialysis that prevent the opportunity for a fistula to mature (4). Fistulae are recommended over grafts and catheters, however, because of their superior long-term patency. It is widely believed that the superior patency of fistulae also should be reflected in lower costs of care because fewer interventions and replacements would be necessary. The empiric evidence for this belief is largely missing. Some have argued that the implementation of DOQI guidelines may result in higher costs (10), but at least one study showed that the aggressive shift from a predominantly graft-based access system to the primary use of fistulae has decreased overall costs (11).

This study presents information on trends in vascular access in the immediate post-DOQI era. The most recent trends in vascular access procedures are examined using data collected through the HCFA Clinical Performance Measures (CPM) project as well as HCFA billing data. This study also compares total Medicare expenditures following placement of fistula, graft, and catheter types of access.

METHODS AND DATA

Data for this study were obtained from two sources. The distribution of vascular access procedures in 1998 was taken from the CPM project, which is an extension of the ESRD Core Indicators Project, started in 1994 (12). The Core Indicators Project was HCFA's first nationwide, population-based study designed to improve the care of patients with ESRD. The project has collected clinical information annually on four key care indicators (i.e., adequacy of dialysis, hematocrit value, nutritional status, and blood pressure control) for a national sample of adult in-center hemodialysis and peritoneal dialysis patients. The ESRD CPMs are similar to the core indicators, with the addition of measures for vascular access. The 1998 sample includes 8,336 dialysis patients, of whom 1,621 began dialysis in 1998 and are defined as *incident patients*.

The expenditure analyses were taken from data from the ESRD Program Management and Medical Information System (PMMIS), which is maintained by the Office of Clinical Standards and Quality (OCSQ) at the HCFA. The ESRD PMMIS is a longitudinal file of patients with ESRD who are entitled to Medicare benefits. In addition to the basic enrollment data available for all Medicare beneficiaries, such as sex, race, date of birth, date of death, and entitlement dates, the PMMIS contains information unique to ESRD beneficiaries. The medical evidence form (HCFA 2728) is used to determine the date and cause of renal failure. The ESRD PMMIS file used in this study was updated through November 1999. This update of the ESRD PMMIS contained more than 967,000 patients, which is the complete count of Medicare ESRD patients ever entitled since 1978.

In addition to entitlement records, HCFA receives billing data on all ESRD persons served by fee-for-service providers. All billing data for ESRD beneficiaries receiving care in the fee-for-service sector were linked to individual ESRD beneficiaries. Services covered by Medicare include short-stay hospitalizations, physician services, outpatient services (largely dialysis and erythropoietin treatment), home health care, skilled nursing care, and hospice. Vascular procedures are coded by the HCFA common procedure coding system (HCPCS). The HCPCS is based on the American Medical Association common procedure coding (CPT) system with additions for durable medical equipment, drugs, ambulance, and other services not provided by physicians. Vascular surgery was defined as fistula (HCPCS = 36821 and 36825), graft (HCPC = 36830), and catheter (HCPC = 36533).

RESULTS

Recent Trends in Vascular Access Surgery

Vascular access results from the CPM are shown in Table 4.1. In 1998, more than a quarter (27%) of hemodialysis patients had a fistula as their access site. More than half were using a synthetic graft (53%), and the remaining 20% were undergoing dialysis via a catheter. Catheter use was greater (25%) for

TABLE 4.1. PERCENT OF SAMPLED PATIENTS WITH DIFFERENT ACCESS TYPES FOR INCIDENT AND PREVALENT SAMPLES: 1998

Characteristic	1998 Incident (n = 1,621)			Prevalent (n = 8,336)		
	Fistula	Graft	Catheter	Fistula	Graft	Catheter
Total	27	48	25	27	53	20
Gender						
Male	34[a]	43	24	36[a]	46	18
Female	19	54	27	17	61	22
Race						
White	28[a]	44	27	30[a]	49	22
African American	20	59	21	22	60	18
Age group (yr)						
18–44	36[a]	37	26	36[a]	45	19
45–64	31	46	24	29	53	18
65 and over	20	54	26	22	56	22
Primary ESRD cause						
Diabetes mellitus	24[a]	52	24	23[a]	57	20
Hypertension	24	51	26	27	55	18
Glomerulonephritis	36	44	20	36	47	16
Other/unknown	31	39	30	31	47	22
Duration of dialysis (yr)						
0.5	NA	NA	NA	21[a]	38	40
0.5–0.9	NA	NA	NA	27	49	24
1–1.9	NA	NA	NA	28	53	19
>2	NA	NA	NA	29	58	13

ESRD, end-stage renal disease; NA, not applicable.
From Vascular Access for In-Center Hemodialysis Patients: Preliminary Findings: Supplemental Report No. 1. 1999 ESRD Clinical Performance Measures Project, with permission; available at: www.hcfa.gov.
[a] $p < .05$.

TABLE 4.2. NUMBER OF MEDICARE BILLINGS FOR VASCULAR ACCESS BY TYPE OF PLACEMENT AND SITE OF SERVICE: 1992–1999

Year	Total (n)	Graft (n)	Fistula (n)	Fistula (%)	Inpatient (n)	Outpatient (n)	Outpatient (%)
1992	68,988	51,841	17,147	25%	55,964	13,024	19
1993	70,023	53,657	16,366	23	54,907	15,116	22
1994	75,021	57,520	17,501	23	56,162	18,859	25
1995	77,855	59,347	18,508	24	54,729	23,126	30
1996	80,132	60,413	19,719	25	52,118	28,014	35
1997	80,873	57,413	23,460	29	48,412	32,461	40
1998	83,638	56,560	27,078	32	45,757	37,881	45
1999	84,948	54,715	30,233	36	41,065	43,883	52

From: Part B extract and summary system (BESS) maintained by the Office of Information Services, Health Care Financing Administration, with permission.

the patients who began dialysis during 1998. Use of fistulae was greater for male patients (36%), for white patients (30%), and for persons in the 18- to 44-year-old age group (36%). Persons whose renal failure was caused by diabetes were less likely (23%) to have a fistula than were other persons. Fistula placement rates varied by region (data not shown) and were highest in the Northeast (36%) and lowest in a number of Southern states and in southern California (20% to 21%).

Table 4.2 shows the number of fistula and graft procedures billed to Medicare for the years 1992 through 1999[1]. In 1992, there were almost 69,000 vascular procedures, of which 17,000 (25%) were fistula placements. The percentage with a fistula remained largely unchanged through 1996. In 1997, 1998, and 1999, the percentage of vascular procedures that were fistulae was 29%, 32%, and 36%, respectively. The increase in fistulae coincides with the publication of the DOQI guidelines in the spring 1997. The promulgation of the guidelines has likely led to more serious efforts to use fistulae for vascular access. The other notable trend evidenced in Table 4.2 is the increasing tendency to perform these surgeries in the outpatient setting. In 1992, less than one fifth (19%) of vascular placements were performed in an outpatient setting. By 1999, more than half of these placements were performed in the outpatient setting, which greatly reduced the costs of these procedures because the costs of an inpatient stay greatly exceed outpatient surgery.

Hospitalization rates for vascular access are shown in Table 4.3. This table represents all vascular procedures, initial placement as well as revisions, declotting procedures, and other repairs. In 1994, there were 48 hospitalizations per 100 dialysis patients for vascular procedures. This rate ranged from a low of 34 per 100 persons aged 15 to 24 years to a rate of 66 hospitalizations per 100 persons aged 75 years and older. Female patients had higher rates than male patients (52 and 44 per 100, respectively), and rates were higher for

African Americans (52 per 100) than for other races. From 1994 to 1998, vascular hospitalizations declined by 16%, to 40 per 100 persons. Declines were greater for elderly, white, and African-American dialysis patients.

The impact of these declines in vascular inpatient hospitalizations on Medicare expenditures is shown in Table 4.4. Per capita Medicare expenditures for inpatient hospital stays for dialysis patients in 1994 were $17,720. This increased to $19,828 by 1997 and then dropped slightly in 1998 to $19,329, for an overall increase of 9%. Per capita expenditures for vascular access hospitalizations, however, dropped by almost $500, or 12%. Expenditures increased by over 20% for circulatory, respiratory, infectious signs and symptoms and related hospitalizations.

Medicare Expenditures after Access Placement

This analysis was designed to compare total Medicare expenditures after placement of a native fistula, an artificial graft, and central venous catheters. The earliest date at which placement (fistula, graft, or catheter) was made during 1997 was used as the starting date. Total Medicare expenditures (including the initial placement) were calculated through the end of 1998. That is, follow-up ranged from 12 months for procedures occurring in December 1997 to 24 months for procedures occurring in January 1997. Patients were censored at either death or transplantation. Expenditures were attributed to the initial type of access placement (i.e., an intent-to-treat fashion) regardless of changes in access type during the observation period.

Table 4.5 shows the number of initial vascular placements[2] in 1997 by various demographic groupings. A total of 75,820 initial placements were performed: 20% fistulas, 48% grafts,

---

[1] Catheters were not included in this table because the source of data, the part B extract and summary system (BESS), does not distinguish between ESRD and other patients. Most of the catheter implants in the Medicare population are for purposes other than dialysis access.

[2] The initial placement was defined as the first placement in 1997. Many of these patients had vascular procedures in previous years not captured in this analysis. As such, these distributions are not directly comparable to the rates shown in Table 4.1, which represent a cross-section of procedures functioning at the end of 1998.

TABLE 4.3. MEDICARE ESRD DIALYSIS PATIENTS INPATIENT HOSPITALIZATION RATES PER 100 PERSONS FOR VASCULAR ACCESS: 1994 TO 1998

	1994	1995	1996	1997	1998	Percent Change
Age, Sex, Race						
All persons	48	48	45	42	40	−16
Age (yr)						
<15	40	44	37	29	33	−17
15–24	34	41	39	35	36	6
25–34	39	40	38	37	36	−7
35–44	38	40	39	36	36	−5
45–54	42	41	39	37	35	−15
55–64	44	44	43	38	37	−15
65–74	55	52	48	45	42	−23
>75	66	58	53	49	46	−31
Sex						
Male	44	44	41	39	37	−16
Female	52	53	49	46	43	−16
Race						
Asian	33	32	31	31	31	−8
African-American	52	53	49	46	43	−17
White	46	46	43	40	38	−18
Native American	44	51	52	43	44	1
Other/unknown	40	50	49	44	44	11

ESRD, end-stage renal disease.
From Health Care Financing Administration (HCFA) ESRD Program Management and Medical Information System and National Claims History, with permission.

and 32% catheters. Fistula placement did not vary greatly by age, but catheters were most common among persons under the age of 25 years (44%) and least common among those aged 65 to 74 years (29%). Male patients were much more likely to have a fistula placement than were female patients (25% and 15%, respectively). Fistula placement was least common among African (16%) and Asian (19%) Americans. Persons with glomerulonephritis are most likely to have fistula placement (23%). Not surprisingly, the longer the person had been on dialysis, the less likely he or she received a fistula.

For persons whose renal failure preceded 1996, the fistula placement rate was only 14%. Conversely, for the 2,823 persons whose vascular placement preceded the start of dialysis (in 1998), the fistula placement rate was 50%, with only 11% receiving a catheter.[3] Fistulae accounted for 18% of the pro-

---

[3] Note that Table 4.1 shows functioning vascular access types in 1998. An unknown number of the fistulae in this table and the expenditure analysis failed to mature. Thus, the comparison of types of access should be considered as "intent to treat."

TABLE 4.4. MEDICARE PER CAPITA EXPENDITURES FOR DIALYSIS PATIENTS FOR INPATIENT CARE BY REASON FOR STAY: 1994 TO 1998

	1994	1995	1996	1997	1998	Change (%)
All causes	$17,720	$18,464	$19,271	$19,828	$19,329	9
Vascular access	4,147	4,131	4,055	3,908	3,657	−12
Circulatory (390–459)	4,333	4,685	5,097	5,362	5,273	22
Digestive (520–579)	1,632	1,618	1,648	1,698	1,639	0
Genitourinary (580–629)	777	868	880	888	801	3
Endocrine/metabolic (240–279)	1,521	1,543	1,551	1,572	1,554	2
Respiratory (460–519)	1,175	1,273	1,375	1,439	1,437	22
Infectious (001–139)	796	902	1,036	1,093	1,025	29
Signs and symptoms (780–799)	700	696	729	786	844	21
All others	2,639	2,748	2,899	3,083	3,099	17

[a] Numbers in parentheses represent ranges of ICD-9 codes. From Health Care Financing Administration (HCFA) ESRD Program Management and Medical Information System and National Claims History, with permission.

TABLE 4.5. FIRST VASCULAR ACCESS PROCEDURE IN 1997 BY AGE, SEX, RACE, CAUSE OF RENAL FAILURE, ESRD INCIDENT YEAR, AND PLACE OF SERVICE

	All Procedures (n)	Fistula (%)	Graft (%)	Catheter (%)
All	75,820	20	48	32
Age group				
0 to 24	894	21	35	44
25 to 44	8,779	21	43	35
45 to 64	20,385	18	49	33
65 to 74	24,523	22	49	29
75+	21,239	20	48	32
Gender				
Male	37,956	25	45	29
Female	37,864	15	50	34
Race				
White	43,949	22	44	33
African-Am.	26,665	16	53	31
Asian	1,427	19	58	23
Native Am.	976	23	43	34
Other	2,803	24	53	23
Cause of ESRD				
Diabetes	31,364	20	50	30
Hypertension	22,636	20	49	31
G. nephritis	7,857	23	45	32
Other	13,963	20	42	38
Incident year				
Pre-1994	16,263	14	50	36
1994	5,980	14	49	37
1995	7,851	14	47	39
1996	11,863	18	48	34
1997	31,040	25	48	28
1998	2,823	50	39	11
Place of service				
Inpatient	47,363	18	48	34
Outpatient	28,457	24	48	28

ESRD, end-stage renal disease.
From Health Care Financing Administration (HCFA) ESRD Program Management and Medical Information System and National Claims History, with permission.

cedures done on an inpatient basis and 24% of those done on an outpatient basis.

Table 4.6 shows Medicare expenditures for the first year after placement of a vascular access. Overall, Medicare expenditures were $77,619 per person-year, considerably greater than the $52,000 per person-year average cost for all dialysis patients (13). This reflects the increased morbidity associated with vascular procedure creation and maintenance. Average expenditures were much greater for patients receiving a graft ($75,611 per person-year) or a catheter ($86,927 per person-year) than for persons receiving a fistula ($68,002 per person-year). Dialysis and erythropoietin costs are largely fixed, and there were no significant differences in outpatient services. Most of the differences were explained by higher costs for hospitalization and physician care. Second-year costs following access placement ($54,206 per person-

year) more nearly approximate average costs for all dialysis patients. As expected, outpatient costs remained fairly unchanged, whereas inpatient costs decreased by more than $10,000 per person-year, and in the case of catheter patients, it decreased by almost $20,000 per person-year. Although expenditures decreased for all types of placements, there still remained a cost advantage to fistulae.

As shown in Table 4.5, there are many differences between the patients who receive the three types of vascular access. To control for these differences, a multivariate analysis was performed on the expenditure levels. The dependent variable was calculated as total Medicare expenditures per day of Medicare eligibility. Variables included in the model were age, sex, race, cause of renal failure, and type of access. In addition, three other variables were added to the model. Because there is usually some excess morbidity

TABLE 4.6. TOTAL PER CAPITA MEDICARE EXPENDITURES FOR 1ST AND 2ND YEAR FOLLOWING 1997 ACCESS PLACEMENT BY TYPE OF SERVICE

	All Procedures	Fistula	Graft	Catheter
1st year				
Total	$77,619	$68,002	$75,611	$86,927
Inpatient	35,037	29,069	32,980	42,108
Outpatient	22,877	22,599	23,528	22,014
Physician	14,304	12,449	13,900	16,126
Home health	2,649	1,836	2,687	3,104
Skilled nursing	2,681	1,997	2,459	3,468
Hospice	71	52	56	107
2nd year				
Total	54,206	49,689	54,555	57,178
Inpatient	19,535	17,067	19,181	22,153
Outpatient	21,688	21,317	22,356	20,765
Physician	10,074	9,096	10,016	10,962
Home health	1,395	984	1,464	1,598
Skilled nursing	1,458	1,174	1,487	1,633
Hospice	55	52	51	66

From Health Care Financing Agency (HCFA) ESRD Program Management and Medical Information System and National Claims History, with permission.

TABLE 4.7. MULTIVARIATE ANALYSIS OF MEDICARE EXPENDITURES FOLLOWING VASCULAR ACCESS PROCEDURES

Variable	Parameter Estimate	Annualized ($)	P value
Intercept	104.89	38,286	0.0001
0–24	1.36	496	0.7073
25–34	4.74	1,731	0.0330
35–44	5.19	1,895	0.0032
45–54	Comparison	—	—
55–64	0.88	322	0.5736
65–74	2.42	883	0.0662
75–84	0.34	124	0.8154
≥85	−3.52	−1,286	0.1778
Female	Comparison	—	—
Male	−6.49	−2,369	0.0001
White	Comparison	—	—
Asian	−1.70	−621	0.5831
African American	7.27	2,654	0.0001
Native American	−7.37	−2,689	0.0506
Other Race	8.32	3,036	0.1589
Glomerulonephritis (GN)	Comparison	—	—
Diabetes	17.28	6,307	0.0001
Secondary GN	8.21	2,996	0.0022
Interstitial nephritis	3.44	1,254	0.1089
Hereditary diseases	−3.98	−1,452	0.0987
Neoplasms	14.97	5,465	0.0001
Other diseases	34.23	12,495	0.0001
Unknown	3.16	1,153	0.1655
Missing	32.95	12,027	0.0001
Incident	21.63	7,895	0.0001
Death	123.67	N/A	0.0001
Hospitalization	34.09	12,442	0.0001
Fistula	Comparison	—	—
Graft	12.23	4,464	0.0001
Catheter	24.73	9,026	0.0001

NA, not applicable.
From the Health Care Financing Administration (HCFA) ESRD Program Management and Medical Information System and National Claims History, with permission.

associated with the initiation of dialysis, a variable was added to indicate incident patients. Hospitalization for the initial procedure also adds greatly to the costs of the procedure, but it does not reflect on the success of the procedure itself. So a variable was added to control for the place of service for the original access placement. Finally, a crude measure of severity was added to the model. Because it is highly unlikely that the access type itself would cause excess mortality, a bivariate indicator of death during the observation period was added to approximate the severity for some patients.

The results of the multivariate analysis are shown in Table 4.7. In addition to daily parameter estimates, estimates of annual expenditures are also shown. There were no consistent age effects, although persons 25 to 34 years of age and 35 to 44 years of age had statistically higher expenditure levels than persons in the 45- to 54-year age group (p <0.05). Expenditures were higher for female patients (p <0.0001), African-American patients (p <0.0001), and persons whose renal failure was attributed to diabetes (p <0.0001), secondary glomerulonephritis (p <0.003), and neoplasms (p <0.0001). Higher expenditures were also associated with incident patients (p <0.0001) and with patients whose initial placement was in an inpatient facility (p <0.0001). Finally, compared with fistula recipients, persons who received a graft had $4,464 in predicted additional annualized expenditures, and catheter recipients had $9,026 greater annualized expenditure levels.

CONCLUSIONS

The importance of vascular access as a source of both morbidity and costs for dialysis patients has received more attention in recent years. The publication of the DOQI guidelines has highlighted the low level of fistula placement in the United States compared with other countries. This study showed that there is evidence that the dialysis community is working to reverse the long-term trend to increased use of artificial grafts. Medicare billing data show that the number of fistula placements in 1999 represents almost a doubling of the number of these procedures since 1993. In addition, the placement of artificial grafts declined from 1997 to 1999. Although this shift in treatment patterns cannot be attributed directly to DOQI guidelines, given the congruence of this trend with DOQI, it is likely that dialysis professionals are working toward this end (14).

Another trend shown by these data is the movement of vascular procedures from the inpatient setting to outpatient settings. Although there are no guidelines recommending a reduction in inpatient procedures, the shift has welcome economic benefits. Previous work has shown that, in 1994, hospitalizations for vascular procedures accounted for about one fourth of all hospital costs for dialysis patients (3). By 1998, the shift in vascular procedures had decreased hospitalization costs by almost $500 per dialysis patient, a 12% decrease.

Finally, these data provide the strongest evidence yet of the economic advantages of fistula placement compared with either graft or catheter access types. Controlling for basic demographic and cause-of-renal-failure variables, fistulae appear to have an annual savings to Medicare of $4,500 over grafts and $9,000 over catheter placement. This last finding needs to be regarded with considerable caution, however. It is almost certain that there is a great deal of patient selection when it comes to access placement, particularly with respect to catheters. It is not possible, using administrative data such as Medicare billing, to discern the intent of catheter placement. People who receive catheters probably fall into one of two categories. First, catheters often are used as a bridge therapy, often while a fistula is maturing. A catheter that is replaced by a functioning fistula within a few weeks or months cannot be considered a failed therapy. In fact, in this case, it probably makes more sense to consider the catheter cost as part of the total cost of the fistula than as a separate procedure. The second group of catheter recipients who are not evident in the billing data are patients whose declining health makes a catheter the only available option. Controlling for patient selection effects probably would attenuate the apparent cost advantage to fistula placement.

Work on the cost-effectiveness of different access procedures can be enhanced by linking the Medicare expenditure data with clinically based data sets or trials. In this manner, selection effects can be mitigated and more accurate assessments of cost advantages and disadvantages can be obtained.

REFERENCES

1. U.S. Renal Data System (USRDS). USRDS 1997 annual data report. Bethesda, MD: National Institutes of Health, National Institute of Diabetes and Digestive and Kidney Diseases; April 1997.
2. Feldman HI, Held PJ, Hutchinson JT, et al. Hemodialysis vascular access morbidity in the United States. *Kidney Int* 1993;43:1091–1096.
3. Eggers PW. Medicare expenditures for vascular access in the ESRD program [syllabus]. The Sixth Biannual Symposium on Dialysis Access. Miami, FL; 1998.
4. Schwab SJ. Vascular access for hemodialysis. *Kidney Int* 1999;55:2078–2090.
5. Pastan S, Bailey J. Dialysis therapy. *N Engl J Med* 1998;338:1428–1437.
6. Hakim R, Himmelfarb J. Hemodialysis access failure: a call to action. *Kidney Int* 1998;54:1029–1040.
7. Rocco MV, Bleyer AJ, Burkart JM. Utilization of inpatient and outpatient resources for the management of hemodialysis access complications. *Am J Kidney Dis* 1996;28:250–256.
8. Hirth RA, Turrenne MN, Woods JD, et al. Predictor of type of vascular access in hemodialysis patients. *JAMA* 1996;276:1303–1308.

9. National Kidney Foundation-Dialysis Outcomes Quality Initiative (NKF-DOQI) clinical practice guidelines for vascular access. New York: National Kidney Foundation; 1997.

10. Wish J, Roberts J, Besarab A, et al. The cost of implementing the dialysis outcomes quality initiative clinical practice guidelines. *Adv Ren Replace Ther* 1999;6:67–74.

11. Becker BN, Breiterman-White R, Nylander W, et al. Care pathway reduces hospitalizations and cost for hemodialysis vascular access surgery. *Am J Kidney Dis* 1997; 30:525–531.

12. Helgerson SD, McClellan WM, Frederick PR, et al. Improve- ment in adequacy of delivered dialysis for adult in-center hemodialysis patients in the United States, 1993 to 1995. *Am J Kidney Dis* 1997;29:851–861.

13. U.S. Renal Data System (USRDS). USRDS 1999 annual data report. Bethesda, MD: National Institute of Health, National Institute of Diabetes and Digestive and Kidney Diseases; April 1999.

14. Ascher E, Gade P, Hingoram A, et al. Changes in the practice of angioaccess surgery: impact of dialysis outcome and quality initiative recommendations *Vasc Surg* 2000;31:84–92.

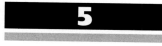

EARLY REFERRAL FOR VASCULAR ACCESS

JACK MOORE, JR.
SUSAN P. LOUGHLIN

Patients with end stage renal disease (ESRD) are afforded several different options for treatment of their chronic kidney disease, among which are hemodialysis, peritoneal dialysis, and kidney transplantation. For a variety of different reasons, most patients either choose or are placed in a maintenance hemodialysis program, in which they usually receive treatment three times a week. In fact, at the end of 1998, more than 320,000 patients were on hemodialysis (1). Medical contraindications and severe shortages of kidneys continue to be barriers against the more widespread use of transplantation. For hemodialysis to be delivered, it is necessary to have access to the circulation.

Vascular access has always been one of the principal problems facing patients on hemodialysis. When dialysis was first made available in the United States in the 1950s, cannulae were surgically placed in juxtaposed arteries and veins, and treatment was delivered for as long as 8 to 10 hours. Because of the limitations of surgical techniques and materials available to achieve access, it was usual that the artery and vein combination could be used only once. Thus, the radial artery and brachiocephalic vein could be used for one treatment; with two treatments, this vascular grouping would be exhausted for the upper extremities. The development and availability of techniques and material that permitted long-term vascular access were the two of the most formidable technical obstacles that had to be overcome to provide long-term maintenance hemodialysis.

With the passage of the ESRD legislation in 1972, a funding mechanism (i.e., Medicare) made dialysis available to most persons who required it in the United States. Under this legislation, the federal government agreed to have patients with ESRD included in the Medicare program; so 80% of the costs of dialysis were funded. This funding mechanism permitted the growth of the ESRD population. With the aging of the population and the increased prevalence of diseases such as diabetes mellitus and hypertension, the growth of the dialysis population has increased at a rate of more than 5% per year. It now has been estimated that more than 600,000 persons will likely be receiving hemo-

dialysis by the end of the first decade of the twenty-first century (1). Given this explosion, it has become axiomatic that kidney transplantation will not be able to support all these patients and that the hemodialysis population will continue to require more effective methods of maintaining vascular access.

At present, there are three methods by which patients on hemodialysis can have vascular access established. The preferred method is by the surgical creation of an autologous fistula, optimally in the nondominant arm. The second method is by the surgical placement of an arteriovenous graft. A variety of materials have been used for grafts. Currently, most grafts are made from a synthetic material known as polytetrafluoroethylene (PTFE), which has been manipulated in a number of different ways to make it more biocompatible, less thrombogenic, and less prone to infectious and hemorrhagic complications. Finally, indwelling catheters, the number and design of which have proliferated, have been used in patients in whom no other form of access could be achieved or who, for a variety of reasons, needed to have dialysis initiated before a fistula or graft could be created or placed. These catheters can be placed percutaneously or surgically, with or without traversing a subcutaneous tunnel, and have been widely used. Both the synthetic arteriovenous graft and percutaneous catheters are fraught with complications, including recurrent thrombosis, occlusion, infection, or malfunction. These complications have played a major role in attenuating adequate dialysis and represent a substantial burden on patients in terms of increasing hospital days, recurrent surgical procedures, and infectious complications. Obviously, such morbidity translates directly into an increased financial impact on the Medicare ESRD program and has resulted in excessive cost overruns in this program, which supports a relatively small number of patients in comparison to the entire Medicare-eligible population. In fiscal year 1998, Medicare expenditures for ESRD patients totaled 12 billion dollars (USRDS), and private insurers spent an additional 4.7 billion dollars on these patients (1). This high per-patient cost led to increasing scrutiny of the ESRD health care system, with attendant efforts to determine methods to reduce costs without decreasing the quality of care.

NATIONAL KIDNEY FOUNDATION-DIALYSIS OUTCOMES QUALITY INITIATIVE

The increased emphasis on health care outcomes initially started because of the need to control costs. More recently, it has become obvious, using evidence-based medicine, that higher quality care often can be demonstrated to be less expensive than suboptimal care. In no group of patients is this more obvious than in the hemodialysis population. Adequate dialysis has been shown to be associated with improved longevity (2). Because complications of vascular access, including inadequate dialysis, recurrent infections, and recurrent access malfunction, whether from thrombosis or occlusion, remain the principal reasons why dialysis patients are hospitalized, it seems logical that an increased utilization of optimal vascular access methods would result in both improved patient outcomes and reduced costs.

To this end, the National Kidney Foundation (NKF), a not-for-profit organization committed to research and patient advocacy, developed a series of clinical practice guidelines known as the Dialysis Outcomes Quality Initiative (DOQI) guidelines. The NKF was supported in this endeavor by its constituent members, including nephrologists, surgeons, nurses, social workers, dietitians, and patients. Recently, an updated and expanded version of the DOQI guidelines, renamed the Kidney Disease Outcomes Quality Initiative, or K-DOQI, was published (3). These guidelines, including those involved with hemodialysis adequacy, peritoneal dialysis adequacy, vascular access, and the anemia of chronic kidney disease, eventually will include guidelines on nutrition as well as the control of cardiovascular disease. The hope of all who have been involved in the generation and dissemination of the K-DOQI guidelines has been that they will result in better care for our patients. This may be achieved through interventions that change the natural history of a particular disease, reduce the burden of comorbid conditions, or provide strategies that improve how we treat and monitor patients with established ESRD.

BENEFITS OF EARLY REFERRAL

Patients with chronic, often progressive, kidney disease usually have a number of comorbid conditions in addition to their kidney disease. Many of these conditions can be managed relatively easily with the judicious use of appropriate diet, lifestyle changes, and pharmaceutical agents. It is important, however, that such conditions be aggressively managed so as to reduce their untoward effects. Thus, patients' survival on hemodialysis is predicated not only on the ade-

quate treatment of kidney failure, but the management of their comorbid conditions. Many nephrologists believe that referral of patients with early kidney disease to their practice might result in enhanced management of these problems.

Although the precise definition of early kidney disease is still under discussion, it is the hope of nephrologists that early detection and therapeutic intervention might decrease the number of patients entering end-stage kidney programs or at least allow these patients to enter such programs better prepared than in the past. This paradigm is based on the concept that patients with early kidney disease have a number of (often subtle) abnormalities that are amenable to prospective intervention and that such intervention would be translated into an improved downstream outcome. Thus, the early detection and treatment of the anemia of chronic kidney disease with recombinant erythropoietin has been shown to result in improved quality of life as well as regression of left ventricular hypertrophy, a major risk factor for cardiovascular morbidity and mortality (3). Rigorous control of hypertension, often with antihypertensive agents that appear to be specifically renoprotective, have been shown to reduce the rate of progression of diabetic kidney disease (4). Another example is the early recognition and treatment of divalent ion abnormalities that lead to renal osteodystrophy.

Nonetheless, vascular access problems remain the principal reason for hospitalization of these patients once they enter dialysis programs, and recurrent problems with vascular access result in enormous costs to both patients and society. We have long believed that the single most powerful intervention available to us is the creation of an appropriate form of vascular access in the patient approaching dialysis. This provides us with the ability to initiate dialysis electively rather than urgently, avoids the myriad of complications associated with temporary catheters, reduces hospitalization rates for access malfunction, facilitates patients' ability to resume a reasonably normal lifestyle while enrolled in a dialysis program, and permits long-term adequate dialysis to be provided as free of complications as possible. There is absolutely no question that the vascular access of choice is a properly created autologous fistula, preferably in the lower forearm of the nondominant extremity.

IMPLEMENTATION OF EARLY REFERRAL

A high-quality vascular access program with an acceptably high proportion of arteriovenous fistulae is dependent on the referral of patients for arteriovenous fistula placement early enough to provide time for the fistula to mature. Our ability to refer early for vascular access creation is fundamentally predicated on the patient being referred to our nephrology practice sufficiently early. Our practice has been immeasurably improved by the Vascular Access Clinical Practice Guidelines contained in the most recent K-DOQI. We have found it useful to disseminate the information contained in the K-DOQI guidelines to our surgical colleagues. Regular communication with our surgeons facilitates better planning and execution of an optimal vascular access strategy.

Our ultimate goal for patients entering dialysis has been to eliminate the need for dialysis catheters entirely, to increase the proportion of patients entering dialysis with a functioning arteriovenous fistula, and to reduce our proportion of patients with synthetic arteriovenous grafts. To accomplish this goal, we found it necessary to identify proactively patients at risk for progressive kidney disease at an early stage, refer suitable patients for vascular access creation when appropriate, and to work closely with our surgical colleagues to plan and execute an appropriate vascular access strategy for all patients in whom hemodialysis is anticipated.

We have operated under a prospective strategy that allows us to identify and implement strategic planning in patients with early kidney disease. To facilitate early referral of patients with kidney disease to our group, we have used continuing medical education efforts to remind internists, endocrinologists, and family physicians that early kidney disease can be identified easily and that there are high-risk populations in which it should be aggressively sought. We have encouraged such physicians to refer patients based on their serum creatinine concentration so that women with a creatinine concentration greater than or equal to 1.2 mg per deciliter should be referred for an initial consultation. Men should be referred when their creatinine is 1.5 mg per deciliter or greater. During this initial evaluation, we review the likely causes for the early kidney disease and recommend strategies to retard the progression of such disease, including the rigorous control of hypertension and diabetes, if present; treatment of dyslipidemias; cessation of smoking; institution of an exercise program; evaluation and treatment of anemia; and avoidance of nephrotoxic medications and diagnostic agents. During the initial visit, we spend a great deal of time with the patient and the family (if appropriate) and work to empower the patient to participate in his or her own medical care. We believe this intervention often makes the patient less fearful of kidney disease and is useful in that it makes the patient more amenable to close follow-up. Although we encourage primary care physicians to use us as consultants and remain as principal providers, we find that many non-nephrology physicians are uncomfortable providing care to patients with clearly progressive chronic kidney disease. Therefore, inevitably, over time, a substantial number of patients gradually will have more and more of their care delivered by us.

We believe patients should be evaluated for vascular access once their serum creatinine has reached 4.0 mg per deciliter, when their creatinine clearance is less than 25 mL per meter, or when the need for dialysis is expected within the year. We use a lower serum creatinine concentration in patients with reduced muscle mass or certain kidney diseases that tend to progress very rapidly. We see little detriment to

early referral because the timing of surgical placement of vascular access is a joint decision among the nephrologist, the surgeon, and the patient. As part of our chronic kidney disease initiative, we use patient-friendly educational materials, including pamphlets and videotapes, to acquaint patients with the different modalities available for renal replacement therapy. Unfortunately, most of our patients will enter hemodialysis programs. When we refer these patients to our access surgeon, he or she performs an initial evaluation of the patient as a potential access candidate. Our surgeons use the Vascular Access Clinical Practice Guidelines to guide their initial evaluation. The guidelines for patient evaluation prior to access placement are simple and require that the surgeon perform a history and physical examination, with particular emphasis on those conditions that may affect longevity on dialysis. In many patients, a simple physical examination is sufficient. In other patients, the initial evaluation may include further diagnostic evaluation before surgery. Venography is indicated in patients who have edema in the extremity of interest, collateral vein development, differential extremity size, prior subclavian vein cannulation, current or prior transvenous pacemaker placement, previous trauma or surgery near the venous drainage area of the proposed site, or multiple or previous accesses. Doppler ultrasound evaluation or magnetic resonance angiography can be used as necessary (5).

Before a surgical procedure is scheduled, we meet with the surgeon and discuss the patient's situation in a multidisciplinary format. We have encouraged the creation of primary arteriovenous fistulae, even if we are not confident that they will mature sufficiently. We have tended to accept this risk, with the understanding that the fistula can always be converted to a synthetic graft if the former does not mature. We also increased the proportion of patients who undergo more creative surgical procedures, such as transposition of the basilic vein, because our patients with arteriovenous fistulae as vascular access have remarkably fewer complications than do those with synthetic grafts. This translates into fewer infections, fewer thromboses, fewer hospitalizations, fewer surgical procedures, and less time lost from work or other activities. Although we have little way to quantify the information, it has been our impression that patient satisfaction is tremendously higher with a fistula rather than a graft because the former patients are aware of the morbidity of their fellow dialysis patients' experiences.

COSTS OF INADEQUATE VASCULAR ACCESS

The costs of improper dialysis vascular access can be divided into several categories. The first categories comprise those borne by the patient, such the immeasurable psychosocial costs associated with never knowing when the graft will clot, when the catheter will malfunction, or when either will become infected and perhaps result in sepsis. Patients who undergo dialysis with catheters tend to receive less adequate dialysis than do those who have a permanent access, and inadequate dialysis is associated with poor hypertension and volume control, less control of anemia, poor nutrition, and a reduced sense of wellness. Finally, employability may suffer because patients may exhaust their sick and vacation days. A properly functioning arteriovenous fistula can last for many years, whereas a graft usually will not last longer than 5 years. The life of a tunneled catheter usually is measured in months.

The second category of costs are those borne by insurers, whether Medicare or private insurers. Declotting of grafts requires operating room facilities, and patients often miss their outpatient dialysis treatment. This may require that they be admitted for volume overload or hyperkalemia and requires utilization of inpatient facilities in many cases. Obviously, the initial cost of an arteriovenous fistula is much less than that of a synthetic graft or catheter because the cost of the graft or catheter itself can be several hundred dollars.

The third category of costs are those borne by the dialysis clinic provider, who is not reimbursed if a patient does not undergo dialysis. Moreover, untoward hours of staff time can be expended in trying to manipulate a catheter to have it work. These efforts, which usually include the use of intra-catheter thrombolytic agents, cost staff time and predispose the patient to infection. From a business perspective, a dialysis clinic is most successful when all of its patients receive all of their treatments in a timely and uncomplicated fashion.

Unfortunately, many patients with ESRD are still insured under a fee-for-service system. Medicare also reimburses surgeons and nephrologists for services rendered during hospitalization so that there is little financial incentive to

place vascular accesses that will work flawlessly for long periods. Declotting of grafts, restoration of catheter patency, and the support of the patient who is hospitalized represent revenue streams for all providers involved in the care of dialysis patients. The institution of a properly funded, prospective capitation reimbursement system undoubtedly would result in an increased emphasis on maintaining patients in a state of optimal health. In our opinion, until insurers uniformly require that the Vascular Access Practice Guidelines promulgated by K-DOQI be adopted, patients will continue to bear the most of the costs of improper and delayed vascular access.

REFERENCES

1. U.S. Renal Data System (USRDS). Excerpts from the United States Renal Data System 2000 Annual Data Report: Atlas of End Stage Renal Disease in the United States. Bethesda, MD: National Institutes of Health, National Institute of Diabetes and Digestive and Kidney Diseases, Precis. A Summary of the United States Renal Data System Report 2000:16–41.
2. Owen WF, Lew NL, Liu Y, et al. The urea reduction ratio and serum albumin concentration as predictors of mortality in patients undergoing hemodialysis. *N Engl J Med* 1993;320:1001–1006.
3. National Kidney Foundation. K/DOQI clinical practice guidelines for hemodialysis adequacy, peritoneal dialysis adequacy, vascular access, and anemia of chronic kidney disease, 2000. *Am J Kidney Dis* 2001;37:S7–S238.
4. Lewis EJ, Hunsicker LG, Bain RP, et al. The effect of angiotensin-converting-enzyme inhibition on diabetic nephropathy. *N Engl J Med* 1993;329:1456–1462.
5. National Kidney Foundation. K/DOQI clinical practice guidelines for vascular access, 2000. *Am J Kidney Dis* 2001;37:S137–S181.

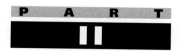

PHYSIOLOGY OF HEMODIALYSIS

PHYSIOLOGIC PRINCIPLES OF HEMODIALYSIS

JUDITH H. VEIS

The dialysis process was designed to approximate closely the functions of a normal kidney, in particular, the removal of waste as well as the regulation of fluid and electrolyte balance. In general, most waste removal is achieved via diffusion across a semipermeable membrane; fluid and sodium balances are attained via convective clearances, that is, bulk flow, across this same membrane. The devices required to achieve these clearances are biocompatible, semipermeable, and provide for adequate solute clearance. Dialysate is devised to maintain electrolyte homeostasis and acid–base balance without concomitantly containing potentially toxic contaminants, such as chloramines, fluoride, and aluminum. Intermittent treatments need to be efficient enough to replace the continuous function of native kidneys. Anticoagulation is necessary to prevent clotting within the tubing and dialyzer. Finally, adequate access to the circulation is paramount to support the hemodialysis process. This chapter provides an overview of hemodialysis given the assumption that a functional vascular access is present with an emphasis on the National Kidney Foundation's Dialysis Outcomes Quality Initiative guidelines.

THE DIALYSIS MACHINE

All dialysis machines consist of several basic components (Fig. 6.1). The first is a blood pump to pull a stream of blood continuously at 200 to 500 mL per minute from the patient via an access device. An infusion pump allows continuous infusion of heparin into the blood path. Tubing then delivers the blood to the dialyzer itself, where it travels through the hollow fibers of the dialysis membranes, which are bathed in dialysate. Dialysate is generated from a source of ultrapurified water (see below) and proportioned with a specified concentrate of electrolytes and sodium bicarbonate, which then is carried via countercurrent flow through the dialysate compartment of the dialyzer at a rate of 500 to 1,000 mL per minute and disposed of subsequently. The blood then travels through an air detector and is returned to the patient.

Multiple safety devices are incorporated into current dialysis machines, such as a blood leak detector, an air detector

to prevent the entry of air into the blood circulation, and a temperature monitor to prevent overheating of dialysate, which could lead to hemolysis. A conductivity monitor assesses the accuracy of the proportioning system to ensure that the dialysate achieves an osmolality near that of serum and so that neither hyponatremia nor hypernatremia ensues during dialysis. Pressure transducers measure the arterial and venous pressures, allowing calculation of a transmembrane pressure with alarms to prevent excessive pressure buildup within the dialyzer that could lead to membrane rupture. This transmembrane pressure, along with the intrinsic ultrafiltration characteristics of the membrane itself, allows calculation of the fluid removal that occurs across the membrane. Volumetric control allows much more precise fluid removal by preventing excessive ultrafiltration from the patient during the use of newer more permeable (high-flux) membranes.

Sodium and bicarbonate levels can be adjusted during therapy to individualize treatments; this is achieved by adjusting the proportion of concentrate with water. Software enhancements have allowed individualized "profiling" of

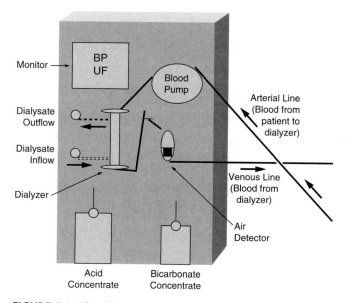

FIGURE 6.1. The dialysis machine. *BP,* blood pressure; *UF,* ultrafiltration.

these parameters during a treatment. For example, dialysate sodium concentrations may be set at a level higher than serum, for example, 150 mEq per liter, at the beginning of a treatment. This helps to mobilize excess fluid from the patient, thereby preventing hypotension. The sodium concentration then can be gradually lowered, in either a stepwise or linear manner, to normal before the end of the treatment; so the serum sodium concentration returns to normal. The amount of fluid removed via ultrafiltration also can be similarly modeled, that is, for more rapid fluid removal at the beginning of a treatment rather than using a flat rate over the entire dialysis session.

Newer innovations include online monitoring of blood volume, generally via measurement of changes in the hematocrit. As fluid volume is removed, refilling occurs from the extravascular space. If this "refilling" occurs more slowly than fluid removal, symptoms such as hypotension and cramping develop. These symptoms of hypovolemia can be predicted by monitoring for changes in hemoconcentration, measured by a rise in hematocrit. Using on-line hematocrit monitoring, adjustments to either the rate of fluid removal or replacement of volume by saline infusion can prevent the development of these symptoms or, conversely, allow more aggressive fluid removal in patients in whom refilling occurs more quickly. On-line urea clearance determinations are beginning to be available on newer machines and can be used to ascertain whether clearance goals are being met in a given treatment. Machines that are easier to operate for use in the home setting for sustained treatments are in development.

DIALYSATE

Dialysate is formulated to approximate serum concentrations of electrolyte concentrations that need to be maintained while facilitating the clearances of substances that accumulate in renal failure as well as correcting the acidosis of uremia (Fig. 6.2). Standardized highly concentrated mixes of sodium chloride, potassium chloride, magnesium chloride, and calcium chloride are available with variable potassium and calcium concentrations. Glucose at a concentration of 200 mg per deciliter can be added to prevent hypoglycemia during dialysis. Acetate can be included as a base equivalent, in which case sodium acetate is utilized. At current rates of dialysate delivery, however, the rate of acetate infusion exceeds the rate of conversion of acetate to bicarbonate, leading to clinical instability during treatments, including hypoxemia, hypotension, nausea, and vomiting. Bicarbonate dialysis has therefore become the standard base used to correct the acidosis of renal failure. The concentration of bicarbonate used is generally higher than plasma bicarbonate to treat the acidosis that occurs in renal failure (1). Bicarbonate dialysate necessitates the use of a separate bicarbonate delivery system, which is proportioned along with the concentrate. The concentrate and bicarbonate are mixed

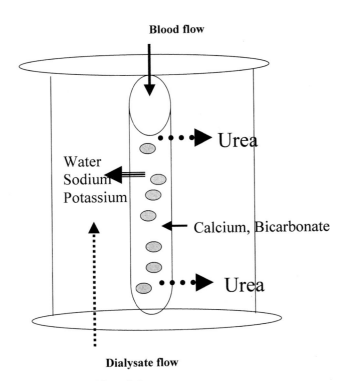

FIGURE 6.2. Inside a dialyzer.

with the appropriate proportion of purified water (see below) to create a final dialysate with a sodium concentration of 135 to 142 mEq per liter, potassium 0 to 4 mEq per liter, chloride 100 to 111 mEq per liter, calcium 2.0 to 3.5 mEq per liter, bicarbonate 35 to 40 mEq per liter, glucose 0 to 200 mg per deciliter, and magnesium 0.75 to 1.5 mEq per liter.

WATER PURIFICATION FOR HEMODIALYSIS

To create purified dialysate, purified water must be generated, which then is mixed with concentrate as described in the preceding section. Tap water contains several types of contaminants that must be removed: particulate matter, chemical contaminants (e.g., trace metals), chemicals (e.g., chlorine, chloramines, alum, or fluoride, which have been added to municipal water systems), and bacteria or bacterial byproducts. These contaminants vary considerably by municipality, leading to a requirement for customization. Water systems to remove these contaminants are set up with several components (2). In general, a carbon filter is used to remove chlorines, chloramines, and other organic substances from tap water. Sediment filters are used to remove particulates. To achieve the highest levels of purity, either a deionizer or a reverse osmosis filter is used. Deionizers exchange cations for hydrogen and anions for hydroxyl ions and remove most electrolytes and minerals from the water; however, they require significant ongoing maintenance. Reverse osmosis (RO) systems are more commonly used and create purified water by forcing the feed water through a semipermeable membrane at high pressures, causing separation of the water and contaminants by sieving and ion exclusion. Most of the feed water is "rejected" and sent either back into the system or to the drain. Bacteria, viruses, and pyrogens also are removed by an RO, but attention to the entire water circuit is necessary to prevent bacterial contamination because endotoxins can pass from the dialysate to the patient when high-flux dialyzers are used. Water entering the RO may require pretreatment to prevent scaling and degradation of the membranes resulting from calcium and magnesium.

Water systems require meticulous attention to detail. Carbon tanks are monitored to ensure that they have not been exhausted, resulting in the release of the previously filtered toxins to the patient. The plumbing that leads from the RO to each dialysis machine must be examined to avoid connections or so-called "blind loops" that can serve as sites for bacterial overgrowth. Dialysis units must have systems in place to monitor the incoming tap water to assess the needs of each individual system. The end-product water also must be screened for chloramines and endotoxin. The Association for the Advancement of Medical Instrumentation (AAMI) has set guidelines for the maximal allowed content of a variety of minerals in end-product water of dialysis systems (3). Microbiologic limits also have been set that require monthly monitoring and total microbial counts not to exceed 200 per milliliter in water used for dialysate or 2,000 per milliliter in proportioned dialysate exiting the dialyzers (4).

DIALYZER CHARACTERISTICS

The clearance characteristics of a dialysis membrane must approximate those of the human kidney as closely as possibly, that is, excellent permeability to small- and middle-weight molecules combined with low permeability to albumin and larger molecules. The artificial membrane must also be biocompatible, that is, not activating inflammatory or clotting mediators present in the bloodstream. This membrane must be large enough to provide effective clearances at achievable blood and dialysate flow rates.

Membranes currently in use are hollow fibers ranging from 0.5 to 2 m^2 total surface area and are made of a variety of materials, such as cellulose acetate or modified cellulose acetate, polysulfone, polyacrylonitrile, polymethylmethacrylate, and others (5). These materials then are modified to form membranes of variable permeabilities, that is, conventional, high efficiency, or high flux. The higher flux membranes can be used only with dialysis machines that have volumetric control; otherwise, volume removal via ultrafiltration will be excessive. Flux characteristics are related to the porosity of the membrane, whereas biocompatibility is related more closely to the type of membrane itself. Less biocompatible membranes, such as cuprophan or unmodified cellulose acetate,

may trigger allergic-type reactions via activation of the complement cascade via the alternative pathway (6). These activated components, especially C5a, then lead to white blood cell (WBC) sequestration in the lungs, which clinically can cause wheezing or hypoxemia within the first 20 minutes of dialysis. Anaphylactic-like reactions, including dyspnea and chest and back pain, also can occur. This so-called first-use syndrome does not occur following reuse of the dialyzer during subsequent treatments. Direct contact of blood with cuprophan membranes during dialysis also has been demonstrated to activate the proinflammatory cytokines interleukin 1 (IL-1), interleukin 6 (IL-6), and tumor necrosis factor alpha (TNF-α), particularly if a second inflammatory stimulus is present (7). This activation has been proposed as one of the mechanisms of chronic immune system dysregulation in end-stage renal disease (ESRD) patients. Long-term use of the less biocompatible membranes also has been demonstrated to lead to a greater incidence of clinical problems related to β-2 microglobulin, a substance that can cause amyloid deposition in the bones and elsewhere in ESRD patients (8).

DIALYSIS PRESCRIPTION

Although many of the parameters already discussed are generally fixed, such as the type of machine and water treatments, dialysis treatments should be individualized to the particular patient. A conventional membrane is necessary if the machine used does not have volumetric control, if long-term survival is less likely, or if a more gentle treatment is required (e.g., a patient's first-ever dialysis). Higher flux, biocompatible membranes are preferred for patients on long-term dialysis, specifically to improve the clearance of larger molecules, such as β-2 microglobulin. The size of the membrane prescribed is determined in general by the size of the patient, the treatment time desired, and the quality of the dialysis access. Access quality can significantly alter the range of blood flow rates that can be achieved, thus dramatically affecting overall clearance. For example, if a higher rate of blood flow cannot be achieved, attempting to use a larger dialyzer will not improve clearances. Instead, longer treatment times are required.

The quantity of dialysis that should be delivered during each treatment in a chronic hemodialysis patient has not been precisely defined. Even though urea itself is not the "uremic toxin" (i.e., the toxin responsible for the symptoms of uremia), it is used a surrogate marker for small-molecular-weight clearances and has been correlated best with long-term outcomes. As a simple guide, the urea reduction ratio (URR) is used:

$$\text{URR} = predialysis\ BUN - postdialysis\ BUN$$
$$\times 100\ /\ predialysis\ BUN$$

where BUN is blood urea nitrogen.

That is, to achieve a specific removal of urea, a greater than 65% reduction in urea should occur during a treatment. This degree of urea removal has been correlated with improved survival among patients on chronic hemodialysis (9,10). When the URR is low, the dialysis prescription must be modified in any of a number of factors; for example, the blood flow or dialysate flow rates may be increased, a larger dialysis membrane used, or treatment time lengthened.

Although the URR is a useful guide, it does not adequately reflect the removal of urea during dialysis. In the shortened treatment times of dialysis, compared with normal kidney function, urea does not freely move from the intracellular to extracellular space; nor are all body "compartments" (i.e., the extremities vs. the abdomen) evenly perfused during dialysis. A simple one-compartment model, which implies free movement of urea across all intracellular and extracellular spaces, therefore cannot describe urea kinetics. Formal urea kinetic modeling (UKM) takes into this into account and also takes into account additional urea removed as water is cleared via convection in the ultrafiltrate. The additional urea removal if several liters of fluid are removed can add significantly to overall dialytic clearances. UKM is expressed by the concept of Kt/V: If the volume of distribution of urea in an individual patient (V, expressed in liters) and clearance characteristics of the dialyzer are known at a given blood flow rate (K, liters per minute), then the time (expressed in minutes) can be prescribed to achieve a certain Kt/V (11). A Kt/V of 1.2 reflects a degree of dialysis comparable to a URR of 65% and more accurately taking into account urea removal via ultrafiltration. Studies are ongoing, however, to determine the optimal Kt/V by comparing a prescription of dialysis to a Kt/V of 1.2 with one of 1.6 (12). Once dialysis is prescribed, validation as to whether the prescribed dialysis has been delivered represents the widest use of UKM. Computer models are required for these calculations and are fully addressed in the DOQI guidelines (13). The largest problem in the determination of Kt/V is the determination of V because V as a fraction of total body weight can differ significantly between patients.

If a URR or Kt/V is obtained that is less than predicted, then a search for factors that contribute to the underdelivery of prescribed dialysis is required. The most frequent problem encountered in clinical practice is that of a poorly functioning vascular access, such as a recirculating arteriovenous graft or poor flows from a dialysis catheter. Additional factors include miscalibration of the dialysis blood pump, which results in underdelivery of blood to the dialyzer or clinical factors such as hypotension or dialyzer clotting. Not completing the prescribed dialysis time is another frequent issue. Abbreviated sessions may result from concomitantly scheduled medical procedures, a patient's arriving late, or shortening or skipping of treatments. Overall, outcomes clearly depend on delivery of the fully prescribed dialysis three times per week (14).

Other prescribed parameters include the dialysate potassium and calcium. In general, dialysate potassium should be set at 2 or 3 mEq per liter because lower values may lead to posttreatment hypokalemia and arrhythmias (15). Calcium prescription is more controversial because with lower calcium baths, there may be negative calcium balance and a concern for the development of hemodynamic instability during dialysis (16). More recently, concerns have arisen over the generation of a positive calcium balance during dialysis, which could contribute to cardiac calcifications, which have a high incidence in the ESRD population and correlate with the development of ischemic coronary disease (17).

Fluid volume removal also requires consistent monitoring. Most patients on chronic hemodialysis have a set "target weight," which is empirically determined at a point where the patient appears euvolemic with a "normal total body water." Edema and hypertension are usually indicators that a patient requires additional fluid removal. Intradialysis or postdialysis hypotension and cramping conversely may suggest either excessive fluid removal or that the fluid removal is overly rapid.

ANTICOAGULATION DURING DIALYSIS

Unfractionated heparin is the most commonly used anticoagulant during hemodialysis because it is both clinically effective and inexpensive. Anticoagulation prevents dialyzer clotting and has been demonstrated to improve urea clearances (18). A bolus of 1,000 to 5,000 U may be given at the start of hemodialysis, allowing systemic anticoagulation during much of the treatment but trailing off toward the end to allow hemostasis when the needles are removed from an arteriovenous fistula or graft. Alternatively, a bolus followed by either a midtreatment bolus dose or a continuous heparin infusion of 500 to 2,000 U per hour may be used, particularly when heparin needs are high. Activated clotting times (ACT) are used to help with adjustment of the heparin dose. An increase in ACT to 1.5 to 2 times baseline is believed to represent adequate anticoagulation. Heparin use, however, is not without its complications and may lead to heparin-induced thrombocytopenia, osteoporosis, and dyslipidemia (19). Thrombocytopenia is uncommon in a general ESRD practice, and the long-term effects of heparin on bones and lipids are not fully appreciated.

Alternatives to unfractionated heparin include heparin-free dialysis, low-molecular-weight heparins (LMWHs), and regional strategies. Many patients at high risk of bleeding will tolerate a heparin-free dialysis. This is most feasible when high blood flow rates are used and is the treatment of choice in patients with active bleeding. LMWHs are used in Europe and less frequently in the United States because they are more expensive and have a longer half-life and thus a potential for increased bleeding postdialysis. Danaproid is a low-molecular weight heparinoid that has been successfully in some patients with heparin-induced thrombocytopenia (20). Other alternatives include regional heparinization with protamine sulfate given in the venous line to reverse anticoagulation or citrate administered similarly with calcium used for reversal; however, the cumbersome nature of needing reversal and complications limit their routine use.

COMPLICATIONS OF HEMODIALYSIS

The complications of the dialysis procedure are characterized in Table 6.1 and must be distinguished from the medical issues that otherwise occur in patients with ESRD. The most frequent complications are related to the volume removal that occurs with each treatment. If a patient is brought below his or her target "dry" weight, then hypotension, muscle cramping, or nausea and vomiting may occur. Some patients experience difficulty in shifting fluid into the intravascular compartment quickly enough during dialysis, despite total body salt and water excess, resulting in similar symptoms. Longer treatment times with slower rates of ultrafiltration may correct this problem. Vasodilation resulting from warming of the blood in the extracorporeal circuit also may be a contributing factor, as can venous pooling in muscles or, in some patients, splanchnic pooling following food intake during the treatment. Other prescriptive changes that have been shown to decrease the severity and incidence of dialysis-induced hypotension include sodium modeling and lowered dialysate temperatures (21). Less often, patients may develop hypertension as a consequence of excessive fluid removal, presumably because of the release of pressor mediators. Fatigue is a nonspecific complaint that also may be related to fluid removal during treatments (22).

Dialysis dysequilibrium generally occurs with the first-ever dialysis treatments, especially in patients who are extremely uremic with high BUN levels. Removal of urea from the blood compartment may be more rapid than the removal of urea from inside the cells. The urea then becomes an osmotically active substance. With a higher osmolality inside compared with outside cells, water then moves into cells. In the brain, cerebral edema then ensues that is clinically manifested by headaches, nausea, vomiting, and reduced levels of consciousness. Prevention by an initially less aggressive dialysis treatment or the use of hypertonic substances such as mannitol to maintain serum osmolality as urea is removed is recommended (23).

Complications of anticoagulation include increased bleeding, usually from access sites following dialysis. Other conditions, such as those that cause gastrointestinal blood loss, may become apparent because of anticoagulation-induced enhancement of bleeding during dialysis. In women, menstrual blood losses may be excessively heavy as well. Anticoagulation is routinely held following most surgical procedures, particularly ophthalmologic procedures.

Contaminants in the dialysate may cross the dialyzer into the bloodstream and cause reactions that vary from acute life-threatening reactions to more subacute or chronic processes because of accumulation over time. The most serious reaction is hemolysis due to chloramines, cadmium, or nickel present in the feed water. Fluoride intoxication resulting from exhaustion of deionization systems can lead to death (24). Long-term high levels of aluminum exposure in dialysate can lead to either dementia or seizures in the subacute setting. Chronic lower-level exposure predisposes to aluminum-induced osteomalacia.

Febrile episodes that occur during or shortly after dialysis may be due to pyrogens present in the dialysate. The source has been considered to be endotoxin movement from a contaminated water treatment system or bicarbonate dialysate across newer higher permeability membranes. These reactions must be distinguished from other much more common causes of fevers in dialysis patients, particularly infections of the dialysis access. Hepatitis B infection was common in the 1970s but has been markedly reduced because of isolation of patients who are hepatitis B surface antigen positive and vaccination of staff and patients. Hepatitis C is more common in dialysis patients with a prevalence of 9.3% noted in U.S. populations (25). The incidence is lower at 0.2% in 1997, with likely transmission occurring at some point in the dialysis setting as suggested by similarity in the virus between patients. Needle-stick injuries or breakdown in usual infection-control measures may represent the most common modes of transmission;

TABLE 6.1. COMPLICATIONS OF HEMODIALYSIS

Consequence of waste removal
    Dialysis dysequilibrium
Dialyzer related
    Anaphylactoid reactions
    Hypoxemia
Volume removal related
    Hypotension
    Nausea, Vomiting,
    Cramps
    Hypertension
Dialysate related
    Cardiac arrhythmias: due to hypokalemia, electrolyte imbalance
    Hemolysis: chloramines, heavy metals, fluoride toxicity
    Pyrogen reactions
    Dialysis dementia: aluminum
    Hypoxemia
Coagulation related
    Blood loss due to clotting
    Bleeding due to anticoagulation
Other
    Infections: hepatitis B, hepatitis C
    Stroke/death: air embolism

however, virus potentially may cross dialysis membranes and has been linked in some outbreaks to sharing of a common machine (26,27). Transmission of human immunodeficiency virus (HIV), other than via needle-stick injury, has not been reported in dialysis units in the United States. There is also the potential for patient-to-patient transmission of antibiotic-resistant bacteria, such as methicillin-resistant *Staphylococcus aureus* or vancomycin-resistant enterococcus. This type of transmission is much more likely to occur in the hospital setting than in outpatient dialysis centers (28).

CARE OF THE PATIENT WITH END-STAGE RENAL DISEASE

More than 240,000 patients in the United States have ESRD requiring renal replacement therapy, with most treated with chronic outpatient hemodialysis. More than 40% of ESRD is now caused by diabetes mellitus, with much of the remainder caused by hypertensive renal disease (29). Cardiovascular disease and infections represent the major causes of illness and death in ESRD patients. The care of these patients requires not only attention to the specific details of the dialysis procedure as outlined already but also to concomitant medical issues, some of which are listed in Table 6.2. These issues include the management of anemia resulting from erythropoietin deficiency, that is, due to

ESRD itself. Hypertension can be a particular problem in ESRD patients because it may be related to underlying renal disease or result from volume overload without adequate fluid removal during dialysis. Other medical issues are related to the underlying disease that led to ESRD, such as diabetes mellitus causing retinopathy and neuropathy. Remaining medical issues may be entirely unrelated to a patient's renal disease and yet may impact on ESRD management and vice versa. In conclusion, the treatment of dialysis patients requires attention to detail, both in the dialysis procedure itself and in concomitant medical care.

TABLE 6.2. FREQUENT MEDICAL PROBLEMS IN ESRD PATIENTS

ESRD or underlying renal disease
  Hypertension
  Hypotension, cramps during dialysis
  Anemia due to erythropoeitin deficiency
  Bone disease
    Secondary hyperparathyroidism
    Osteomalacia
    Adynamic bone disease
    Amyloidosis due to β-2 microglobulin
  Malnutrition
Secondary disease
  Diabetes Mellitus-related
    Neuropathy
    Retinopathy
    Gastroparesis
  Cardiac disease (related to risk factors frequent in ESRD: diabetes, hypertension, hyperlipidemia, smoking)
    Coronary artery disease
    Congestive heart failure
    Hyperlipidemia
Unrelated disease (potential impact on ESRD care)
  Adjustment of medication doses for renal failure and drug removal during dialysis
  Adjustment of anticoagulation during dialysis

ESRD, end-stage renal disease.

REFERENCES

1. Oettinger CW, Oliver JC. Normalization of uremic acidosis in hemodilaysis patients with a high bicarbonate dialysate. *J Am Soc Nephrol* 1993;3:1804–1807.
2. Ismail N, Becker BN, Hakim RM. Water treatment for hemodialysis. *Am J Nephrol* 1996;16:60–72.
3. Association for the Advancement of Medical Instrumentation. *Hemodialysis systems. 2nd edition.* ANSI/AAMI RD5–1992. Arlington, VA: AAMI, 1993a. The American Standard.
4. Bland LA. Microbiological and endotoxin assays of hemodialysis fluids. *Adv Ren Replace Ther* 1995;2:70–79.
5. Clark WR. Quantitative characterization of hemodialyzer solute and water transport. *Seminars in Dialysis* 2001;14:32–36.
6. Hakim RM. Fearon DT. Lazarus JM. Biocompatibility of dialysis membranes: effects of chronic complement activation. *Kidney Int* 1984;26:194–200.
7. Pertosa G, Grandaliano G, Gesauldo L, et al. Clinical relevance of cytokine production in hemodialysis. *Kidney Int* 2000;58:S104–S111.
8. Koda Y, Nishis S, Miyazake S, et al. Switch from conventional to high-flux membrane reduces the risk of carpal tunnel syndrome and mortality of hemodialysis patient. *Kidney Int* 1997;52:1096–1101.
9. Owen WF, Lew NL, Liu Y, et al. The urea reduction ratio and serum albumin concentration as predictors of mortality in patients undergoing hemodialysis. *N Engl J Med* 1993;329:1001–1006.
10. Held PJ, Port FK, Wolfe RA, et al. The dose of hemodialysis and patient mortality. *Kidney Int* 1996;50:550–556.
11. Daugirdas JT. Dialysis adequacy and kinetics. *Curr Opin Nephrol Hypertens* 2000;9:599–605.
12. Eknoyan G, Levey AS, Beck GJ, et al. The Hemodialysis (HEMO) Study: rationale for selection of interventions. *Semin Dial* 1996;9:24–33.
13. Anonymous. I. NKF-K/DOQI clinical practice guidelines for hemodialysis adequacy: update 2000. *Am J Kidney Dis* 2001;37(1 Suppl 1):S7–S64.
14. Kimmel PL, Weihs KA, Peterson R, et al. Behavioral compliance with dialysis prescription in hemodialysis patients. *J Am Soc Nephrol* 1995;5:1826–1834.
15. Munger MA, Ateshkadi A, Cheung AK, et al. Cardiopulmonary events during hemodialysis: effects of dialysis membranes and dialysate buffers. *Am J Kidney Dis* 2000;36:130–139.
16. Palmer BF. Dialysate composition in hemodialysis and peritoneal dialysis. In: Henrich WL, ed. *Principles and practice of dialysis.* Baltimore: Williams & Wilkins, 1999:22–40.
17. Goodman WG, Goldin J, Kuizon BD, et al. Coronary-artery calcification in young adults with end-stage renal disease who are undergoing dialysis. *N Engl J Med* 2000;342:1478–1483.

18. Wei SS, Ellis PW, Magnusson MO, et al. Effect of heparin modeling on delivered hemodialysis therapy. *Am J Kidney Dis* 1994; 23:389–393.

19. Ouseph R, Ward RA. Anticoagulation for intermittent hemodialysis. *Semin Dial* 2000;13:181–187.

20. Magnani HN. Heparin-induced thrombocytopenia: an overview of 230 patients treated with Orgaran (ORG 10172). *Thomb Haemostas* 1993;70:554–561.

21. Dheenan S, Henrich WL. Preventing dialysis hypotension: a comparison of usual protective maneuvers. *Kidney Int* 2001;59: 1175–1181.

22. Sklar A, Newman N, Scott R, et al. Identification of factors responsible for postdialysis fatigue. *Am J Kidney Dis* 1999;34:464–470.

23. Mahoney CA, Arieff AI. Uremic encephalopathies: clinical, biochemical, and experimental features. *Am J Kidney Dis* 1982;2: 324–336.

24. Bland LA, Arnow PM, Arduino MJ, et al. Potential hazards of deionization systems used for water purification in hemodialysis. *Artif Organs* 1996;20:2–7.

25. Tokars JI, Miller ER, Alter MJ, et al. National surveillance of dialysis-associated diseases in the United States, 1997. *Semin Dial* 2000;13:75–85.

26. Pereira BJG. Hepatitis C in Dialysis. *Semin Dial* 1998;11:113–118.

27. Fabrizi F, Martin P, Dixit V, et al. Acquisition of hepatitis C virus in hemodialysis patients: a prospective study by branched DNA signal amplification assay. *Am J Kidney Dis* 1998;31:647–654.

28. Anonymous. Recommendations for preventing transmission of infections among chronic hemodialysis patients. *MMWR Morb Mortal Wkly Rep* 2001;50RR-5:1–43.

29. Excerpts from the United States Renal Data System's 2001 annual data report: atlas of end-stage renal disease in the United States. *Am J Kidney Dis* 2001;38:S1–S248.

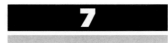

IS QUANTITATIVE MEASUREMENT OF DIALYSIS ADEQUACY A USEFUL OUTCOME MEASURE?

GERALD SCHULMAN

Dialysis is a life-saving treatment for more than 300,000 patients with end-stage renal disease (ESRD) in the United States and more than a million patients worldwide. Despite this enviable record extending over more than a quarter of a century of treatment, the annual mortality rate of dialysis patients in the United States over the past decade remains in excess of 20% (1). Multiple lines of evidence implicate inadequate dialysis prescriptions and the underdelivery of the prescribed dose of dialysis as central factors responsible for the high mortality rate (2–7). This chapter examines the evidence supporting the use of quantitative assessment of dialysis adequacy both as an outcome measure as well as a method of improving the care of patients with ESRD.

HISTORICAL PERSPECTIVE

It is instructive to review the evolution of the methods that have been used to determine the adequacy of the dose of hemodialysis. One might pose a question regarding adequate dialytic therapy that is similar to the one asked by Dr. Henry Stubb centuries ago concerning the practice of blood transfusions: "What regulation shall we have for the operation? Shall a man transfuse [*dialyze*] he knows not what, to correct he knows not what, God knows how?" (8).

The maintenance of homeostasis and of fluid balance and the elimination of toxins generated from dietary protein catabolism and other sources are chief functions of the kidneys. The accumulation of toxins results in manifestations of the uremic syndrome. In chronic renal failure, uremic symptoms are worsened by excessive protein intake and may be ameliorated by restriction of protein intake. This clearly indicates that nitrogenous compounds are central in the pathogenesis of uremia. A quandary exists, however, as to which specific substance or combinations of compounds produce symptoms. This makes difficult the task of assessing treatment adequacy by indexing the dose of dialysis to a simple plasma level or removal rate of particular compound.

Easily measured substances, such as urea or creatinine, are themselves not major toxins. Furthermore, the plasma levels of these substances are influenced by many factors beyond clearance by the artificial kidney. Thus, generation rates and removal rates must be used to describe the fate of the substance being used to describe the efficiency of the treatment.

Low-Molecular-Weight Substances and Middle Molecules

The use of compounds like urea to judge adequacy rests on the assumption that the clearance rate of low-molecular-weight solutes correlates with well-being. This is contradictory to the observation that long treatment sessions with the Kiil dialyzer, a relatively inefficient device with a large surface area, could mitigate the severity of peripheral neuropathy. Long dialysis time and large membrane surface area are characteristics that enhance the removal of high-molecular-weight substances. The finding that these features improved neuropathy led to the square meter-hour hypothesis (9). This hypothesis holds that solutes with molecular weights in the range of 300 to 12,000 daltons, termed *middle molecules*, play a role in the pathogenesis of the uremic syndrome (10).

The subject of middle molecules as uremic toxins was reviewed recently (11). Compounds resulting from protein catabolism as well as peptides such as parathormone (PTH) and β_2-microglobulin are among the larger solutes that are retained in renal failure. The latter two high-molecular-weight substances have been given roles as mediators of uremic toxicity (12–17). Vanholder suggested that low-molecular weight also may behave as middle molecules by virtue of their physical properties, such as charge, steric configurations, or ability to bind to plasma proteins or because of their high generation rates (11). These properties result in a reduction in their clearance rate by dialysis that would not have been predicted by size alone. Candidates for this designation include methylguanidine, indoxyl sulfate, hippuric acid, and inorganic phosphate. On the other hand, Teschan

TABLE 7.1. THE IDEAL MARKER OF DIALYSIS ADEQUACY

Retained in renal failure
Eliminated by dialysis
Proven dose-related toxicity
Generation and elimination representative of other toxins
Easily measured

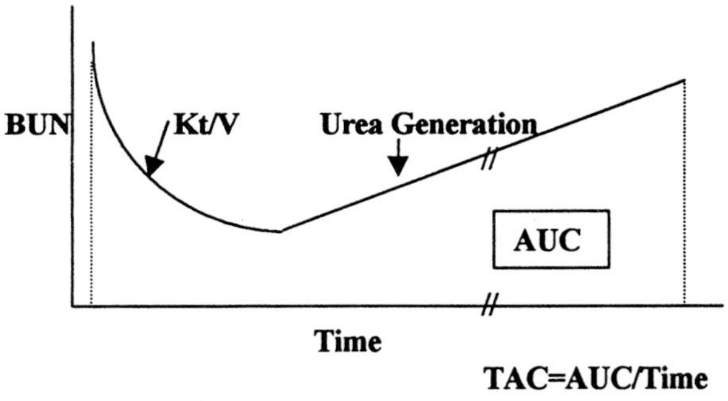

FIGURE 7.1. The hemodialysis cycle and elements of kinetic modeling. *AUC*, area under the curve; *BUN*, blood urea nitrogen; *TAC*, timed average concentration.

and colleagues and the results of the National Cooperative Dialysis Study (NCDS) suggested that a low-molecular-weight compound, urea, can serve as a legitimate surrogate for uremic toxins (18,19).

The attributes of an ideal marker of the adequacy of dialysis that have been suggested by Vanholder and are listed in Table 7.1 (11). No single marker meets all the requirements. Unresolved issues preclude the use of middle molecules to determine adequacy. PTH secretion is not directly dependent on the dialysis treatment. Many putative uremic toxins are not routinely measured in a clinical chemistry laboratory. Levels of these substances never have been indexed to measures of well-being. The use of hemodialysis membranes with high permeability and the implementation of longer dialysis times would be required to enhance the removal of substances with high molecular weight, if indeed these substances determine uremic toxicity. Yet no evidence has been forthcoming to substantiate conclusively that long hemodialysis sessions with high-flux membranes improves patient survival independently of changes attributable to the simultaneously enhanced removal of low-molecular-weight substances (Table 7.2).

National Cooperative Dialysis Study

The NCDS was initiated in 1976. The study applied pharmacokinetic principles to urea concentrations as they varied during the intradialytic and interdialytic periods of the hemodialysis session (20). For purposes of the analysis, a single pool volume of distribution for urea was assumed. Developed by Gotch and Sargent, changes in serum urea concentrations are measured over time, so that "average" concentration of urea for the treatment session can be expressed as timed average urea concentration (TAC_{urea}). From the intradialytic curve, the index related to the ele-

ments of the dialysis treatment and the size of the patient or Kt/V can be calculated, and from the interdialytic curve, urea generation can be determined, as seen in Figure 7.1.

The NCDS was a multicenter prospective, randomized 2 $\times$ 2 factorial trial (Table 7.3). The study participants were hemodialysis patients randomized to one of four groups based on short or long dialysis treatment times and high and low TAC_{urea}. Based on the design, groups I and III received a higher level of dialysis delivered over a longer or shorter time, respectively; groups II and IV received a lower level of dialysis delivered over a longer or shorter time, respectively. The goals were achieved by manipulation of dialyzer size and T_D. If groups I and III have a good outcome, this would suggest that the dose of hemodialysis could be indexed to low-molecular-weight compounds such as urea.

Two measures of outcome were analyzed: subjects who withdrew from the study for medical reasons or death (F1) and those who withdrew from the study for hospitalization within the first 6 months of the experimental phase (F2). Of 160 randomized patients, about 50% completed the study protocol. Importantly, group IV (high TAC, short dialysis time) was discontinued before the study was completed because of excessive hospitalizations and medical withdrawal.

The index of dialysis adequacy used in the analysis of the primary outcome of the NCDS, TAC, was the best predictor of failure. A much weaker but statistically significant relation also was found for dialysis time: Short time was associated with a greater incidence of F2 failure. Not all adverse medical events or hospitalizations were those commonly associated with too little dialysis, such as episodes of volume overload, hyperkalemia, or pericarditis. Although only three patients died during the actual study, an additional 13 died during a 12-month follow-up after withdrawal from the study. Ten were assigned to groups II and IV. In many instances, these patients were returned to a higher level of therapy at completion of the study, and yet the adverse effects of what was shown to be an inadequate level of therapy were difficult to correct. The NCDS suggested that removal of small molecules strongly predicted morbidity and that urea kinetic modeling (determination of TAC) could be

TABLE 7.2. FACTORS AFFECTING DIALYZER CLEARANCE (DECREASING IMPORTANCE)

Small Molecules	Large Molecules
Blood flow	Membrane
Dialysate flow	Dialysis time
Surface area	Surface area
Dialysis time	Blood and dialysate flows
Membrane	

TABLE 7.3. DESIGN OF THE NATIONAL COOPERATIVE DIALYSIS STUDY

	Intensive	Less Intensive
Long duration	Group I TAC = 51.3 +/− 1.1 mg/dL T_D = 269 min	Group II TAC = 87 +/− 1.4 mg/dL T_D = 271 min
Short duration	Group III TAC = 54.1 +/− 1.1 mg/dL T_D = 199 min	Group IV TAC = 89.6 +/− 1.2 mg/dL T_D = 194 min

TAC, timed average concentration; T_D, treatment duration.

used to index the level of therapy delivered, despite the fact that urea does not fulfill all the criteria listed in Table 7.1.

The primary results of the NCDS were expressed in terms of TAC_{urea}, with this index serving as a global parameter of both interdialysis and intradialysis events. A particular value for TAC_{urea} is influenced by many variables: dialyzer size, ultrafiltration, blood and dialysate flow rates, dialysis time, patient size, residual renal function, and rate of urea generation. The former six factors are important intradialytic variables whereas the last three are important interdialytic variables. When dialysis dose and residual renal function remain constant, AC_{urea} will be influenced to the greatest extent by the interdialytic variable of urea generation rate (Fig. 7.1). Thus, poor protein intake associated with a low urea generation rate would tend to lower TAC_{urea} and mask a simultaneously inadequate dialysis dose: A relatively "normal" TAC would result from the combination of poor dialysis and low urea generation. This finding is similar to the finding that very low predialysis urea values actually are associated with high mortality rates (21). Using TAC alone as an index of adequacy of treatment may be hazardous. One must be careful to interpret the TAC with either the knowledge of the urea generation or of the actual delivered dose of dialysis.

Subsequent analysis of the NCDS suggested that it would be informative to analyze separately the components of the dialysis cycle (Fig. 7.1). The dimensionless term, Kt/V, describes aspects directly related to the hemodialysis treatment dialyzer clearance × dialysis time factored by the volume of urea distribution in the patient (22). Morbidity could be indexed to this term. The advantage of using Kt/V as a marker of adequacy is that it allows one to focus on the elements of the intradialytic period. This is the part of the dialysis cycle that is amenable to manipulation of the prescription: blood and dialysate flow, ultrafiltration rate, size of the artificial kidney, and dialysis time, in the case of hemodialysis, or dialysate volume in the case of peritoneal dialysis. The initial analysis of data from the NCDS indicated that a Kt/V greater than 0.8 was associated with a good outcome.

By design, the prescriptions in the NCDS were manipulated to achieve high or low TAC_{urea} goals for the study. The TAC_{urea} covers the entire dialysis cycle; thus, it will be influenced by urea generation, an index of dietary protein intake in the stable hemodialysis patient (Fig. 7.1). Thus, for the TAC goal to be reached, the dialysis dose (Kt/V) was determined partially by the subject's protein intake (urea generation). The implication of this design is that adequacy in the NCDS has been defined by Kt/V levels that have been interpreted in the context of protein intake of the subject (Fig. 7.2).

Although the initial interpretation from the NCDS suggested that there was little to be gained by increasing Kt/V to values beyond 0.8 to 1.0, subsequent analysis of the data indicated that the relationship between morbidity and Kt/V may be continuous. Improved outcome is found at higher doses of Kt/V (23).

ASSESSMENT OF DIALYSIS ADEQUACY AND THE DERIVATIVES OF THE NATIONAL COOPERATIVE DIALYSIS STUDY OUTCOME MEASURES

Since conclusion of the NCDS, the principles of urea kinetic modeling have been applied to the assessment of the

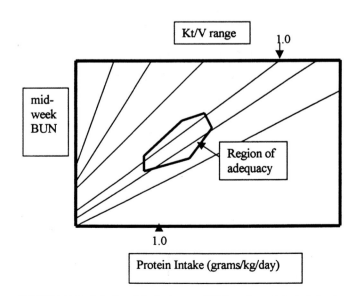

FIGURE 7.2. Relationship between Kt/V and protein intake in the National Cooperative Dialysis Study.

adequacy of both hemodialysis and peritoneal dialysis. The impetus behind this practice has been the suggestion that improving the clearance of low-molecular-weight substances would impact favorably on the unacceptably high mortality rate experienced by dialysis patients in the United States. Subsequently, three retrospective and observational studies provided further evidence that patient outcome correlated with the dose of hemodialysis as measured by Kt/V (5–7). A 5% and 7% decrease in the relative risk of mortality can be demonstrated for each 0.1 increase in Kt/V in nondiabetic and diabetic patients, respectively. In all these studies, patient survival improved as Kt/V was increased (Fig. 7.3).

The benefits of high levels of hemodialysis delivered by conventional cellulosic membranes over extremely long sessions of 6 to 8 hours resulted in remarkable survival statistics (24). In patients achieving a mean Kt/V of 1.67 delivered in this fashion, the *10-year* survival ranges from 88% for patients initiating hemodialysis at 35 years of age or younger to 64% for patients older than 65 years of age. The 15-year survival for all patients in this dialysis center is 55%. These studies, along with data gathered from other dialysis registries, provide strong circumstantial evidence that Kt/V$_{urea}$, an index of removal of low-molecular-weight substances, is a predictor of mortality in hemodialysis.

The principles of urea kinetic modeling also have been applied to peritoneal dialysis as well (25). The Canada/United States (CANUSA) study demonstrated that the expected 2-year survival on peritoneal dialysis is 78% with a weekly Kt/V of 2.1, whereas the 2-year survival rates falls to 67% at a weekly Kt/V of 1.5. As with hemodialysis, an increase of 0.1 U of Kt/V per week is associated with a decrease in the relative risk of death of 5% in peritoneal dialysis patients.

The compelling evidence from these studies has served to make urea kinetic modeling a key outcome measure in the United States and part of the evidence use by the Dialysis Outcome Quality Initiative (DOQI) guidelines for determining the adequacy of hemodialysis and peritoneal dialysis (26,27). Indeed, it is likely that documentation of the dose of dialysis delivered to ESRD patients will be mandated by governmental regulatory agencies and may be tied to reimbursement for treatment. Quality assurance programs in most dialysis centers already use kinetic modeling as part of the assessment of the care delivered to patients.

DIALYSIS ADEQUACY: APPLICABILITY AND LIMITATIONS OF THE NATIONAL COOPERATIVE DIALYSIS STUDY

The NCDS remains the only prospective study conducted to examine *hemodialysis* outcome indexed to the clearance of low-molecular-weight substances. The remaining studies, described in the previous section (5–7) are retrospective and observational. The same is true for studies that that have been used to support the application of Kt/V$_{urea}$ to determine adequate levels of peritoneal dialysis. The improvement in outcome for dialysis patients that occurred following the application of the principles of urea kinetic modeling is the ultimate proof that the clearance of low-molecular-weight substances has had an important impact

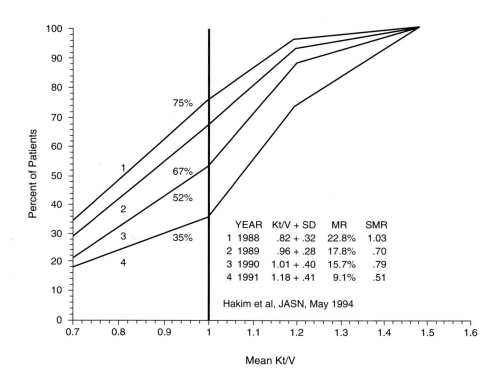

YEAR		Kt/V + SD	MR	SMR
1	1988	.82 + .32	22.8%	1.03
2	1989	.96 + .28	17.8%	.70
3	1990	1.01 + .40	15.7%	.79
4	1991	1.18 + .41	9.1%	.51

Hakim et al, JASN, May 1994

FIGURE 7.3. The improvement in standardized mortality rate (SMR) as Kt/V is increased over 4 years. The percentage of patients receiving higher doses of dialysis was increased during each year of the study.

on survival. Nevertheless, the limitations of the NCDS also should be appreciated to understand the unresolved issues regarding kinetic modeling.

The subjects eligible to enter the NCDS differed substantially from the current hemodialysis population. They were younger, compliant, and free of comorbid conditions. Only 20% of the current hemodialysis population would meet the NCDS entry criteria (28). The follow-up period of the study was short. Thus, the influence of factors such as age and comorbid conditions that occur over a longer period could not be assessed by the NCDS. The NCDS was able to define a dose of dialysis below which an unacceptable number of complications occur, but it was not designed to define an optimal level of dialysis beyond which no further improvement was realized.

Technical advances in dialysis delivery also have occurred since the NCDS was completed. Thus, it may not be possible to generalize the methods used in that study to our current practice. So biocompatible, synthetic, high-efficiency or high-flux dialyzers have largely replaced low-flux cellulosic dialyzers used in the NCDS. Acetate-buffered dialysate has been universally replaced with bicarbonate-buffered dialysate. Hemodialysis treatments have been more stable with the use of dialysate with higher sodium concentration and with volumetric machines capable of changing ultrafiltration rate and sodium concentration during treatment.

Increasing evidence points to nutrition as an important independent determinant of survival for dialysis patients (29). In the NCDS, the level of protein intake influenced the dialysis dose: By design, the levels of dialysis determined by Kt/V and protein intake were *inter*dependent rather than *in*dependent variables.

The dose of dialysis in the study was adjusted by alterations in blood flow, dialyzer size, and length of time. Indeed, time was an independent variable in the design. Dialyzer surface area and time will impact on middle molecule clearance as well as on the clearance of low-molecular-weight substances. Longer dialysis time and dialyzers of greater surface areas introduced a confounding variable, enhanced middle molecule clearance, when these techniques were used to increase Kt/V_{urea}. Group IV (short time, low Kt/V) fared most poorly of all groups, and it remains possible that reduced middle molecule clearance played a role in this outcome.

The National Cooperative Dialysis Study and Dialysis Time

The effect of the length of the dialysis treatment on outcome was not determined in the NCDS, and it is yet to be included as an independent variable in any study of the dialysis prescription to date. As mentioned, the issue remains unsettled because time was partially confounded with the effects of Kt/V_{urea}: An increase or a decrease in time was one of the methods used to change the TAC to meet the goals to

which the study participants were assigned. The current practice of using large-surface-area dialyzers at blood flows greater than 400 mL per minute and at dialysate flows of 600 to 800 mL per minute allows a Kt/V to be reached far in excess of values in NCDS groups I or III in many patients without increasing time. Indeed, many small- to medium-sized patients reach high levels of dialysis in times that are shorter than those used in group III.

Whether time is an important factor remains to be proven. Increased time may have a direct effect, or it may be a surrogate marker for the removal of larger substances. A decrease in cardiovascular instability and greater ease of ultrafiltration to a dry weight that is associated with a reduction or absence in the requirement of antihypertensive medications might be outcomes associated with increased dialysis time. In this regard, it should be remembered that the best survival statistics for hemodialysis patients, not withstanding somewhat favorable demographic features of the population, have been reported in a group of patients undergoing long, slow hemodialysis of 6 to 8 hours' duration against cellulosic membranes (27). Although this form of treatment is associated with very high Kt/V_{urea}, analysis of the data suggests that excellent blood pressure control *without the need for antihypertensive medication* is central to the favorable outcome experienced by the patients.

The superior control of hypertension with long dialysis also is supported by the experience from daily nocturnal hemodialysis (30,31). Preliminary studies showed that fluid balance is better maintained and that fewer antihypertensive agents are required to maintain normotension. In addition, the control of phosphorus appears to be excellent with nocturnal hemodialysis. Given the developing evidence that accelerated vascular calcification occurs in patients on dialysis, likely because of the use of calcium containing phosphate binders, nocturnal dialysis eventually may be shown to reduce cardiovascular morbidity associated with ESRD. This would be an effect of high-dose dialysis that is disassociated from urea kinetics. In this regard, despite its relatively low molecular weight, phosphorus behaves much more like a high-molecular-weight substance that is dependent on the length of treatment rather than on blood and dialysate flow.

Finally, long dialysis times would be more forgiving of errors such as poor needle placement or incorrect or unachievable blood flow rates that lead to disparities between prescribed and delivered levels of dialysis. The optimal length of dialysis time needs to be defined by further investigation.

Effect of Dialysis with High-efficiency and High-flux Dialysis

In the NCDS, cellulosic membranes with a low-molecular-weight solute cutoff were exclusively used. The introduction of high-efficiency and high-flux membranes has added more complexity to the quantification of hemodialysis. The kinetic modeling used in the NCDS and in most of the observational studies assumed that urea would instantly equilibrate across all body-fluid compartments: the single-pool model. This model did not account for the finding of an immediate rapid increase in the postdialysis urea level that occurs at the termination of dialysis. This rapid rise, termed *urea rebound*, is caused by three factors: dialysis access recirculation, cardiopulmonary recirculation, and urea compartmentalization (32–34). The first two phases occur within the 2 minutes after the termination of hemodialysis. The rebound that results from urea compartmentalization occurs over 60 minutes. It is caused by a delay in urea equilibration between tissue stores and blood. This delay is due to a slower than expected removal of urea from the intracellular fluid compartment (35–38). Alternatively, reduced perfusion of regions of the body containing high amounts of urea could explain the delay in equilibration (33). Rebound is enhanced under conditions of high-efficiency dialysis, lower-access blood flow, during hypotension, and in states of low cardiac output (39–41). Single-pool Kt/V may overestimate the equilibrated Kt/V by more than 0.2 U. An equation that allows the equilibrated Kt/V to be estimated from single-pool Kt/V has been developed (42). Thus, equilibrated Kt/V = single-pool Kt/V − 0.6 × K/V + 0.03.

THE HEMODIALYSIS (HEMO) STUDY

Although multiple lines of evidence indicate that kinetic modeling is an important index of dialysis adequacy and that the degree of removal of low-molecular-weight substances correlates with survival, these relationships have not been proven by prospective studies. It is important to confirm the impression of the observational studies that high doses of dialysis will have a favorable impact on patient outcome. The time, effort, and costs associated with providing high doses of dialysis are substantial. The DOQI guidelines already have made recommendations regarding a dose of dialysis below which poor patient outcomes are likely to occur. What is completely lacking is prospective data regarding the effects of increasing Kt/V to very high levels. Consequently, the National Institutes of Health initiated a multicenter, prospective, randomized trial to assess the impact of the dialysis prescription on the morbidity and mortality rate of hemodialysis patients (43).

The study is a two-by-two factorial design that will assess the effect of hemodialysis dose and membrane flux on outcome. In this study, an equilibrated Kt/V of 1.05 will be compared with an equilibrated Kt/V of 1.45, comparable on average to single-pool Kt/V of 1.25 and 1.65, respectively. In addition, the effect on the mortality and morbidity rates of high-flux versus low-flux dialyzers will be compared. All-cause mortality is the primary outcome; morbidity assessed from hospitalization, time to hospitalization for cardiovascular and infectious causes, and time to a decline in serum albumin concentration are secondary outcome measures. A concurrent sample size of 900 patients from 15 clinical centers with replacement of those participants who die or drop out will be used. The study concluded at the end of 2001.

ALTERNATIVE APPROACHES TO QUANTIFICATION OF DIALYSIS

The use of Kt/V$_{urea}$ in determining the adequacy of dialysis is based on mathematical models and is supported by clinical experience. Numerous paradoxic observations led some to question the validity of Kt/V$_{urea}$ as the best index of judging adequacy. One paradox is that the curve relating dialysis dose and survival is J-shaped (44). Low dialysis dose is associated with large declines in the mortality and mortality rates with increased doses of dialysis, but mortality again trends upward at the highest levels of dialysis. A second observation is that survival of black Americans on dialysis is better than that of white Americans, despite the finding that the latter group generally receives a higher dose of dialysis (45–47). It *is* important to note that these observations do not necessarily invalidate the practice of indexing adequacy against low-molecular-weight substances. Rather, the issue is whether Kt/V$_{urea}$ is the best measure of low-molecular-weight solute removal.

A common feature that may explain these observations relates to patient size (48). At the same $K \times t$, smaller patients are more likely to receive higher Kt/V$_{urea}$ than larger patients because their urea volume is smaller. Black Americans tend to have a greater body mass than whites (47,49,50). A low body mass is an independent risk factor for death in dialysis patients (47,50–53). *V*, the urea volume, may be an independent variable of survival because it tends to vary directly with body mass. Thus, when the work of dialysis, $K \times t$, is divided by *V*, a parameter that also may correlate with survival, in the computation of Kt/V, "these elements may offset each other, producing a complex quantity that does not reflect a true relationship between dialysis exposure and clinical outcome" (48). Proponents of this concept have demonstrated that when patient survival is examined as a function of Kt, the J-shaped curve disappears and mortality declines over the entire range of Kt.

Further analysis along these lines provides clarification of this complex relationship (52). From the U.S. Renal Data System database, 9,165 patients treated between 1990 and 1995 were studied. A Cox proportional hazards model, adjusting for patient characteristics, was used to calculate the relative risk for death. Hemodialysis dose (equilibrated Kt/V) and various indices of body size (body mass index, body weight, and body volume) were independently inversely related to mortality. Thus, the mortality rate was lower in patients with larger body size or volume and decreased as a function of hemodialysis dose (Fig. 7.4). The relationship between Kt/V and declining mortality is valid,

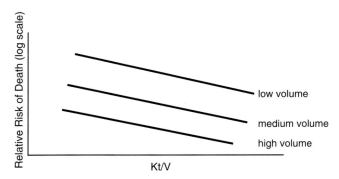

FIGURE 7.4. The interaction between hemodialysis dose and volume on relative risk of death.

but patient size also must be considered. The implication of this analysis is that the indices of body size may be surrogates for nutritional status. Nutritional status is clearly an important predictor of survival.

Urea Reduction Ratio and Solute Removal Index

There are alternative methods to the quantification of the dose of hemodialysis. Urea reduction rate (URR) (predialysis blood urea nitrogen, or BUN; postdialysis BUN/predialysis BUN) and solute removal index (SRI), based on dialysate urea measurements (total dialysate urea in grams $\times$ 100/predialysis BUN $\times$ V). URR depends exclusively on the changes that occur in urea levels during intermittent hemodialysis. The urea removed by convection is not accounted for by URR. Although URR correlates with survival in a fashion similar to Kt/V and is recognized by DOQI guidelines as a valid index of hemodialysis adequacy, Kt/V is a more precise index. Unlike URR, Kt/V also permits rational adjustments to the dialysis prescription to be made. Furthermore, URR cannot be used to judge the adequacy of peritoneal dialysis because urea levels are essentially in a steady state (URR about 0).

The SRI measures the *amount* of urea removed rather than the *fractional change* in urea. It is not influenced by compartmental distribution of urea. Measurement of dialysate urea requires special techniques, however, and is not routinely done. There have been few studies that validated SRI as an index of adequacy.

CONCLUSION

The NCDS was designed to ascertain prospectively which determinants of the dialysis prescription had an impact on patient outcome. The study was able to validate urea removal, a surrogate for low-molecular-weight substances, as an index of morbidity. Based on urea kinetics, the *minimum level* of hemodialysis below which increased morbidity resulted was a key finding that has stood the test of time. More importantly, the NCDS provided the stimulus for a large

number of observational studies that has resulted in the recommendations of the DOQI guidelines. At this writing, the question of whether an *optimal dose* of dialysis can be determined awaits the conclusion of the HEMO study.

Other issues remain. The small differences in time did not permit any conclusions to be made with respect to the importance of the removal of middle molecule in outcome. Indeed, the poor outcome of group IV suggested that further examination of this question was necessary. The importance of the removal of higher-molecular-weight substances or related substances, such as phosphorus, that are associated with them also has been suggested by studies of long hemodialysis and nocturnal dialysis. The interaction between body size and dose of dialysis also pointed out the complexity in interpreting the relationship between urea kinetic and survival. Despite the uncertainty, the preponderance of evidence suggests that the answer to the question, "Is quantitative measurement of dialysis adequacy a useful outcome measure?" must be in the affirmative.

REFERENCES

1. U.S. Renal Data System (USRDS). *USRDS 1999 annual data report*. Bethesda, MD: The National Institutes of Health, National Institute of Diabetes and Digestive and Kidney Disease, 1999.
2. Hakim RM. Assessing the adequacy of dialysis. *Kidney Int* 1990;37:822–832.
3. Gotch FA, Yarian S, Keen M. A kinetic survey of U.S. hemodialysis prescriptions. *Am J Kidney Dis* 1990;5:511–515.
4. Sargent JA. Shortfalls in the delivery of dialysis. *Am J Kidney Dis* 1990;15:500–510.
5. Hakim RM, Breyer J, Ismail N, et al. Effects of dose of dialysis on morbidity and mortality. *Am J Kidney Dis* 1994;23:661–669.
6. Parker TF, Husni L, Huang W, et al. Survival of hemodialysis patients in the United States is improved with a greater quantity of dialysis. *Am J Kidney Dis* 1994;23:670–680.
7. Collins AJ, Ma JZ, Umen A. Urea index (Kt/V) and other predictors of hemodialysis patient survival. *Am J Kidney Dis* 1994;23:272–282.
8. Stubbs H [quoted by Dau PC]. Plasmapheresis therapy in myasthenia gravis. *Muscle Nerve* 1980;3:468–482.
9. Babb A, Farrell P, Uvelli D, et al. Hemodialyzer evaluation by examination of solute molecular spectra. *Trans Am Soc Artif Intern Organs* 1972;18:98–105.
10. Schoots A, Mikkers F, Cramers C, et al. Uremic toxins and the elusive middle molecules. *Nephron* 1984;38:1–8.
11. Vanholder R. Middle molecules as uremic toxins: still a viable hypothesis. *Semin Dial* 1994;7:65–68.
12. Malachi T, Bogin E, Gafter U, et al. Parathyroid hormone effect on the fragility of human young and old red blood cells in uremia. *Nephron* 1986;42:52–57.
13. Bogin E, Massry SG, Harary I. Effect of parathyroid hormone on rat heart cells. *J Clin Invest* 1981;67:1215–1227.
14. Hajjar SM, Fadda GZ, Thanakitcharu P, et al. Reduced activity of Na+ -K+ ATPase of pancreatic islets in chronic renal failure: role of secondary hyperparathyroidism. *J Am Soc Nephrol* 1992;2:1355–1359.
15. Perna AF, Smogorzewski M, Massry SG. Effects of verapamil on the abnormalities in fatty acid oxidation of myocardium. *Kidney Int* 1989;36:453–457.

16. Fadda GZ, Akmal M, Premdas FH, et al. Insulin release from pancreatic islets: effects of CRF and excess PTH. *Kidney Int* 1988; 33:1066–1072.

17. Gejyo F, Odani S, Yamada T, et al. β$_2$-microglobulin: a new form of amyloid protein associated with chronic hemodialysis. *Kidney Int* 1986;30:385–390.

18. Teschan PE, Ginn HE, Bourne Jr, et al. Neurobehavioral probes for adequacy of dialysis. *Trans Am Soc Artif Intern Organs* 1977; 23:556–560.

19. Lowrie EG, Laird NM, Parker TF, et al. Effect of the hemodialysis prescription on patient morbidity: report from the National Cooperative Dialysis Study. *N. Engl J Med* 1981;305:1176–1180.

20. Sargent JA, Gotch FA. The analysis of concentration dependence of uremic lesions in clinical studies. *Kidney Int* 1975;7(Suppl 2):S35–S44.

21. Lowrie EG, Lew NL. Death risk in hemodialysis patients: the predictive value of commonly measured variables and an evaluation of death rate differences between facilities. *Am J Kidney Dis* 1990; 15:458–482.

22. Gotch F, Sargent J. A mechanistic analysis of the National Cooperative Dialysis Study (NCDS). *Kidney Int* 1985;28:526–534.

23. Keshaviah P. Urea kinetic and middle molecule approaches to assess adequacy of hemodialysis and CAPD. *Kidney Int* 1993;43 (Suppl 40):S28–S38.

24. Charra B, Calelmard E, Ruffet M, et al. Survival as an index of adequacy of dialysis. *Kidney Int* 1992;41:1286–1291.

25. Canada USA (CANUSA) Peritoneal Dialysis Study Group. Adequacy of dialysis and nutrition in continuous peritoneal dialysis: association with clinical outcomes. *J Am Soc Nephrol* 1996;7:198.

26. NKF-DOQI Clinical Practice Guidelines for Hemodialysis Adequacy. V. Prescribed dose of hemodialysis. *Am J Kidney Disease* 1997;30(Suppl 2):S86.

27. NKF-DOQI Clinical Practice Guidelines for Peritoneal Dialysis Adequacy. V. Adequate dose of peritoneal dialysis. *Am J Kidney Dis* 1997;30(Suppl 2):S86.

28. Eggers PW. Mortality rates among dialysis patients in Medicare's end-stage renal disease program. *Am J Kidney Dis* 1990;15:414–421.

29. Owen WF Jr, Lew NL, Liu Y, et al. The urea reduction ratio and serum albumin concentration as predictors of mortality in patients undergoing hemodialysis. *N Engl J Med* 1993;329:1001–1006.

30. Pierratos A, Ouwendyk M, Francoeur R. Nocturnal hemodialysis: three-year experience. *J Am Soc Nephrol* 1988;9:859.

31. Mucsi I, Hercz G, Vldall R. Central of serum phosphate without any phosphate binders in patients treated with nocturnal hemodialysis. *Kidney Int* 1978;53:1399–1404.

32. Schneditz D, Kaufman AM, Polaschegg H, et al. Cardiopulmonary recirculation during hemodialysis. *Kidney Int* 1992;42: 1450–1456.

33. Schneditz D, Van Stone JC, Daugirdas JT. A regional blood circulation alternative to in-series two-compartment urea kinetic modeling. *ASAIO J* 1993;39:M573–M577.

34. Van Stone JC, Daugirdas JT. Physiologic principles. In: Daugirdas JT, Ing TS, eds. *Handbook of dialysis*, 2nd ed. Boston: Little, Brown, and Company, 1994:13–29.

35. Shackman R, Chisholm GD, Holden AJ, et al. Urea distribution in the body after haemodialysis. *BMJ* 1962;34:817–824.

36. Schleifer CR, Snyder S, Jones K. The influence of urea kinetic modelling on gross mortality in hemodialysis. *J Am Soc Nephrol* 1991;2:349(abst).

37. Frost TH, Kerr DNS. Kinetics of hemodialysis: a theoretical study of the removal of solutes in chronic renal failure compared to normal health. *Kidney Int* 1977;12:41–50.

38. Heineken FG, Evans MC, Keen MI, et al. Intercompartmental fluid shifts in hemodialysis patients. *Biotechnol Prog* 1987;3:69–73.

39. Tsang HK, Leonard EF, Lefavour GS, et al. Urea dynamics during and immediately after dialysis. *ASAIO J* 1985;8:251–260.

40. Kjellstrand C, Kjellstrand P, Skroder R, et al. Dialysis kinetics using pre- and post-concentrations of BUN are not accurate. *J Am Soc Nephrol* 1992;3:375.

41. Spiegel DM, Paker PL, Babcock S, et al. Hemodialysis urea rebound: the effect of increasing dialysis efficiency. *Am J Kidney Dis* 1994 (*in press*).

42. Daugirdas JT, Schneditz D. Overestimation of hemodialysis dose (delta Kt/V) depends on dialysis efficiency (K/V) by regional blood flow and conventional 2-pool urea kinetic analyses. *ASAIO J* 1995;41 (*in press*).

43. Eknoyan G, Levey A, Beck G, et al. The hemodialysis (HEMO) study: rationale for selection of interventions. *Seminars in Dialysis* 1996;9:24–33.

44. Chertow GM, Owen WF, Lazarus JM, et al. The interplay of uremia and malnutrition: a hypothesis for the reverse J-shaped curve between URR and mortality. *Kidney Int* 1999;56:1872–1878.

45. Frankenfield DL, McClellan WM, Helgerson SD. Urea reduction ratio, demographic characteristics, and body weight in the 1996 National ESRD Core Indicators Project. *Am J Kidney Dis* 1999;33:584–591.

46. Owen WF, Price D. African-Americans on maintenance dialysis: a review of racial differences in incidence, treatment, and survival. *Adv Ren Replace Ther* 1997;4:2–12.

47. Owen WF, Chertow GM, Lazarus JM, et al. Dose of hemodialysis and survival: differences by race and sex. *JAMA* 1998;280: 1764–1768.

48. Zhensheng L, Lew N, Lazarus M, et al. Comparing the urea reduction ratio and the urea product as outcome-based measures of hemodialysis dose. *Am J. Kidney Dis* 2000;35:598–605.

49. Lowrie EG, Zhu X, Lew NL. Primary associates of mortality among dialysis patients: trends and reassessment of Kt/V and urea reduction ratio as outcome-based measures of dialysis dose. *Am J Kidney Dis* 1998;32(Suppl 4):S16–S32.

50. Kopple JD, Zhu X, Lew NL, et al. Body weight-for-height percentile relationships predict mortality in maintenance hemodialysis patients. *Kidney Int* 1999;56:1136–1148.

51. Fleischmann E, Teal N, Dudley J, et al. Influence of excess weight on mortality and hospital stay. I. 1346 hemodialysis patients. *Kidney Int* 1999;55:1560–1567.

52. Wolfe, RA, Ashby VB, Daugirdas JT, et al. Body size, dose of hemodialysis and mortality. *Am J Kidney Dis* 2000;35:80–88.

53. Lowrie EG, Chertow GM, Lew NL, et al. The {clearance X time} product (Kt) as an outcome-based measure of dialysis dose. *Kidney Int* 1999;56:729–737.

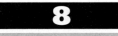
PATHOPHYSIOLOGY OF ARTERIOVENOUS GRAFT FAILURE

ALAN B. LUMSDEN
CHANGYI CHEN

Hemodialysis access grafts are the most frequently implanted type of prosthetic graft in vascular surgery. Their mean patency is only 18 months. Despite such widespread use, no improvement in their patency has been made since they were first introduced in 1976 (1,2). Failure in more than 90% of cases is due to venous anastomotic stenosis (3–6). Histologic analysis of this venous anastomotic lesion demonstrates that it is identical to the restenotic lesion, which occurs following coronary angioplasty or arterial-to-arterial bypass. The pathophysiology of arteriovenous (AV) graft failure, therefore, is largely the pathophysiology of neointima formation at the venous anastomosis.

Once graft failure has occurred, thrombectomy or graft revision or percutaneous transluminal angioplasty results in an additional 3 months of patency. Thus, once graft occlusion occurs, prolonged patency is unusual (7). The inability to prolong graft patency after occlusion has occurred is reflective of several factors: difficulty in correcting the primary lesion for graft failure, alteration in graft thrombogenicity, persistence of secondary lesions, or a combination of one or more of these factors.

In this chapter, we examine the data for the causes of primary and secondary graft failure.

DISTRIBUTION OF NEOINTIMAL HYPERPLASTIC LESIONS

Color duplex imaging (CDI) provides a quantitative, noninvasive method for examining functioning AV grafts. It provides both anatomic imaging (B-mode ultrasound) and functional data (Doppler ultrasound) (Fig. 8.1). In a cross-sectional study of all patients at a single dialysis center, we used CDI to survey ePTFE grafts for the presence of stenoses greater than or equal to 50%. The duplex findings were compared with contrast angiography. During the period from December 1993 to January 1995, all patients on chronic hemodialysis were screened as candidates for enroll-

ment in this trial. Of 150 patients within the dialysis center, 110 had ePTFE bridge grafts. Stenoses of greater than 50% diameter were identified in 41 patients. Of the 41 patients, 54 stenoses were identified by CDI. Angiography demonstrated a total of 64 stenoses in the same patient cohort. Per CDI, 29 (54%) of the lesions were located at the venous anastomosis compared with 31 (48%) observed at the venous anastomosis by angiography. The mean percent stenosis of these lesions was 60% by CDI and 67% by angiography. Our study demonstrated that 37% of patients in a single dialysis center with functioning ePTFE AV grafts have graft stenoses of greater than 50%. The average number of stenoses per graft was 1.38 per CDI and 1.61 per angiography. This difference was accounted for largely by the increased number of central venous stenoses detected by angiography (see Chapter 25). CDI effectively detected stenoses within the graft and at the arterial and venous anastomoses but was ineffective in detecting central venous lesions. Similar data have been reported previously, although others note an even higher incidence of venous anastomotic lesions (8–10).

One important finding worth emphasis is that most grafts have more than one stenosis, the implication being that function may be compromised by more than one lesion and that identification and correction of both lesions are essential to prolonging graft patency. Also, we do not know what degree of stenosis should be regarded as physiologically significant. Furthermore, lesions that are insignificant at baseline can become important during or after dialysis, when major fluid shifts are occurring.

Physically, the venous anastomotic lesion is regarded as one of the most difficult lesions to dilate, with high rates of recurrence. Special high-pressure balloons are necessary to stretch this resistant lesion. In addition, it has much more elastic recoil than does an arterial lesion or indeed other venous lesions. It is this combination of physical characteristics along with the perpetually elevated proliferation rate of smooth-muscle cells that leads to the dismal results in both primary and secondary graft patencies.

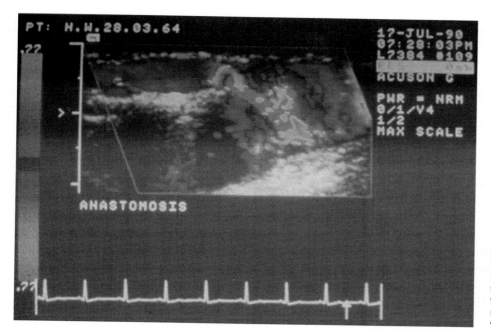

FIGURE 8.1. Color flow duplex image showing increased flow velocities within a venous anastomotic stenosis. Increasing flow velocities occur as the stenosis becomes progressively more severe. The gray scale image also can be used to measure the diameter of the vessel directly.

CHARACTERIZATION OF NEOINTIMAL HYPERPLASTIC LESIONS

To characterize neointimal hyperplastic lesions, we performed histologic analysis on 12 human dialysis graft venous anastomotic explants. All venous segments as well as adjacent portions of ePTFE graft material exhibited marked neointimal hyperplastic lesions. Often the original lumen was nearly completely occluded.

Several specific features were observed within the neointimal lesion. Widespread vascularization (60 ± 8 microvessels/mm^2) of the neointima by capillary-sized vessels was seen in all specimens. Identification of cell types was facilitated by specific immunocytochemical staining. The vast majority of neointimal cells were smooth-muscle cells (α-actin-positive cells). Endothelial cells (factor VIII–related antigen-positive cells) covered the luminal surface of the neointima and lumens of most microvessels. T-lymphocytes (CD43-positive cells) and macrophages (HAM56-positive cells) were ubiquitous, with a tendency toward distribution near the anastomoses or in close association with the ePTFE graft material. B-lymphocytes were not present in the neointima. A small proportion of cells in the neointima (about 10%) were negative for the individual cell type-specific antibodies used. Those cells were most likely fibroblasts, whereas the origin of the nonreactive cell population was not clear.

All the neointimal lesions studied were hypocellular, and extracellular matrix (ECM) constituted the bulk of the lesions (Fig. 8.2). Verhoeff–Masson's trichrome stain demonstrated that collagen was widespread in the lesions, whereas elastin fibers were rarely found. Mucopolysaccharides were overproduced in the luminal one-third layer of the neointima. The cellular and ECM volumes were analyzed as three layers, each of which was one third of the thickness of the neointima. The luminal layer consisted of $34 \pm 13\%$ cells and $66 \pm 13\%$ ECM in volume. The middle layer was made up of $14 \pm 3\%$ cells and $86 \pm 3\%$ ECM in volume. The deep layer near the grafts comprised $21 \pm 14\%$ cells and $79 \pm 14\%$ ECM in volume. Statistical analysis showed that ECM volume percentage was significantly lower in the luminal layer of neointima than in the middle and deep layers of neointima ($p < 0.05$). No significant difference was found, however, between the ECM volume percentages in the middle and deep layers of neointima ($p > 0.05$).

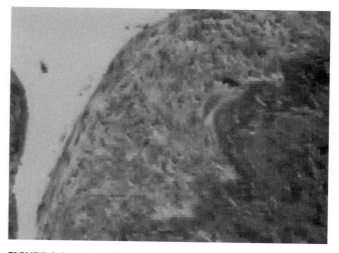

FIGURE 8.2. Verhoeff–Masson's staining of vein adjacent to the venous anastomosis demonstrating smooth-muscle cells, which stain red within the intima (*arrow*) surrounded by large quantities of extracellular matrix (mucopolysaccharides) produced by the smooth-muscle cells.

Cell proliferation was assayed by proliferating cell nuclear antigen (PCNA) index. Very few PCNA-positive cells were found in normal artery and vein, in agreement with previous reports (11,12). PCNA indices in the normal artery and vein ranged from 0.01% to 0.1%. In contrast, higher PCNA indices were observed in the neointimal lesions, which reflected increased cell proliferation. Those indices were as follows: luminal layer, 29 ± 11%; middle layer, 9 ± 5%; deep layer near the graft, 9 ± 7%; and microvessel-containing intimal fields, 67 ± 4% (Fig. 8.3). The cell proliferation rate was significantly higher in the luminal layer than in the middle or deep layers of neointima ($p < 0.05$). The PCNA index in microvessel-containing intimal fields was three to eight times that of avascular fields ($p < 0.001$).

Tenascin (TN) is a recently characterized hexameric ECM glycoprotein that is composed of six similar subunits joined together at their amino termini by disulfide bonds. This molecule is made up of several epidermal growth factor (EGF)-like repeats, followed by fibronectin type III homology repeats and a domain with a sequence similar to the β and γ fibrinogen chains. Originally, TN was thought to play a role in embryogenesis and oncogenesis (13–16). Recently, TN has been observed in the neointima formed by proliferating SMCs 2 weeks after balloon catheter injury of the rat carotid artery (17). We also have reported that TN is markedly increased in human neointimal hyperplastic lesions (18,19). TN was not detected in the normal arteries and veins. TN was found in all the venous anastomotic neointimal hyperplastic lesions of AV ePTFE grafts from 12 patients. The strongest immunoreactivity was observed in the luminal layer of neointima and periendothelial layer of microvessels. Specifically, TN was distributed in the neointima as follows: (a) in the luminal layer, all lesions were intensely stained; (b) in the middle layer, nine of 12 (75%) lesions had moderate reactivity, and three of 12 (25%) had occasional positive fibers; (c) in the deep layer near the ePTFE grafts, three of 12 (25%) lesions were strongly stained, five of 12 (42%) had moderate reactivity, and four of 12 (33%) had weak positive staining; and (d) 90 ± 6% of microvessels within the neointima showed intense pe-

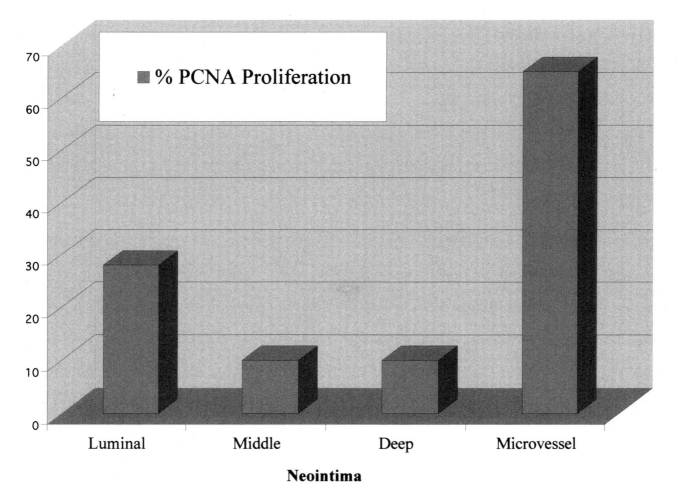

FIGURE 8.3. This graph shows that using proliferating cell nuclear antigen staining, nearly 30% of smooth-muscle cells in the luminal third of the intima are actively dividing. This rate is only exceeded by the very high proliferation rate within the walls of newly formed microvessels within the intima.

riendothelial staining. These data demonstrate that TN is distributed in a pattern similar to cell proliferation in human neointimal hyperplastic lesions. The results suggest that TN expression may have a potential role in neovascularization and neointimal growth in human AV PTFE graft failure.

Furthermore, we conducted a time-course study of intimal hyperplasia in a canine model of femoral AV ePTFE grafts and found that the lesions produced in this animal model are very similar to those seen in humans (20–23). Neointimal hyperplasia at the venous anastomoses developed more rapidly than did that at the arterial anastomoses over a 3-month study (0.37 ± 0.27 mm versus 0.20 ± 0.21 mm of neointimal thickness; $p < 0.05$), supporting the clinical evidence that venous anastomotic lesions are a primary cause of AV graft failure.

We also attempted to determine TN distribution and cell proliferation in the anastomoses of AV loop grafts in a dog model. ePTFE grafts were implanted bilaterally between the femoral artery and vein in five mongrel dogs. Histologic analysis at the mid-anastomotic level was carried out at 1 week. Immunohistochemical staining was used to identify TN and proliferating cells that incorporated bromodeoxyuridine (BrdU). The results indicate that TN production is increased at both arterial and venous anastomoses in the early stages of graft healing, that TN is distributed mainly in the intima–inner media and adventitia at both arterial and venous anastomoses, and that TN distribution has a pattern similar to cell proliferation. This study supports the findings that TN may be involved in the development of anastomotic neointimal hyperplasia in human lesions.

This lesion differs from that of arterial neointima in the marked degree of ongoing cell proliferation identified in the luminal third of the lesion. Typically, peak proliferation after arterial injury occurs at approximately day 5, with little persistent proliferation after 2 to 3 weeks. The marked ongoing proliferation at the venous anastomosis would suggest an ongoing injury, and it also may have important implications for intervention: It is unlikely that a one-time mechanical intervention would provide significant long-term improvement in patency. Therefore, repeated interventions may be an absolute requirement unless we can profoundly alter the functional behavior of the vessel wall at the same time.

THROMBOSIS MARKERS AND PLATELET DEPOSITION IN FUNCTIONING ARTERIOVENOUS GRAFTS

A possible reason for the propensity of AV grafts to develop venous neointimal hyperplasia is that chronic platelet aggregation occurring in the midportion of the prosthetic graft leads to the release of SMC mitogens, which bathe the distal anastomosis. We studied several markers of thrombosis in patients with ePTFE bridge grafts: (a) platelet activation was

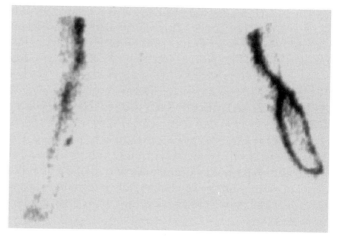

FIGURE 8.4. Indium-labeled platelet deposition onto a 5-year-old left-forearm loop graft in a patient with end-stage renal disease compared with the right forearm.

evaluated via serum concentrations of platelet factor 4 (PF4) and β-thromboglobulin (BTG); (b) stimulation of individual platelets was determined by expression of ligand-induced binding sites (LIBS) on the glycoprotein IIb/IIIa receptor; and (c) thrombin generation was measured by assay of serum fibrinopeptide-A (FPA) and thrombin–antithrombin (TAT) complexes. Platelet aggregation on chronic grafts was quantitated by measurement of indium[111]-labeled platelet deposition (Fig. 8.4). The serum levels of PF4 (21.9 ± 35.2 IU/mL), BTG (155.1 ± 36.8 IU/mL), FPA (13.5 ± 12.9 nM), and TAT peptide (8.0 ± 4.1 ng/mL) were increased compared with normal values in adults ($p < 0.05$). LIBS expression also was increased ($7,444 \pm 4,809$ epitopes per platelet versus $2,569 \pm 1,328$ epitopes per platelet in controls, $p < 0.01$). Platelet deposition on each graft at 2 hours was $10.94 \pm 1.76 \times 10^9$. The graft-to-blood ratio of radioactivity remained significantly ($p < 0.05$) elevated at 24 and 36 hours, with ratios of 33.0 and 49.6, respectively. We concluded that platelet activation occurs in patients with ePTFE grafts as demonstrated by increased circulating platelet markers and expression of LIBS and that significant platelet deposition continues to occur in chronically implanted grafts. Strategies designed to inhibit platelet deposition may prolong graft patency.

We also quantitatively analyzed platelet deposition on 21 AV ePTFE grafts in a canine model. Autologous canine platelets were labeled with 500 mmCi indium[111] oxine and reinjected at least 1 hour before imaging. Scintillation camera images were performed at 30, 60, and 90 minutes after establishing flow in the grafts. Graft platelet deposition was 3.00×10^9, 3.19×10^9, and 3.23×10^9 at 30, 60, and 90 minutes, respectively. We similarly demonstrated that even in chronically implanted human grafts, platelets continue to be deposited onto the graft, although a steady state of platelet deposition and elution from the graft most likely develops.

These data demonstrate that platelets are rapidly accumulated on ePTFE grafts. Thrombogenicity of graft material and hemodynamic factors contribute to platelet deposition on AV ePTFE grafts.

HEMODYNAMICS OF THE ARTERIOVENOUS GRAFT

Anastomotic SMC proliferation complicates all grafts, and it has been widely claimed that the addition of a cuff at the distal anastomosis of lower-extremity bypass grafts prolongs patency. This observation, together with that of Dr.

Fredrick Scholtz, of the Queen Elisabeth Hospital in Berlin, who used a self-made AV patch, led to the development of a one-piece ePTFE AV bridge graft the Venaflo graft (Impra, Tempe, AZ, U.S.A.) (Fig. 8.5). The Venaflo graft concept was based on these observations and supported by complex hemodynamic modeling suggesting that the cuffed anastomosis would lead to reduced oscillating and low-shear areas within the anastomosis and, consequently, could reduce restenosis if hemodynamic factors were the inciting event.

A prospective randomized clinical study was conducted at six different institutions that performed vascular access surgery. Life-table primary patencies were as follows: stan-

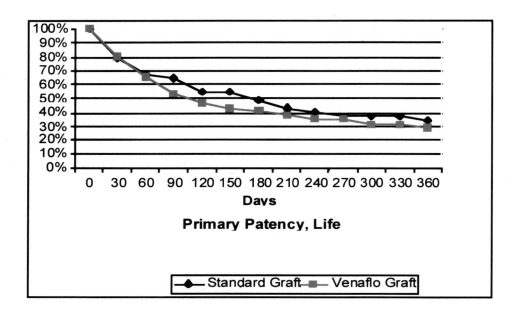

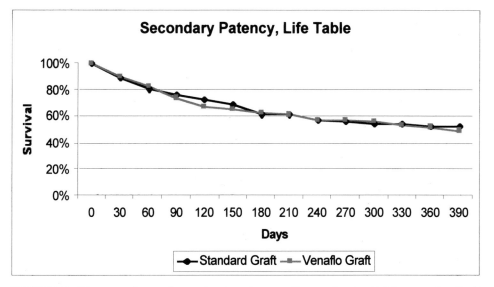

FIGURE 8.5. Primary and secondary patencies of prospective randomized trial comparing the Venaflo (modified venous anastomosis) versus standard grafts.

dard 48.84% versus Venaflo 41.74% (6 months) and standard 34.4% versus (Fig. 8.1) Venaflo 28.6% ($p = 0.2706$; 12 months); these did not differ significantly. Secondary patencies were standard 61.8% versus Venaflo 62.8% at 6 months, and standard 53.28% versus Venaflo 49.47% ($p = 0.6068$; 12 months); these also did not differ significantly (Fig. 8.2). As expected, graft thrombosis was the most common complication in both graft types, but the rates were equivalent for both devices: 2.1 per patient for Venaflo versus 1.9 per patient for standard type.

A feature of AV graft function used to determine patency on clinical examination is the presence of a thrill. When viewed using color flow duplex imaging, this represents turbulent flow within the graft, which is transmitted to the surrounding tissues as perigraft vibration. This pronounced vibration is detected as a thrill on palpation. It has long been speculated, but remains to be proven, that this degree of turbulence with its associated areas of low-shear, high-shear vortex formation promotes venous anastomotic neointima.

SUMMARY

There are 220,000 patients with end-stage renal disease in the United States and at least 20,000 new cases diagnosed yearly (24). Failure of AV grafts represents an enormous clinical burden. The mechanism of venous neointimal hyperplasia development and graft failure is complex and multifactorial, including local release of growth factors, compliance mismatch, turbulence, and platelet deposition. Unlike other models of vascular injury, SMC proliferation rates of AV grafts are high and continuous. Interventions utilizing balloon angioplasty provide short-term benefit and are unlikely to be efficacious. In this chapter, we analyzed the composition of neointimal hyperplastic lesions and outlined strategies that are potentially useful in controlling this aggressive lesion.

REFERENCES

1. Baker LD Jr, Johnson JM, Goldfarb D. Expanded polytetrafluoroethylene (PTFE) subcutaneous arteriovenous conduit: an improved vascular access for chronic hemodialysis. *ASAIO Trans* 1976;22:382–387.
2. Windus DW. Permanent vascular access: a nephrologist's view. *Am J Kidney Dis* 1993;21:457–471.
3. Palder SB, Kirkman RL, Whittemore AD, et al. Vascular access for hemodialysis. *Ann Surg* 1986;202:235–239.
4. Zibari GB, Rohr MS, Landreneau MD, et al. Complications from permanent hemodialysis vascular access. *Surgery* 1988;104:681–686.
5. Imparato AM, Bracco A, Kim GE, et al. Intimal and neointimal fibrous proliferation causing failure of arterial reconstruction. *Surgery* 1972;72:1007–1017.
6. Bell DD, Rosenthal JJ. Arteriovenous graft life in chronic hemodialysis. *Arch Surg* 1988;123:1169–1172.
7. Feldman HI, Held PJ, Hutchinson JT, et al. Hemodialysis vascular access morbidity in the United States. *Kidney Int* 1993;43:1091–1096.
8. Daniels ID, Berlyne GM, Barth RH. Blood flow rates and access recirculation in hemodialysis. *Int J Artif Organs* 1992;15:470–474.
9. Swedberg SH, Brown BG, Sigley R, et al. Intimal fibromuscular hyperplasia at the venous anastomosis of PTFE grafts in hemodialysis patients: clinical, immunocytochemical, light and electron microscopic assessment. *Circulation* 1989;80:1726–1736.
10. Scottiurai VS. Biogenesis and etiology of distal anastomotic intimal hyperplasia. *Int Angiol* 1990;9:59–69.
11. Salmivirta M, Elenius K, Vainio S, et al. Syndecan from embryonic tooth mesenchyme binds tenascin. *J Biol Chem* 1991;266:7733–7740.
12. End P, Panayotou G, Entwistle A, et al. Tenascin: a modulator of cell growth. *Eur J Biochem* 1992;209:1041–1130.
13. Erickson HP, Inghesias JL. A six-armed oligomer isolated from cell surface fibronectin preparations. *Nature* 1984;311:267–270.
14. Inaguma Y, Kusakabe M, Mackie EJ, et al. Epithelial induction of stromal tenascin in the mouse mammary gland: from embryogenesis to carcinogenesis. *Dev Biol* 1988;128:245–262.
15. Steindler DA, Cooper NGF, Faissner A, et al. Boundaries defined by adhesion molecules during development of the cerebellar cortex: the J1/tenascin glycoprotein in the mouse somatosensory cortex barrel field. *Dev Biol* 1989;131:243–251.
16. Riou JF, Shi DL, Chiquet M, et al. Expression of tenascin in response to neural induction in amphibian embryos. *Development* 1989;104:511.
17. Hedin U, Holm J, Hansson G. Induction of tenascin in rat arterial injury: relationship to altered smooth muscle cell phenotype. *Am J Pathol* 1991;139:649–657.
18. Mackie EJ, Chiquet-Ehrismann R, Pearson CA, et al. Tenascin is a stromal marker for epithelial malignancy in the mammary gland. *Proc Natl Acad Sci USA* 1987;84:4621–4625.
19. Chen C, Suwyn C, Mattar SG, et al. Distribution of tenascin in human neointimal hyperplastic lesions. *Surg Forum* 1994;XLV:382–395.
20. Chen C, Mattar SG, Allen AC, et al. Tenascin distribution and cell proliferation in the early stage of arteriovenous loop graft. *J Am Soc Nephrol* 1994;5:411(abst).
21. Lumsden AB, Chen C, Ku DN. Neovascularization in the venous neointimal hyperplastic lesions of arteriovenous grafts. *J Am Soc Nephrol* 1994;5:421(abst).
22. Lumsden AB, Chen C. Arteriovenous fistula for dialysis access: clinical use and pathophysiologic changes. In: Brockbank KGM, ed. *Principles of autologous, allogenic, and cryopreserved venous transplantation.* Austin, TX: R.G. Landes Company, 1995:135–144.
23. Chen C, Allen RC, Jaffe MB, et al. Quantitative study of neointimal hyperplasia in a canine model of arteriovenous polytetrafluoroethylene grafts. Presented at The 5th Annual Winter Meeting of the Peripheral Vascular Surgery Society, Breckenridge, CO; Jan. 27–29, 1995.
24. Prevalence and cost of ESRD therapy. In: *U.S. Renal Data System, USRDS 1994 Annual Data Report.* Bethesda, MD; NIH, National Institute of Diabetes and Digestive and Kidney Diseases, 1994:23–42.

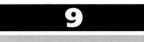

MANAGEMENT OF BLEEDING AND CLOTTING DISORDERS IN DIALYSIS PATIENTS

BARBARA ALVING

Dialysis patients may be at increased risk for bleeding because of inherited or acquired coagulation abnormalities in addition to hemostatic defects associated with renal failure. Patients also may be at increased risk for thrombosis if they have inherited or acquired hypercoagulable states. The use of anticoagulants, such as low-molecular-weight (LMW) heparin, danaparoid, and hirudin, all require special consideration in patients who are receiving dialysis. This chapter discusses the management of bleeding and clotting disorders in dialysis patients, including the role of renal failure in modification of drug treatment.

BLEEDING DISORDERS IN DIALYSIS PATIENTS

Uremia

Patients who are uremic usually will have a normal prothrombin time (PT), activated partial thromboplastin time (aPTT), and platelet count. They may have prolonged bleeding times; however, the degree of prolongation appears to correlate with clinical bleeding (1). The platelet dysfunction is due to multiple causes, including excess formation of nitric oxide, which inhibits platelet function (2). In addition, platelets may have a storage pool defect, reduced production of prostaglandin, and decreased adhesion resulting from a decrease in expression of the receptor glycoprotein (GP) IIb/IIIa, which is a binding site for von Willebrand factor (vWF) as well as fibrinogen (3). The vessel wall in patients with uremia may produce an increased amount of prostaglandin I_2 (PGI_2), which impairs platelet adhesion (4). Plasma factors, which are not well characterized, also may inhibit platelet adhesion and aggregation *in vivo* (5).

Multiple strategies can be used to reduce the excessive bleeding associated with uremia (Table 9.1). Platelet function in patients with uremia can be maximized rheologically by maintaining the hematocrit at 30% (6). The prolonged bleeding time can be corrected by administration of desmopressin (DDAVP) intravenously at a dose of 0.3 µg per kilogram of body weight. The effect begins 1 hour after infusion and persists for about 4 hours (6,7). DDAVP should not be used more frequently than once in 24 hours; repeated doses are not efficacious and can result in hyponatremia and seizures.

In a double-blind randomized trial of intravenous conjugated estrogens administered at a dose of 0.6 mg per kilogram of body weight daily to six patients with uremia, a prolonged bleeding time was partially corrected by 6 to 48 hours after the first dose; peak effect was at 5 to 7 days and duration was as long as 14 days (8). Transdermal estrogen was efficacious in reducing or stopping bleeding in a series of six patients with renal failure, prolonged bleeding times, and excessive bleeding from telangiectasia of the gastrointestinal tract (9). The estrogen was administered as 17 β-estradiol (Estraderm: Novartis Pharmaceuticals Corporation, East Hanover, NJ, U.S.A.) in a skin patch that delivered 50 or 100 µg daily. In these patients, the mean bleeding time decreased from 14 to 7 minutes. The effects were noted at 24 hours and persisted at 17 days (total duration of administration was 2 months). No adverse effects were noted (9). Vigano and colleagues (10) postulate that the prolonged effect of estrogens is due to their ability to enter endothelial cells, which are known to have estrogen receptors, and alter their function such that improved hemostasis occurs. Other studies have shown that administration of estrogen inhibits nitric oxide production (2).

In the surgical setting, a realistic goal is to provide sufficient hemostatic support to allow the patient to undergo surgery or other invasive procedures without undue risk. Thus, complete correction of coagulation laboratory abnormalities may not be possible or even desirable. For example,

This chapter was written by Dr. Alving in her private capacity. The views expressed in this article do not necessarily represent the views of the National Institutes of Health, DHHS, or the United States.

TABLE 9.1. HEMOSTATIC OPTIONS FOR PATIENTS WITH UREMIA

Goal	Treatment	Comments
Maintain hematocrit 27%–32%	Erythropoietin	Monitor for hypertension; check iron stores if patient is resistant to erythropoietin
Acutely enhance platelet function	DDAVP, 0.3 μg/kg i.v.	Administer no more frequently than once in 24 h. Monitor for hyponatremia to avoid seizures
Chronic enhancement of platelet function	Conjugated estrogens (0.6 mg/kg day i.v. for 4–5 days or transdermal 17β-estradial at a dose of 50–100 μg/24 h applied as patch every 3–5 days	Adverse effects: fluid retention, hot flashes

DDAVP, desmopressin; i.v., intravenous.

replacement of factor VII, which has a half-life of 2 to 6 hours, by infusion of plasma could lead to excessive volume expansion and pulmonary edema.

A critical factor for patients who require invasive procedures such as line placement is the skill of the operator. In one retrospective review of patients who had received arterial, pulmonary artery, or central venous lines, the researchers found that hemostatic complications were rare and were related more to the experience of the operator than to the underlying hemostatic defect (11). They concluded that only patients with severe hemostatic defects require correction of the abnormalities before line placement.

Fibrin sealant can be used to provide localized hemostasis. In the United States, one commercial product is now available (Tisseel; Baxter-Immuno, Vienna, Austria; marketed in the United States by Baxter Healthcare, Deerfield, IL, U.S.A.). The indication is for patients who are undergoing redo coronary artery bypass surgery or who have bleeding from sites not controlled by sutures, such as splenic trauma. The product comprises human fibrinogen (75–115 mg/mL) and human thrombin (500 IU/mL), both of which are virally inactivated (12). The thrombin is solubilized in calcium chloride (40 mM), which stimulates cross-linking of the clot by factor XIII in the product (or patient). The product also contains aprotinin, a bovine-derived protein that directly inhibits plasmin. This is included to increase clot stability. A much less expensive form of this product can be made by mixing cryoprecipitate in one syringe (fibrinogen concentration, 10–15 mg/mL) and bovine thrombin (1,000 IU/mL) in the second syringe. This preparation contains a lower concentration of fibrinogen and has not undergone viral inactivation. Furthermore, the bovine thrombin may be contaminated with bovine factor V, which can stimulate production of antibodies in the recipient which cross react with human factor V, inducing a potentially severe bleeding disorder several days after surgery (13–15). Currently, the bovine thrombin preparation with the lowest degree of contamination with factor V is that produced for Jones Pharma Incorporated (St. Louis, MO, U.S.A.) (16).

Although randomized, blinded studies have not been done, fibrin sealant has been applied to sites of dental extractions in individuals with hemophilia; this treatment, combined with the use of an antifibrinolytic agent, has reduced or eliminated the need for systemic factor VIII replacement (17,18). This combined therapy is potentially efficacious in patients with coagulation factor inhibitors as well as those with severe thrombocytopenia who require dental extraction. The sealants potentially could be used outside the operating room to provide local hemostasis in the critical care setting in patients with coagulopathies attributable to uremia and who have a localized site of bleeding.

Common Inherited Bleeding Disorders

Patients with von Willebrand disease (vWD), which is the most common of the inherited bleeding disorders, can be treated with DDAVP at an intravenous dose of 0.3 μg per kilogram of body weight or by intranasal spray (at a tenfold higher dose) to increase the concentration of vWF before a surgical procedure or if minor bleeding is occurring (19). If more sustained levels of vWF are required, patients can undergo infusion with virally inactivated intermediate-purity factor VIII concentrates that contain functional vWF (either Humate-P, Aventis Behring, Kankakee, IL, U.S.A. or Alphanate, Alpha Therapeutic, Los Angeles, CA, U.S.A.). Thus, cryoprecipitate is no longer used for patients with vWD. For patients with hemophilia A or hemophilia B, recombinant products are available. The consultation of a hematologist should be sought for treatment of patients who have bleeding disorders such as vWD or hemophilia.

Bleeding Associated with Liver Disease

Patients with liver disease may have a complex coagulopathy consisting of impaired coagulation factor synthesis, increased fibrinolytic activity, and thrombocytopenia (20). In patients with splenomegaly due to cirrhosis and portal hypertension, 90% of the circulating platelets can be sequestered in the spleen with platelet counts decreasing to as low as 30,000/μL. A further reduction in platelet counts is usually due to additional factors such as coexisting immune thrombocytopenia (20). Patients may have an acquired dysfibrinogenemia, which is due to the synthesis of a fibrinogen molecule that has impaired polymerization because of an increased sialic acid content (21). The fibrinogen levels are usually normal; however the PT, aPTT, and thrombin time are prolonged. The acquired dysfibrinogenemia is not associated with a bleeding diathesis, and patients with this abnormality do not need any treatment before invasive procedures.

The assessment of bleeding risk in a patient with liver disease includes measurement of the platelet count, PT, aPTT, fibrinogen level, and D-dimer. Liver disease is associated with hyperfibrinolysis as defined by increased activity of tissue plasminogen (tPA) and elevation of D-dimer. Although measurement of tPA or the euglobulin clot lysis time is desirable, these tests are usually not available in a hospital setting. The PT is also reported as an international normalized ratio (INR), which originally was developed to standardize anticoagulation among patients taking warfarin. INRs are not well standardized for patients with liver disease and can vary depending on the reagent. This is also true for the measurement of the PT with the different reagents. Patients with liver disease may have only a prolonged PT (normal aPTT and thrombin time), reflecting a decrease in factor VII, which is the first to be reduced in liver disorders, because of its short half-life of 2 to 6 hours.

Guidelines for prophylaxis in patients with liver disease who are undergoing invasive procedures are summarized in Table 9.2. These suggestions are empiric and are based on

TABLE 9.2. MANAGEMENT OF PATIENTS WITH LIVER DISEASE

Prophylaxis before procedures	
Platelet count	
<50,000/μL	Administer platelets to increase to 50–75,000/μL
Fibrinogen	
<100 mg/dL	Administer cryoprecipitate to maintain fibrinogen >100 mg/dL
Prolonged PT and aPTT	Vitamin K, 10 mg daily subcut for 3 d, then FFP if factor VII <10% or other factors <50%
Prolonged PT, nl aPTT	Give only vitamin K if factor VII is >10%
Prolonged thrombin time	No treatment if fibrinogen >100 mg/dL

PT, prothrombin time; a PTT, activated partial thromboplastin time; FFP, fresh frozen plasma; Prothrombin complex concentrates and epsilon aminocaproic acid are not recommended since they may increase the risk for thrombosis. DDAVP (desmopressin) can be used to shorten the bleeding time, but its clinical significance in reducing bleeding in patients with liver disease has not been demonstrated.

many factors as described subsequently herein. In a retrospective study of patients undergoing percutaneous liver biopsy, McVay and Toy found that mild elevations of the PT or aPTT were not associated with bleeding or with platelet counts greater than 50,000 per microliter (22). Risks for bleeding were malignancy (hepatoma) and multiple passes. These investigators concluded that patients with liver disease who have a PT and aPTT that are prolonged to less than 1.5 times the midnormal range do not require treatment with plasma infusions and that a platelet count of greater than 50,000 per microliter is satisfactory. Controlled studies in patients with cirrhosis have shown that desmopressin at a dose of 0.3 μg per kilogram of body weight significantly shortens the prolonged bleeding time for up to 4 hours; however, these patients did not have renal disease as well. Nonetheless, DDAVP is an effective therapy for uremia and also has been shown to be active, as assessed by shortening of the bleeding time, in the setting of liver disease as well. It is an obvious choice for a hemostatic agent if there are concerns about the platelet function (23,24).

For patients in whom standard percutaneous biopsy is contraindicated, such as those who have ascites, portal hypertension, and also a coagulopathy, laparoscopic liver biopsy can be successfully performed using direct pressure and topical Gelfoam and thrombin to achieve hemostasis (25). In these patients, there appears to be no correlation between the risk of bleeding and the prophylactic administration of fresh frozen plasma (FFP) or platelets. The advantage of laparoscopic liver biopsy technique is the ability to place direct pressure along with hemostatic agents.

There is usually little or no need to infuse FFP in a patient who has only a prolonged PT and normal aPTT because factor VII levels of 10% or greater are sufficient for hemostasis. If the PT and aPTT are prolonged and the patient has not responded to empiric treatment with vitamin K at a dose of 10 mg per day subcutaneously for 3 days (20), measurement of factor levels IX, X, and V (a non–vitamin K dependent factor) provides a good assessment of liver function with respect to synthesis of coagulation factors. On occasion, abnormalities are simply due to dysfibrinogen, which can be detected by a prolonged thrombin time and reptilase time. If the latter is the case, then no plasma treatment is needed (26). Preoperative replacement for patients with severe factor VII deficiency consists of infusion of plasma at a dose of 5 to 10 mL per kilogram beginning preoperatively (in time to achieve a level of 10%) and continued during and after surgery for at least 1 to 2 days.

For patients who have hemostatic defects and are bleeding or are to undergo a major procedure, the goal of therapy is to maintain the platelet count greater than 50,000 to 75,000 per microliter and the fibrinogen concentration greater than 100 mg/dL. This is achieved by infusion of cryoprecipitate. The quantity of fibrinogen in each bag of cryoprecipitate is approximately 250 mg and the volume of distribution for the fibrinogen is 30% greater than the intravascular volume. Thus, to increase the fibrinogen level by 50 mg per deciliter in a 70-kg patient, seven bags of cryoprecipitate would be required.

For patients undergoing rapid blood loss, recombinant factor VIIa (NovoSeven, NovoNordisk, Princeton, NJ, U.S.A.), which has just been approved for use in hemophiliacs with inhibitors, can be combined with FFP. In one preliminary study, factor VIIa was effective in transiently reversing the prolonged PT in a group of nonbleeding cirrhotic patients (27). It is expensive, however, and has not been tried in a larger clinical trial. Prothrombin complex concentrates and antifibrinolytic agents such as epsilon aminocaproic acid are not recommended because they may be associated with thrombosis (20). The bovine protein aprotinin, which is an inhibitor of plasmin, has been shown to reduce blood loss in the setting of orthotopic liver transplantation (28).

Disseminated Intravascular Coagulation

Disseminated intravascular coagulation (DIC) is associated with clinical conditions such as sepsis, acute brain injury, or abruption placentae, that induce expression of tissue factor and overwhelming activation of the coagulation system with a resulting fibrinolytic response. The clinical manifestations of DIC are variable and depend on whether microvascular thrombosis with fibrin formation is the prominent feature or if the major component is the fibrinolytic response to fibrin formation (29,30). The laboratory evaluation of DIC includes measurement of the platelet count, PT, aPTT, D-dimer, and examination of the peripheral blood smear for schistocytes. Abnormalities in any one of these tests are not specific for DIC. Rather, the test results are combined with the clinical setting to make a diagnosis. Treatment should be directed at the underlying cause of the DIC (e.g., sepsis, leukemia).

Coagulopathies due to Anticoagulants

Warfarin

The frequency of bleeding for patients who are receiving warfarin ranges from 8 to16 per hundred patient-years, with major bleeding occurring in 1.3 to 2.7 patients per hundred years (31). The main strategies for treating warfarin overdose, based on the degree of over anticoagulation and the clinical site of bleeding, include administration of vitamin K, prothrombin complex concentrates (PCCs), possibly recombinant factor VIIa, or FFP (Table 9.3). PCCs, which contain factors II, VII, and X in addition to factor IX and are virally inactivated, are efficacious in persons who have a major bleed and are anticoagulated with warfarin (32). The potential side effect in using the concentrates is unwanted thrombosis.

About 50% to 90% of intracranial hemorrhages in patients anticoagulated with warfarin occur at a time when the INR is within the target range (33). The mortality from an intracranial bleed is 16% to 68% and is influenced by the ra-

TABLE 9.3. GUIDELINES FOR REVERSAL OF WARFARIN ANTICOAGULATION

Major bleeding (INR >2)	Stop warfarin
	Infuse PCC[a] (50 U/kg) or FFP (15 mL/kg)
	Give vitamin K 5 mg (s.c.)
INR 6–8 (With no or minor bleeding)	Stop warfarin
	Restart with INR <3
	Give 1.0–2.5 mg vitamin K orally if reversal within 24–48 h needed
INR >8 (With no or minor bleeding)	Stop warfarin
	Restart warfarin when INR <3
	Give 3–5 mg vitamin K orally if reversal within 24–48 h needed

INR, international normalized ratio; PCC, prothrombin complex concentrate; FFP, fresh frozen plasma; s.c., subcutaneous (original guidelines recommend i.v. but this is usually not necessary).
[a] The efficacy of recombinant factor VIIa in treatment of patients with warfarin overdose and major bleeding is under investigation.

pidity with which normalization of the coagulation factor deficiencies occur. The preferred replacement therapy in intracranial hemorrhage is PCCs (25–50 U/kg). When this dose was compared with infusion of 800 mL of FFP in a small study of patients with intracranial hemorrhage who also were anticoagulated with warfarin, the coagulation factor levels were raised into normal range with the PCCs but not with FFP. Correction of the INR can be achieved four to five times more quickly with the PCCs than with FFP. The elimination half-lives of the coagulation factors are as follows: II (58 hours), VII (5 hours), IX (19 hours), and X (35 hours); thus, repeat infusion may be necessary if the factor deficiency has not been reversed by the administration of vitamin K in 24 hours. Factor VII is in very low concentration in some PCCs relative to the other coagulation factors, and it has a very short half-life. The importance of replacing the factor VII level to values less than 10% is unknown. FFP can be used to achieve minimal levels of 10% if this is deemed necessary. Recombinant factor VIIa is also undergoing study in this setting.

Unfractionated Heparin and Low-Molecular-Weight Heparin

Unfractionated heparin does not require dose-adjustment when used in patients on dialysis. Reversal of anticoagulant activity can be achieved by slow infusion (over 10 minutes) of protamine sulfate, which will neutralize 100 U of heparin for every milligram of protamine administered. Assuming that heparin has a half-life of 60 minutes, the protamine dose could be calculated by adding the heparin dose infused in the last hour to 50% of the dose in the previous hour and 25% of the dose infused three hours earlier (34). The risk for anaphylaxis with protamine sulfate is approximately 1% and may be higher in diabetics who have taken neutral protamine Hagedorn (NPH) insulin.

Protamine does not neutralize the anti-factor Xa activity of LMW heparin, and at present there is no satisfactory neutralizing agent for this form of heparin (35). LMW heparin is cleared principally by the renal route and therefore has a prolonged half-life in patients with renal impairment (36). Randomized trials of LMW heparin have not included patients with renal failure, and therefore the pharmacokinetics of the drug in this patient population has not been well established. According to one report in which a single dose of enoxaparin (40 mg) was administered to patients with renal insufficiency, the half-life was prolonged 1.7 times above that of the volunteers with normal renal function (37). Therefore, if LMW heparin is to be used in patients with renal failure, periodic monitoring with anti-factor Xa assays is recommended. (36). LMW heparin, when administered subcutaneously, has a plasma half-life of 3 to 6 hours in normal subjects.

In persons with normal renal function who are receiving prophylactic LMW heparin, published guidelines have emphasized that placement for epidural or spinal anesthesia should occur no sooner than 12 hours after the last dose (38–40). Subsequent dosing should be delayed for at least 2 hours after needle placement. Epidural catheters should be removed 12 to 24 hours after the last LMW heparin dose, with subsequent dosing delayed by at least 3 hours (38,39). These time spans probably should be doubled (combined with monitoring the antifactor Xa activity) in patients with renal failure who are to undergo invasive procedures. In addition, enoxaparin should be used whenever possible as a once-daily dose (40), and other antiplatelet agents or anticoagulant agents should not be administered at the same time.

Use of Argatroban, Hirudin, and Danaparoid in the Treatment of Heparin-induced Thrombocytopenia

Three agents are now available for the treatment of established or suspected heparin-induced thrombocytopenia (HIT); they are danaparoid and the two thrombin-specific inhibitors known as argatroban and lepirudin. Argatroban is the only agent that is not cleared through the kidneys and therefore does not need dose adjustment in patients with renal disease. The thrombin-specific inhibitors, unlike unfractionated heparin, prolong the PT as well as the aPTT. If patients are undergoing conversion to warfarin while receiving argatroban or hirudin, the agents can be discontinued several hours before a PT is drawn to ensure an accurate indication of the INR. Clinical experience with these agents in critically ill patients who are receiving multiple other drugs as well as anesthetic agents is limited and is not well described in the literature. Thus, dosing in critically ill patients should be established with caution. The agents are described in greater detail in the following sections.

Argatroban (GlaxoSmithKline, Research Triangle Park, NC, U.S.A.) has a half-life of 40 minutes in normal subjects. Argatroban, which is cleared by the liver, requires dose reduction in patients with significant hepatic dysfunction (Table 9.4). It is administered on weight-based dosing and is monitored with the aPTT with the goal of maintaining the aPTT at 1.5 to 3 times the baseline value. Argatroban has been used successfully in one patient with HIT who required repeated dialysis (41) and in a patient with HIT and thrombosis who required coronary stent implantation (42).

Lepirudin (Refludan, Aventis Pharmaceuticals, Parsippany, NJ, U.S.A.), which is a recombinant protein, is approved for use in patients with HIT and associated thrombosis to prevent further complications (Table 9.4). It is similar to the 65 amino acid natural thrombin inhibitor known as hirudin. For patients with normal renal function, current dosing recommendations are for 0.4 mg per kilogram of body weight as a bolus with 0.15 mg per kilogram hourly (up to a weight of 110 kg). The dose can be monitored with the aPTT; recommendations are to maintain the aPTT at 1.5 to 2.5 times the median value for the normal range. In normal volunteers, lepirudin, which is excreted and also perhaps metabolized by the kidneys, has a half-life of approximately 2 hours. Pharmacokinetic studies in patients with renal failure who were undergoing dialysis showed that

TABLE 9.4. PROPERTIES OF ANTICOAGULANTS USED IN PATIENTS WITH HEPARIN-INDUCED THROMBOCYTOPENIA

Property	Danaparoid	Argatroban	Lepirudin
Composition	Dermatan sulfate, heparin sulfate, chondroitin sulfate	Synthetic arginine analog	Recombinant protein
Molecular wt	6,000	506	6,979
Action	Inhibits factor Xa and thrombin through AT-III	Direct thrombin inhibitor	Direct thrombin inhibitor
Half-life	22 h	40 min	1.5 h (terminal)
Monitoring	None or anti factor Xa assay	APTT	APTT
Effect of PT	None	Prolongation	Prolongation
Neutralization	None	None	None
Excretion	Renal	Liver	Renal
Caution	Prolonged half-life in renal disease	Prolonged half-life in liver disease	Prolonged half-life in renal disease

MW, molecular weight; AT-III, antithrombin III; APTT, activated partial thromboplastin time; PT, prothrombin time.

after a single dose of lepirudin (0.08–0.2 mg/kg) followed by five additional dialyses without further dosing, the half-life was increased to 52 hours) (43). The distribution volume was also lower in hemodialysis patients than for normal volunteers. Lepirudin has been used successfully to maintain anticoagulation during dialysis when given one time before dialysis at a dose of 0.08 mg per kilogram (44). Subsequent dosing, however, would need adjustment because of the prolonged half-life. The manufacturer recommends that dosing be reduced by 50% for both bolus and infusion for patients with a creatinine of 1.5 to 2.0 mg per deciliter. Reductions would be even greater for more severe renal impairment.

Danaparoid (Orgaran, Organon, Inc., West Orange, NJ, U.S.A.) is a LMW heparinoid composed of heparan sulfate, dermatan sulfate, and chondroitin sulfate (45). The U.S. Food and Drug Administration (FDA)–approved indication for danaparoid is prophylaxis of venous thromboembolism, usually at a dose of 750 anti-factor Xa units twice daily administered subcutaneously (46). It is used primarily in patients suspected of having HIT. Danaparoid has an anti-factor Xa–antifactor II activity of 28:1 (compared with a 1:1 ratio for heparin). Thus, it cannot be neutralized by protamine. The elimination half-life of the anti-factor Xa activity is 24 hours and that of the minor component of anti-factor factor II is approximately 4 hours (Table 9.4) (45). The steady state of anti-factor Xa activity is reached after 4 to 5 days of dosing. Because about 40% to 50% of the plasma clearance is by the renal route, after an initial dose in patients with real insufficiency, subsequent doses should be reduced. Danaparoid can be monitored by its anti-factor Xa activity; however, the assay for the anti Xa activity should contain danaparoid as the standard.

Danaparoid has been used in many different clinical settings with adjustment of the dose. For example, danaparoid has been used as a continuous infusion in patients undergoing hemofiltration with an initial bolus of 2,500 U followed by a dose of 200 to 600 U per hour (47). Even lower doses, however, such as 50 to 100 U per hour, may be safer in the critically ill patient. Danaparoid also has been used at a dose of 3,750 U for patients undergoing hemodialysis (47). Ideally, if danaparoid is to be used at doses higher than those used for prophylaxis in the intensive care setting, assays should be readily available for monitoring anticoagulation, and the lowest effective dose should be used to reduce the risk for bleeding. Furthermore, a minimum of 24 hours should be allowed between the last dose and a planned invasive procedure.

Bleeding Induced by Antiplatelet Agents

Agents Directed against the Platelet GPIIb/IIIa Receptor (Abciximab, Tirofiban, and Eptifibatide)

The most potent antiplatelet agents in clinical practice today are those that block the interaction between fibrinogen and platelet GPIIb/IIIa, thus mimicking the bleeding diathesis seen in patients with Glanzmann thrombasthenia. Abciximab (ReoPro, Centocor, Malvern, PA, U.S.A.) is an Fab frag-

ment of chimeric human-murine monoclonal antibody c7E3, which is used in patients undergoing percutaneous transluminal angioplasty (PTCA) and unstable angina with PTCA planned in 24 hours (48). Two newer GPIIb/IIIa inhibitors include tirofiban (Aggrastat, Merck & Co. Inc., West Point, PA, U.S.A.), a nonpeptide tyrosine derivative that is indicated for patients with unstable angina/non–Q-wave myocardial infarction (with or without PTCA), and eptifibatide (Integrilin, COR Therapeutics, Inc., South San Francisco, CA, U.S.A.), a cyclic heptapeptide that is indicated for patients with unstable angina/non–Q-wave myocardial infarction (with or without PTCA) and for patients undergoing PTCA (49).

The risk for bleeding with these agents is due in part to their pharmacokinetics. Abciximab, which has a high affinity for GPIIb/IIIa, has a biologic half-life of 8 hours; by comparison, after completion of the infusion of eptifibatide, the bleeding time normalizes within 1 hour (50). The antiplatelet effect of tirofiban is also short-lived after completion of infusion, although in patients with renal failure, the biologic effect is more prolonged. Platelet function is inhibited when more than 80% of the GPIIb/IIIa receptors are blocked. For patients who are bleeding, the drugs should be discontinued immediately and 8 to 10 U of platelets administered. The drug will redistribute to the receptors of the infused platelets, thus lowering the degree of occupancy of the receptors of the entire platelet pool and causing normalization of platelet function. In patients who have received abciximab within 12 hours of requiring an emergent bypass procedure, platelet infusions should be administered prophylactically to prevent excessive bleeding (51). The recommendation for preoperative platelet infusions probably does not apply for tirofiban or eptifibatide because of their shorter duration of action.

All the agents that interact with the GPIIb/IIIa receptor have been associated with induction of thrombocytopenia, with the incidence ranging from 1% to 5.6% in published reports (52). The mechanism may be that the binding of the agents to the receptors induces exposure of an epitope that can be recognized by preexisting anti GPIIb/IIIa antibodies. Berkowitz and colleagues developed an algorithm and recommendations for evaluation and treatment of thrombocytopenia (52,53). They recommend monitoring the platelet count within 2 to 4 hours of starting treatment; if thrombocytopenia is found, a pseudothrombocytopenia needs to be ruled out by examination of the peripheral smear. The drug should be discontinued (although aspirin can be continued), and platelet infusions should be given for platelet counts below 20,000 per microliter to decrease the risk for intracranial hemorrhage or other major bleeds.

Agents Directed against the Platelet Adenosine Diphosphate Receptor (Clopidogrel and Ticlopidine)

The thienopyridines ticlopidine and clopidogrel inhibit platelet function by blocking the adenosine diphosphate (ADP) receptor (54). Adverse events in patients receiving ticlopidine have included neutropenia, agranulocytosis, aplastic anemia, and thrombotic thrombocytopenic purpura (TTP) and have resulted in diminished use (55). In contrast, clopidogrel appears to have a more acceptable safety profile, although cases of TTP have been reported for this drug as well. Clopidogrel is indicated for the reduction in atherosclerotic events (myocardial infarction, stroke, and vascular death) in patients with atherosclerosis documented by recent stroke, myocardial infarction, or peripheral vascular disease.

Both clopidogrel and ticlopidine require metabolism by the hepatic cytochrome P450-1A enzyme system to acquire activity (54). When clopidogrel is given at a dose of 300 to 400 mg orally, it causes maximal inhibition of platelet function within 2 hours (56). With a daily dose of 75 mg, this same degree of inhibition is achieved at 3 to 7 days. Recovery of platelet function occurs over 3 to 5 days after discontinuation of either drug. Specific treatment for bleeding due to these agents is not well described. Administration of DDAVP, however, may shorten the bleeding time and provide temporary hemostasis (57). Otherwise, supportive care and infusion of platelets might be needed in patients who are taking clopidogrel or ticlopidine and have a major bleeding episode.

ASSESSMENT AND TREATMENT OF DISORDERS THAT PROMOTE VENOUS OR ARTERIAL THROMBOSIS

Inherited Disorders

Acquired and inherited hypercoagulable disorders may be suspected in dialysis patients who have a past history of venous thromboembolism or arterial thrombosis. Documentation of these disorders may be helpful in determining the best way to approach patients who are to undergo invasive procedures or kidney transplantation. The disorders that are often considered and that can be documented only by specialized laboratory testing are listed in Table 9.5. Inheri-

tance of an abnormal factor V (known as factor V Leiden), which is relatively resistant to inhibition by activated protein C, is also known as resistance to activated protein C. The resistance to inhibition of factor Va is due to a single amino acid change in factor V (arginine to glutamine at position 506) (58–60). The risk for venous thrombosis is also increased in patients who have the mutation in the prothrombin gene (a guanine to adenine change in the base 20,210, which is in the 3′-untranslated region of the prothrombin gene (61–63). This mutation results in elevated levels of prothrombin and is associated with a threefold increase in the risk for venous thrombosis. In prospective studies, factor V Leiden is the most common of the inherited disorders, accounting for 14% of cases of inherited thrombophilia in white populations (62). The prothrombin gene mutation may be second in frequency.

The most common presentation of patients with inherited thrombophilia is deep venous thrombosis, usually of the lower extremities, although patients may have recurrent episodes of superficial phlebitis. In symptomatic patients, those with deficiencies of protein C, protein S, or antithrombin III (AT III) tend to develop their first thrombosis at a younger age compared to those with factor V Leiden. For example, 60% to 80% of patients deficient in protein C, protein S, and AT III who develop thrombosis will do so before the age of 45 years, and approximately half of these will recur if appropriate anticoagulation is not provided (64). Approximately half of the episodes of venous thrombosis occur when patients are at increased risk for thrombosis from additional factors, such as surgery or pregnancy (65). Arterial thrombosis is rare in patients with deficiency of AT III, protein S or protein C, or factor V Leiden. All the inherited disorders are transmitted in an autosomal dominant fashion.

Testing for patients with thrombosis can be based on whether or not the thrombotic event was arterial or venous and by the age at which the patient first became symptomatic. Thus, patients who were younger than 45 years of

TABLE 9.5. APPROACH TO LABORATORY TESTING FOR HYPERCOAGULABILITY

Venous thromboembolism Patient <45 yr with first episode	Patient >45 yr for first episode and has no family history
1. Factor V Leiden (DNA test)	1. Factor V Leiden
2. Prothrombin gene mutation (DNA test)	2. Prothrombin gene mutation (DNA test)
3. Antithrombin III deficiency	3. Homocysteine level
4. Protein C deficiency	4. Lupus anticoagulant
5. Protein S deficiency	5. Anticardiolipin antibody
6. Homocysteine level	
7. Lupus anticoagulant	
8. Anticardiolipin antibody	
Arterial thrombosis	
Homocysteine level	
Lupus anticoagulant	
Anticardiolipin antibody	

age at the time of the first thrombosis would undergo testing as listed in Table 9.5. Factor V Leiden is much less common in African Americans (1% incidence) than in whites (5%) (66); the prothrombin gene mutation is present in 1% to 2% of whites and African Americans. It is possible that these abnormalities can be present in any patient with hypercoagulability; therefore, testing probably should not be based on ethnicity.

The treatment for acute thrombosis in patients with a hereditary clotting disorder is the same as for patients in a similar situation without this condition. Patients receive intravenous heparin (preferably according to a weight-based nomogram) to achieve an aPTT that correlates with an antifactor Xa activity of 0.3 to 0.7 U per milliliter. This should be standardized with the aPTT reagents used for each hospital. Warfarin is started when the heparin levels are therapeutic and is monitored with INR maintained between 2 and 3 if the patient has no evidence for antiphospholipid syndrome. LMW heparin also may be satisfactory for such patients, although they have been excluded from many of the trials of the use of outpatient LMW heparin. Frequently, such patients are treated with LMW heparin because the diagnosis of an underlying hypercoagulable state has not been made. Patients who have had more than one thrombosis probably should receive life-long anticoagulation if the benefits outweigh the risk. Such decisions need to be made on an individual basis.

Acquired Disorders

Hyperhomocysteinemia in Dialysis Patients

Hyperhomocysteinemia, which is common in dialysis patients, is associated with an increased risk for venous thrombosis, stroke, myocardial infarction, and peripheral arterial disease (67–70). Nygard and colleagues (70) found that in nondialysis patients with established coronary artery disease, fasting homocysteine levels were predictors of mortality. The relationship between plasma homocysteine levels and cardiovascular death was linear between 5 to 20 μM, with the slope increasing at 15 μM. The tendency for hyperhomocystinemia may be inherited or may be acquired (i.e., dietary deficiency of folate) or renal failure (71).

According to one study, elevated homocysteine levels confer a graded independent risk for thrombosis of hemodialysis access (fistula or graft) (72). This has not been confirmed by any other study, however (73). Lowering of homocysteine levels is not easily achieved in dialysis patients. Administration of folate at a daily dose of 5 mg does not appear to reduce homocysteine levels in this population (74). In one 12-week study, 39 dialysis patients who had homocysteine levels ranging from 14.4 to 24.9 μM received daily doses of folic acid (15 mg) or an equivalent amount of reduced folate as well as vitamin B_6 (50 mg) and B_{12} (1 mg) (75). At the end of the study, only two of 39 had achieved homocysteine levels below 12μM. In another study, 37 patients undergoing hemodialysis received intravenous folinic acid (50 mg weekly) and intravenous pyridoxine (250 mg three times weekly) for 11 months (range, 7–17 months) (76). Mean pretreatment homocysteine levels were 37 μM; at the end of the study, 78% of the patients had homocysteine levels that were <14 μM. No adverse effects of the treatment were reported. Although this latter report is promising, the best therapy for lowering homocysteine levels in hemodialysis patients has not been established.

Antiphospholipid Syndrome

Patients with the antiphospholipid syndrome may have venous thrombosis, arterial thrombosis (stroke, myocardial infarction, gangrene), recurrent pregnancy loss, or thrombocytopenia (Table 9.6) (77–79). The diagnosis of antiphospholipid syndrome is substantiated in such patients if they test positive for antiphospholipid–protein antibodies (APA), known also as antiphospholipid antibodies. Immunoglobulin G (IgG), IgM, or IgA antibodies are directed against a complex of phospholipid with a protein such as prothrombin or β2-glycoprotein I (β2-GPI) (80–82). APA can be detected as lupus anticoagulants (LA) in a clotting assay or in an immune-based assay (enzyme-linked immunosorbent assay, or ELISA). For the antiphospholipid syndrome to be confirmed in a patient with the appropriate symptoms, one or both of the tests for APA should be positive when performed on two separate occasions at least six weeks apart (83).

Major issues in the management of patients with the antiphospholipid syndrome and thrombosis are the intensity of anticoagulation that should be given, the duration of an-

TABLE 9.6. MAJOR FEATURES OF THE ANTIPHOSPHOLIPID SYNDROME

Clinical
  Venous thromboembolism
    Deep venous thrombosis
    Pulmonary embolism
  Arterial thromboses
    Myocardial infarction
    Neurologic (vascular dementia, cerebral infarction, transient ischemic attack, amaurosis fugax, retinal vessel infarction)
  Recurrent fetal loss
Laboratory
  Thrombocytopenia
  Moderate to high positive titer of anticardiolipin antibodies (IgG or IgM) or positive lupus anticoagulant on two occasions (6 weeks apart)[a]

IgG, immunoglobulin G; IgM, immunoglobulin M.
[a] Antiphospholipid-protein antibodies (APA) or formerly antiphospholipid antibodies: Antibodies of the IgG, IgM, or IgA isotype directed against phospholipid-binding proteins such as prothrombin or β_2-glycoprotein I (β_2-GPI). When measured by an enzyme-linked immunosorbent assay (ELISA), the antibodies are called *anticardiolipin antibodies* because assays contain the phospholipid cardiolipin (the phospholipid to which β_2-GP I binds). If the antibodies are detected in a phospholipid-dependent clotting assay, they are described as *lupus anticoagulants.*

ticoagulation, and the appropriate monitoring. One goal is to reduce other risk factors for thrombosis, such as uncontrolled hypertension, smoking, and use of oral contraceptives (84). Treatment of asymptomatic patients with LA or with moderate or high titers of ACA is controversial. Some physicians will prescribe low-dose aspirin (81 mg/day) and then use anticoagulation with warfarin or heparin at times of increased risk for thrombosis (84).

Patients with the antiphospholipid syndrome and venous thromboembolism are at high risk for recurrence if anticoagulation is discontinued after a first episode of venous thrombosis (85–87). The rate of recurrence is highest in the first 6 months after discontinuation of anticoagulation (86). In one study, continuation of warfarin (INR 2.5–4.0) resulted in 100% freedom from thrombosis during an 8-year follow-up period (86).

The intensity of anticoagulation required may depend on whether or not the patient has underlying systemic lupus erythematosus (SLE); however, this issue has not been resolved. In the meantime, for patients with antiphospholipid syndrome and thrombosis who are receiving warfarin, an INR of 2 to 3, with an attempt to maintain the INR nearer to 3, is recommended if there are no contraindications; furthermore, anticoagulation should be continued on an indefinite basis as long as the risks of bleeding are lower than the risk of thrombosis (88,89). Low-dose aspirin may be added, depending on the whether thrombotic manifestations such as superficial thrombophlebitis persist.

The role of corticosteroids or plasmapheresis has not been documented for patients with the antiphospholipid syndrome. These treatments are reserved for patients with a "catastrophic antiphospholipid syndrome," defined as acute multiorgan failure in patients with antiphospholipid antibodies (90). In this rare syndrome, mortality is 60%; plasmapheresis may be beneficial in patients who have not responded to heparin, corticosteroids, or immunosuppressive agents (90).

Rarely, the antiphospholipid syndrome can be associated with a bleeding diathesis resulting from the association with antiprothrombin antibodies that induce severe prothrombin deficiency by causing increased clearance of the protein. The antibody against prothrombin can develop anytime during the clinical course of a patient with the antiphospholipid syndrome. If a patient is receiving warfarin and the INR becomes progressively prolonged, development of a prothrombin-neutralizing antibody should be considered. This can be determined by measurement of the factor II activity, which then can be compared with the activity of the other vitamin K dependent factors, such as factor X or factor IX. The antibody production usually can be easily suppressed by the administration of corticosteroids and azathioprine, as was demonstrated in one patient in whom the PT was normal 7 days after initiation of treatment (91). If a patient is actively bleeding, treatment with FFP or PCC, or possibly recombinant factor VIIa, may be required.

SUMMARY

In general, for patients who present with arterial thrombosis, included in the evaluation should be measurement of fasting homocysteine levels and testing for LA and anticardiolipin antibody. In addition, more extensive testing for lipid disorders and vascular abnormalities should be undertaken, based on the patient's family and personal history. Acquired causes of thrombosis, such as malignancy and myeloproliferative syndromes such as polycythemia vera, should be excluded. When an initial evaluation is being performed, testing for all the appropriate potential abnormalities, based on the preceding outline, is recommended because patients with more than one risk factor have a greatly increased chance for recurrent thrombosis (65). Furthermore, some of these risks can be altered by medications other than warfarin (i.e., treatment for hyperhomocysteinemia).

REFERENCES

1. Steiner RW, Coggins SC, Carvalho ACA. Bleeding time in uremia: a useful test to assess clinical bleeding. *Am J Hematol* 1979; 7:107–117.
2. Noris M, Remuzzi G. Uremic bleeding: closing the circle after thirty years of controversies. *Blood* 1999;94:2569–2574.
3. Sreedhara R, Itagaki I, Hakim RM. Uremic patients have decreased shear-induced platelet aggregation mediated by decreased availability of glycoprotein IIb-IIIa receptors. *Am J Kidney Dis* 1996;27:355–364.
4. Zachee P, Vermylen J, Boogaerts MA. Hematologic aspects of end-stage renal failure. *Ann Hematol* 1994;69:33–40.
5. Rabelink TJ, Zwaginga JJ, Koomans HA, et al. Thrombosis and hemostasis in renal disease. *Kidney Int* 1994;46:287–296.
6. Bolan CD, Alving BM. Pharmacologic agents in the management of bleeding disorders. *Transfusion* 1990;30:541–551.
7. Mannucci PM. Desmopression (DDAVP) in the treatment of bleeding disorders: the first 20 years. *Blood* 1997;90:2515–2521.
8. Livio M, Mannucci PM, Vigano G, et al. Conjugated estrogens for the management of bleeding associated with renal failure. *N Engl J Med* 1986;315:731–735.
9. Sloand JA, Schiff MS. Beneficial effect of low-dose transdermal estrogen on bleeding time and clinical bleeding in uremia. *Am J Kidney Dis* 1995;26:22–26.
10. Vigano G, Gaspari F, Locatelli M, et al. Dose-effect and pharmacokinetics of estrogens given to correct bleeding time in uremia. *Kidney Int* 1988;34:853–858.
11. DeLoughery TG, Liebler JM, Simonds V, et al. Invasive line placement in critically ill patients: do hemostatic defects matter. *Transfusion* 1996;36:827–831.
12. Alving BA, Weinstein MJ, Finlayson JS, et al. Fibrin sealant: summary of a conference on characteristics and clinical uses. *Transfusion* 1995;35:783–790.
13. Rapaport SI, Zivelin A, Minow RA, et al. Clinical significance of antibodies to bovine and human thrombin and factor V after surgical use of bovine thrombin. *Am J Clin Pathol* 1992;97:84–91.
14. Zehnder JL, Leung LK. Development of antibodies to thrombin and factor V with recurrent bleeding in a patient exposed to topical bovine thrombin. *Blood* 1990;76: 2011–2016.
15. Ortel TL, Charles LA, Keller FG, et al. Topical thrombin and acquired factor coagulation inhibitors: clinical spectrum and laboratory diagnosis. *Am J Hematol* 1994;45:128–135.

16. Christie RJ, Carrington L, Alving BA. Postoperative bleeding induced by topical bovine thrombin: report of two cases. *Surgery* 1997;121:708–710

17. Martinowitz U, Schulman S. Fibrin sealant in surgery of patients with hemorrhagic diathesis. *Thromb Haemost* 1995;74:486–492.

18. Rakocz M, Mazar A, Varon D, et al. Dental extractions in patients with bleeding disorders: the use of fibrin glue. *Oral Surg Oral Med Oral Pathol* 1993;75:280–282.

19. Scott JP, Montgomery RR. Therapy of von Willebrand disease. *Semin Thromb Hemost* 1993;19:37–47.

20. Martinez J, Barsigian C. Coagulopathy of liver failure and vitamin K deficiency. In: Loscalzo J, Schafer AL, eds. *Thrombosis and hemorrhage*, 2nd ed. Philadelphia: Williams & Wilkins, 1998: 987–1004.

21. Gralnick HR, Givelber H, Abrams E. Dysfibrinogenemia associated with hepatoma: increased carbohydrate content of the fibrinogen molecule. *N Engl J Med* 1978;299:221–226.

22. McVay PA, Toy PTCY. Lack of increased bleeding after liver biopsy in patients with mild hemostatic abnormalities. *Am J Clin Pathol* 1990;94:747–753.

23. Mannucci PM, Vicento V, Vianello L, et al. Controlled trial of desmopressin in liver cirrhosis and other conditions associated with a prolonged bleeding time. *Blood* 1986;67:1148–1153.

24. Burroughs AK, Matthews K, Qadiri M, et al. Desmopressin and bleeding time in patients with cirrhosis. *BMJ* 1985;291:1377–1381.

25. Inabet WB, Deziel DJ. Laparoscopic liver biopsy in patients with coagulopathy, portal hypertension, and ascites. *Am Surg* 1995;61:603–606.

26. Dawson NA, Barr CF, Alving BM. Acquired dysfibrinogenemia: paraneoplastic syndrome in renal cell carcinoma. *Am J Med* 1985;78:682–686.

27. Bernstein DE, Jeffers L, Erhardtsen E, et al. Recombinant factor VIIa corrects prothrombin time in cirrhotic patients: a preliminary study. *Gastroenterology* 1997;113:1930–1937.

28. Porte RJ, Molenaar IQ, Begliomini B, et al. Aprotinin and transfusion requirements in orthotopic liver transplantation: a multicenter randomised double-blind study. *Lancet* 2000;355:1303–1309.

29. Levi M, ten Cate H. Disseminated intravascular coagulation. *N Engl J Med* 1999;341:586–592.

30. Levi M, de Jonge E, van der Poll T, et al. Disseminated intravascular coagulation. *Thromb Haemost* 1999;82:695–705.

31. Baglin T. Management of warfarin (Coumadin) overdose. *Blood Rev* 1998;12:91–98.

32. Roberts HR, Bingham MD. Other coagulation factor deficiencies. In: Loscalzo J, Schafer AI, eds. *Thrombosis and hemorrhage*, 2nd ed. Philadelphia: Williams & Wilkins, 1998:773–802.

33. Butler AC, Tait RC. Management of oral anticoagulant-induced intracranial haemorrhage. *Blood Rev* 1998;12:35–44.

34. Hirsh J, Warkentin KE, Raschke R, et al. Heparin and low-molecular-weight heparin: mechanisms of action, pharmacokinetics, dosing considerations, monitoring, efficacy, and safety. *Chest* 1998;114:489s–510s.

35. Wolzt M, Weltermann A, Nieszpaur-Los M, et al. Studies on the neutralizing effects of protamine on unfractionated and low molecular weight heparin (Fragmin^R) at the site of activation of the coagulation system in man. *Thromb Haemost* 1995;73:439–443.

36. Hirsh J, Warkentin TE, Shaughnessy SG, et al. Heparin and low-molecular-weight heparin mechanisms of action, pharmacokinetics, dosing, monitoring, efficacy, and safety. *Chest* 2001;119:64s–94s.

37. Cadroy Y, Pourrat J, Baladre M-F, et al. Delayed elimination of enoxaparin in patients with chronic renal insufficiency. *Thromb Res* 1991;63:385–390.

38. Vandermeulen EP, Van Aken H, Vermylen J: Anticoagulants and spinal-epidural anesthesia. *Anesth Analg* 1994;79:1165–1177.

39. Horlocker TT, Heit JA. Low molecular weight heparin: biochemistry, pharmacology, perioperative prophylaxis regimens, and guidelines for regional anesthetic management. *Anesth Analg* 1997;85:874–875.

40. Horlocker TT, Wedel DJ. Spinal and epidural blockade and perioperative low molecular weight heparin: smooth sailing on the *Titanic*. *Anesth Analg* 1998;86:1153–1156.

41. Matsuo T, Kario K, Chikahira Y, et al. Treatment of heparin-induced thrombocytopenia by use of argatroban, a synthetic thrombin inhibitor. *Br J Haematol* 1992;82:627–629.

42. Lewis BE, Iaffaldano R, McKiernan TL, et al. Report of successful use of argatroban as an alternative anticoagulant during coronary stent implantation in a patient with heparin-induced thrombocytopenia and thrombosis syndrome. *Cathet Cardiovasc Diagn* 1996;38:206–209.

43. Vanholder R, Camez A, Veys N, et al. Pharmacokinetics of recombinant hirudin in hemodialyzed end-stage renal failure patients. *Thromb Haemost* 1997;77:650–655.

44. Vanholder R, Camez A, Veys N, et al. Recombinant hirudin: a specific thrombin inhibiting anticoagulant for hemodialysis. *Kidney Int* 1994;45:1754–1759.

45. Danhof M, deBoer A, Magnani HN, et al. Pharmacokinetic considerations on orgaran (Org 10172) therapy. *Hemostasis* 1992;22:73–84.

46. *Medical Letter* 1997;39:94.

47. Chong BH, Magnani HN. Orgaran in heparin-induced thrombocytopenia. *Hemostasis* 1992;22:85–91.

48. The EPISTENT Investigators. Randomised placebo-controlled and balloon-angioplasty-controlled trial to assess safety of coronary stenting with use of platelet glycoprotein-IIb/IIIa blockade. *Lancet* 1998;352:87–92.

49. The PURSUIT Trial Investigators. Inhibition of platelet glycoprotein IIb/IIIa with eptifibatide in patients with acute coronary syndromes. *N Engl J Med* 1998;339:436–443.

50. Kleiman NS. Pharmacokinetics and pharmacodynamics of glycoprotein IIb-IIIa inhibitors. *Am Heart J* 1999;13:S263–275.

51. Ferguson JJ, Kereiakes DJ, Adgey AAJ, et al. Safe use of platelet GP IIb/IIIa inhibitors. *Am Heart J* 1998;135:s77–89.

52. Madan M, Berkowitz SD. Understanding thrombocytopenia and antigenicity with glycoprotein IIb-IIIA inhibitors. *Am Heart J* 1999;138:S317–S326.

53. Berkowitz SD, Harrington RA, Rund MM, et al. Acute profound thrombocytopenia after c7E3 Fab (abciximab) therapy. *Circulation* 1997;95:809–813.

54. Quinn MJ, Fitzgerald DJ. Ticlopidine and clopidogrel. *Circulation* 1999;100:1667–1672.

55. Bennett CL, Weinberg PD, Rozenberg-Ben-Dror K, et al. Thrombotic thrombocytopenic purpura associated with ticlopidine: a review of 60 cases. *Ann Intern Med* 1998;128:541–544.

56. Savcic M, Hauert J, Bachmann F, et al. Clopidogrel loading dose regimens: kinetic profile of pharmacodynamic response in healthy subjects. *Semin Thromb Hemost* 1999;25(Suppl 2):15–19.

57. Cattaneo M, Gachet C. ADP receptors and clinical bleeding disorders. *Arterioscler Thromb Vasc Biol* 1999;19:2281–2285.

58. Greengard J, Eichinger S, Griffin J, et al. Brief report: variability of thrombosis among homozygous siblings with resistance to activated protein C due to an Arg→Gln mutation in the gene for factor V. *N Engl J Med* 1994;331:1559–1562.

59. Rosendaal FR, Koster T, Vandenbroucke JP, et al. High risk of thrombosis in patients homozygous for factor V Leiden (activated protein C resistance). *Blood* 1995;85:1504–1508.

60. Ridker PM, Hennekens CH, Lindpaintner K, et al. Mutation in the gene coding for coagulation factor V and the risk of myocardial infarction, stroke, and venous thrombosis in apparently healthy men. *N Engl J Med* 1995;332:912–917.

61. Poort SR, Rosendaal FR, Reitsma PH, et al. A common genetic variation in the 3'-untranslated region of the prothrombin gene is associated with elevated plasma prothrombin levels and an increase in venous thrombosis. *Blood* 1996;88:3698–3703.

62. Cumming AM, Keeney S, Salden A, et al. The prothrombin gene G20210A variant: prevalence in a U.K. anticoagulant clinic population. *Br J Haematol* 1997;98:353–355.

63. Brown K, Luddington R, Williamson D, et al. Risk of venous thromboembolism associated with a G to A transition at position 20210 in the 3'-untranslated region of the prothrombin gene. *Br J Haematol* 1997;98:907–909.

64. De Stefano V, Leone G, Mastrangelo S, et al. Clinical manifestations, and management of inherited thrombophilia: retrospective analysis and follow up after diagnosis of 238 patients with congenital deficiency of antithrombin III, protein C, protein S. *Thromb Haemost* 1994;72:352–358.

65. Rosendaal FR. Risk factors for venous thrombosis: prevalence, risk, and interaction. *Semin Hematol* 1997;34:171–187.

66. Ridker PM, Miletich JP, Hennekens CH, et al. Ethnic distribution of factor V Leiden in 4047 men and women: implications for venous thromboembolism screening. *JAMA* 1997;277:1305–1307.

67. Den Heijer M, Koster T, Blom HJ, et al. Hyperhomocysteinemia as a risk factor for deep-vein thrombosis. *N Engl J Med* 1996;334:759–762.

68. Graham IM, Daly LE, Refsum HM, et al. Plasma homocysteine as a risk factor for vascular disease: the European concerted action project. *JAMA* 1997;277:1775–1781.

69. Malinow MR. Homocyst(e)ine and arterial occlusive diseases. *J Intern Med* 1994;236:603–617.

70. Nygard O, Nordrehaug JE, Refsum H, et al. Plasma homocysteine levels and mortality in patients with coronary artery disease. *N Engl J Med* 1997;337:230–236.

71. Frosst P, Blom HJ, Milos R, et al. A candidate genetic risk factor for vascular disease: a common mutation in methylenetetrahydrofate reductase. *Nat Genet* 1995;10:111–113.

72. Shemin D, Lapane KL, Bausserman L, et al. Plasma total homocysteine and hemodialysis access thrombosis: a prospective study. *J Am Soc Nephrol* 1999;10:1095–1099.

73. Sirrs S, Duncan L, Djurdjev O, et al. Homocyst(e)ine and vascular access complications in haemodialysis patients: insights into a complex metabolic relationship. *Nephrol Dial Transplant* 1999;14:738–743.

74. Spence JD, Cordy P, Kortas C, et al. Effect of usual doses of folate supplementation on elevated plasma homocyst(e)ine in hemodialysis patients: no difference between 1 and 5 mg daily. *Am J Nephrol* 1999;19:405–410.

75. Bostom AG, Shemin D, Gohh RY, et al. Treatment of mild hyperhomocysteinemia in renal transplant recipients versus hemodialysis patients. *Transplantation* 2000;69:2128–2131.

76. Touam M, Zingraff J, Jungers P, et al. Effective correction of hyperhomocysteinemia in hemodialysis patients by intravenous folinic acid and pyridoxine therapy. *Kidney Int* 1999;56:2292–2296.

77. Sammaritano LR, Gharavi AE, Lockshin MD. Antiphospholipid antibody syndrome: immunologic and clinical aspects. *Semin Arthritis Rheum* 1990;20:81–96.

78. Asherson RA, Khamashta MA, Ordi-Ros J, et al. The "primary" antiphospholipid syndrome: major clinical and serological features. *Medicine* 1989;68:366–374.

79. McNeil HP, Chesterman CN, Krilis SA. Immunology and clinical importance of antiphospholipid antibodies. *Adv Immunol* 1991;49:193–280.

80. McNeil HP, Simpson RJ, Chesterman CN, et al. Anti-phospholipid antibodies are directed against a complex antigen that includes a lipid-binding inhibitor of coagulation: B_2-glycoprotein I (apolipoprotein H). *Proc Natl Acad Sci USA* 1990;87:4120–4124.

81. Galli M, Comfurius P, Maassen C, et al. Anticardiolipin antibodies (ACA) directed not to cardiolipin but to a plasma protein cofactor. *Lancet* 1990;335:1544–1547.

82. Matsura E, Igarashi Y, Fujimoto M, et al. Anticardiolipin cofactor(s) and differential diagnosis of autoimmune disease. *Lancet* 1990;38:177–178.

83. Wilson WA, Gharavi AE, Koike T, et al. International consensus statement on preliminary classification criteria for definite antiphospholipid syndrome: report of an international workshop. *Arthritis Rheum* 1999;42:1309–1311.

84. Khamashta MA. Management of thrombosis in the antiphospholipid syndrome. *Lupus* 1996;5:463–466.

85. Rosove MH, Brewer PMC. Antiphospholipid thrombosis: clinical course after the first thrombotic event in 70 patients. *Ann Intern Med* 1992;117:303–308.

86. Khamashta MA, Cuadrado MJ, Mujic F, et al. The management of thrombosis in the antiphospholipid-antibody syndrome. *N Engl J Med* 1995;332:993–997.

87. Kearon C, Gent M, Hirsh J, et al. A comparison of three months of anticoagulation with extended anticoagulation for a first episode of idiopathic venous thromboembolism. *N Engl J Med* 1999;340:901–907.

88. Vianna JL, Khamashta MA, Ordi-Ros J, et al. Comparison of the primary and secondary antiphospholipid syndrome: a European multicenter study of 114 patients. *Am J Med* 1994;96:3–9.

89. Ginsberg JS, Wells PS, Brill-Edwards P, et al. Antiphospholipid antibodies and venous thromboembolism. *Blood* 1995;86:3685–3691.

90. Asherson RA, Piette J-C. The catastrophic antiphospholipid syndrome 1996: acute multi-organ failure associated with antiphospholipid antibodies: a review of 31 patients. *Lupus* 1996;5;414–417.

91. Bajaj SP, Rapaport SI, Fierer DS, et al. A mechanism for the hypoprothrombinemia of the acquired hypoprothrombinemia-lupus anticoagulant syndrome. *Blood* 1983;61:684–692.

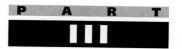

PART

III

HEMODIALYSIS ACCESS CREATION

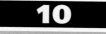

PREOPERATIVE ULTRASONOGRAPHY

MICHAEL R. JAFF

Successful renal replacement therapy mandates comprehensive planning and institution of appropriate therapy. Hemodialysis is a mainstay of renal replacement therapy. Although synthetic "bridge" grafts are commonly used, limitations include recurrent graft thrombosis and the need for repeated "declotting" procedures and ultimately multiple graft reconstruction procedures. The Dialysis Outcomes Quality Initiative provided by the National Kidney Foundation urges a shift in access to the use of autologous arteriovenous fistulae, such as the radial artery to cephalic vein procedure (Brescia–Cimino fistula) (1).

Rationale for use of the "bridge" synthetic grafts include a lack of obviously suitable superficial veins, a need for immediate dialysis, and the relative surgical ease of constructing these grafts compared with autologous arteriovenous fistulae.

The shift toward the use of autologous arteriovenous fistula requires a change in practice patterns and philosophy. There are, however, practical aspects to this paradigm shift that can be utilized. A cornerstone of this is appropriate preoperative planning. Classically, this has centered around physical examination and, in certain circumstances, contrast venography.

The first step in preoperative assessment is the patient history. Certain key questions must be asked (Table 10.1). The physical examination is potentially helpful and can aid in planning the ideal surgical procedure (2) (see Chapter 18).

Venography has its limitations, including the invasive nature of the examination, the potential for allergic contrast reactions, and the risk of inducing superficial or deep venous thrombophlebitis. One important reason for contrast venography is in an effort to identify central venous stenosis, which may be a culprit for graft thrombosis. Venography is quite helpful in uncovering this pathology (see Chapter 11 and the section on diagnosis in Chapter 25).

Duplex ultrasonography has been used by some dialysis centers to follow the patency of the access, either when problems with dialysis are identified or in a surveillance program (3). Duplex ultrasonography has determined that more than 35% of functioning bridge grafts have significant (>50%) stenosis (4). Duplex scanning, however, is also ideally suited as the preoperative management test of choice (5). It is noninvasive, painless, and, performed by a qualified vascular diagnostic laboratory, is accurate and highly reproducible. In one series of 50 consecutive patients requiring dialytic support, duplex ultrasonography identified only 33% of patients with normal upper-extremity venous and arterial anatomy. When duplex ultrasonography was used, primary and secondary graft patency rates were superior to the reported rates of other series in which physical examination was the sole preoperative evaluation method (6).

Standard protocols exist for preoperative assessment of the nondominant upper extremity. The superficial veins are imaged with the use of a proximal tourniquet, and the size of the veins, along with patency, are documented. The deep veins of the upper arm are identified and interrogated through the subclavian vein to identify central venous stenosis.

Following venous evaluation, upper-extremity arterial blood pressures are measured, ensuring that the pressure in the nondominant arm is not lower than 20 mm Hg of the

TABLE 10.1. HISTORICAL DATA REQUIRED PRIOR TO DIALYSIS ACCESS SURGERY

Which is the dominant arm?
Prior history of vascular access
Pacemaker, implantable defibrillator
Prior central venous catheter placement
Coagulopathy, bleeding diathesis
Hemodynamically important comorbid illness
    Diabetes mellitus
    Congestive heart failure
    Prosthetic heart valve

Adapted from the National Kidney Foundation's Dialysis Outcomes Quality Initiative. Clinical practice guidelines for vascular access. New York: National Kidney Foundation, 1997:18–21, with permission.

contralateral arm. The radial artery is imaged with duplex ultrasonography to determine patency, presence of atherosclerotic plaque, and continuity with the palmar arch. If the radial artery does not appear suitable, imaging of the ulnar, brachial, and axillary arteries is routinely performed.

Criteria for the suitability of the venous and arterial structures of the upper extremities have been developed and are useful in superficial venous transposition procedures in patients in whom the classic single incision radial artery–

cephalic vein arteriovenous fistula cannot be used (Table 10.2) (5) (see Chapter 14).

In an aging and ill population where dialysis access is challenging, and in the face of an initiative urging the use of autogenous arteriovenous fistulae, preoperative duplex ultrasonography represents an effective, economical, and simple method of planning appropriate and durable surgical access procedures.

TABLE 10.2. DUPLEX ULTRASONOGRAPHY PREOPERATIVE CRITERIA FOR DIALYSIS ACCESS

Venous anatomy
    For arteriovenous fistula: venous diameter ≥2.5 mm
    For bridge grafts: venous diameter ≥4.0 mm
    Patent venous segments without stenosis/thrombosis
    Continuity with the deep veins of the upper arm
    Absence of central venous stenosis
Arterial anatomy
    Symmetric upper-extremity blood pressures (discrepancy <20 mm Hg)
    Arterial inflow lumen ≥2.0 mm
    Patent palmar arch

Adapted from Silva MB, Simonian GT, Hobson RW. Increasing use of autogenous fistulas: selection of dialysis access sites by duplex scanning and transposition of forearm veins. *Semin Vasc Surg* 2000;13:44–48, with permission.

REFERENCES

1. National Kidney Foundation Dialysis Outcome Quality Initiative (NKF-DOQI). *Clinical practice guidelines for vascular access.* New York: National Kidney Foundation, 1997:18–21.
2. Trerotola SO, Scheel PJ, Powe NR, et al. Screening for dialysis access graft malfunction: comparison of physical examination with US. *J Vasc Interv Radiol* 1996;7:15–20.
3. Villemarette PA, Kornick AL, Rosenberg DM, et al. Use of color flow Doppler to evaluate vascular access graft function. *J Vasc Technol* 1989;13:164–170.
4. MacDonald MJ, Martin LG, Hughes JD, et al. Distribution and severity of stenoses in functioning arteriovenous grafts: a duplex and angiographic study. *J Vasc Technol* 1996;20:131–136.
5. Silva MB, Simonian GT, Hobson RW. Increasing use of autogenous fistulas: selection of dialysis access sites by duplex scanning and transposition of forearm veins. *Semin Vasc Surg* 2000;13:44–48.
6. Comeaux ME, Bryant PS, Harkrider WW. Preoperative evaluation of the renal access patient with color Doppler imaging. *J Vasc Technol* 1993;17:247–250.

VENOGRAPHY BEFORE ANGIOACCESS CREATION

ALAIN C. RAYNAUD

Good knowledge of the anatomy of veins of the upper limb is necessary for performing and reading venography examinations. Deep veins run beside arteries. They are double and easily identified in the forearm. They follow the brachial artery in the upper arm. These veins are thin-walled, deep veins that have many collaterals, and they cannot be used to create an autologous fistula. They should be differentiated from the superficial veins, which are the most suitable veins for access creation.

Three superficial veins can be used in the forearm: the basilic, cephalic, and accessory cephalic veins. In the upper arm, the cephalic vein remains superficial, in contrast to the basilic vein, which becomes deep. Both veins are suitable for access creation. One difficulty in phlebography reading is to differentiate the basilic vein from the brachial veins because both veins are superimposed. The basilic vein, however, is formed by superficial veins, in contrast to the brachial veins, which are formed by the convergence of deep forearm veins.

An autologous fistula for hemodialysis requires a feeding artery that can provide sufficient flow (at least 500 mL/ minute), a good-quality superficial vein able to develop and to be punctured three times a week, and normally patent proximal veins to avoid too high access pressure and limb edema.

Before creating an angioaccess, arterial patency and quality are easily assessed by clinical examination and ultrasonography. (See Chapter 18 for a description of the preoperative physical examination.) The patency and quality of superficial and proximal veins are much more difficult to evaluate. Their assessment is based on their past history, clinical examination, ultrasonography, nuclear magnetic resonance imaging, and venography. The last technique remains the gold standard; however, regular venography requires injection of iodine contrast material, which is contraindicated in cases of renal failure. Thus, indications for iodine venography are very wide in patients who have already undergone hemodialysis and are very limited in patients with severe renal failure who have not been previously dialyzed. Little has been published on the topic of venogra-phy in the evaluation of upper-limb veins before the creation of an angioaccess for hemodialysis, although it is a routine examination in many institutions. We will therefore set out our approach to performing this examination in a European country in which more than 80% of accesses are native venous accesses. Readers interested in angiographic evaluation of established grafts or autologous fistulas are referred to Chapters 23 and 24.

One major value of venography is avoiding attempts to create a fistula using a vein that is not suitable for access creation or detecting a clinically unsuspected suitable vein. Venography technique should therefore be faultless. Venography should satisfactorily visualize all the superficial veins in the upper limb and the deep veins from the basilic vein to the superior vena cava (Fig. 11.1).

The following are the main indications for preoperative venography:

- An insufficient clinical examination, which occurs frequently in children, obese patients, and in patients with limb edema;
- Past history of central vein line placement, which may have compromised the patency of proximal veins (Fig.11.1D);
- Failure to create a first access

Another less frequent indication for venography is when clinical examination detects a superficial vein, but some doubt remains about its quality. The aim of venography is then to opacify that vein selectively.

IODINE UPPER-LIMB VENOGRAPHY

Vein puncture should be performed into a vein on the dorsum of the hand. Puncture of a vein close to the thumb allows better opacification of the cephalic vein and close to the little finger provides better opacification of the basilic vein. Puncture should never be attempted into a vein that can be used for creation of an angioaccess. The upper limb should be placed in anatomic position (upper limb abducted 45 degrees with the palm facing anteriorly) to allow identification of the veins.

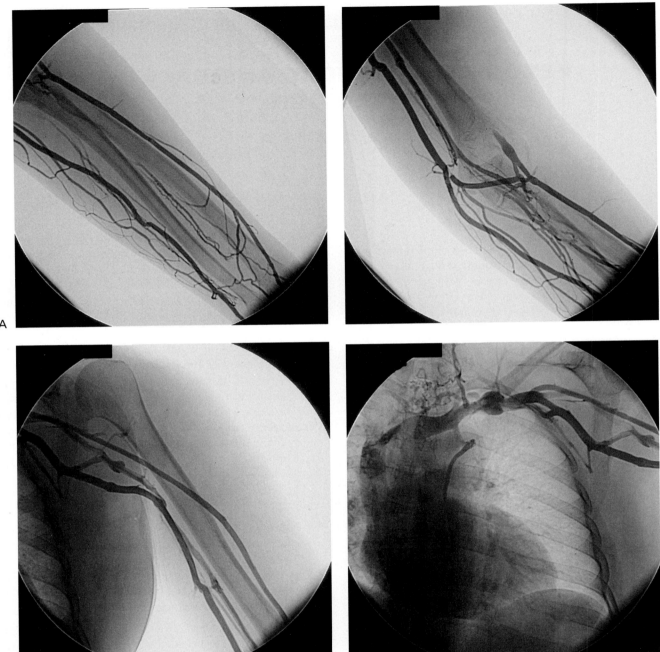

FIGURE 11.1. Left upper-limb iodine venography of a patient on chronic hemodialysis with a past history of central venous catheter. **A:** Forearm. Basilic and main cephalic veins are of normal appearance. **B:** Elbow. The cephalic vein appears to be occluded, but the tourniquet is still tightened. **C:** Upper arm. Following removal of the tourniquet, cephalic and basilic veins are of normal patency. **D:** Central veins. There is significant stenosis of the brachiocephalic vein preventing access creation in the entire limb.

Opacification

All the superficial veins of the upper limb should be opacified by the contrast material, not only those located on the direct drainage from the puncture site. The deep proximal veins also should be visualized. A large amount of contrast material is therefore required. To reduce the amount, the contrast material can be pulsed by 5% glucose solution. We routinely use 35 to 40 mL of contrast material pulsed by 40 to 50 mL of 5% glucose solution.

Veins should be distended to allow evaluation of their real size and quality. This can be achieved by using a tourniquet placed on the arm at least a few minutes before injection. A tourniquet encourages filling of the deep veins, how-

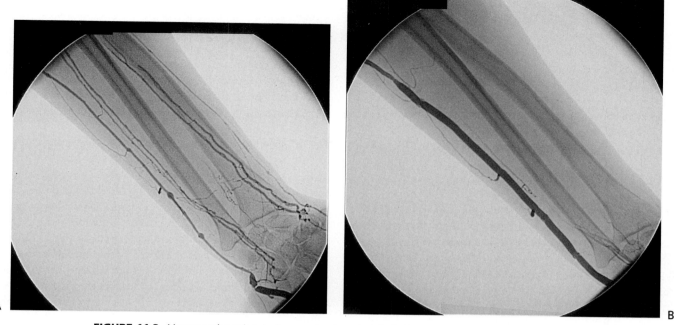

FIGURE 11.2. Venography using iodine contrast material. **A:** Forearm. Despite tourniquet, only one superficial vein is visible: the basilic vein. This vein is very thin with short zones of enlargement around the valves. This appearance is very suggestive of spasm. **B:** Forearm. The basilic vein appears to be of normal patency and of good caliber following injection of 0.5 mg of molcidomine.

ever, and may lead to nonvisualization of the cephalic vein in the arm (Fig 11.1B). We therefore recommend removing it when two thirds of the contrast material has been injected. Another factor that favors vein distension is injection of a large volume of fluid upstream from the tourniquet. Occasionally, injection of nitroglycerin is helpful when differentiation of spasm from a real venous lesion is not possible despite tourniquet and fluid injection (Fig. 11.2). Nitroglycerine should be injected while the tourniquet is tightened. This increases the time of contact between vein walls and the drug and thus improves its efficacy. The drug we use in Europe is chlorhydrate de linsidomine (0.5 mg per limb diluted in 20 mL of saline solution). (*Editor's note*: We use 200 μg nitroglycerine in 2 mL saline, which is available in the United States. Others dilute nitroglycerine into a larger volume.)

Images of the entire limb and proximal veins from the wrist to the right atrium should be obtained. Some false images of stenosis should be borne in mind:

- Despite removal of the tourniquet during the injection, the imprint of the tourniquet on the cephalic vein often remains during image acquisition. The same mechanism explains disparity in the caliber of the cephalic vein upstream and downstream from the tourniquet site (Fig 11.3).
- When the arm is in anatomic position, compression by soft tissues can cause false stenosis or occlusion of the deep vein at the brachioaxillary junction (Fig 11.3). A new injection, with the arm in abduction, will confirm the normal patency of the deep veins.

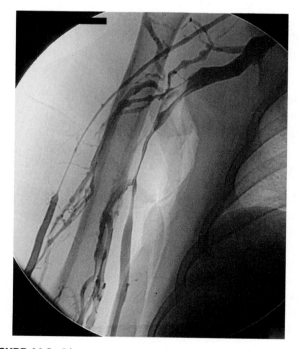

FIGURE 11.3. Discrepancy in size of encephalic and basilic veins remaining despite tourniquet removal. Compression by soft tissue due to the patient's position is another cause for the decreased size of the axillary vein.

- Washout due to nonopacified flow coming from cerebral veins, particularly the internal jugular vein, can cause a false image of stenosis; however, the appearance of such a false lesion is often different from one frame to another. When there is doubt, the absence of collateral circulation is sufficient to rule out a hemodynamically significant stenosis for normal venous flows. A moderate stenosis may become significant with the increase in flow after access creation.

SELECTIVE VENOGRAPHY

In the case of selective venography, the aim is to define the quality of one vein segment. This examination is requested when the clinical examination shows a vein but there is some doubt about the quality of one segment of this vein. For example, is a basilic vein that can be felt at the elbow normally patent above the elbow? Similarly, is a cephalic vein, which is palpable in the lower part of the forearm but disappears above the elbow, occluded or simply becoming deep?

The venography technique is completely different. The puncture site should not be located on a vein potentially suitable for access creation but should be on one of its roots. Venous dilatation by tourniquet, with or without nitroglycerin, is often required. Frames should be taken in the region of interest. When digital subtraction angiography is used, highly diluted iodine contrast material (up to 90%) can be injected. Severe renal failure does not contraindicate this examination because of the very minimal amount of iodine contrast material used, with 1 or 2 mL often sufficient.

Selective venography is simple and effective. It competes with ultrasonography, which is less invasive, and also is effective for the same indications.

UPPER-LIMB CO_2 VENOGRAPHY

The absence of contraindication in cases of severe renal failure is the major advantage of CO_2 venography, which also can be performed in cases of severe allergy to iodine contrast material. This examination can thus be attempted easily before angioaccess creation. It is currently used in the Paris area when clinical examination is not sufficient and doubts remain about the patency or quality of veins. To our knowledge, nothing has been published about this examination. Nevertheless, the technique of CO_2 venography in our institute is close to that of iodine. Frames should be acquired at a higher rate (i.e., six images per second), and filling of superficial veins is more difficult to obtain. Injection of a compressible gas does not cause sufficient venous distension (in contrast to injection of a liquid) upstream from a tourniquet. Nitroglycerin injection is therefore systematically required (0.5 mg chlorhydrate de linsidomine per limb diluted in 20 mL of saline solution) (Fig. 11.4).

Previously, we injected CO_2 manually using a 50-mL syringe. Too fast an injection of CO_2 is painful and causes the patient to move. Too slow an injection is insufficient to fill the superficial veins. Injection of CO_2 at a satisfactory rate therefore requires an experienced operator.

Patients tolerate CO_2 venography well, although they often complain of dizziness during the 30 minutes following the examination. We therefore keep the patient lying down for half an hour after this examination.

Major complications are due mainly to overinjection of CO_2, which may even cause patient death. This may occur when a stopcock remains open and the CO_2 goes directly from the cylinder to the patient. To avoid this complication, we open the tap of the CO_2 cylinder for only a few seconds to fill the pressure reducer. All the examinations then are performed with the CO_2 contained between the two manometers of the pressure reducer. When both arms are studied, it is usually necessary to refill the pressure reducer. For the same reason, the injection should be reduced to the minimum necessary. At least three injections are needed to study an upper limb (Fig. 11.5): one for the forearm with the tourniquet tightened, one in the upper arm, and one in the central veins and the superior vena cava, both without a tourniquet.

When the cephalic vein is not sufficiently opacified in the forearm, another injection without a tourniquet or with compression of the vein preferentially draining the CO_2 may be indicated such as compression of the basilic vein at the elbow. When the cephalic vein is not opacified in the upper arm because of preferential opacification of the basilic vein, a new injection should be performed with compression of the basilic vein. Placing the arm along the body is often sufficient to squash the basilic vein at the humeroaxillary junction; in lean patients, placing a hard object in the axillary fossa should reinforce this maneuver. In obese patients, a new injection with the arm in abduction may be indicated to opacify the basilic vein (Fig. 11.5).

In our experience, the results of CO_2 venography are similar to those of iodine venography. Between February 2, 1998, and July 15, 1998, we performed 21 bilateral and 9 unilateral CO_2 venography examinations of the upper limbs and one of the lower limbs. The results of upper limb venography are reported in Table 11.1. The indications for CO_2 venography rapidly increased in our institution during the year 2000; we performed 280 CO_2 venography examinations without any severe complications.

Analysis of proximal veins was satisfactory in all cases. Visualization was insufficient in only 9 of the 153 forearm veins; in eight of these nine cases, the insufficient visualization was explained by preferential filling of another normally patent forearm vein with CO_2 (Fig. 11.5A). In the only lower limb CO_2 venography we performed, opacification of the internal saphenous, superficial femoral, and iliac veins was satisfactory, and these veins were of normal patency. (*Editor's note*: CO_2 and gadolinium angiography in established grafts and fistulas is discussed in Chapter 23).

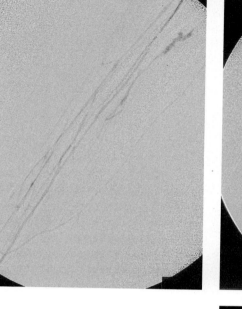

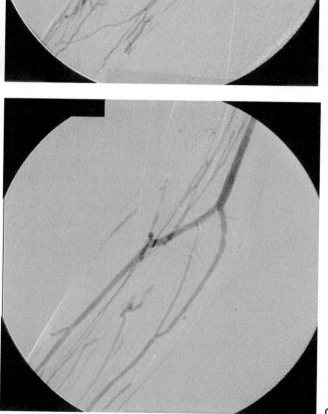

FIGURE 11.4. CO_2 venography before creation of an angioaccess. **A:** Forearm level. Despite a tourniquet tightened for few minutes, all superficial veins are spastic and barely visible. **B,C:** After injection of 0.5 mg of molcidonine, main cephalic and basilic veins are clearly visible and of normal patency.

GADOLINIUM VENOGRAPHY

Gadolinium can be used as vascular contrast. It provides a third or a quarter of the contrast provided by iodine contrast material.

The nephrotoxicity of gadolinium is very low at the doses used for magnetic resonance imaging. Higher doses are required for angiography and then gadolinium nephrotoxicity must be compared with diluted iodine contrast material, providing the same contrast (10 mL of iodine contrast material provides as much contrast as 30 to 40 mL of gadolinium). The nephrotoxicity of diluted iodine contrast material does not appear to be higher than gadolinium contrast material.

Thus, in our opinion, gadolinium is of no interest in venography except maybe as an alternative to CO_2 in certain cases of severe allergy to iodine contrast material.

MAGNETIC RESONANCE VENOGRAPHY

Venography serves two purposes for access creation: (a) evaluation of the patency of central veins and (b) detection of superficial veins suitable to develop and transform into an angioaccess.

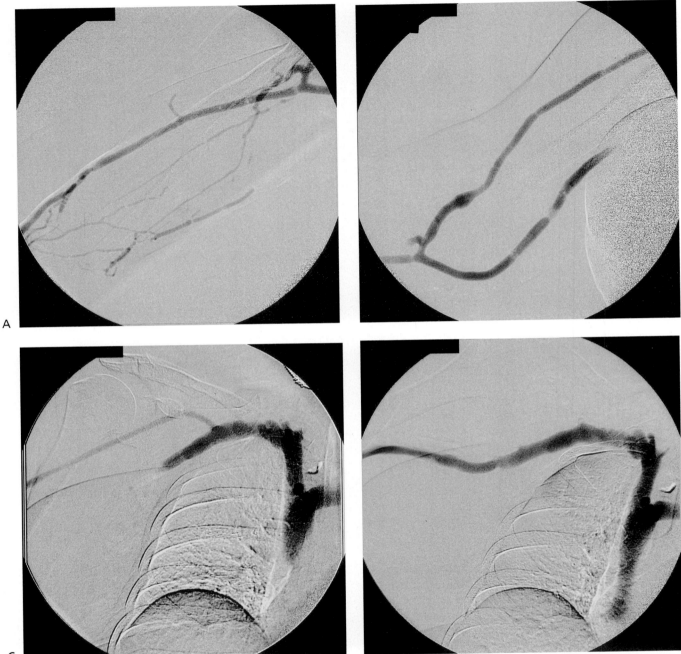

FIGURE 11.5. Patient with severe renal failure not yet under hemodialysis. CO_2 venography. **A:** Forearm. A large main cephalic vein drains all the CO_2. **B:** Upper arm. Normal-appearing cephalic vein. Upper third of the basilic vein not opacified. **C:** Central vein. Normal appearance of cephalic arch and central veins. However, the upper basilic and axillary veins are not opacified. **D:** When the arm is placed in abduction, basilic and axillary veins appear normal, but the cephalic vein is no longer visible.

Central Veins

In contrast to regular venography, magnetic resonance venography is not contraindicated in cases of allergy to iodine contrast material or in cases of poor renal function. It is very effective for evaluation of the patency of central veins (1–3) and is as effective as regular iodine venography for detection of stenoses and thromboses.

Peripheral Veins

Venography also must be used to detect superficial veins and appreciate their ability to develop. Little has been published about magnetic resonance imaging for this indication (4), and its suitability remains to be proved for satisfactory evaluation of the superficial veins of the upper limbs.

TABLE 11.1. RESULTS OF UPPER-LIMB VENOGRAPHY

Vein Quality	Forearm			Arm		Proximal Vein
	Cephalic	Accessory Cephalic	Basilic	Cephalic	Basilic	
Usable for access	8	4	8	20	35	48
Intermediate	9	2	6	6	6	3
Thrombosed or unusable	33	42	32	24	9	0
Poorly opacified	1[a]	3[a]	5[a]	1	1	0

[a] Eight of the nine insufficiently opacified forearm veins were explained by preferential filling of another wide and normal appearing forearm superficial vein which drained all the CO_2.

There are two aspects of such evaluation: the detection of superficial veins and appreciation of the quality of their walls. According to Menegazzo et al. (4), the detection of superficial veins is possible when veins are more than 3 mm in diameter. Magnetic resonance venography therefore requires placement of a tourniquet at the root of the limb to dilate veins. A tourniquet is not always sufficient, however, and superficial veins may remain spastic despite correct placement and tightening. A tourniquet may completely stop the flow into superficial veins (especially the cephalic vein in the upper arm) and impair vein detection by magnetic resonance. The sensitivity of magnetic resonance venography may be inadequate because many veins smaller than 3 mm in diameter may develop satisfactorily and be used for access creation. This is particularly evident for access creation in children.

Detection of a large superficial vein is not sufficient to assess whether a vein is suitable for angioaccess creation. The quality of the wall also should be appreciated. Wall irregularities revealed on iodine venography and wall thickening on ultrasonography often represent a diseased vein wall and the inability of the vein to develop. The geometric resolution of magnetic resonance venography is clearly insufficient to evaluate venous wall quality. Magnetic resonance imaging is improving very fast, however, and remains a promising technique for the evaluation of upper limb veins for native vein access creation.

REFERENCES

1. Finn JP, Zisk JHS, Edelman RR, et al. Central venous occlusion: MR angiography. *Radiology* 1993;187:245–251.
2. Shinde TS, Lee VS, Rofsky NM, et al. Three dimensional gadolinium enhanced MR venographic evaluation of patency of central veins in the thorax: initial experience. *Radiology* 1999;213:555–560.
3. Thornton MJ, Ryan R, Varghese JC, et al. A three dimensional gadolinium enhanced MR venography technique for imaging central veins. AJR Am J Roentgenol 1999;173:999–1003.
4. Menegazzo D, Laissy JP, Dürrbach A. Hemodialysis access fistula creation: proeoperative assessment with MR venography and comparison with conventional venography. *Radiology* 1998;209:723–728.

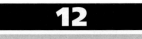

NEW NOMENCLATURE FOR ARTERIOVENOUS HEMODIALYSIS ACCESSES

ANTON N. SIDAWY
MICHAEL B. SILVA, JR.

Various investigators report on the patency and complications of arteriovenous (AV) access. It is rather difficult, however, to compare outcomes because of the wide variety of access materials, configurations, and locations. Although there have been reporting standards for dialysis access endovascular interventions as well as central venous access placement (1,2), standards regarding surgical access placement and its configurations were lacking. It is important to note that reporting standards are different from "practice guidelines" or "best practices." *Best practices* provide recommendations for optimal clinical practices aimed at improving patient care and ultimately survival. In the case of dialysis, we refer the reader to an important document published by the National Kidney Foundation (NKF), "Dialysis Outcomes Quality Initiative" (DOQI) (3). Reporting standards serve to guide authors and readers of vascular literature to report, analyze, and use clinical data in a comprehensive and uniform manner. To recommend reporting standards dealing with AV dialysis accesses, the American Association for Vascular Surgery and the Society for Vascular Surgery (AAVS/SVS) appointed a committee that included vascular surgeons, interventional radiologists, a nephrologist, and a transplant surgeon. The committee published a reporting standards document in the *Journal of Vascular Surgery* (4).

cess, including location (snuff box) (6,7), configuration (forearm loop graft) (8), anatomy (Brach-Ax), or a combination of the preceding. For example, although the name *forearm loop graft* gives a good idea of the location of the access in the forearm, its "loop" configuration, and the material used to construct it, it does not provide specifics related to the artery of origin or the target vein. The inflow artery in a loop graft can be the brachial, proximal radial, or proximal ulnar. The target vein can be the antecubital, the brachial, the cephalic, or the basilic vein (above or below the elbow). When comparing various accesses, the artery of origin or the vein may influence complications and patency. For example, a larger artery will provide higher flow into the access; conceivably, higher flow leads to better patency but an increase in the possibility of steal syndrome.

Additionally, there is lack of consensus among practitioners in defining even broad categories of access procedures as either fistulas or grafts. These terms are used inconsistently and often inaccurately. Therefore, the Reporting Standards Committee recommended the following system to report the types of access procedure placed or studied. Although it is unfamiliar at present and more detailed in its scope, adoption of this system will have the benefit of allowing accurate standardization and comparison of access procedures by category.

RATIONALE

It is important in reporting and reading the literature to have a consensus on how to define various terms and configurations related to hemodialysis accesses because the current literature is replete with a myriad of eponyms (Cimino, Snuff box fistula, Forearm loop graft, Brach-Ax graft, Bridging graft) used to describe different types of dialysis access procedures. Names are based on the author who described the access (Brescia-Cimino) (5) or the attributes of the ac-

RECOMMENDATIONS

The system is component based, with three essential categories to be included in describing each procedure: conduit, location, and configuration. The need for additional descriptive adjectives may be indicated by study design or intent and can be included at the discretion of the reporting authors. Although the use of additional modifiers is not precluded by this system, they should be supplemental to the three essential components, described below.

TABLE 12.1. FOREARM ACCESS PROCEDURES

Recommended Nomenclature	Traditional Nomenclature
Autogenous	
Autogenous posterior radial branch-cephalic direct access	Snuff box fistula
Autogenous radial-cephalic direct wrist access	Brescia-Cimino arteriovenous fistula
Autogenous ulnar-basilic forearm transposition	Superficial venous transposition in the forearm, basilic vein to ulnar artery
Autogenous radial-cephalic forearm transposition	Superficial venous transposition in the forearm, cephalic vein to radial artery
Autogenous brachial-cephalic forearm looped transposition	Superficial venous transposition in the forearm, cephalic vein to brachial artery, looped
Autogenous radial-brachial indirect saphenous vein translocation	Greater saphenous vein reversed and translocated radial artery to brachial vein
Prosthetic	
Prosthetic brachial-antecubital forearm loop access	e-PTFE forearm loop graft
Prosthetic radial-median cubital forearm straight access	e-PTFE forearm straight graft

e-PTFE, expanded polytetrafluoroethylene.

TABLE 12.2. UPPER-ARM ACCESS PROCEDURES

Recommended Nomenclature	Traditional Nomenclature
Autogenous	
Autogenous brachial-cephalic upper arm direct access	Cephalic vein to brachial artery
Autogenous brachial-basilic upper arm transposition	Basilic vein transposition
Autogenous brachial-axillary indirect translocation	Greater saphenous vein reversed and translocated Brachial artery to axillary vein
Prosthetic	
Prosthetic brachial-axillary access	Brachial-axillary bridging graft

TABLE 12.3. LOWER-EXTREMITY ACCESS PROCEDURES

Recommended Nomenclature	Traditional Nomenclature
Autogenous	
Autogenous femoral-greater saphenous loop access	Greater saphenous vein end to side to femoral artery fistula transposition
Prosthetic	
Prosthetic femoral-femoral loop inguinal access	Femoral artery to femoral vein looped e-PTFE graft

e-PTFE, expanded polytetrafluoroethylene.

TABLE 12.4. BODY WALL ACCESS PROCEDURES

Recommended Nomenclature	Traditional Nomenclature
Prosthetic axillary-axillary chest access	Collar graft or axillary artery to axillary vein with e-PTFE graft
Prosthetic axillary-axillary chest loop access	Axillary artery to ipsilateral axillary vein loop with e-PTFE graft
Prosthetic axillary-internal jugular chest loop access	Axillary artery to ipsilateral internal jugular e-PTFE graft
Prosthetic femoral-femoral supra-inguinal access	Femoral artery to contralateral femoral vein e-PTFE graft
Prosthetic axillary-femoral body wall access	Axillary artery to femoral vein e-PTFE graft

e-PTFE, expanded polytetrafluoroethylene.

Conduit

Autogenous is used to describe a native vein, whether it is *in situ*, transposed or translocated. *Prosthetic* is used to describe any of the available man-made material access products. Although expanded polytetrafluorethylene (ePTFE) is the most commonly used prosthetic material at this time, other materials also can be used, and therefore the type of prosthetic graft material and the manufacturer should be included. Other nonautogenous products, such as biografts (i.e., bovine heterograft, human umbilical vein) should be labeled as such in this portion of the component description process. Additional *prosthetic* descriptors, such as *tapered*, *ringed*, or *thin walled*, are optional and may be used if indicated.

Location

The specific vascular anatomic sites of origination and termination of the access should be included in this component. Arterial inflow site is reported first, followed by a hyphen, and then the venous outflow site. Examples of possible arteries of origin are radial, ulnar, brachial, axillary, and femoral arteries. Examples of target veins are cephalic, basilic, median cubital, or antecubital, brachial vein, axillary, subclavian, femoral vein, internal jugular, and external jugular veins.

In instances where such a descriptor may be ambiguous, the addition of a broader anatomic reference should be included. Typically, this is reported as the anatomic site where the access procedure is located and cannulation will occur. Common examples include *forearm* and *upper arm*. Less common examples include *inguinal* and *body wall* (e.g., brachial-cephalic autogenous access should be described as either a forearm brachial-cephalic or an upper-arm brachial-cephalic access).

Configuration

This component gives descriptive information regarding the anastomotic connection and the course of the conduit. Essential descriptors include either *direct* or *indirect*. Additional descriptors such as *transposed, translocated, straight,* or *looped* may be used. A *direct* access refers to a connection between native artery and vein and includes end-to-side, side-to-side, and end-to-end anastomoses. An *indirect* access is one in which either prosthetic or autogenous material is inserted between the artery and vein to establish the connection.

An access performed using a transposed vein is a *transposition*; it is a subtype of the *direct* descriptor and may be used in its place. This type of access is used when the peripheral portion of the vein is moved from its original position, typically through a more superficial tunnel, and is connected to the artery while the more central portion remains intact in its native location. The much less commonly used *translocation* access is a subtype of the *indirect* descriptor and may be used in its place. It describes a vein that has been disconnected both proximally and distally, removed from its bed, and inserted in a position remote from its origin, requiring anastomoses to both the arterial and venous segments of the access. *Looped* and *straight* refer to the course of the conduit and may be included at the reporting researcher's discretion. It should be noted that their inclusion is not essential if the configuration can be inferred from the anatomic location descriptors.

All access procedures using prosthetic material are necessarily *indirect* procedures. The use of the descriptor *prosthetic* implies an *indirect* configuration; the *indirect* descriptor may be omitted in these instances at the discretion of the reporting investigators.

Tables 12.1 through 12.4 give examples of access procedures described using both the traditional nomenclature and the recommended system. The use of the recommended nomenclature will help to make reporting, analyzing, and reading AV access data more comprehensive and uniform.

REFERENCES

1. Gray RJ, Sacks D, Trerotola S, et al. Reporting standards for percutaneous interventions in dialysis access. *J Vasc Interv Radiol* 1999;10:1405–1415.

2. Silberzweig JE, Sacks D, Khorsandi AS, et al. Reporting standards for central venous access: Technology Assessment Committee. *J Vasc Interv Radiol* 2000;11:391–400.
3. Dialysis Outcome Quality Initiative (DOQI). *Am J Kidney Dis* 1997;30(Suppl 3):150–189.
4. Sidawy AN, Gray R, Besarab A, et al. Recommended standards for reports dealing with arteriovenous hemodialysis accesses. *J Vasc Surg* 2002;35:603–610.
5. Brescia MJ, Cimino JE, Appel K, et al. Chronic hemodialysis using venipuncture and a surgically created arteriovenous fistula. *N Engl J Med* 1966;275:1089–1092.
6. Bonalumi U, Civalleri D, Rovida S, et al. Nine years' experience with end-to-end arteriovenous fistula at the 'anatomical snuffbox' for maintenance haemodialysis. *Br J Surg* 1982;69:486–488.
7. Mehigan JT, McAlexander RA. Snuffbox arteriovenous fistula for hemodialysis. *Am J Surg* 1982;143:252–253.
8. Savader SJ, Lund GB, Scheel PJ. Forearm loop, upper arm straight, and brachial-internal jugular vein dialysis grafts: a comparison study of graft survival utilizing a combined percutaneous endovascular and surgical maintenance approach. *J Vasc Interv Radiol* 1999;10:537–545.

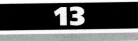

13

TECHNIQUES AND OUTCOMES AFTER POLYTETRAFLUOROETHYLENE GRAFT CREATION

AMER RAJAB
MITCHELL L HENRY

More than 250,000 patients are treated for chronic renal failure yearly. About 5% will undergo renal transplantation, but for the remainder, dialysis remains the only option. A decision must be made between peritoneal dialysis and hemodialysis. Many patients, for reasons of preference, motivation, compliance, intellect, absence of family support, or previous multiple abdominal surgeries with severe adhesions, are not candidates for peritoneal dialysis, and hemodialysis is the only option. Hemodialysis access should be achieved early, before indiscriminate phlebotomy and venous infusions deplete the veins. Temporary hemodialysis access via the subclavian vein should be avoided to decrease the risk of venous stenosis.

IMPORTANT RULES

Native arterial venous fistulae have been demonstrated to be superior to the access graft, especially regarding long-term patency and morbidity. Therefore, strategies to increase the percentage of arteriovenous (AV) fistula and conversely to decrease the use of PTFE graft need to be implemented to achieve these long-term goals. Planning strategies aimed at the first attempt to place the forearm AV fistula (Brescia–Cimino), subsequently the cephalic upper arm native fistula, and finally consideration of performing transposed basilic vein AV fistula in the upper arm should be entertained. If these options are exhausted, then an AV polytetrafluoroethylene (PTFE) graft is placed. Also, it is important to stress instructing all medical staff about avoiding peripheral vein depletion by indiscriminant use of intravenous lines as well as not to use the subclavian vein for temporary dialysis.

The limiting factor in obtaining access is usually an adequate vein. In general, access should be performed as low in the arm as possible because revision at a higher site is usually feasible, whereas revision at a lower point may not be available if the upper arm has been used. The arm is preferred to the leg for access because of the lower incidence of infection in prosthetic shunts of the arm. In addition, the incidence of atherosclerosis is greater in the lower extremity, and an attempted access there may yield inadequate arterial inflow or produce ischemia.

PREOPERATIVE EVALUATION

Most centers do not use radiologic and vascular laboratory methods on a routine basis before vascular access placement. Physical examination is traditionally thought to be adequate. Nevertheless, Koksoy and colleagues (1) found abnormal results in 5 of 17 patients studied by preoperative duplex scan. Two of these five patients had an insufficient brachial artery flow rate, and three had obstruction of the subclavian vein. The opposite extremity was therefore used, and no early graft failure occurred in this group. In contrast, 3 of 22 patients who underwent access placement without prior study developed early thrombosis. Their workup revealed proximal venous stenosis in two patients and atherosclerotic narrowing of the brachial artery in the third patient. Silva and colleagues (2) used duplex ultrasonography preoperatively to identify arteries and veins suitable for hemodialysis access and to increase the number of primary fistulas. Their results showed a significant increase in the number of primary fistulas from 14% to 63%. One-year patency rate also improved from 48% to 83% for primary fistulas and from 63% to 74% for grafts.

Schuman and colleagues (3) used magnetic resonance angiography (MRA) and ultrasonography for preoperative vascular evaluation prior to hemodialysis access placement in 24 patients. Their results showed improved primary patency rates (182 days versus 134 days) with preoperative vascular evaluation.

ANESTHESIA

Most end-stage renal disease patients are elderly or anemic, and up to 50% are diabetic. General anesthesia should be therefore avoided, especially in overweight patients, even though adequate regional anesthesia is more difficult to achieve in these patients. Regional anesthesia works very well in expert hands but may require supplementation with local anesthesia. Because of the condition of these patients (severe cardiopulmonary disease, anticoagulated), local anesthesia alone is occasionally the only option. It, however, requires attention to detail plus a potentially large amount of anesthetic drug, especially in an obese arm, and for passing the tunneler.

PROSTHETIC CHOICES

The perfect AV graft has been sought since the inception of hemodialysis. In the past, various access options have been used, including external AV shunt, saphenous vein, bovine heterograft, Dacron, and PTFE. Saphenous vein has been reserved for coronary bypass in these high-risk patients for heart disease. Bovine grafts have been abandoned because of the tendency for aneurysm formation and difficulty in performing thrombectomy. Dacron grafts are not suitable for hemodialysis access. Currently, expanded PTFE (ePTFE) is thought to be the graft material of choice for hemodialysis patients in whom autogenous fistulae cannot be constructed. PTFE grafts are available in standard and thin walls. Lenz and colleagues (4) prospectively randomized 108 patients to receive either standard (56 patients) or thin-wall (52 patients) grafts. Both primary and secondary patency rates were better for the standard wall grafts than for the thin wall grafts. So far, it is mainly surgeon and institute preference. Schuman and colleagues (5) evaluated both reinforced and nonreinforced PTFE grafts for hemodialysis in 632 grafts. They found that the primary patency rate was significantly better for nonreinforced PTFE than for reinforced. The secondary patency rates were similar, with 80% of the nonreinforced and 77% of the reinforced functioning at 1 year. They concluded that nonreinforced PTFE performs better than reinforced PTFE as a hemodialysis conduit.

Distal-hand ischemia, or arterial steal syndrome, is a potentially devastating complication of vascular access. Tapered grafts have been introduced to prevent steal syndrome. Davidson and colleagues reported on the long-term outcome of 446 (4–7 mm) tapered (6) PTFE grafts. They found the clot-free survival rate to be 85%, 81%, and 79% at 1, 3, and 5 years, respectively. Schaffer (7) prospectively randomized 59 diabetic patients to receive 6 mm (33 patients) or 4- to 7-mm (26 patients) tapered PTFE grafts for hemodialysis. Schaffer found that in this group of patients, tapered graft did not reduce the risk of ischemic complications and was associated with a significantly higher risk of thrombosis.

TECHNICAL CONSIDERATIONS

Forearm Loop Shunt Graft

After the induction of adequate axillary block anesthesia, and again confirming that the patient is not a candidate for a primary fistula, the upper extremity is prepared and draped in the usual fashion. A transverse incision almost 2 cm distal to the antecubital fold is made with electrocautery, and homeostasis is obtained. The vein is usually dissected first. The cephalic vein is our choice for outflow. If the cephalic vein is missing or inadequate, we usually check for the basilic vein, which would be the second best choice before using a deep concomitant vein. It is usually recommended not to bypass the elbow joint during the first PTFE graft placement. By using the superficial vein, later revision usually is easier because many PTFE grafts will return for declotting procedures requiring venous outflow reconstruction or angioplasty. During vein dissection, it is important to leave all significantly sized branches so as not to restrict the venous outflow (Fig. 13.1). A sufficient length of the vein is usually dissected free. Because of spasm, the vein may appear smaller after dissection. Vessel loops are used for proximal and distal control. A small longitudinal opening in the vein is made at a selected site for the anastomosis. A dilator is passed proximally to ensure patency.

The artery is addressed next. At this point, the subcutaneous tissue has been divided down to the biceps aponeurosis. The fibrous aponeurosis then is divided to expose the vascular sheath containing the artery and concomitant veins. The artery is dissected from the veins. Extreme care is taken during dissection of these thin wall veins. Usually the brachial artery and radial and ulnar branches (Fig. 13.1) can be dissected and exposed appropriately to facilitate the anastomosis. Always remember that in this patient population, arterial disease is common, and aggressive manipulation of

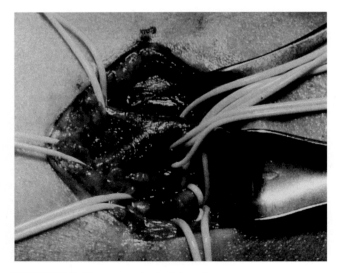

FIGURE 13.1. Venous and arterial anatomy.

the artery may dislodge atherosclerotic emboli, damage the artery, or result in dissection and future stenosis, obstruction, or pseudoaneurysm.

Different tunnelers are available to create the subcutaneous tunnel: the Noon (Codman, A Johnson & Johnson Co., MA, U.S.A.) tunneler, the Kelly–Weck (Impra, Tempe, AZ, U.S.A.) tunneler, and the Gore Sheath (W.L. Gore & Associates, Tempe, AZ, U.S.A.) tunneler. The Noon tunneler is a 6-mm dilator head at either end of a 25-cm-long flexible steel rod. The graft is tied to one end and pulled through the subcutaneous tissue. The Kelly–Weck tunneler comes in various degrees of curvature and head size. The tunneler first is passed to create the tunnel; the graft is tied to its head and pulled through. The Gore sheath tunneler consists of three parts: a semicircular sheath containing a rod to which a bullet or head is screwed. The graft is attached to the rod and passed though the sheath. Surgeons who prefer this tunneler argue that it eliminates dragging the graft through the subcutaneous tissue, which potentially damages the graft and causes kinking and rotation. We use the Kelly–Weck tunneler and believe that twisting or kinking can be avoided by proper position of the graft and also that pulling the graft directly through the tissue creates a tight fit that prevents hematoma and bleeding around the graft.

Regardless of the tunneling device used, the main objective is an atraumatic procedure placing the graft at an appropriate depth while avoiding pinching and twisting the graft. The longitudinal blue line indicator on the graft helps to align the graft between the first and second portion of the loop to avoid twisting. If the graft is placed too deep, it will be difficult for cannulation later on for dialysis. On the other hand, if the graft is placed superficially, it can cause skin necrosis from the pressure. Also, the dome on the loop should not be very narrow because an acute angle can result in a kink. Further, the graft should be placed several centimeters proximal to the wrist crease. Usually the tunneler is passed in a semicircular loop toward the wrist (Fig. 13.2). A counterincision is made toward the wrist. The tunneler again is passed from the elbow toward the counter incision to complete the loop (Fig. 13.3).

The vascular anastomoses are constructed in an end-to-side fashion. The venous anastomosis is completed first, followed by the arterial anastomosis. One should attempt to make the venotomy right over one or more side branches (if available), which will optimize the venous outflow. Also, the venotomy should be placed on the side of the vein from where the graft comes. A common mistake is to make the venotomy directly on the top of the vein, which would create a 90-degree turn or twist the vein 90-degree on the anastomotic side. The graft is next cut at the appropriate angle. For the anastomosis, we use a CV-6 Gore-Tex suture on a TT 9 needle because we believe this causes less needle-hole bleeding (Fig. 13.4). After completion of venous anastomosis and before arterial occlusion, the patient is given heparin. The arterial anastomosis then is completed in similar fashion (Fig. 13.5). After the anastomosis is complete, the arte-

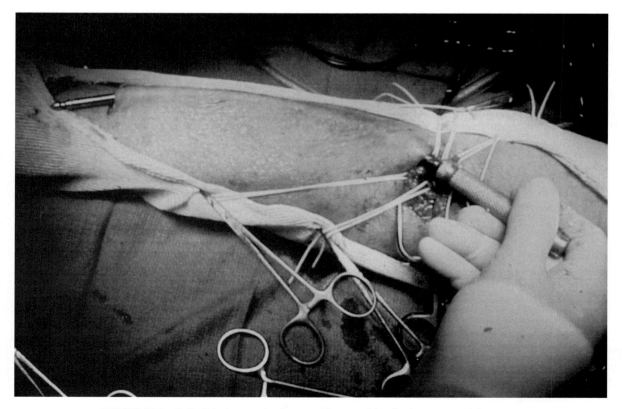

FIGURE 13.2. Kelly–Weck tunneler is passed in a semicircular loop toward the wrist.

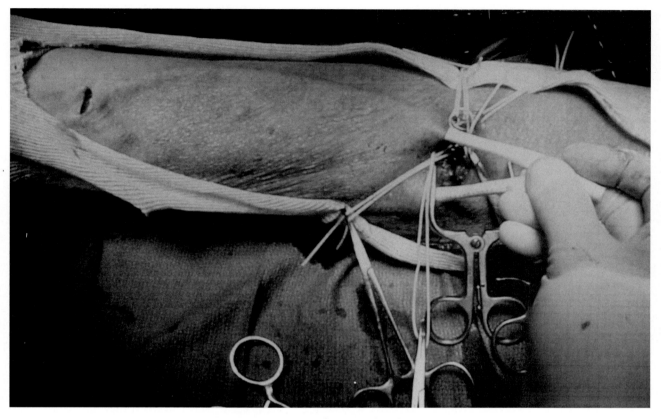

FIGURE 13.3. The graft is passed in the tunnel.

rial anastomosis is opened first to fill the graft and to allow all the graft air to be removed. When blood reaches the venous anastomosis, the venous anastomosis is opened and homeostasis is achieved. The graft as well as the venous outflow then is palpated to search for thrill. The thrill is an important sign of a successful outcome. After homeostasis is

achieved, the incision is closed in multiple layers (Fig. 13.6). A loose dressing is placed.

Upper-arm Shunt Graft

If the forearm is already exhausted, upper-arm graft placement is the next choice. One should always evaluate the

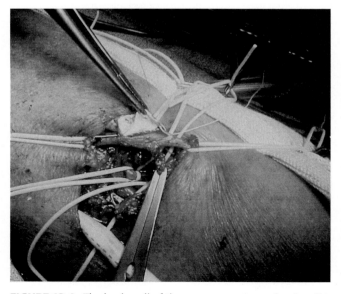

FIGURE 13.4. The back wall of the venous anastomosis using CV-6 Gore-Tex suture.

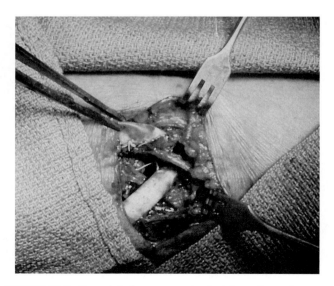

FIGURE 13.5. Completed venous and arterial anastomosis.

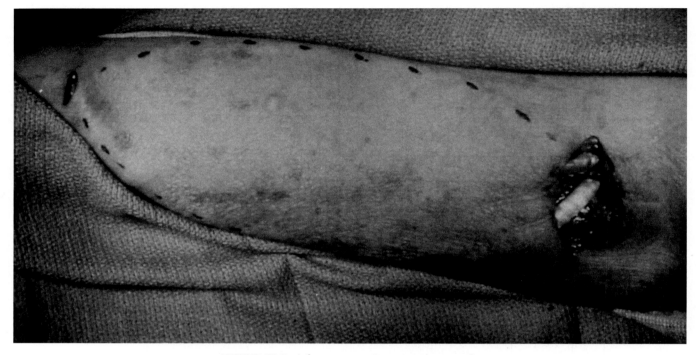

FIGURE 13.6. A forearm arteriovenous shunt graft.

cephalic vein or the basilic vein for an upper-arm native fistula before placing a PTFE upper-arm graft. A longitudinal incision is made in the medial aspect of the upper arm in the groove between the biceps and triceps muscles. For venous outflow, the basilic vein is our first choice, followed by the brachial/axillary vein. After an adequate vein exposure is achieved, a segment of the distal brachial artery is dissected for inflow. A subcutaneous tunnel is created and the PTFE graft is placed. Venous and arterial anastomoses are designed as described already. It is always important to preserve as much proximal vein as possible for future revision.

Other Sites

After all sites in the upper extremities (forearm followed by upper arm in the nondominant arm, forearm and upper arm in the dominant arm) are exhausted, other sites are used. The options here are center preference. A subclavian artery to ipsilateral subclavian vein shunt graft placed in the anterior chest wall is an option. At our institute, we use thigh AV graft. For a thigh graft, the greater saphenous or femoral veins are used as outflow; superficial or common femoral arteries are used as inflow. The graft is placed subcutaneously in the medial aspect of the thigh.

SURVEILLANCE

Early detection of dialysis access dysfunction and timely intervention may result in prolongation of access function. Whereas impending graft thrombosis may be heralded by ris-

ing venous pressure or poor flow characteristics on dialysis prompting intervention, many such episodes occur without warning. The ability to predict imminent graft failure more accurately would allow elective revision in a greater number of patients. In fact, Sands and Miranda (8) followed up on 153 hemodialysis accesses (56 fistulas and 97 PTFE grafts) and found that elective access revision prior to thrombosis improved the longevity of the access in both primary fistulas (999 days versus 358 days) and PTFE grafts (1023 days versus 689 days). In addition, early revision prior to thrombosis significantly decreased the number of clotting episodes for primary fistula (0.5 clots per patient-year versus 4.8) and PTFE grafts (1.1 clots per patient-years versus 3.6).

Several methods are available for the diagnosis of the failing access. (See Chapter 28 for detailed presentations of these methods.) Physical examination and simple clinical parameters, such as difficult needle insertion, are of questionable value. Although angiography is considered the gold standard for vascular assessment, it is expensive, invasive, and demonstrates hemodynamic changes poorly. Doppler ultrasound has the advantage of evaluating both anatomic and flow parameters; however, ultrasound is associated with potential problems, including availability, need for trained personnel, variability of data between machines, and high cost. Venous pressure (static or dynamic) monitoring and access flow measurement have important diagnostic implications; however, the technology is still evolving. Regardless of the method used, the aim should be AV graft placement, surveillance, early detection of a failing graft, and elective intervention prior to thrombosis.

NATURAL HISTORY

Several studies have outlined the natural history of prosthetic vascular access grafts. The best outcomes were reported by Davidson and colleagues (6) in 446 patients with PTFE grafts. The primary patency rate was 85%, 81%, and 79% at 1, 3, and 5 years, respectively (6). The secondary patency rate was 92%, 88%, and 84% at 1, 3, and 5 years, respectively (6). Miller and colleagues (9) evaluated prospectively the outcomes of 256 grafts placed at a single institution during a 2-year period. A salvage procedure to maintain graft patency (thrombectomy, angioplasty, or surgical revision) was required in 29% of the grafts at 3 months, 52% at 6 months, 77% at 12 months, and 96% at 24 months. Thus, primary graft survival (time from graft placement to the first intervention) was only 23% at 1 year and 4% at 2 years. Leapman and colleagues (10) followed up on 387 grafts, which required a total of 261 revisions. Of these, 36% never required a repair, whereas 64% did require surgical intervention. The mean time to revision was 10.5 months postplacement, and the 1-year secondary patency rate was 93%. Sicard and colleagues (11) described a 1-year secondary patency rate for PTFE grafts of 87% (n = 613). These patients underwent 894 revisions, or a revision rate of 1.46 per patient. Of these, 33% required one or two interventions, whereas 31% required three or more procedures to maintain patency. Sabanayagam (12) observed in 1,229 patients receiving 526 PTFE grafts that only one third of PTFE grafts were primarily patent (no revisions) after 5 years, but the secondary patency rate in the same population was 67%.

REFERENCES

1. Koksoy C, Kuzu A, Erden I, et al. Predictive value of color Doppler ultrasonography in detecting failure of vascular access grafts. *Br J Surg* 1995;82:50–52.
2. Silva MB, Hobson RW, Pappas PJ, et al. A strategy for increasing use of autogenous hemodialysis access procedures: impact of preoperative noninvasive evaluation. *J Vasc Surg* 1998;27:302–308.
3. Schuman ES, Quinn SF, Standage BA, et al. Magnetic resonance angiography in evaluation of central and peripheral vasculature prior to dialysis surgery. In: Henry ML, ed. *Vascular access for hemodialysis-VI*. Chicago: W.L. Gore & Associates and Precept Press, 1999:103–110.
4. Lenz BJ, Veldenz HC, Dennis JW, et al. A three-year follow-up on standard versus thin wall ePTFE grafts for hemodialysis. *J Vasc Surg* 1998;28:464–470.
5. Schuman ES, Standage BA, Ragsdale JW, et al. Reinforced versus nonreinforced polytetrafluoroethylene grafts for hemodialysis access. *Am J Surg* 1997;173:407–410.
6. Davidson IJA, Ar'Rajab A, Balfe P, et al. Long-term outcome of PTFE arteriovenous grafts. In: Henry ML, Ed. *Vascular access for hemodialysis VI*. Chicago: W.L. Gore & Associates and Precept Press, 1999:155–162.
7. Schaffer D. A prospective randomized trail of 6 mm versus 4–7 mm PTFE grafts for hemodialysis access in diabetic patients. In: Henry ML, Ferguson RM, eds. *Vascular access for hemodialysis-V*. Chicago: W.L. Gore & Associates and Precept Press, 1997:91–94.
8. Sands JJ, Miranda CL. Prolongation of hemodialysis access survival with elective revision. *Clin Nephrol* 1995;44:329–333.
9. Miller PE, Carlton D, Deierhoi MH, et al. Natural history of arteriovenous grafts in hemodialysis patients. *Am J Kidney Dis* 2000;36:68–74.
10. Leapman, SB, Pescovitz, MD, Thomalla JV, et al. Salvage surgery for arteriovenous conduits: does it make sense? In: Henry ML, Ferguson RM, eds. *Vascular access for hemodialysis-III*. Chicago: W.L. Gore & Associates and Precept Press, 1993:169–185.
11. Sicard GA, Allen BT, Anderson CB. Polytetrafluoroethylene grafts for vascular access. In: Sommer BG, Henry ML, eds. *Vascular access for hemodialysis*. Chicago: W.L.Gore & Associates and Precept Press, 1989:51–64.
12. Sabanayagam P. 15-year experience with tapered (4–7mm) and straight (6 mm) PTFE angio-access in the ESRD patient. In: Henry ML, Ferguson, RM, eds. *Vascular access for hemodialysis-IV*. Chicago: W.L. Gore & Associates and Precept Press, 1995:159–168.

14

TECHNIQUES AND OUTCOMES AFTER BRACHIOCEPHALIC AND BRACHIOBASILIC ARTERIOVENOUS FISTULA CREATION

ENRICO ASCHER
ANIL P. HINGORANI
WILLIAM R. YORKOVICH

The National Kidney Foundation has identified the use of arteriovenous grafts (AVGs) and the interventions required to maintain their patency as two important causes of increased expenditure in the management of hemodialysis access in end-stage renal disease (ESRD) patients. They have issued an appeal for the increased use of native arteriovenous fistulae (AVF) (1). Based on these recommendations, we, as well as others, have initiated an all-autogenous policy for the placement of AVF; 95% of patients undergoing access procedures have undergone placement of an AVF (2). Although the radiocephalic AVF is considered the procedure of choice for these patients, the nature of its construction makes it unfeasible for a number of patients because of the poor quality of the distal cephalic vein resulting from prior venipuncture, thrombosis, or small size. Consequently, we suggest the use of other veins to maintain this all-autogenous AVF policy.

Two alternatives are using the upper-arm veins to form a brachiocephalic AVF (BCAVF) or a brachiobasilic AVF (BBAVF); however, scant data exist that compare the BCAVF and BBAVF to guide surgeons as to which type of fistula should be placed (3–8). Most researchers have focused on one type of AVF compared with AVGs (9,10). Because the literature examining radiocephalic AVF is already extensive, we examine our experience by using arm veins that were transposed to the brachial artery in the context of an all-autogenous AVF policy implemented at our institution.

PATIENT CHARACTERISTICS

From December 1997 to May 2000, 109 BCAVFs and 63 BBAVFs were placed in 163 patients with chronic renal failure and inadequate distal cephalic veins or radial arteries. During this period, an additional 139 radiocephalic AVFs

were placed. Of the 163 patients who had BBAVF or BCAVF placed, three additional patients underwent upper-arm AVF placement but were not included in this group because hemodialysis was not required. In each group (BCAVF and BBAVF), there were 40 (37%) and 25 (40%) males, respectively. Twenty-nine (27%) of the BCAVF and 16 (25%) of the BBAVF had previously undergone placement of an AVF. Twenty of the BCAVF patients (18 %) and six of the BBAVF patients (10 %) had prior placement of AVGs. In each respective group, ages ranged from 29 to 88 years (mean 67 ± 1.4 years) and 37 to 84 years (mean 69 ± 2.0 years). Diabetic patients constituted 56% and 65 % of each group, and hypertensive patients constituted 73% and 75% of each group. Data collection was via chart review, personal interviews, and review of the dialysis records.

UPPER-EXTREMITY VENOUS MAPPING WITH DUPLEX ULTRASONOGRAPHY

Preoperative duplex imaging of the veins was used selectively in patients with poor visualization of the veins on clinical examination or patients with multiple prior access procedures or venipuncture. The deep venous system was imaged using a 7-5 MHz linear transducer while the patient was in supine position. Brachial veins of the arm and the subclavian vein were studied to rule out thrombosis and stenosis. This was particularly relevant in patients who had previous access procedures or central lines (11). For obese patients, a lower frequency scanner (3-2 MHz phased array or 5-2 MHz curvilinear) was used to visualize the subclavian vein.

Imaging of the superficial venous system was primarily performed with a high frequency scanner (12-10 or 10-5 MHz) which affords better B-mode resolution and greater accuracy in the detection of intraluminal webs and synechiae. The superficial system was assessed for compressibility and diameter measurement of the vein in cross section at several levels. The cephalic vein was evaluated from the wrist to the cephalic-subclavian junction. If the cephalic vein at the wrist was <2 mm in diameter with outflow occlusion, it was not considered large enough to be used. The basilic vein was studied at the upper forearm, elbow, and arm. Upper-arm veins greater than 3 mm in diameter were considered adequate for placement of AVF. Additionally, the length of the basilic vein from antecubital fossa to the junction with the deep venous system was measured to evaluate whether the basilic vein length was acceptable for transposition. Visualization of the superficial venous system was facilitated by application of a tourniquet at the upper arm. Segments of poorly compressible segments of vein or veins with intraluminal webs in the antecubital fossa were not considered for creation of AVF. Preoperative skin marking was performed in obese patients, particularly for brachial–basilic or brachial–cephalic fistulae and for those with previous AVGs.

ANESTHESIA

Because of the overall general medical condition of these patients, we attempted to use general anesthesia as little as possible. Instead, local or, more recently, regional anesthesia has been emphasized. Regional anesthesia consisted of a combination axillary and interscalene block (AXIS). The department of anesthesia performed the block by using a nerve stimulator set at below 0.5 mA to localize the brachial plexus. Thirty milliliters of a mixture of lidocaine 1.5% and ropivacaine 0.5% in equal portions was injected at each site. After the block, the arm was completely anesthetic and paralyzed for 3 to 6 hours, and the patient required minimal sedation. Rarely, if the block was not complete, minimal additional local anesthesia was required. We have noted that the venodilatation that occurs as a result of the sympathetic block resulted in a 50% to 100% increase in the diameter of the veins of the entire arm as documented by duplex. This venodilatation facilitated visualization of more distal veins that were not appreciated and that might be acceptable for formation of a fistula. We have noted no instances of systemic toxicity, hematomas, or nerve injury from the block.

TECHNIQUE OF BRACHIOCEPHALIC ARTERIOVENOUS FISTULAE

The cephalic vein at the level of the elbow was mobilized and the brachial artery exposed using a separate incision or through the same incision, depending on whether the biceps muscle was small enough to allow the brachial artery to be easily accessible through the same incision. The cephalic vein was gently dilated with heparinized saline. The vein was passed through a subcutaneous tunnel, maintaining its axial orientation, and an end-to-side anastomosis was created. In cases where the overlying subcutaneous tissue was greater than 1 cm, the cephalic vein was mobilized up to the shoulder and transposed to a more superficial position to make it more accessible for access. The fistula was allowed to mature for 4 to 6 weeks before cannulation.

TECHNIQUE OF BRACHIOBASILIC ARTERIOVENOUS FISTULAE

The basilic vein of the upper arm was exposed through a medial longitudinal incision. Care was taken not to injure the medial cutaneous nerve of the arm during vein dissection. All branches of the vein were isolated, ligated, and divided. Occasionally, broad and short communicating veins required transection and repair with fine vascular sutures to avoid compromising the lumen of basilic or brachial veins The basilic vein was mobilized up to its junction with the brachial vein. In cases where the basilic vein joined the brachial vein in the middle upper arm and a second brachial vein was patent and of adequate caliber, the basilic and brachial veins were used in combination to form the fistula. The brachial artery at the level of the elbow was exposed using the same incision (12). The basilic vein was transected close to the elbow and distended with heparinized saline solution. A subcutaneous tunnel was created using an aortic cross clamp on the anterior aspect of the arm, maintaining its axial orientation; the vein was passed through this tunnel. An end-to-side anastomosis was created using 6-0 polypropylene suture using a four-quadrant technique. Additional care was taken to secure hemostasis at the end of the procedure.

Patients were followed with duplex ultrasonography and physical examinations. Hospital, office, and dialysis center charts and the Social Security Death Index were reviewed. Follow-up was obtained by telephone interviews. Because of incomplete data, two patients were not included in the analysis.

STATISTICAL ANALYSIS

Fistula patency rates were determined by the life-table method of analysis using the statistical formulae recommended by the Ad Hoc Committee on Reporting Standards, Society for Vascular Surgery/North American Chapter, and International Society for Cardiovascular Surgery (13). Log-rank comparison for statistically significant differences ($p < 0.05$) between life-table groups was performed with SPSS (version 9.0, SPSS Science, Inc., Chicago, IL, U.S.A.). Log-rank test was performed in conjunction with Kaplan-Meier survival analysis.

TABLE 14.1. PRIMARY PATENCY OF BRACHIOBASILIC ARTERIOVENOUS FISTULA

Interval Start Time	No. Entering this Interval	No. Withdrawn during Interval	No. Exposed to Risk	No. of Terminal Events	Proportion Terminating	Cumulative Proportion Surviving	Proportion Surviving at End	Probability Density	Hazard Rate	SE of Cumulative Surviving	SE of Probability Density	SE of Hazard Rate
0.0	63.0	11.0	57.5	5.0	0.0870	0.9130	0.9130	0.0290	0.0303	0.0372	0.0124	0.0135
3.0	47.0	9.0	42.5	5.0	0.1176	0.8824	0.8056	0.0358	0.0417	0.0558	0.0151	0.0186
6.0	33.0	4.0	31.0	1.0	0.0323	0.9677	0.7796	0.0087	0.0109	0.0597	0.0085	0.0109
9.0	28.0	6.0	25.0	0.0	0.0000	1.0000	0.7796	0.0000	0.0000	0.0597	0.0000	0.0000
12.0	22.0	5.0	19.5	2.0	0.1026	0.8974	0.6997	0.0267	0.0360	0.0758	0.0180	0.0254
15.0	15.0	7.0	11.5	0.0	0.0000	1.0000	0.6997	0.0000	0.0000	0.0758	0.0000	0.0000
18.0	8.0	4.0	6.0	0.0	0.0000	1.0000	0.6997	0.0000	0.0000	0.0758	0.0000	0.0000
21.0	4.0	0.0	4.0	1.0	0.2500	0.7500	0.5248	0.0583	0.0952	0.1618	0.0509	0.0943
24.0	3.0	2.0	2.0	0.0	0.0000	1.0000	0.5248	0.0000	0.0000	0.1618	0.0000	0.0000
27.0	1.0	1.0	0.5	0.0	0.0000	1.0000	0.5248	0.0000	0.0000	0.1618	0.0000	0.0000

SE, standard error.

INTRAOPERATIVE FINDINGS

Five patients underwent exploration of the cephalic veins that were found to be inadequate and underwent placement of a BBAVF (Table 14.1). Two patients had a phlebitic basilic vein and underwent placement of a BCAVF. Three patients had attempted placement of a radial–cephalic AVF; however, the distal cephalic veins were found to be inadequate in these patients intraoperatively, and therefore a BCAVF was performed.

COMPLICATIONS

During the postoperative period, hematoma evacuation was required in five and seven patients in the BCAVF and BBAVF groups, respectively. One patient required hematoma drainage after revision of a BCAVF. One additional BCAVF patient had a repair of a pseudoaneurysm (Table 14.2).

Three patients, all diabetic women who underwent BBAVF placement, developed steal syndrome that was severe enough to necessitate intervention. Two of these patients underwent revascularization; one of these underwent eventual ligation of the fistula. An additional patient underwent ligation of the fistula (Table 14.3).

PATENCY

Follow-up was up to 30 months (mean 364 ± 20 days, 347 ± 28 days for each group, $p > 0.05$). No thrombosed AVF underwent thrombolysis or thrombectomy. In each group, 12% and 6% of the patients had thrombosis of their AVF during the follow-up ($p = 0.2$), respectively. To maintain patency and adequate flows during dialysis, five BBAVF patients required balloon angioplasties, and two required patch angioplasties. Of the BCAVF patients, four required a balloon angioplasty, four required a patch angioplasty, two underwent transposition to a more superficial location, and one

TABLE 14.2. LIFE TABLE FOR BRACHIOCEPHALIC ARTERIOVENOUS FISTULA

Interval Start Time	No. Entering this Interval	No. Withdrawn during Interval	No. Exposed to Risk	No. of Terminal Events	Proportion Terminating	Cumulative Proportion Surviving	Proportion Surviving at End	Probability Density	Hazard Rate	SE of Cumulative Surviving	SE of Probability Density	SE of Hazard Rate
0.0	108.0	18.0	99.0	4.0	0.0404	0.9596	0.9596	0.0135	0.0137	0.0198	0.0066	0.0069
3.0	86.0	9.0	81.5	5.0	0.0613	0.9387	0.9007	0.0196	0.0211	0.0316	0.0085	0.0094
6.0	72.0	12.0	66.0	2.0	0.0303	0.9697	0.8734	0.0091	0.0103	0.0360	0.0063	0.0073
9.0	58.0	18.0	49.0	7.0	0.1429	0.8571	0.7487	0.0416	0.0513	0.0535	0.0147	0.0193
12.0	33.0	9.0	28.5	1.0	0.0351	0.9649	0.7224	0.0088	0.0119	0.0577	0.0086	0.0119
15.0	23.0	3.0	21.5	5.0	0.2326	0.7674	0.5544	0.0560	0.0877	0.0793	0.0224	0.0389
18.0	15.0	4.0	13.0	1.0	0.0769	0.9231	0.5117	0.0142	0.0267	0.0839	0.0138	0.0266
21.0	10.0	3.0	8.5	1.0	0.1176	0.8824	0.4515	0.0201	0.0417	0.0932	0.0191	0.0416
24.0	6.0	3.0	4.5	0.0	0.0000	1.0000	0.4515	0.0000	0.0000	0.0932	0.0000	0.0000
27.0	3.0	3.0	1.5	0.0	0.0000	1.0000	0.4515	0.0000	0.0000	0.0932	0.0000	0.0000

SE, standard error.

TABLE 14.3. SURVIVAL VARIABLE FOR DIABETES MELLITUS

Interval Start Time	No. Entering this Interval	No. Withdrawn during Interval	No. Exposed to Risk	No. of Terminal Events	Proportion Terminating	Cumulative Proportion Surviving	Proportion Surviving at End	Probability Density	Hazard Rate	SE of Cumulative Surviving	SE of Probability Density	SE of Hazard Rate
0.0	70.0	6.0	67.0	5.0	0.0746	0.9254	0.9254	0.0249	0.0258	0.0321	0.0107	0.0115
3.0	59.0	6.0	56.0	5.0	0.0893	0.9107	0.8428	0.0275	0.0312	0.0458	0.0118	0.0139
6.0	48.0	5.0	45.5	1.0	0.0220	0.9780	0.8242	0.0062	0.0074	0.0484	0.0061	0.0074
9.0	42.0	13.0	35.5	5.0	0.1408	0.8592	0.7081	0.0387	0.0505	0.0636	0.0162	0.0225
12.0	24.0	3.0	22.5	3.0	0.1333	0.8667	0.6137	0.0315	0.0476	0.0749	0.0172	0.0247
15.0	18.0	6.0	15.0	2.0	0.1333	0.8667	0.5319	0.0273	0.0476	0.0844	0.0183	0.0336
18.0	10.0	2.0	9.0	0.0	0.0000	1.0000	0.5319	0.0000	0.0000	0.0844	0.0000	0.0000
21.0	8.0	1.0	7.5	0.0	0.0000	1.0000	0.5319	0.0000	0.0000	0.0844	0.0000	0.0000
24.0	7.0	4.0	5.0	0.0	0.0000	1.0000	0.5319	0.0000	0.0000	0.0844	0.0000	0.0000
27.0	3.0	3.0	1.5	0.0	0.0000	1.0000	0.5319	0.0000	0.0000	0.0844	0.0000	0.0000

SE, standard error.

underwent both patch angioplasty and balloon angioplasty of two separate lesions. One additional patient underwent balloon angioplasty of the junction of the cephalic vein and the subclavian vein, and one underwent extension to the internal jugular vein for subclavian vein thrombosis.

Log-rank analysis failed to reveal any statistical differences between BAVF and BCAVF primary patency (Fig. 14.1). The primary patency rates of BCAVF and BBAVF were 72% and 70%, respectively, at 12 months postoperatively ($p = 0.54$). The data for primary assisted patency consisted of very limited numbers and were not able to yield significant results. The patients without diabetes did seem to have better patency compared with those with diabetes

(Fig. 14.2) ($p = 0.01$). In these sets of data, no statistical differences in patency were found for sex or age and presence of hypertension. If the patients had undergone a prior fistula placement, they seemed to have a worse patency (Fig. 14.3) ($p = 0.02$). No clear differences could be found with BBAVF and BCAVF with and without diabetes mellitus or hypertension.

Although large published series have described experience with the management of failed or failing prosthetic AVGs for hemodialysis, there are scant data regarding failing AVF. To analyze the management of nonfunctioning or nonmaturing (AVFs), we recently reviewed our experience with salvage procedures for all AVF in a separate series.

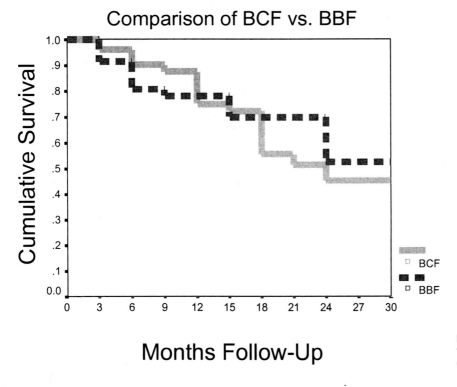

FIGURE 14.1. Brachial–basilic arteriovenous fistula (BBAVF) versus brachial–cephalic arteriovenous fistula (BCAVF) primary patency.

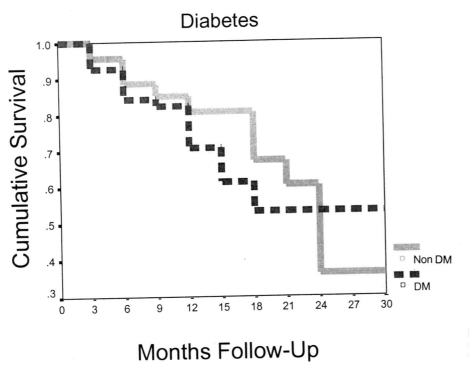

FIGURE 14.2. Diabetes mellitus (*DM*) versus non-DM for upper-arm arteriovenous fistula.

These included radiocephalic AVFs. Of the 378 AVFs placed at our institution in 338 patients from June 1997 to June 2000, 47 (12%) have undergone revisions. Twenty-one patients have undergone vein patch angioplasty, and 12 have undergone balloon angioplasty. Three underwent vein interposition, and four underwent revision of the fistula to a more proximal level. Extended salvage procedures consisted of four turndowns to the basilic vein for proximal cephalic vein thrombosis or stenosis and three extension bypasses to the jugular vein or the contralateral axillary for subclavian vein thrombosis. Follow-up ranged from 1 to 36 months (mean of 13 months). Primary patency of the vein

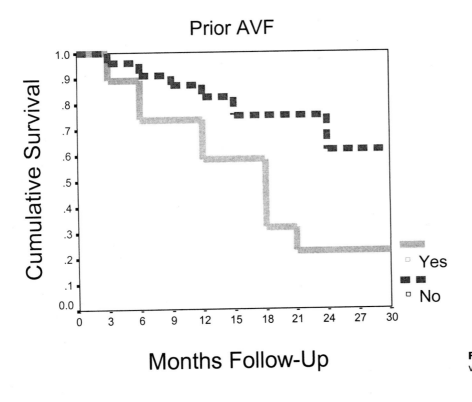

FIGURE 14.3. Prior arteriovenous fistula (*AVF*) versus non-prior AVF.

patch angioplasty was significantly better compared with balloon angioplasty ($p = 0.002$) by life-table analysis. The patency rates after revision of a forearm fistula and upper-arm fistula were not statistically different. One interposition failed during the follow-up, and all four revisions to a more proximal level are functional. Two of the turndown procedures had thrombosed at 2 and 11 months. The remaining two have remained functional at 1 and 24 months. One extension thrombosed at 8 months, whereas the two others have remained functional at 5 and 10 months.

DISCUSSION

As the ESRD population continues to grow (14) and an increasing emphasis is focused on the placement of autogenous accesses for hemodialysis, surgeons can anticipate evaluating more and more patients in the future in whom the distal cephalic veins are not available. These trends suggest that alternative options need to be explored. Whereas the distal basilic vein can be transposed to the volar forearm to form a fistula (15), there are times when these veins also have been damaged by thrombosis or repeated cannulation.

Other options, such as the BCAVF and BBAVF, were first described in 1970 and 1976, respectively (16,17). Despite the length of time since these first descriptions, scant current information exists describing a large series that compares the two fistulae with a detailed analysis. The few prior investigators who have compared BBAVF and BCAVF suggested that these AVFs have similar 1- and 2-year patencies ranging from 60% to 80% (6,8,12). These studies, however, consisted of a limited number of patients in each group.

During our AVF placement experience, we noted some advantages and disadvantages of each type of fistula. On the one hand, the basilic vein tends to be of a larger diameter compared with the cephalic vein. Furthermore, the basilic vein is less accessible for venipuncture before transposition because of its deep location. Consequently, the basilic vein tends to be involved with less thrombosis and postphlebitic state compared with the cephalic vein. On occasion, patients have stated that they prefer, from a cosmetic viewpoint, the medial incision on the upper arm for the BBAVF compared with the anterior–lateral incision of the BCAVF.

The basilic vein is shorter than the cephalic vein, especially if it joins the brachial vein very low in the upper arm. We also found, in our experience, that steal syndrome tends to be more prevalent with BBAVF compared with BCAVF ($p = 0.02$), most probably because of the larger diameter of the vein. In addition, more severe atherosclerotic arterial disease in these patients that may have resulted in multiple prior failed access procedures and led these patients to now undergo a BBAVF placement also may be a contributing factor to steal syndrome.

On the other hand, the BCAVF also allows a long length of vein for access. Additionally, placement of a BCAVF entails less dissection unless a long segment of cephalic vein needs to be mobilized to translocate the vein closer to the skin as is the case in obese patients.

In addition, because some of these AVFs will fail and ESRD patients have an increasing life span, future options for placement of access need to taken into account when considering placement of access. Placement of a BBAVF may make future access procedures much more difficult in the upper arm because of scar formation over the length of the brachial artery and vein. Conversely, initial construction of a BCAVF still allows enough undissected brachial artery to allow the later placement of a BBAVF. Based on these observations, one may chose to place a BCAVF before a BBAVF.

Placement of these upper-arm fistulae does not preclude future placement of an AVG if the AVF fails. We found that placement of upper-extremity AVGs often results in thrombosis or stenosis of the upper-arm superficial and deep veins making future placement of an AVF more demanding. Therefore, we preferentially place an autogenous AVF pending exhaustion of all other options before AVG placement, as occurred in three patients during this experience.

The analysis of the patency rates suggests equivalency between these two types of fistulae; however, this needs to be confirmed with longer-term follow-up. The subgroup analysis suggested an advantage to patients without diabetes correlating with prior data for radial–cephalic AVFs and AVGs (18,19) (Table 14.4). These data are in contrast to prior reviewers who were unable to identify subgroups of patients with upper-arm AVF with improved patencies (20,21). This may have been due to the relatively small sample size of these studies. The inferior patency of patients with prior AVF may represent patients with more severe atherosclerotic disease, smaller arteries, or more damaged veins.

Although follow-up is limited in these data, they do suggest that simple and extended salvage procedures may allow maturation and add to the life span of arteriovenous AVF for hemodialysis. Based on this experience of revisions of AVF, we do suggest that screening for occult stenosis in a functional AVF with regularly scheduled duplex imaging may be a future area for investigation. Despite the fact that we tended to perform balloon angioplasty on the shorter focal lesions and reserve patch angioplasty for the longer lesions, these data also suggest an advantage for patch angioplasty compared with percutaneous techniques. This led us to discontinue using percutaneous techniques for easily accessible lesions.

These patency data do not necessarily offer guidelines to which type of AVF is superior in each situation; however, based on the experience that we have gained, we can make some suggestions. If a radial–cephalic AVF is not feasible, we attempt to place a BCAVF. If this is not possible or has failed, then a BBAVF is placed before an AVG is placed. In this manner, we try to maximize future options, increase the patency of the access, and minimize the complications and costs (Table 14.5).

TABLE 14.4. LIFE TABLE FOR NON–DIABETES MELLITUS

Interval Start Time	No. Entering this Interval	No. Withdrawn during Interval	No. Exposed to Risk	No. of Terminal Events	Proportion Terminating	Cumulative Proportion Surviving	Proportion Surviving at End	Probability Density	Hazard Rate	SE of Cumulative Surviving	SE of Probability Density	SE of Hazard Rate
0.0	101.0	23.0	89.5	4.0	0.0447	0.9553	0.9553	0.0149	0.0152	0.0218	0.0073	0.0076
3.0	74.0	12.0	68.0	5.0	0.0735	0.9265	0.8851	0.0234	0.0254	0.0364	0.0101	0.0114
6.0	57.0	11.0	51.5	2.0	0.0388	0.9612	0.8507	0.0115	0.0132	0.0423	0.0080	0.0093
9.0	44.0	11.0	38.5	2.0	0.0519	0.9481	0.8065	0.0147	0.0178	0.0504	0.0102	0.0126
12.0	31.0	11.0	25.5	0.0	0.0000	1.0000	0.8065	0.0000	0.0000	0.0504	0.0000	0.0000
15.0	20.0	4.0	18.0	3.0	0.1667	0.8333	0.6721	0.0448	0.0606	0.0823	0.0238	0.0348
18.0	13.0	6.0	10.0	1.0	0.1000	0.9000	0.6049	0.0224	0.0351	0.0978	0.0214	0.0350
21.0	6.0	2.0	5.0	2.0	0.4000	0.6000	0.3629	0.0807	0.1667	0.1449	0.0461	0.1141
24.0	2.0	1.0	1.5	0.0	0.0000	1.0000	0.3629	0.0000	0.0000	0.1449	0.0000	0.0000
27.0	1.0	1.0	0.5	0.0	0.0000	1.0000	0.3629	0.0000	0.0000	0.1449	0.0000	0.0000

SE, standard error.

Because the Dialysis Outcome Quality Initiative (DOQI) guidelines do advocate that each patient be evaluated for placement of AVF after AVG thrombosis (1), it must be appreciated that placement of an AVF in the ipsilateral extremity after AVG thrombosis does entail certain nuances. Preoperative duplex imaging was used to assess the axillosubclavian vein. Although none of these studies revealed areas of stenosis or thrombosis of the axillosubclavian vein, which might have contributed to AVG thrombosis, we believe it should continue to be an integral part of the preoperative evaluation of patients with thrombosed angioaccess undergoing placement of a new angioaccess in the same extremity. Occasionally, a portion of an overlying prior thrombosed AVG was resected to obtain an adequate length of the upper-arm cephalic vein for angioaccess. In these instances, the overall results of these patients did not vary significantly from that of the overall group of AVF. Whereas this information base is limited, it does suggest that patients with prior AVG placement can enter this protocol and enjoy good results (Table 14.6).

The placement of a tunneled dialysis catheter allows time for maturation of the fistula or revision of the fistula, if needed, but the catheter placement also adds a small but not insignificant risk to the procedure in both the short and long term. These catheters should be placed on the contralateral side whenever possible because of the small incidence of innominate vein stenosis that we have noted in our series. The DOQI guidelines recommend that patients be referred for angioaccess placement when their creatinine level is greater than 4.0 mg per deciliter, their creatinine clearance rate is below 25 mL per minute, or when they are within 1 year of anticipated need for dialysis (1). In the data presented, only 9% of the patients did not need a catheter placed for dialysis prior to fistula maturation. This obviously indicates that patients are not being referred early enough in their disease process to avoid the use of a dialysis catheter. Greater emphasis on these guidelines by primary care providers for earlier referrals clearly needs to be undertaken to initiate the protocol before urgent dialysis is needed.

TABLE 14.5. LIFE TABLE FOR NON–PRIOR ARTERIOVENOUS FISTULA

Interval Start Time	No. Entering this Interval	No. Withdrawn during Interval	No. Exposed to Risk	No. of Terminal Events	Proportion Terminating	Cumulative Proportion Surviving	Proportion Surviving at End	Probability Density	Hazard Rate	SE of Cumulative Surviving	SE of Probability Density	SE of Hazard Rate
0.0	133.0	26.0	120.0	5.0	0.0417	0.9583	0.9583	0.0139	0.0142	0.0182	0.0061	0.0063
3.0	102.0	14.0	95.0	5.0	0.0526	0.9474	0.9079	0.0168	0.0180	0.0279	0.0073	0.0081
6.0	83.0	14.0	76.0	3.0	0.0395	0.9605	0.8721	0.0119	0.0134	0.0336	0.0068	0.0077
9.0	66.0	22.0	55.0	3.0	0.0545	0.9455	0.8245	0.0159	0.0187	0.0415	0.0089	0.0108
12.0	41.0	13.0	34.5	3.0	0.0870	0.9130	0.7528	0.0239	0.0303	0.0548	0.0132	0.0175
15.0	25.0	6.0	22.0	0.0	0.0000	1.0000	0.7528	0.0000	0.0000	0.0548	0.0000	0.0000
18.0	19.0	7.0	15.5	0.0	0.0000	1.0000	0.7528	0.0000	0.0000	0.0548	0.0000	0.0000
21.0	12.0	2.0	11.0	2.0	0.1818	0.8182	0.6159	0.0456	0.0667	0.0984	0.0294	0.0469
24.0	8.0	5.0	5.5	0.0	0.0000	1.0000	0.6159	0.0000	0.0000	0.0984	0.0000	0.0000
27.0	3.0	3.0	1.5	0.0	0.0000	1.0000	0.6159	0.0000	0.0000	0.0984	0.0000	0.0000

SE, standard error.

TABLE 14.6. LIFE TABLE FOR PRIOR ARTERIOVENOUS FISTULA

Interval Start Time	No. Entering this Interval	No. Withdrawn during Interval	No. Exposed to Risk	No. of Terminal Events	Proportion Terminating	Cumulative Proportion Surviving	Proportion Surviving at End	Probability Density	Hazard Rate	SE of Cumulative Surviving	SE of Probability Density	SE of Hazard Rate
0.0	38.0	3.0	36.5	4.0	0.1096	0.8904	0.8904	0.0365	0.0386	0.0517	0.0172	0.0193
3.0	31.0	4.0	29.0	5.0	0.1724	0.8276	0.7369	0.0512	0.0629	0.0757	0.0210	0.0280
6.0	22.0	2.0	21.0	0.0	0.0000	1.0000	0.7369	0.0000	0.0000	0.0757	0.0000	0.0000
9.0	20.0	2.0	19.0	4.0	0.2105	0.7895	0.5818	0.0517	0.0784	0.0912	0.0236	0.0389
12.0	14.0	1.0	13.5	0.0	0.0000	1.0000	0.5818	0.0000	0.0000	0.0912	0.0000	0.0000
15.0	13.0	4.0	11.0	5.0	0.4545	0.5455	0.3173	0.0881	0.1961	0.1005	0.0322	0.0838
18.0	4.0	1.0	3.5	1.0	0.2857	0.7143	0.2267	0.0302	0.1111	0.1050	0.0273	0.1096
21.0	2.0	1.0	1.5	0.0	0.0000	1.0000	0.2267	0.0000	0.0000	0.1050	0.0000	0.0000
24.0	1.0	0.0	1.0	0.0	0.0000	1.0000	0.2267	0.0000	0.0000	0.1050	0.0000	0.0000
27.0	1.0	1.0	0.5	0.0	0.0000	1.0000	0.2267	0.0000	0.0000	0.1050	0.0000	0.0000

SE, standard error.

These data do suggest that these types of AVF compare favorably to AVGs and should be constructed for hemodialysis access whenever feasible. They also suggest that the decreased need for intervention for AVFs compared with AVGs may have an impact on overall cost of the access and quality of life of these patients, although these issues have not been addressed specifically. In this manner, these data also support the guidelines issued by the National Kidney Foundation's DOQI (1). Several differences do exist, however. Based on these data, a goal of greater than 50% of new placement of AVF for access and a prevalence of AVF of 40% suggested by DOQI can be easily surpassed with an aggressive program focused on an all-autogenous policy as documented by multiple studies (17,19,22). In contrast to DOQI, we suggest that a BBAVF should be performed before placement of an AVG because BBAVFs seem to have a lower complication rate and fewer thromboses (2,23). Finally, venography for preoperative evaluation of upper-extremity veins was used in none of the patients in our review. In our opinion, venography entails a risk of damage to veins that are being studied, is expensive, and does not always fully evaluate the upper-arm veins well. We have used duplex ultrasonography and magnetic resonance imaging for upper-extremity veins and central veins with good results and believe that venography is very rarely indicated.

REFERENCES

1. The Vascular Access Work Group. NKF-DOQI clinical practice guidelines for vascular access. *Am J Kidney Dis* 1997;30(Suppl 3):S150–S191.
2. Ascher E, Gade P, Hingorani A, et al. Changes in the practice of angioaccess surgery: impact of dialysis outcome and quality initiative recommendations. *J Vasc Surg* 2000;31:84–92.
3. Rivers SP, Scher LA, Sheehan E, et al. Basilic vein transposition: an underused autologous alternative to prosthetic dialysis angioaccess. *J Vasc Surg* 1993;18:391–396.
4. Rubens F, Wellington JL. Brachiocephalic fistula: a useful alternative for vascular access in chronic hemodialysis. *Cardiovasc Surg* 1993;1:128–130.
5. Butterworth PC, Doughman TM, Wheatley TJ, et al. Arteriovenous fistula using transposed basilic vein. *Br J Surg* 1998;85:653–654.
6. Elcheroth J, de Pauw L, Kinnaert P. Elbow arteriovenous fistulas for chronic haemodialysis. *Br J Surg* 1994;81:982–984.
7. Humphries AL Jr, Colborn GL, Wynn JJ. Elevated basilic vein arteriovenous fistula. *Am J Surg* 1999;177:489–499.
8. Livingston CK, Potts JR 3rd. Upper arm arteriovenous fistulas as a reliable access alternative for patients requiring chronic hemodialysis. *Am Surg* 1999;65:1038–1042.
9. Matsuura JH, Rosenthal D, Clark M, et al. Transposed basilic vein versus polytetrafluoroethylene for brachial-axillary arteriovenous fistulas. *Am J Surg* 1998;176:219–221.
10. Coburn MC, Carney W. Comparison of basilic vein and polytetrafluoroethylene for brachial arteriovenous fistula. *J Vasc Surg* 1994;20:896–902.
11. Silva MB Jr, Hobson RW 2nd, Pappas PJ, et al. A strategy for increasing use of autogenous hemodialysis access procedures: impact of preoperative noninvasive evaluation. *J Vasc Surg* 1998;27: 302–307.
12. Hakaim AG, Nalbandian M, Scott T. Superior maturation and patency of primary brachiocephalic and transposed basilic vein arteriovenous fistulae in patients with diabetes. *J Vasc Surg* 1998; 27:154–157.
13. Ad Hoc Committee on Reporting Standards, Society for Vascular Surgery/North American Chapter, International Society for Cardiovascular Surgery. Suggested standards for reports dealing with lower extremity ischemia. *J Vasc Surg* 1986 Jul;4: 80–94.
14. Excerpts from United States Renal Data System 1999 Annual Data Report. The National Institutes of Health, National Institute of Diabetes and Digestive and Kidney Diseases. *Am J Kidney Dis* 1999;34:S1–S176.
15. Silva MB Jr, Hobson RW 2nd, Pappas PJ, et al. Vein transposition in the forearm for autogenous hemodialysis access. *J Vasc Surg* 1997;26:981–986.

16. Dagher F, Gelber R, Ramos E, et al. The use of basilic vein and brachial artery as an A-V fistula for long term hemodialysis. *J Surg Res* 1976;20:373–376.

17. Carcardo S, Acchiardo S, Beven E. Proximal arteriovenous fistulas for hemodialysis when radial arteries are not available. *Proc Eur Dial Transplant Assoc* 1970;7:42.

18. Lazarides MK, Iatrou CE, Karanikas ID, et al. Factors affecting the lifespan of autologous and synthetic arteriovenous access routes for haemodialysis. *Eur J Surg* 1996;162:297–301.

19. Windus DW. The effect of comorbid conditions on hemodialysis access patency. *Adv Ren Replace Ther* 1994;1:148–154.

20. Bender MH, Bruyninckx CM, Gerlag PG. The brachiocephalic elbow fistula: a useful alternative angioaccess for permanent hemodialysis. *J Vasc Surg* 1994;20:808–813.

21. Zibari GB, Rohr MS, Landreneau MD, et al. Complications from permanent hemodialysis vascular access. *Surgery* 1988;104:681–686.

22. Burger H, Kootstra G, de Charro F, et al. A survey of vascular access for haemodialysis in The Netherlands. *Nephrol Dial Transplant* 1991;6:5–10.

23. Coburn MC, Carney WI Jr. Comparison of basilic vein and polytetrafluoroethylene for brachial arteriovenous fistula. *J Vasc Surg* 1994;20:896–902.

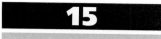

15

OVERVIEW OF COMPLICATIONS AND MANAGEMENT AFTER VASCULAR ACCESS CREATION

HARRY SCHANZER

For a patient on hemodialysis, vascular access is an essential aspect of his or her well-being and survival. Technically, creation of these accesses may be simple, but their long-term function often is threatened by varying and frequent complications. Handling these problems is challenging and requires knowledge in the management of vascular complications, good judgment, creativity, and technical proficiency. The goal of long-term patency can be achieved only by properly treating the expected complications.

The following chapter deals with complications of native arteriovenous (AV) fistulas and prosthetic bridge AV fistulas. The complications of central dialysis catheters are covered in Chapters 35 and 36. It is the aim of the present section to explore these complications, understand their etiology and pathophysiology, get to know the subtleties of their clinical presentation, and based on all of this knowledge, help to decide the best therapy. (See also Chapter 18 for physical findings of complications.)

COMPLICATIONS OF NATIVE ARTERIOVENOUS FISTULAS

Complications of autologous AV fistulas (see also Chapter 31) include the following:

1. Thrombosis
2. Infections
3. Aneurysms
4. Hand edema
5. Hand ischemia

Fistula Thrombosis

This is the most common AV fistula complication. Early thrombosis within 4 weeks after surgical construction is usually due to error in technique or judgment. Common problems are inadequate anastomosis, kinking of the vein just proximal to the anastomosis, or undetected occlusion of the venous outflow. An inadequate arterial inflow due to proximal arterial disease can also produce early failure. Simple thrombectomy of the fistula, without correcting the primary problem that produced the failure, inevitably will result in rethrombosis. Late occlusion is most commonly due to progressive stenosis at the anastomosis or in the vein as it leaves the anastomosis, secondary to intimal hyperplasia. Another common cause of venous stenosis is fibrosis of the vein in an area that has been abused by repeated traumatic needle punctures. Correction of this problem usually can be accomplished by doing a new AV fistula just proximal to the area of stenosis. This can be done as long as the proximal vein remains patent.

Infection

Primary infection of the wound is extremely rare. If it occurs, it has to be treated aggressively because it poses the potential danger of anastomotic breakdown and massive bleeding. Superficial erythema and cellulitis can be treated with intravenous antibiotics. The presence of frank pus involving the anastomosis requires open drainage and ligation of the fistula (proximal and distal arterial ligation). Late infections are usually due to a break in aseptic technique during cannulation of the fistula. Because there is no foreign body, these infections usually respond well to drainage and antibiotic therapy.

Aneurysm Formation

Aneurysmal dilatation of the vein is quite common in AV fistulas. The high-pressure flow present in a vein weakened by repeated punctures is responsible for this abnormality. This complication produces little in terms of symptoms or potential problems. The main problem is a cosmetically unappealing appearance. An aneurysmatic fistula can continue to provide excellent hemodialysis access for many years. If possible, cannulation should be avoided in the area of the aneurysm. Correction by excision or exclusion should be attempted only if there is erosion of the covering skin or significant progressive growth.

Hand Edema

This is a rare complication of AV fistula. Previously, hand edema occurred more commonly with the use of side-to-side anastomoses for AV fistula creation. Usually, it occurs late in the course of AV fistula and is due to distal venous hypertension secondary to obstruction of the outflow vein with persistence of flow in the distal vein. Often, venous tributaries that have dilated and become incompetent perfuse toward the hand, producing capillary hypertension. If this problem is not treated, development of a classic chronic venous stasis syndrome of the hand with edema, pigmentation, and ulceration can occur. Treatment is simple and consists of repair of the fistula outflow and, if not possible, ligation of the fistula. A dramatic and immediate improvement occurs after performing these corrections.

Hand Ischemia

Symptoms and signs of arterial insufficiency in the distal extremity after AV fistula are rare (about 1%). It is more common after upper-arm AV fistula creation. Its clinical presentation, pathophysiology, and treatment are discussed extensively in the following section on bridge AV fistulas (See also Chapter 18).

COMPLICATIONS OF PROSTHETIC BRIDGE ARTERIOVENOUS FISTULAS

Complications of prosthetic bridge AV fistulas include the following:

1. Thrombosis
2. Swelling
3. Infection
4. Aneurysm
5. Seroma
6. Cardiac failure
7. Ischemia

Thrombosis

Thrombosis is the most common complication of bridge AV fistulas. Systemic causes such as hypotension and hypercoagulability can produce thrombosis anytime in the life of the access. Early thrombosis usually is due to technical errors in the performance of the access (poor anastomosis, kinking of the graft, poor in-flow or out-flow). In a well-established access, the most common cause of thrombosis is stenosis at the venous anastomosis site and occasionally stenosis of the vein several centimeters beyond the anastomosis, secondary to intimal hyperplasia (see Chapter 8). Stenoses of the arterial anastomosis or graft defects due to the trauma produced by multiple punctures are less common. Successful treatment must include correction of the original defect that caused the thrombosis.

Swelling

Early postoperative swelling is a very common finding following creation of a prosthetic bridge AV fistula. It results from venous hypertension and, as collaterals develop and outflow improves, it rapidly disappears. Arm elevation and patient reassurance are usually enough. Persistence of very severe swelling suggests obstruction of a major outflow vein (axillary–subclavian–innominate vein). An angiogram will document this clinical impression. This condition can be treated by primary balloon angioplasty, balloon angioplasty plus stenting, extending the graft to a vein beyond the obstruction (i.e., internal jugular vein in case of subclavian obstruction), or by ligating the graft. Late swelling is usually due to central vein (axillary, subclavian, or innominate vein) stenosis or obstruction. In this particular situation, the causative factor is intima hyperplasia that results from either the turbulent flow draining the bridge AV fistula or trauma to the vein wall induced by previously placed indwelling catheters. The clinical presentation can vary from simple swelling to advanced changes of chronic venous stasis with pigmentation, indurated swelling, and ulcerations. Diagnosis is supported by the presence of venous collaterals around the shoulder and is documented by fistula angiography. Treatment again consists of balloon angioplasty alone or with stenting, extension of the graft to an unobstructed vein, or access ligation [the Dialysis Outcome Quality Initiative (DOQI) guidelines recommend only angioplasty and stents for central lesions. See treatment in Chapter 25].

Infection

This is a serious and potentially lethal complication of access surgery. In bridge AV fistulas, the presence of a foreign material makes the complication even more difficult to treat. The infection can result from a breakdown in sterility during surgery or as a consequence of poor sterile technique during cannulation. Agents most commonly responsible are skin pathogens (*Staphylococcus aureus, Staphylococcus epidermidis*). The surgical-wound infection can be superficial or deep. The former can be treated successfully with aggressive local treatment (debridement of all infected and necrotic tissue and systemic antibiotics). If the infection is deep, involves the graft, and occurs soon after surgery (the graft is not well incorporated yet), treatment requires opening of the wound, debridement, systemic antibiotics, and excision of the whole graft with ligation of the artery. In the upper extremity, because of rich collaterals, ligation of the artery

AV fistula is to eliminate reversal of flow. The addition of the arterial bypass provides the distal vascular bed with normal perfusion pressure and flow. This technique has given excellent results, with immediate reversal of the ischemic condition while maintaining function of the access (25,26). In our view, it is the procedure of choice for the correction of ischemic steal induced by AV fistula/bridge AV fistula.

REFERENCES

1. Ayus JC, Sheikh-Hamad D. Silent infection in clotted hemodialysis access grafts. *J Am Soc Nephrol* 1998;9:1–6.
2. Bolton W, Cannon J. Seroma formation associates with PTFE vascular grafts used as arteriovenous fistulae. *Dialysis & Transplantation* 1981;10:60–63.
3. LeBlanc J, Albus R, Williams W, et al. Serous fluid leakage: a complication following the modified Blalock-Taussig shunt. *J Thorac Cardiovasc Surg* 1984;88:259–262.
4. Blumenberg RM, Gelfand M, Dale W. Perigraft seromas complicating arterial grafts. *Surgery* 1985;97:192–203.
5. Buche M, Schoevaerdts JC, Jaumin P, et al. Perigraft seroma following axillofemoral bypass: report of three cases. *Ann Vasc Surg* 1986;1:374–377.
6. Ahn S, Machleder H, Gupta R, et al. Pathogenesis of perigraft seroma: Evidence of a humoral fibroblast inhibitor. *Surg Forum* 1986;37:460–461.
7. Sladen J, Mandl M, Grossman L, et al. Fibroblast inhibition: a new and treatable cause of prosthetic graft failure. *Am J Surg* 1985;149:588–590.
8. Maitland A, Williams W, Coles JG, et al. A method of treating serous fluid leak from a polytetrafluoroethylene Blalock-Taussig shunt. *J Cardiovasc Surg* 1985;90:791–793.
9. Bosanac P, Bilder B, Grunberg RW, et al. Post-permanent access neuropathy. *Trans Am Soc Artif Intern Organs* 1977;23:162–167.
10. Kwun KB, Schanzer H, Finkler N, et al. Hemodynamic evaluation of angioaccess procedures for hemodialysis. *Vasc Surg* 1979;13:170–177.
11. Schanzer H, Schwartz M, Harrington E, et al. Treatment of ischemia due to "steal" by arteriovenous fistula with distal artery ligation and revascularization. *J Vasc Surg* 1988;7:770–773.
12. Duncan H, Ferguson L, Faris I. Incidence of the radial steal syndrome in patients with Brescia fistula for hemodialysis: its clinical significance. *J Vasc Surg* 1986;4:144–147.
13. Haimov M, Burrows L, Schanzer H, et al. Experience with arterial substitutes in the construction of vascular access for hemodialysis. *J Cardiovasc Surg* 1980;21:149–154.
14. Porter JA, Sharp WV, Walsh EJ. Complications of vascular access in a dialysis population. *Curr Surg* 1985;42:298–300.
15. Zibari GB, Rohr MS, Landreneau MD, et al. Complications from permanent hemodialysis vascular access. *Surgery* 1988;104:681–686.
16. Winsett OE, Wolma FJ. Complications of vascular access for hemodialysis. *South Med J* 1985;78:513–517.
17. Barnes RW. Hemodynamics for the vascular surgeon. *Arch Surg* 1980;115:216–223.
18. Bussell JA, Abbott JA, Lim RC. A radial steal syndrome with arteriovenous fistula for hemodialysis. *Ann Intern Med* 1971;75:387–394.
19. Corry RJ, Natvarlal PP, West JC. Surgical management of complications of vascular access for hemodialysis. *Surg Gynecol Obstet* 1980;51:49–54.
20. Drasler WJ, Wilson GJ, Jenson ML, et al. Venturi grafts for hemodialysis access. *ASAIO Trans* 1990;36:M753–M760.
21. Khalil IM, Livingston DH. The management of steal syndrome occurring after access for dialysis. *J Vasc Surg* 1988;7:572–573.
22. Mattson WJ. Recognition and treatment of vascular steal secondary to hemodialysis prostheses. *Am J Surg* 1987;154:198–201.
23. West JC, Bertsch DJ, Peterson SL, et al. Arterial insufficiency in hemodialysis access procedures: correction by "banding" technique. *Transplant Proc* 1991;23:1838–1840.
24. West JC, Evans RD, Kelley SE, et al. Arterial insufficiency in hemodialysis access procedures: reconstruction by an interposition polytetrafluoroethylene graft conduit. *Am J Surg* 1987;153:300–301.
25. Jendrisak MD, Anderson CB. Vascular access in patients with arterial insufficiency. *Ann Surg* 1990;212:187–193.
26. Schanzer H, Skladany M, Haimov M. Treatment of angioaccess-induced ischemia by revascularization. *J Vasc Surg* 1992;16:861–866.
27. Schanzer H, Skladany M, Knight R, et al. Ischemia following angioaccess surgery. In: Veigh F, ed. *Current critical problems in vascular surgery*, vol 7. Quality Medical Publishing, 1996:484–486.

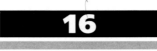

MANAGEMENT OF HEMODIALYSIS VASCULAR ACCESS INFECTIONS

KURT B. STEVENSON

The annual mortality rate reported among hemodialysis patients is 28% (1,2). Infections are the second most common cause of death, after cardiovascular disease, accounting for 15% of all deaths. Direct and repeated access to the vascular system to provide rapid extracorporeal blood flow is a required element for all chronic hemodialysis patients. Standard types of vascular access include native arteriovenous (AV) fistulae, synthetic AV bridge grafts, permanent tunneled cuffed central catheters, and temporary central catheters. Many hemodialysis-associated infections directly involve vascular access sites and account for increased hospitalizations and significant morbidity in addition to significant mortality (2–5). In one French study, 28% of all infections in the hemodialysis population involved the vascular access site (6). Other reports have demonstrated that the vascular access site may be responsible for 27% to 73% of all the bacteremias in hemodialysis patients (2,5,7–9). These often are associated with complicated and other metastatic infections (see section on "Complications" to follow). In addition, local infections (exit site, tunnel, and cellulitis) can occur without associated bacteremia.

This chapter reviews the risk factors and epidemiology, microbiologic etiology, complications, and management of infections associated with hemodialysis vascular access. Information on the importance of surveillance for vascular access infections by hemodialysis personnel is also presented. The reader is also referred to Chapter 35.

RISK FACTORS AND EPIDEMIOLOGY

Several studies over the past decade have examined the risk factors for developing infections, particularly bacteremia, in hemodialysis patients (4,10–15). A prospective study from March 1988 to September 1989 was conducted in 18 hemodialysis centers in 13 Canadian cities (4). Hospitalization from any infectious cause was more likely among patients with a low serum albumin level [relative risk (RR) 2.86, 95% confidence interval (CI) 1.57–5.23] and those with an AV graft (RR 2.49, 95% CI 1.18–5.25). Initial vascular access infections requiring antibiotic treatment were evaluated prospectively in 347 patients with either fistulae (227, 65.4%) or AV grafts (120, 34.6%). No catheter infections were evaluated. The survival curves showed that the probability of an access infection by 12 months was 4.5% for AV fistulae and 19.7% for AV grafts. Analysis of a number of risk factors by Cox proportional hazards regression modeling indicated only the type of access as significant (RR 3.41, $p = 0.002$ for grafts versus fistulae). Thirty-four patients with septicemia also were evaluated. The RR for development of septicemia for AV grafts relative to AV fistulae was 5.85 (95% CI 1.85–18.48). Additional significant risk factors for septicemia were low serum albumin level (RR 2.66, 95% CI 1.31–5.39) and aboriginal race (RR 3.83, 95% CI 1.78–8.24).

Powe and colleagues conducted a longitudinal cohort study using data from the U.S. Renal Data System (USDRS) consisting of follow-up data from hospitalization and death records (10). Patients who had a primary diagnosis of septicemia were identified by discharge coding. Risk factors for septicemia were determined subsequently in both peritoneal

The analyses on which this publication is based were performed under contract 500-99-ID02 entitled "Utilization and Quality Control Peer Review Organization for the State of Idaho," sponsored by the Centers for Medicare & Medicaid Services (CMS, formerly Health Care Financing Administration), Department of Health and Human Services. The content of this publication does not necessarily reflect the views or policies of the Department of Health and Human Services, nor does mention of trade names, commercial products, or organizations imply endorsement by the U.S. government. The author assumes full responsibility for the accuracy and completeness of the ideas presented. This chapter is a direct result of the Health Care Quality Improvement Program initiated by CMS, which has encouraged identification of quality improvement projects derived from analysis of patterns of care and, therefore, required no special funding on the part of this contractor. The author welcomes ideas and contributions concerning experience in engaging with the issues presented.

The guidelines outlined in this chapter, although based on published reports and clinical experience, are intended only as general recommendations. The final decision for treatment of an individual patient is ultimately dependent on the clinical judgment and expertise of the prescribing physician.

and hemodialysis patients and evaluated by multivariate Poisson regression. Older age and diabetes were independent risk factors for all patients. Over the 7-year study period, 11.7% of 4,005 hemodialysis patients were identified with a diagnosis of septicemia. Among hemodialysis patients, low serum albumin (RR 1.66, 95% CI 1.38–1.99) and dialyzer reuse (RR 1.28, 95% CI 1.05–1.56) were associated with increased risk. Among vascular access types, only temporary catheters (RR 1.48, 95% CI 1.16–1.89) and AV grafts (RR 1.34, 95% CI 1.04–1.71) had a statistically significant relative risk for septicemia compared with AV fistulae.

In a similar study using USRDS data, these same researchers looked at additional risk factors for septicemia in diabetic versus nondiabetic hemodialysis patients (14). Older age and low serum albumin levels were risk factors for all patients. Among patients with diabetes, white race (RR 1.31, 95% CI 1.00–1.70), peripheral vascular disease (RR 1.44, 95% CI 1.10–1.89), and hemodialyzer reuse (RR 1.38, 95% CI 1.04–1.84) were independent risk factors. Among patients without diabetes, coronary artery disease (RR 1.48, 95% CI 1.18–1.84), cerebrovascular disease (RR 1.56. 95% CI 1.14–2.14), and temporary (RR 1.78, 95% CI 1.29–2.44) and permanent catheters (RR 1.79, 95% CI 1.16–2.75) were associated with an increased risk.

In two prospective 6-month cohort analyses, Hoen and colleagues evaluated the risk for bacterial infections and bacteremia in chronic hemodialysis patients by multivariate logistic regression analysis (5,16). In the first study, consisting of 607 patients in 13 centers, the vascular access device was an independent risk factor for the development of bacterial infection. The odds ratio (OR) was 31 (95% CI 3.39–283, $p = 0.003$) for central venous catheters compared with AV fistulae. A previous history of a bacterial infection (OR 3.90, 95% CI 2.26–6.72) and high serum ferritin (OR 1.79, 95% CI 1.06–3.00) were also independent risk factors. The second study, consisting of 988 patients in 19 centers, demonstrated a RR for bacteremia of 7.6 (95% CI 3.7–15.6) for catheters compared with AV fistulae. A previous history of bacteremia (RR 7.3, 95% CI 3.2–16.4), immunosuppressive therapy (RR 3.0, 95% CI 1.0–6.1), and anemia (RR 0.7 per 1 g per deciliter increment, 95% CI 0.6–0.9) also were risk factors. In both studies, the infection risk for AV grafts did not differ significantly from that for AV fistulae, and the type of catheter was not indicated.

From December 1997 to June 1998, the U.S. Centers for Disease Control and Prevention (CDC) performed an infection surveillance study of 796 patients at seven centers looking specifically at risk for vascular access infection (12). Independent risk factors for first vascular access infection were identified using a multivariate model. These risk factors included specific dialysis center [relative hazard (RH) 1.0–4.10, p <0.0001], catheter versus fistula or graft (RH 2.07, p =0.0006), low albumin (RH 2.37, p =0.013), low urea reduction level (RH 2.22, p =0.0042), and number of hospitalizations within the past 90 days

(3–4, RH 4.13, p =0.0038). This study specifically demonstrated the variability of infection rates among different dialysis centers.

A retrospective study performed in 94 male patients at a Veterans Affairs hemodialysis unit specifically examined risk factors for permanent access site (AV fistulae and grafts) infections (11). Fifty-one permanent access infections were identified in 31 patients. In a logistic regression analysis, only graft type and number of graft revisions were associated independently with vascular access site infection. The OR for infection with AV grafts compared with endogenous AV fistulae was 7.8 (95% CI 2.1–30).

Clinical experience and published reports have suggested that, among vascular access types, native AV fistulae have the lowest rates of infection, synthetic AV bridge grafts have intermediate risk, and central catheters have the highest risk (17–19). A 36-month prospective cohort study has confirmed that risk of vascular access infection is highly dependent on the type of type of access used (15). Relative to AV fistulae, the risk for all infections (bacteremia, local, or clinical sepsis) was 2.2 ($p = 0.002$) for AV grafts, 13.6 (p<0.0001) for permanent tunneled catheters, and 32.6 (p <0.0001) for temporary catheters. This high impact of central venous catheters on hemodialysis-related infections has been confirmed by others (13,20–31). Poor patient hygiene and poor needle insertion technique also have been implicated as potential risk factors (9,32).

MICROBIOLOGY

Because infections usually begin at the cutaneous site of vascular access, most implicated pathogens are gram-positive skin flora (19). These are most commonly *Staphylococcus aureus* and coagulase-negative staphylococcal species. Indeed, gram-positive cocci represent the most common organisms associated with hemodialysis-related bacteremia (2,5,7–9, 33,34). Other less commonly associated organisms are gram-negative bacilli, nonstaphylococcal gram-positive cocci (including enterococci), and fungi (32). Most of the *S. aureus* isolates causing infections in hemodialysis patients come from the patient's own endogenous flora (35,36).

Antimicrobial resistance among bacterial species has been increasing steadily and has become a major public health concern (37). Clinically important resistant organisms include methicillin-resistant *S. aureus* (MRSA), methicillin-resistant coagulase-negative staphylococcal (MRCNS) species, vancomycin-resistant enterococci (VRE), and multidrug-resistant gram-negative bacilli (32). MRSA and VRE often are associated with infections in dialysis patients (38–48).

Hemodialysis patients have been central in the development of vancomycin resistance. One of the first cases of VRE was reported from a dialysis unit (49). In other studies, many hospitalized patients with VRE infections were receiving dialysis (50,51). Vancomycin is commonly used in the dialysis setting because of frequent MRSA or MRCNS infections and because of its ease of administration in the setting of decreased renal clearance of the drug. Recent concern has been raised about the development of intermediate resistance to vancomycin in *S. aureus* (52,53). These strains are known as vancomycin-intermediate *S. aureus*, or VISA. Risk factors for developing an infection with VISA, based on the few reported cases, are prior MRSA infections with prolonged vancomycin therapy, long-term or temporary dialysis, and poor clinical responses to vancomycin therapy (52). Vancomycin resistance is also becoming increasingly common among coagulase-negative staphylococci, another common cause of infections in dialysis (54–56). A new trend of resistance is being recognized with newer antibiotics specifically developed to treat vancomycin-resistant strains (57).

Understanding the profile of organisms usually encountered in a specific dialysis center influences the antimicrobial choices made for management of vascular access infections. In centers where the prevalence of MRSA is low, nafcillin, oxacillin, or cefazolin should be used for *S. aureus* in place of vancomycin. These drugs may not be as convenient to dose as vancomycin but avoid its overuse and the potential promotion of vancomycin resistance. The importance of monitoring infections and antimicrobial use is discussed further in the section on "Surveillance and Prevention" to follow.

COMPLICATIONS

Complications occur in many patients with an infected vascular access, most likely due to the high incidence of bacteremia and the frequency of *S. aureus* infections. These organisms have a propensity to adhere to cardiac valves, bones, and joints and result in endocarditis, septic arthritis, osteomyelitis, septic pulmonary emboli, and clinical sepsis syndrome. Some researchers recommend a search for metastatic infections in any dialysis patients with *S. aureus* bacteremia (58). In another study of catheter-related bacteremia, 22% of patients developed some significant complication (22). In a subsequent study, these same researchers further confirmed the incidence and outcome of complications, especially endocarditis, in hemodialysis patients with *S. aureus* bacteremia (90). They recommended the use of sensitive echocardiographic techniques to assist in determining the length of antibiotic therapy for bacteremia and also recommended removal of hardware to improve outcomes.

In addition to catheters, infective endocarditis has been associated with infected AV grafts but rarely with AV fistulae (59,60). In the published studies, most cases were due to staphylococcal species, but enterococci and streptococcal species were also responsible. The mitral valve was most commonly involved; many patients required valve-replace-

ment surgery, and the mortality rate was high. Septic arthritis also appears to be most commonly associated with *S. aureus*, is often monoarticular, and can be fatal (61,62). Other complications include osteomyelitis (58) and metastatic abscesses, the most significant of which are spinal epidural abscesses (63,64). Spinal epidural abscesses may be rare events but can lead to permanent neurologic deficits or death. In one series of 12 cases, *S. aureus* was implicated in all, with catheters and AV grafts as the source (63).

The high frequency of bacteremia associated with vascular access infections and the significance of infectious complications warrant a careful examination of all hemodialysis patients with a suspected or confirmed vascular access infection. Blood cultures should be performed routinely to document the presence of bacteremia, the condition most commonly associated with serious complications. Sensitive echocardiographic techniques and careful clinical examination should be used to evaluate for endocarditis. Radionuclide scans and magnetic resonance imaging are critical in detecting osteomyelitis or spinal epidural abscesses. Invasive diagnostic procedures to diagnose abscesses or septic arthritis are necessary when these conditions are suspected.

MANAGEMENT

Recommendations for optimal management of the infected hemodialysis vascular access currently come from expert consensus guidelines and clinical experience from small series of patients (19,34,65–68). No data from large randomized, controlled trials are available to specifically guide all recommendations. Conservative application of basic principles of infectious diseases management, however, has been combined with available guidelines and clinical experience to develop some general recommendations for the management of infected tunneled catheters (Fig. 16.1), AV grafts (Fig. 16.2), and AV fistulae (Fig. 16.3) (see also Chapter 35).

Basic management principles for infections considered when developing these recommendations were that (a) bacteremia, specifically due to *S. aureus*, often results in metastatic and complicated infections and requires adequate length of treatment with parenteral therapy (usually 4–6 weeks) (69,70); (b) infections involving the endovasculature (such as endocarditis, septic thrombosis, or native vessel AV fistulae) or other complications such as osteomyelitis also require long courses of intravenous antibiotics to cure infection; (c) eradication of significant infections involving foreign material (such as catheters or polytetrafluoroethylene, or PTFE grafts) usually require removal of the infected foreign material; and (d) abscesses require surgical drainage for optimal management. The recommendations for management outlined can be generally applied by nephrologists, but specific complications, unique presentations, or infections with unusual organisms may require input from an infectious diseases specialist for optimal management.

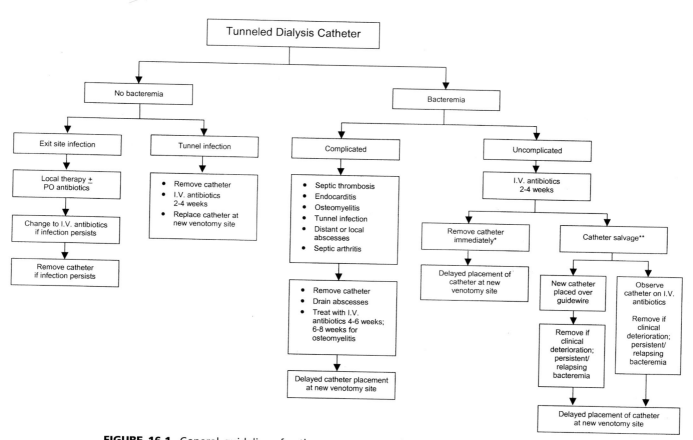

FIGURE 16.1. General guidelines for the management of infections of permanent, tunneled hemodialysis catheters.*, *Staphylococcus aureus* or *Candida* infections; **, Coagulase-negative staphylococci or gram-negative bacilli.

Optimal management for all vascular access infections requires adequate microbiologic information to make therapeutic decisions. Cultures of blood typically should be obtained when vascular access infections are suspected. When a catheter is involved, blood cultures should be obtained from both the catheter and peripheral blood (67). Paired quantitative cultures may be particularly helpful in determining that the catheter is the source of the bacteremia. Cultures through catheters yielding a fivefold to tenfold higher colony count than cultures from peripheral blood are predictive of catheter infections (71). Cultures of the catheter tip also should be obtained if the catheter is removed (72). Efforts to obtain cultures of local drainage from catheters or other access sites should also be made.

Catheter exit-site infections are defined as erythema, induration, or tenderness within 2 cm of the catheter exit site (67) and usually are successfully treated by cleansing with a topical antiseptic and placement of topical antibiotics (34,65). Exit-site infections may require either oral or parenteral antibiotics if topical therapy is unsuccessful. Ultimately, the catheter may need to be removed to eradicate difficult exit site infections (Fig. 16.1).

Tunnel infections are defined as tenderness, erythema, or induration greater than 2 cm from the catheter exit site with or without concomitant bloodstream infection (67). These infections are best treated with catheter removal and lengthy parenteral antibiotic therapy (65,73) (Fig. 16.1). The catheter should be replaced at a new venotomy site.

Catheter-related bacteremia in the setting of complications (septic thrombosis, endocarditis, septic arthritis, osteomyelitis, or distant/local abscesses) requires aggressive therapy with removal of the catheter, drainage of abscesses, excision of infected, thrombosed vessels, and lengthy parenteral antibiotics (67) (Fig. 16.1). In some cases of uncomplicated catheter-related bacteremia, attempts to salvage the catheter or catheter site may be considered. This generally is reserved for infections with coagulase-negative staphylococcal species and gram-negative bacilli that, unlike *S. aureus*, are less likely to cause metastatic or complicated infections (69,70). One study suggested that treatment can be successful while leaving the catheter in place (74). Other investigators demonstrated a high failure rate with this approach (22). Additional studies have examined cure rates of catheter infections when the catheter is replaced over a guidewire (73–75). This approach may be a viable option when combined with parenteral antibiotics in some cases (65). If catheter salvage is attempted but bacteremia persists or the patient clinically deteriorates, the catheter should be removed, followed by delayed placement of a new catheter at a new venotomy site (Fig. 16.1).

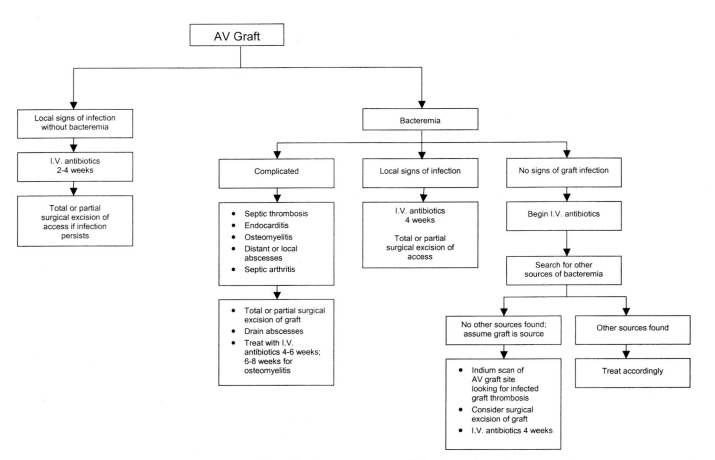

FIGURE 16.2. General guidelines for the management of infections of arteriovenous grafts.

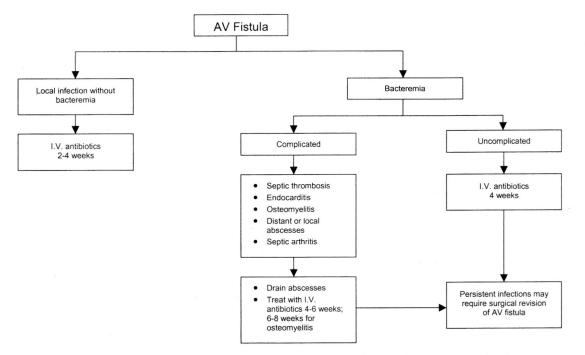

FIGURE 16.3. General guidelines for the management of infections of arteriovenous fistulae.

Infections in synthetic AV grafts containing PTFE material are treated similarly to catheters (Fig. 16.2). Local infections consist of pain, erythema, warmth, swelling, serous or purulent drainage, and skin breakdown (34). In the absence of bacteremia, they can be approached with initial parenteral antibiotics, followed by partial or complete excision of the graft material if the infection persists (19,34,68). Local infections with associated bacteremia and those with systemic complications should be treated with prolonged parenteral antibiotics and partial or complete removal of the graft material (Fig. 16.2). Complications should be treated aggressively as outlined for catheters. If bacteremia presents without obvious AV graft infection, appropriate parenteral antibiotics are begun after cultures are obtained and a search for other sources of bacteremia is undertaken (Fig. 16.2). If another source is found, then appropriate therapy is completed. The graft may become secondarily infected from other sources of bacteremia and ultimately may need to be removed if bacteremia fails to resolve.

If no other sources of bacteremia are identified, then the AV graft, especially if it is an old clotted graft no longer in use, should be considered the most likely source. Several investigators have identified these nonfunctioning grafts as a source for infection (76–78). Radionuclide scans using granulocytes labeled with indium-111 have been shown to localize in occult infections (79,80) and were beneficial in verifying silent AV graft infections in a small series of patients (76). These scans should be considered when looking for the source of occult bacteremia in the setting of existing AV grafts. When the graft is suspected, surgical excision and lengthy parenteral antibiotics are likely to yield the highest cure rates (Fig. 16.2).

Native AV fistulae do not contain foreign material that requires surgical excision for cure of associated infections. Both local infections (pain, erythema, warmth, swelling, serous or purulent drainage, and skin breakdown) and those associated with bacteremia are treated with parenteral antibiotics (Fig. 16.3). Those associated with bacteremia should be considered an endovascular infection requiring a much longer course of treatment. Complications from AV fistula infections with bacteremia should be treated aggressively as outlined already. Persistent infections may ultimately require surgical revision to achieve a clinical and microbiologic cure.

Staphylococcal species, followed by enterococci and gram-negative bacilli, cause most infections of hemodialysis access (see "Microbiology" section). Vancomycin and gentamicin, given parenterally, are popular choices for empiric antimicrobial therapy in this setting. This combination covers the suspected pathogens, including MRSA and enterococci, and is convenient to dose given the long half-lives of both drugs in the setting of end-stage renal disease. In settings of low prevalence rates of MRSA, however, empiric therapy with cefazolin and gentamicin may be adequate and preferable to prevent the development of resistance (81,82). The serious issues of evolving vancomycin resistance among hemodialysis patients has been already been reviewed above. Regardless of the initial empiric antibiotic choice, therapy should rapidly be switched to specific therapy when the culture results are finalized. The length of therapy can be determined by application of the general recommendations outlined in this section. Unusual presentations, unique organisms, or infections that fail to readily respond to therapy should prompt timely consultation with an infectious diseases specialist.

SURVEILLANCE AND PREVENTION

Hemodialysis vascular access, especially those made of foreign material, can be considered medical devices, and medical devices used for medical therapy can be major sources of adverse events. One of the most common adverse events, as outlined in this chapter, is infection (83,84). These adverse events often are not attributed to human cognitive error and may not always be preventable. Nevertheless, failure to implement systems designed to recognize such events and instigate appropriate changes when events are documented does constitute a form of medical error (85,86).

Surveillance for vascular access infections in the chronic hemodialysis setting supports critical patient care functions in the hemodialysis unit including detection of outbreaks, promotion of patient safety, and monitoring the impact of infection control and quality improvement activities. Continuous surveillance establishes the endemic rates of infection in a hemodialysis facility and allows detection of a significant increase in these rates, typically classified as an *outbreak* (15,17). To prevent increases in morbidity and mortality rates, outbreaks require early detection with rapid intervention. Surveillance also establishes the prevalence of bacterial pathogens and antimicrobial resistance associated with vascular access infections in a specific hemodialysis center and can guide empiric antimicrobial therapy. Implementation of surveillance systems seems to be a prudent part of any program designed to manage hemodialysis vascular access complications.

Strategies for preventing vascular access infections have been proposed by the CDC (66) and the National Kidney Foundation (Dialysis Outcomes Quality Initiative, or DOQI) (87). The primary objective for DOQI is to improve patient outcomes and survival by providing recommendations and guidelines for optimal clinical practice (87). The DOQI guidelines, published in 1997, have been based on published evidence whenever possible (88). Furthermore, the guidelines have been the subject of numerous quality improvement activities and have been the focus of clinical performance measures being developed by the Centers for Medicare & Medicaid Services (formerly Health Care Financing Administration) (87,88).

Among potential quality-of-care standards for vascular access, two significant guidelines (Guidelines 29 and 30) outline goals for maximizing the use of native AV fistulae and limiting the use of permanent central catheters for chronic hemodialysis. Both these key guidelines are currently based on opinion and not published evidence. A recent study of 36 months of standardized vascular access infection surveillance from an integrated hemodialysis care system provides epidemiologic support for both of these key guidelines and enhances our understanding of the relative infection risk among different vascular access types (15). This study predicts that encouraging the optimal use of low-risk AV fistulae (Guideline 29), and actively reducing the use of high-risk tunneled catheters (Guideline 30) will result in significant reductions in infectious complications.

Infection control activities recommended in hemodialysis centers have focused on exogenous and endogenous sources of infection (32). Exogenous pathogens acquired from contaminated dialysis fluid, equipment, or medication vials have caused outbreaks but are relatively uncommon. Endogenous pathogens colonize body surfaces and may cause invasive infections. Efforts have been made to decrease colonization with topical antibiotics or prevent infection using aseptic technique (87,89). Sterilization, disinfection, cleaning, and appropriate dialyzer reprocessing have likewise been the target of infection control efforts (32). Additionally, specifically monitoring the type of access utilized and deliberately promoting those types with the lowest complication rates (AV fistulae and grafts) while avoiding those with the highest rates (catheters) also can be expected to result in a significant reduction in infectious problems.

REFERENCES

1. National Institutes of Health. 1999 Annual Report. U.S. Renal Data System. U.S. Department of Health and Human Services, National Institute of Health, National Institute of Diabetes and Digestive and Kidney Diseases; 1999.
2. Bloembergen B, Port F. Epidemiological perspective on infections in chronic dialysis patients. *Adv Ren Replace Ther* 1996;3: 201–207.
3. U.S. Renal Data Systems: VI. Causes of death. *Am J Kidney Dis* 1995;26:S93–S102.
4. Churchill D, Taylor D, Cook R, et al. Canadian hemodialysis morbidity study. *Am J Kidney Dis* 1992;19:214–234.
5. Hoen B, Paul-Daupin A, Hestin D, et al. EPIBACDIAL: a multicenter prospective study of risk factors for bacteremia in chronic hemodialysis patients. *J Am Soc Nephrol* 1998;9:869–876.
6. Kessler M, Hoen B, Mayeux D, et al. Bacteremia in patients on chronic hemodialysis: a mulicenter prospective study. *Nephron* 1993;64:95–100.
7. Quarles LD, Rutsky EA, Rostand SG. *Staphylococcus aureus* bacteremia in patients on chronic hemodialysis. *Am J Kidney Dis* 1985;6:412–419.
8. Dobkin JF, Miller MH, Steigbigel NH. Septicemia in patients on chronic hemodialysis. *Ann Intern Med* 1978;88:28–33.
9. Kaplowitz LG, Comstock JA, Landwehr DM, et al. A prospective study of infections in hemodialysis patients: patient hygiene and other risk factors for infection. *Infect Control Hosp Epidemiol* 1988;9:534–541.
10. Powe N, Jaar B, Furth S, et al. Septicemia in dialysis patients: incidence, risk factors, and prognosis. *Kidney Int* 1998;55:1081–1090.
11. Bonomo RA, Rice D, Whalen C, et al. Risk factors associated with permanent access-site infections in chronic hemodialysis patients. *Infect Control Hosp Epidemiol* 1997;18:757–761.
12. Tokars JI, Light P, Anderson J, et al. A prospective study of vascular access infections at seven outpatient hemodialysis centers. *Am J Kidney Dis* 2001;37:1232–1240.
13. Taylor G, McKenzie M, Buchanan-Chell M, et al. Central venous catheters as a source of hemodialysis-related bacteremia. *Infect Control Hosp Epidemiol* 1998;19:643–646.
14. Jaar BG, Hermann JA, Furth SL, et al. Septicemia in diabetic hemodialysis patients: comparison of incidence, risk factors, and mortality with nondiabetic hemodialysis patients. *Am J Kidney Dis* 2000;35:282–292.
15. Stevenson KB, Hannah EL, Lowder CA, et al. Epidemiology of hemodialysis vascular access infections from longitudinal infection surveillance data: predicting the impact of NKF-DOQI clinical practice guidelines for vascular access. *Am J Kidney Dis* 2002; 39:549–555.
16. Hoen B, Kessler M, Hestin D, et al. Risk factors for bacterial infections in chronic hemodialysis acult patients: a multicentre prospective survey. *Nephrol Dial Transplant* 1995;10:377–381.
17. Stevenson KB, Adcox MJ, Mallea MC, et al. Standardized surveillance of hemodialysis vascualr access infections: 18-month experience at an outpatient, multifacility hemodialysis center. *Infect Control Hosp Epidemiol* 2000;21:200–203.
18. Tokars JI. Description of a new surveillance system for bloodstream and vascular access infections in outpatient hemodialysis centers. *Seminars in Dialysis* 2000;13:97–100.
19. Butterly DW, Schwab SJ. Dialysis access infections. *Curr Opin Nephrol Hypertens* 2000;9:631–635.
20. Cheesebrough JS, Finch RG, Burden RP. A prospective study of the mechanisms of infection associated with hemodialysis catheters. *J Infect Dis* 1986;154:579–589.
21. Capdevila JA, Segarra A, Pahissa A. Catheter-related bacteremia in patients undergoing hemodialysis. *Ann Intern Med* 1998;128: 600.
22. Marr KA, Sexton DJ, Conlon PJ, et al. Catheter-related bacteremia and outcome of attempted catheter salvage in patients undergoing hemodialysis. *Ann Intern Med* 1997;127:275–280.
23. Pezzarossi HE, Ponce de Leon RS, Calva JJ, et al. High incidence of subclavian dialysis catheter-related bacteremias. *Infect Control* 1986;7:596–599.
24. Suchoki P, Conlon PJ, Knelson M, et al. Silastic cuffed catheters for hemodialysis vascular access: thrombolytic and mechanical correction of HD catheters malfunction. *Am J Kidney Dis* 1996; 28:379–386.
25. Almirall J, Gonzalez J, Rello J. Infection in hemodialysis catheters: incidence and mechanisms. *Am J Nephrol* 1989;9:454–459.
26. Blake PG, Huraib S, Uldall PR. The use of the dual lumen jugular venous catheters as definitive long term access for haemodialysis. *Int J Artif Organs* 1990;13:26–31.
27. Tanriover B, Carlton D, Saddekni S, et al. Bacteremia associated with tunneled dialysis catheters: comparison of two treatment strategies. *Kidney Int* 2000;57:2151–2155.
28. Oliver MJ, Callery SM, Thorpe KE, et al. Risk of bacteremia from temporary hemodialysis catheters by site of insertion and duration of use: a prospective study. *Kidney Int* 2000;58:2543–2545.
29. Dryden MS, Samson A, Ludlam HA, et al. Infective complications associated with the use of Quinton "Permcath" for long-term central vascular access in haemodialysis. *J Hosp Infect* 1991; 19:257–262.

30. Hung KY, Tsai TJ, Yen CJ, et al. Infection associated with double lumen catheterization for temporary haemodialysis: experience of 168 cases. *Nephrol Dial Transplant* 1995;10:247–251.

31. Saad TF. Bacteremia associated with tunneled, cuffed hemodialysis catheters. *Am J Kidney Dis* 1999;34:1114–1124.

32. Alter MJ, Lyeria RL, Tokars JI, et al. Recommendations for preventing transmission of infections among chronic hemodialysis patients. *MMWR Morb Mortal Wkly Rep* 2001;50(RR-5):19–31.

33. Marr KA. *Staphylococcus aureus* bacteremia in patients undergoing hemodialysis. *Seminars in Dialysis* 2000;13:23–29.

34. Nassar GM, Ayus JC. Infectious complications of the hemodialysis access. *Kidney Int* 2001;60:1–13.

35. Ena J, Boelaert JR, Boyken BA, et al. Epidemiology of *Staphylococcus aureus* infections in patients on hemodialysis. *Infect Control Hosp Epidemiol* 1994;15:78–81.

36. Kirmani N, Tuazon CU, Murray HW, et al. *Staphylococcus aureus* carriage rate of patients receiving long-term hemodialysis. *Arch Intern Med* 1978;138:1657–1659.

37. Goldmann DA, Weinstein RA, Wenzel RP, et al. Strategies to prevent and control the emergence and spread of antimicrobial-resistant microorganisms in hospitals: a challenge to hospital leadership. *JAMA* 1996;275:234–240.

38. Lye WC, Leong SO, Lee EJ. Methicillin-resistant *Staphylococcus aureus* nasal carriage and infections in CAPD. *Kidney Int* 1993;43:1357–1362.

39. Wanten GJ, van Oost P, Schneeberger PM, et al. Nasal carriage and peritonitis by *Staphylococcus aureus* in patients on continuous ambulatory peritoneal dialysis: a prospective study. *Perit Dial Int* 1996;16:352–356.

40. Tokars JI, Gehr T, Jarvis WR, et al. Vancomycin-resistant enterococci colonization in patients at seven hemodialysis centers. *Kidney Int* 2001;60:1511–1516.

41. Atta MG, Eustace JA, Song X, et al. Outpatient vancomycin use and vancomycin-resistant enterococcal colonization in maintenance dialysis patients. *Kidney Int* 2001;59:718–724.

42. D'Agata EM, Green WK, Schulman G, et al. Vancomycin-resistant enterococci among chronic hemodialysis patients: a prospective study of acquisition. *Clin Infect Dis* 2001;32:23–29.

43. Korff A, Larson E, Kumar P, et al. Vancomycin resistant enterococcus in a hospital-based dialysis unit. *ANNA J* 1998;25:381–386.

44. Brady JP, Snyder JW, Hasbargen JA. Vancomycin-resistant enterococcus in end-stage renal disease. *Am J Kidney Dis* 1998;32:415–418.

45. Osono E, Takahashi M, Kurihara S, et al. Effects of "isolating hemodialysis" on prevention of methicillin-resistant *Staphylococcus aureus* cross-infection in a hemodialysis unit. *Clin Nephrol* 2000;54:128–133.

46. Casewell MW. The nose: an underestimated source of *Staphylococcus aureus* causing wound infection. *J Hosp Infect* 1998;40 (Suppl B):S3–S11.

47. Kluytmans J, van Belkum A, Verbrugh H. Nasal carriage of *Staphylococcus aureus*: epidemiology, underlying mechanisms, and associated risks. *Clin Microbiol Rev* 1997;10:505–520.

48. Tokars JI, Miller ER, Alter MJ, et al. *National surveillance of dialysis associated diseases in the United States, 1995. ASAIO J* 1998;44:98–107.

49. Uttley AHC, George RC, Naidoo J, et al. High-level vancomycin resistant enterococci causing hospital infections. *Epidemiol Infect* 1989;103:173–181.

50. Shay DK, Maloney SA, Montecalvo M, et al. Epidemiology and mortality risk of vancomycin-resistant enterococcal bloodstream infections. *J Infect Dis* 1995;172:993–1000.

51. Stroud L, Edwards J, Danzing L, et al. Risk factors for mortality associated with enterococcal bloodstream infections. *Infect Control Hosp Epidemiol* 1996;17:576–580.

52. Smith TL, Pearson ML, Wilcox KR, et al. Emergence of vancomycin resistance in *Staphylococcus aureus*: glycopeptide-intermediate *Staphylococcus aureus* Working Group. *N Engl J Med* 1999;340:493–501.

53. Centers for Disease Control and Prevention (CDC). *Staphylococcus aureus* with reduced susceptibility to vancomycin—Illinois, 1999. *MMWR Morb Mortal Wkly Rep* 2000;48:1165–1167.

54. Schwalbe RS, Stapleton JT, Gilligan PH. Emergence of vancomycin resistance in coagulase-negative staphylococci. *N Engl J Med* 1987;316:927–931.

55. Raad I, Alrahwan A, Rolston K. *Staphylococcus epidermidis*: emerging resistance and need for alternative agents. *Clin Infect Dis* 1998;26:1182–1187.

56. Garrett DO, Jochimsen E, Murfitt K, et al. The emergence of decreased susceptibility to vancomycin in *Staphylococcus epidermidis*. *Infect Control Hosp Epidemiol* 1999;20:167–170.

57. Tsiodras S, Gold HS, Sakoulas G, et al. Linezolid resistance in a clinical isolate of *Staphylococcus aureus*. *Lancet* 2000;358:207–208.

58. Nicholls A, Edward N, Catto GR. Staphylococcal septicaemia, endocarditis, and osteomyelitis in dialysis and renal transplant patients. *Postgrad Med J* 1980;56:642–648.

59. Robinson DL, Fowler VG, Sexton DJ, et al. Bacterial endocarditis in hemodialysis patients. *Am J Kidney Dis* 1997;30:521–524.

60. McCarthy JT, Steckelberg JM. Infective endocarditis in patients receiving long-term hemodialysis. *Mayo Clin Proc* 2000;75:1008–1014.

61. Slaughter S, Dworkin RJ, Gilbert DN, et al. *Staphylococcus aureus* septic arthritis in patients on hemodialysis treatment. *West J Med* 1995;163:128–132.

62. Mathews M, Shen FH, Lindner A, et al. Septic arthritis in hemodialyzed patients. *Nephron* 1980;25:87–91.

63. Obrador GT, Levenson DJ. Spinal epidural abscess in hemodialysis patients: report of three cases and review of the literature. *Am J Kidney Dis* 1996;27:75–83.

64. Kolmos HJ. Spinal epidural abscess in patients on maintenance haemodialysis (a presentation of two cases). *Int Urol Nephrol* 1979;11:249–253.

65. Favero MS, Alter MJ, Tokars JI, et al. Dialysis-associated infections and their control. In: Bennett JV, Brachman PS, eds. *Hospital infections*. Philadelphia: Lippincott–Raven Publishers, 1998:357–380.

66. Pearson ML. The Hospital Infection Control Practices Advisory Committee. Guidelines for preventions of intravascular device-related infections. *Am J Infect Control* 1996;24:262–293.

67. Mermel LA, Farr BM, Sherertz RJ, et al. Guidelines for the management of intravascular catheter-related infections. *Infect Control Hosp Epidemiol* 2001;22:222–242.

68. Alpers FJ. Clinical considerations in hemodialysis vascular access infections. *Adv Ren Replace Ther* 1996;3:208–217.

69. Sheagren JN. *Staphylococcus aureus*: the persistent pathogen (first of two parts). *N Engl J Med* 1984;310:1368–1373.

70. Sheagren JN. *Staphylococcus aureus*: the persistent pathogen (second of two parts). *N Engl J Med* 1984;310:1437–1442.

71. Fan ST, Teoh-Chan CH, Lau KF. Evaluation of central venous catheter sepsis by differential quantitative blood culture. *Eur J Clin Microbiol Infect Dis* 1989;8:142–144.

72. Maki DG, Weise CE, Sarafin HW. A semi-quantitative method for identifying intravenous catheter infection. *N Engl J Med* 1977;296:1305–1309.

73. Beathard GA. Management of bacteremia associated with tunneled-cuffed hemodialysis catheters. *J Am Soc Nephrol* 1999;10:1045–1049.

74. Schaffer D. Catheter related sepsis complicating long term tunneled central venous catheters: management by guidewire exchange. *Am J Kidney Dis* 1995;25:593–596.

75. Robinson D, Suhocki PV, Schwab SJ. Treatment of infected tunneled venous access hemodialysis catheters with guidewire exchange. *Kidney Int* 1998;53:1792–1794.

76. Ayus JC, Sheikh-Hamad D. Silent infection in clotted hemodialysis access grafts. *J Am Soc Nephrol* 1998;9:1314–1317.

77. Sheikh-Hamad D, Ayus JC. The patient with the clotted PTFE graft developing fever. *Nephrol Dial Transplant* 1998;13:2392–2393.

78. Nassar GM, Ayus JC. Clotted arteriovenous grafts: a silent source of infection. *Semin Dial* 2000;13:1–3.

79. Syrjala MT, Valtonin V, Liewendahl K, et al. Diagnostic significance of indium-111 granulocyte scintigraphy in febrile patients. *J Nucl Med* 1987;28:155–160.

80. Schmidt KG, Rasmussen JW, Sorensen PG, et al. Indium-111 granulocyte scintigraphy in the evaluation of patients with fever of undetermined origin. *Scand J Infect Dis* 1987;19:339–345.

81. Fogel MA, Nussbaum PB, Feintzberg ID, et al. Cefazolin in chronic hemodialysis patients: a safe and effective alternative to vancomycin. *Am J Kidney Dis* 1998;32:401–409.

82. Marx MA, Frye RF, Matzke GR, et al. Cefazolin as empiric therapy in hemodialysis-related infections: efficacy and blood concentrations. *Am J Kidney Dis* 1998;32:410–414.

83. Jansen B, Peters G. Foreign body associated infection. *J Antimicrob Chemother* 1993;32(Suppl A):69–75.

84. Lew DP, Pettit D, Waldvogel FA. Infections that complicate the insertion of prosthetic devices. In: Mayhall CG, ed. *Hospital epidemiology and infection control.* Lipincott Williams & Wilkins, 1999:937–957.

85. Nolan TW. System changes to improve patient safety. *BMJ* 2000;320:771–773.

86. *To err is human: building a safer health system.* Washington, D.C.: National Academy Press, 2000.

87. National Kidney Foundation. Dialysis outcomes quality initiative. Clinical practice guidelines. *Am J Kidney Dis* 1997;30:S137–S240.

88. Steinberg E, Eknoyan G, Levin N, et al. Methods used to evaluate the quality of evidence underlying the National Kidney Foundation-Dialysis Outcomes Quality Initiative Clinical Practice Guidelines: Description, findings, and implications. *Am J Kidney Dis* 2000;36:1–11.

89. Jarvis WR. The epidemiology of colonization. *Infect Control Hosp Epidemiol* 1995; 17:47–52.

90. Marr KA, Kong L, Fowler VG, et al. Incidence and outcome of *Staphylococcus aureus* bacteremia in hemodialysis patients. *Kidney Int* 1998;54:1684–1689.

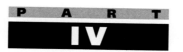

P A R T

IV

MONITORING FOR HEMODIALYSIS ACCESS FAILURE

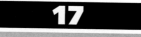

VASCULAR ACCESS SURVEILLANCE: AN OVERVIEW

JEFFREY J. SANDS

Hemodialysis access failure remains a major source of morbidity and hospitalization for patients with end-stage renal disease (ESRD). Currently, access failure is the second leading cause of hospitalization for ESRD patients and results in yearly Medicare expenditures of approximately one billion dollars (P. Eggers, personal communication, from the annual report on ESRD clinical performance measures, December 1999). Over the past 15 years, there has been a growing realization that access failure can be predicted and prevented by elective intervention. Numerous studies demonstrated that techniques, including measurement of access recirculation (1), dynamic venous pressure (2), static venous pressure (3), access flow volume (4), and Doppler ultrasound (5,6), can select a subset of patients at increased risk of developing hemodialysis access failure (thrombosis) and that thrombosis rates can be decreased with elective correction of access stenosis. For these reasons, the Dialysis Outcome Quality Initiative (DOQI) (7) recommends that all vascular accesses undergo a program of regular monitoring for the identification of hemodynamically significant stenosis.

Access monitoring is based on the premise that identification of patients at high risk of developing future access failure, coupled with elective correction of stenotic lesions, will decrease the incidence of hemodialysis access failure and improve patient outcome. Studies have clearly demonstrated the ability of monitoring–intervention programs to decrease the incidence of thrombosis and prolong access life (8) and to decrease the need for emergency interventions (4,6). The impact of these programs on total procedure rates and an analysis of their cost-to-benefit ratio is currently being evaluated. Hemodialysis access monitoring takes many forms, ranging from physical examination (10) to measurements of access recirculation (1), static (3) and dynamic venous pressure (2), access flow volume (4), and vascular access imaging (5,6). Programs based on these techniques have been able to achieve thrombosis rates lower than those targeted by the DOQI [≤0.25 thrombosis/patient-year in arteriovenous (AV) fistulas; ≤0.5 thrombosis/patient-year in polytetrafluoroethylene (PTFE) grafts]. This clearly represents improved care for patients and should become a routine part of care for all hemodialysis patients.

Despite all the evidence that access monitoring coupled with elective intervention improves patient outcomes, access monitoring has not been routinely incorporated into ESRD care in the United States. There continue to be significant barriers to the routine implementation of access monitoring. In particular, the lack of reimbursement to cover the cost of vascular access monitoring, coupled with the more than 20-year decline in the real value of the composite rate (the per-treatment payment for hemodialysis treatments and the basket of services included has only risen in absolute dollars by approximately $3 in 25 years, despite inflationary pressures on costs) has significantly limited the implementation of access monitoring. Other barriers include tight staffing patterns, lack of adequate data systems to facilitate collection and tracking of outcome data, and the lack of coordinators to ensure that abnormal monitoring studies are followed by appropriate interventions. These difficulties with the delivery system have contributed in part to a tacit acceptance of extraordinary high access failure rates.

Access failure and repair continue to cause a tremendous physical and emotional burden for patients and a staggering expense to the health care system. Currently in the United States, PTFE grafts fail at approximately 80 to 120 per 100 patient-years (J. Eggers, personal communication, 1999). Even AV fistulas fail at rates of approximately 20 to 25 per hundred patient-years. This is unacceptable, especially in light of extensive data that clearly demonstrate the ability to cut these failure rates at least in half. Despite this, there has been little if any public funding of monitoring programs or research aimed at the prevention of hemodialysis access failure. For these reasons, a reappraisal of our reimbursement policies and their negative impact on preventative care and a review of our research priorities must be explored.

In the next four sections, experts will present in-depth reviews of the preeminent access monitoring methods, including the role of physical examination, venous pressure monitoring, access flow measurement, and the use of Doppler ultrasound. Although of historic significance, the measurement of access recirculation by urea-based methods will not be addressed directly. More recent work has shown that access recirculation is only present by online methods when the access flow is less than the prescribed dialysis blood flow (QB) (10). Access recirculation is otherwise zero. The use of online techniques to measure recirculation will be discussed in the section on access flow measurement.

In conclusion, access-monitoring programs offer the promise of improved patient care with fewer complications. Access monitoring should be incorporated into the routine treatment of all hemodialysis patients.

REFERENCES

1. Sherman RA. The measurement of dialysis access recirculation. *Am J Kidney Dis* 1993;22:616–621.
2. Schwab SJ, Raymond JR, Saeed M, et al. Prevention of hemodialysis arteriovenous fistulas and grafts. *Radiographics* 1993;13:983–989.
3. Besarab A, Sullivan KL, Ross RP, et al. Utility of intra-access pressure monitoring in detecting and correcting venous outlet stenoses prior to thrombosis. *Kidney Int* 1995;47:1364–1373.
4. Schwab SJ, Oliver MJ, Suhocki P, et al. Hemodialysis arteriovenous access: detection of stenosis and response to treatment by vascular access blood flow. *Kidney Int* 2001;59:358–362.
5. Sands J, Young S, Miranda C. The effect of Doppler flow screening studies and elective revisions on dialysis access failure. *ASAIO J* 1992;38:M524–M527.
6. Mayer DA, Zingale RG, Tsapogas MJ. Duplex scanning of expanded polytetrafluorethylene dialysis shunts: impact on patient management and graft survival. *Vasc Surg* 1993;27:647–658.
7. National Kidney Foundation K/DOQI clinical practice guidelines for vascular access 2000. *Am J Kidney Dis* 2001;37(Suppl 1):S137–S181.
8. Sands JJ, Miranda CL. Prolongation of hemodialysis access survival with elective revision. *Clinical Nephrol* 1995;44:329–333.
9. Trerotola SO, Scheel PJ, Powe NR, et al. Screening for access graft malfunction: comparison of physical examination with US. *J Vasc Interv Radiol* 1996;7:15–20.
10. MacDonald J, Sosa M, Krivitski N, et al. Identifying a new reality: Zero vascular access recirculation using ultrasound dilution. *ANNA J* 1996;23:603–635.

PHYSICAL EXAMINATION: THE FORGOTTEN TOOL

GERALD A. BEATHARD

The examining physician often hesitates to make the necessary examination because it involves soiling the finger.

William J. Mayo *Lancet* 1915;35:339.

PHYSICAL EXAMINATION OF THE DIALYSIS VASCULAR ACCESS

Physical examination (i.e., the use of the hands, eyes, and ears) as diagnostic instruments is a skill that has been basic to medicine from its earliest origins. Unfortunately, in many disciplines of medicine, it is one that has been largely abandoned in favor of more elaborate and costly technical approaches to diagnosis. In the evaluation of the dialysis vascular access, one could argue that it never existed. Nevertheless, physical examination is easily performed, inexpensive to apply, and provides a high level of accuracy (1–4) to the physician who understands its principles and is inclined toward the art of medicine as well as its science.

PHYSICAL EXAMINATION RELATED TO ARTERIOVENOUS FISTULAE

Evaluation Prior to Access Placement

Evaluation of the new end-stage renal disease (ESRD) patient in preparation for the placement of a peripheral venous access is extremely important. Proper patient selection will materially enhance the opportunity to place an arteriovenous fistula (AVF). To determine the type of access most suitable for an ESRD patient, a general physical examination and a detailed focused medical history are important (5). Emphasis should be placed on aspects that might affect the placement of the vascular access. Any physical evidence (i.e., scars) that the patient has had previous central venous catheters should be documented. In most instances, a patient will give a positive history for such an occurrence, but this is not always the case (6). The patient's chest, breast, and upper arms should be evaluated for the presence of swelling or collateral veins. In patients with normal venous pressure, central venous occlusion may not be associated with swelling; however, the presence of collateral veins will alert the examiner to the problem. The presence of scars indicating previous neck or thoracic surgery or trauma should also raise the possibility of a venous anomaly that might affect access creation. Specially directed evaluations of both the arterial and venous anatomy must be completed.

Arterial Evaluation

In relation to the arterial system, two issues are important. The vessel must be capable of delivering blood flow at a rate adequate to support dialysis, and utilization of the vessel for the creation of an access must not jeopardize the viability of the digits and hand. Arterial narrowing and calcification are relatively common in ESRD patients, especially those that are diabetic and hypertensive. This problem usually can be diagnosed before the patient is sent for surgery.

Optimally, three conditions relative to the arterial system (Table 18.1) should be present for the creation of an AVF (7). First, the patient should have less than 20 mm Hg differential in blood pressure between the two arms; a greater difference suggests the presence of arterial disease that should be evaluated before access placement. Second, the palmar arch should be patent. The palmar arch can be tested for patency using the Allen test (Table 18.2). Use of vascular Doppler can increase the effectiveness of the Allen test in predicting collateral arterial perfusion of the hand. Given adequate collateral flow, the Doppler should detect augmented pulsation in the palmar arch during occlusion of ei-

TABLE 18.1. ARTERIAL REQUIREMENTS FOR ARTERIOVENOUS FISTULA

Pressure differential <20 mm Hg between arms
Patient palmar arch
Arterial lumen diameter ≥2.0 mm at point of anastomosis

TABLE 18.2. THE ALLEN TEST

1. Position the patient so that he or she is facing you with their arm extended with the palm turned upward.
2. Compress both the radial and ulnar arteries at the wrist.
3. With the arteries compressed firmly, instruct the patient to create a fist repetitively to cause the palm to blanch.
4. When the patient's hand is blanched, release your compression of the ulnar artery and watch the palm to determine if it becomes pink. Then release all compression.
5. Repeat steps 2–4 for the radial artery.

Interpretation: When color returns to the blanched palm on release of the arterial compression, it indicates arterial patency and reflects upon adequacy of flow. Rapid return of a color that is intense is indicative of an artery that is at least relatively normal. Return of color is referred to as a *negative* Allen Test.

ther the radial or ulnar artery (8). Failure of palmar arch pressures to increase during this maneuver suggests inadequate collateral circulation in the hand and predicts a higher risk for vascular steal if the dominant artery is used for access creation. Third, the arterial lumen should be 2 mm or greater in diameter at the point proposed for the anastomosis. This can best be determined using color flow Doppler.

Venous Evaluation

Venous anatomy is extremely important for access creation, either an AVF or an arteriovenous graft (AVG). Most problems incurred with access creation are actually venous problems. The primary goal when evaluating any patient for a dialysis vascular access should be the identification of a venous anatomy conducive to the creation of an AVF.

The cephalic vein is ideal for an AVF because it is located on ventral surface of the forearm and the lateral surface of the upper arm. These features allow easy access in the dialysis facility with the patient in a sitting position. Ideally, the cephalic should have a straight segment long enough to allow for rotation of cannulation sites and lie within 1 cm of the surface.

To evaluate a patient for these optimum characteristics, venous mapping should be performed. In many patients, this can be done by physical examination. It is essential that the patient be evaluated with outflow obstruction so as to dilate the veins of the arm adequately for evaluation. This is best done using a blood pressure cuff inflated to a pressure about 5 mm Hg above diastolic pressure. This should be left in place for periods of no more than 5 minutes at a time. Although this provides excellent information in many patients, most surgeons will want more detailed information obtained using color flow Doppler ultrasound or venography prior to surgery. Optimum features (Table 18.3) for the creation of an AVF are a luminal diameter at the point of anastomosis of 2 mm or greater, a straight segment of vein, absence of obstruction and continuity with the proximal central veins (7). (See Chapter 11 for detailed information on preoperative venographic techniques.)

TABLE 18.3. VENOUS REQUIREMENTS FOR AVF

Luminal diameter ≥2 mm at anastomosis point
Absence of obstruction
Straight segment for cannulation
Within 1 cm of surface
Continuity with central veins

Evaluation of Early Arteriovenous Fistula Failures

Not all attempts at AVF creation are successful; this is especially true if the surgeon is appropriately aggressive in attempting to create an AVF. Fistulae that never develop adequately for use or those that fail within the first 3 months of use are classified as *early failures*. Whereas there are multiple causes of early failure, the two most frequent causes, if the patients were adequately evaluated prior to placement, are juxta-anastomotic venous stenosis and the presence of cephalic vein side branches referred to as *accessory veins* (9). Both these anomalies can be easily diagnosed by physical examination.

Juxta-anastomotic Venous Stenosis

The most common site for venous stenosis to occur in relation to an AVF is in the segment of vein that is immediately adjacent to the anastomosis (9,10). The cause of this juxta-anastomotic lesion (Fig. 18.1) is not clear, but this segment of vein is mobilized and manipulated by the surgeon in creating the fistula. It may be related to stretching, torsion, or other types of trauma. The effect of the lesion is to obstruct fistula inflow. Since it occurs early, it results in early access failure.

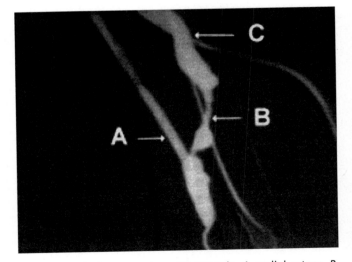

FIGURE 18.1. Juxta-anastomotic stenosis. *A*, radial artery. *B*, stenotic lesion. *C*, cephalic vein.

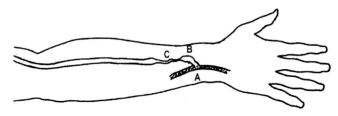

FIGURE 18.2. Radial artery (*A*). Physical examination of juxta-anastomotic stenosis. A strong pulse and thrill are present at the anastomosis (*B*). It disappears as one moves up the fistula to the level of the lesion (*C*).

This lesion can be easily diagnosed by palpation of the anastomosis and distal vein (11). Normally, a prominent thrill is present at the anastomosis. In the absence of abnormalities, the pulse is soft and easily compressible. With juxta-anastomotic stenosis, a water-hammer pulse is felt at the anastomosis. The thrill, which is normally continuous, is present only in systole. As one moves up the vein from the anastomosis with the palpating finger (Fig. 18.2), the pulse goes away rather abruptly as the site of stenosis is encountered. Above this level, the pulse is very weak and the vein is poorly developed. The stenosis itself frequently can be felt as an abrupt diminution in the size of the vein, almost like a shelf. Once these typical physical findings are detected, the cause for poor fistula development becomes obvious. (For more on physical examination of autologous AVFs, see Chapter 24).

Accessory Veins

As previously stated, the optimum venous anatomy for AVF development is a single cephalic vein stretching from the wrist to the antecubital space. In many instances, however, this is not the case. The cephalic vein may have one or several side branches (Fig. 18.3). Each of these accessory veins diverts blood flow from the main channel, which has the effect of reducing resistance and reducing blood flow to the vein above the branch(es). This in turn reduces the pressure on the vein wall that is essential for expansion, dilation, and arterialization to occur. In many cases, this is not a problem; in fact, it can be an advantage, permitting the development of multiple venous sites for access cannulation. In the case where flow is less than optimum, however, the accessory vein(s) can result in early fistula failure. It is important to realize that an upstream stenosis always aggravates the effects of an accessory vein.

If the AVF is created using a side-to-side anastomosis, an abnormal flow pattern in the venous system beyond the fistula over the back of the hand can occur and is yet another potential cause of early access failure (Fig. 18.4). Additionally, this retrograde flow into veins of the hand may cause pain, edema, and limitation of motion.

Accessory veins can be identified easily through physical examination (11). Frequently, they are visible. If not, they can be detected by palpating the fistula. Normally, the thrill

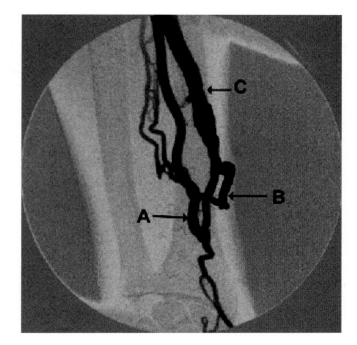

FIGURE 18.3. Accessory vein. Radial artery (*A*) accessory branch (*B*) coming off of the cephalic vein (*C*).

that is palpable over the arterial anastomosis disappears when the upstream fistula is manually occluded. If it does not disappear, an outflow channel (accessory vein) is present below the point of occlusion. Palpation of the fistula below the occlusion point generally reveals the location of the accessory vein by the presence of a thrill over its trunk. As long as the main channel can be identified for occlusion, the entire length of the vein can be evaluated by moving the point of fistula occlusion progressively upward (Fig. 18.4). Ligation of these accessory veins will redirect flow to the main channel and promote the development of a usable AVF (12).

Evaluation of Late Fistula Problems

Once an AVF is functional, it is associated with far fewer problems than is seen with arteriovenous grafts. Nevertheless, problems can occur. In general, physical examination

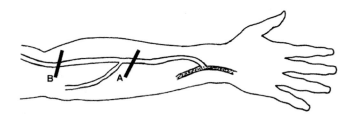

FIGURE 18.4. Physical examination of accessory vein. When the fistula is occluded at point *A*, the thrill will disappear at the anastomosis. As the point of occlusion is moved upward past the accessory vein to point *B*: The thrill will continue when the fistula is occluded.

TABLE 18.4. PHYSICAL FINDINGS OF VENOUS STENOSIS

Parameter	Normal	Stenosis[a]
Thrill	Only at the arterial anastomosis	At site of stenotic lesion
Pulse	Soft, easily compressible	Water hammer
Bruit	Low pitch	High pitched
	Continuous	Discontinuous
	Diastolic and systolic	Systolic only

[a] Abnormalities listed are for the two extremes: completely normal and severe stenosis. With lesser degrees of stenosis, the changes will be intermediate. Significant stenosis tends toward the characteristics of a severe lesion.

plays a major role in the evaluation of these problems. The most common complications associated with the established AVF are venous stenosis, thrombosis, ischemia, aneurysm formation, and infection.

Venous Stenosis of the Arteriovenous Fistula

The details of physical diagnosis of venous stenosis are discussed later in this chapter in detail and in conjunction with the AVG; these details are listed in Table 18.4. They are basically the same for the AVF, with only a few unique differences. Normally, the mature AVF has a soft pulse and the entire structure is easily compressed. When the extremity is elevated, the entire fistula will generally collapse, at least partially. With upstream stenosis, the AVF becomes more forcibly pulsatile and firm. It also enlarges rapidly, often taking on aneurysmal or near-aneurysmal proportions. When the extremity is elevated, that portion of the fistula peripheral to a stenosis remains distended, while the central portion collapses in the normal fashion (Fig. 18.5). This phenomenon allows localization of the site of obstruction. In addition, the pulse diminishes abruptly, as does the caliber of the vessel. Changes in the location and character of thrills and bruits also occur, as described later in association with the AVG.

Aneurysm Formation

An aneurysm in an AVF is recognized as a localized ballooning of the vein. This is very much analogous to the

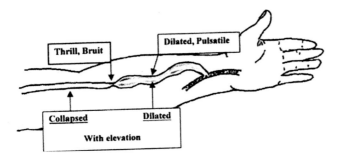

FIGURE 18.5. Physical examination of venous stenosis affecting an arteriovenous fistula.

pseudoaneurysm seen with the AVG, the difference being that with a graft there is no vessel wall involved, thus the term *pseudoaneurysm*. With time, flow in an otherwise normal AVF continues to increase, and the vein may continue to enlarge. Eventually, the AVF may become quite large and somewhat tortuous. It can reach aneurysmal proportions. Aneurysms are more likely to develop upstream to a venous stenosis, especially at sites of repetitive needle insertion. The examiner can recognize these easily. Their progress should be monitored, and any associated skin changes should be noted.

Surgical intervention is indicated when the skin overlying the fistula is compromised with signs suggesting danger of rupture such as marked thinning, ulceration, or evidence of bleeding. Limited cannulation sites resulting from the size of the aneurysm represents another indication for surgical repair. This, too, is should be apparent with routine physical examination.

Ischemia Related to the Arteriovenous Fistula

Ischemia is not as frequent with AVFs as it is with AVGs (13). Susceptibility for the development of ischemia usually can be diagnosed before surgery is performed through physical examination and the procedures already described. In examining the patient with an AVF, skin temperature, gross sensation, movement, and distal arterial pulses in comparison to the contralateral side should also be assessed. The physical changes that may be seen are described in detail later in this chapter, under the section dealing with ischemia associated with grafts. Patients with an established AVF should be assessed monthly. Patients demonstrating abnormalities on physical examination should be further evaluated immediately. Once ischemia occurs, immediate treatment is important.

Infection of Arteriovenous Fistula

Infection associated with an AVF occurs at a rate of about one tenth that seen in AVGs (14). Most infections are actually perivascular cellulitis recognized by localized erythema, swelling, and tenderness on physical examination. These are usually easily treated. Much more serious are the occasional infection-associated anatomic abnormalities, such as aneurysms, perigraft hematomas, or associated abscesses from infected needle puncture sites. These lesions frequently are associated with drainage and may be fluctuant to palpation. Such perivascular abscesses require surgical drainage or excision with access revision (14).

PHYSICAL EXAMINATION RELATED TO ARTERIOVENOUS GRAFTS

Detection of Direction of Flow

Most AVGs are created with a standard configuration; however, occasionally it is necessary to deviate from the usual pattern of placement to accomplish the task. When this occurs, the orientation of the dialysis needles must correspond to the direction of blood flow or gross recirculation will result. To avoid this occurrence, the direction of blood flow should be determined and documented for each patient in the dialysis facility. This can be accomplished easily by occluding the AVG with the tip of the finger and palpating on each side of the occlusion point for a pulse (Fig. 18.6). The side without a pulse is the downstream side of the graft. The upstream pulse will increase in intensity during the occlusion. Although it is easier to accomplish this when the patient is not on dialysis, the maneuver generally can be adequately performed with needles in place if they are not placed too closely together.

Arteriovenous Graft Compression to Detect Recirculation

Recirculation occurs when the blood flow of the AVG falls below the rate demanded by the blood pump. This results in varying degrees of reversal of flow between the needles, depending on the severity of the problem. If the degree of recirculation is more than minimal, it frequently can be detected by physical examination. To perform this maneuver, simply occlude the graft between the two needles during dialysis and observe the venous and arterial pressure gauges

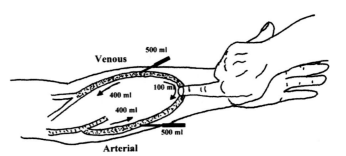

FIGURE 18.7. Technique of graft occlusion to detect recirculation. When the graft that is recirculating is occluded as shown, the venous pressure will quickly rise causing the alarm to sound and the blood pump to stop. The arterial pressure may go down slightly in this instance.

(Fig. 18.7). A hard object, such as a closed hemostat, seems to work more efficiently than a finger in affecting occlusion. With a normal AVG, little or no change is seen in either the venous or arterial pressure readings. If recirculation is secondary to outflow obstruction (venous stenosis), the pressure will rise in the venous return because the lower-resistance, recirculation route has been occluded. As pressure limits are exceeded, the alarm will sound and the blood pump will stop. The arterial pressure may become slightly more negative as the pressure head generated by the venous side is no longer transmitted through the occluded point of the graft. If recirculation is due to poor inflow (arterial stenosis or insufficiency), the major pressure change observed will be a drop (become more negative) as the blood pump demands more blood than is available with the recirculation route cutoff. In this instance, the venous pressure may change very little. If the needles are too close together, this examination will not be possible. This maneuver also can be used to detect reversed placement of needles because malposition of needle sites results in gross recirculation.

Diagnosis of Venous Stenosis

Significant venous stenosis causes hemodynamic changes in the AVG. These changes result in abnormalities that can be detected by physical examination. Unfortunately, venous stenosis is such a common occurrence that many nephrologists do not recognize these changes as being abnormal. A strong pulse or a vigorous thrill often is misinterpreted as evidence of a good access with excellent flow rather than as a sign of a pathologic lesion. A properly functioning AVG has a soft, easily compressible pulse with a continuous thrill palpable (without compression) only at the arterial anastomosis. The normal AVG has a low-pitched bruit, which is continuous with both systolic and diastolic components (Table 18.4). A second thrill downstream from the arterial anastomosis is a sign of pathology (see below).

With the development of significant venous stenosis, upstream resistance is increased. This causes an increase in the

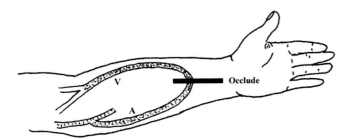

FIGURE 18.6. Detection of direction of flow in an arteriovenous graft. When the graft is occluded, the upstream portion (*A*, arterial) will continue to be pulsatile while the downstream portion (*V*, venous) will be nonpulsatile.

force of the pulse within the graft below the stenosis. As resistance increases, the pulse will eventually develop a "water-hammer" character. Narrowing within the blood flow channel causes turbulence. Turbulent blood flow results in a palpable thrill. The greater the turbulence, the stronger the thrill. Both the turbulence and the thrill are localized to the site of the stenotic lesion. By palpating over the venous anastomosis and the course of the veins that drain the graft, a stenotic site can be identified by detecting the thrill. Even the thrill generated by a central venous stenosis may be palpable, especially in thin-chested patients. These abnormal thrills are generally not continuous; they are only systolic.

The examiner should listen to the graft with a stethoscope paying attention to both the auditory frequency (*pitch*) and the duration of the bruit. As the degree of stenosis increases, the velocity of flow increases and the pitch of the bruit rises. As the resistance to flow increases, the duration of the diastolic component decreases. With severe stenosis, the bruit is high pitched, and only a short systolic component is audible. The entire length of the veins draining the graft also should be examined with the stethoscope. Normally, it is difficult to hear a bruit in the upper arm unless there is some degree of compression of the vein. Normally, if a bruit is heard, it is of low pitch and decreases in pitch as one moves up the arm and the velocity of flow decreases. Because the velocity of flow increases over an area of stenosis, a localized bruit or a localized increase in the pitch of the bruit suggests narrowing. To aid in localizing stenoses, Depner (15) suggested removing the head of the stethoscope and listening with the open end of the tubing. Continuing to listen high into the upper arm or even into the axilla or subclavian area sometimes reveals a venous stenosis at that point as a localized bruit or increase in the pitch of a bruit.

By examining the AVG and draining veins to determine the character of the pulse, the location and intensity of thrills, and the duration and pitch of the bruit, it is possible to detect the graft at risk for thrombosis secondary to venous stenosis. The degree to which these changes occur are dependent on the severity of the stenotic lesion (Table 18.4).

Intragraft stenosis can cause confusion. Abnormal thrills are generally not present. In some instances, it is possible to detect a change in pulsation within the graft as one crosses the stenotic lesion. In many cases, however, the intragraft lesion is so diffuse that this is not possible. In these instances, the graft may be relatively pulseless. Normally, if the outflow of the graft is manually occluded, there is considerable augmentation of the pulse. In cases of diffuse intragraft stenosis, this augmentation does not occur. The bruit does reflect the hemodynamic changes characteristic of a stenotic lesion: It is high pitched and of short duration.

Many cases of central vein stenosis present a feature generally not seen with more peripheral stenosis. In cases of severe stenosis, gross swelling of the access arm is frequently seen. This physical finding is virtually pathognomonic for central vein stenosis. When it is associated with a catheter scar over the subclavian or a cardiac pacemaker, both the disease and its cause become obvious. It is important for the examiner to realize that not all central venous lesions cause arm swelling and not all cases are associated with central venous catheters.

Arteriovenous Graft Infection

Infection of the graft is a serious complication. It has been reported to account for 20% of all dialysis access complications (16) and to be the second leading cause of graft loss. Not all inflammation associated with the graft is indicative of infection. Occasionally, immediately following graft placement, a cutaneous inflammatory reaction occurs. This is characterized by a bright red flare that is restricted to the skin immediately overlying the graft. Typically, it is generalized to the entire course of the graft. With a loop graft, this erythematous flare does not spread to the skin lying within the loop; only the immediate course of the graft itself. There is generally little to no swelling, it is not fluctuant, and frequently there is no pain. This is probably a dermal reaction related to the graft being placed more superficially than usual.

Infection associated with an AVG may be classified as *superficial* or *deep*. Superficial infections do not involve the graft itself. These are generally related to a cannulation site and present with a pustule or a localized area of cellulitis. On physical examination, they are recognized as small pustular lesions with minimal or no inflammation, swelling or pain. They are not fluctuant.

Deep infections involve the graft and are serious problems. Surgical treatment is always required. These infections are recognized on physical examination by the classic combination of erythema, (frequently localized but not just to the skin overlying the graft) and swelling, which on occasion is also fluctuant. Pain may be present but is variable. The area generally feels warm, but this is not a very reliable sign because the skin overlying a flowing graft is always warmer than normal.

Ischemia Associated with an Arteriovenous Graft

Two distinct clinical variants of hand ischemia are recognized following the placement of an AVG (see Chapter 15 for a discussion of treatment): vascular steal syndrome, in which ischemic changes affect all tissues of the hand to a varying degree of severity; and ischemic monomelic neuropathy, where change is confined to the nerves of the hand (17).

Ischemic Monomelic Neuropathy

Ischemic monomelic neuropathy is an underrecognized ischemic complication of vascular access creation related to nerve ischemia or infarction (18). It is most commonly seen in diabetic patients who have severe peripheral artery disease, especially when the brachial artery is used for the creation of the vascular access. When this occurs, the patient complains of profound weakness of the hand immediately postoperatively and frequently associated severe pain and paraesthesia. On physical examination, it is characterized by weakness in the distal muscle groups and a sensory defect characterized by reduced or absent responses to pinprick and vibration. These findings may be located in the distribution of the median, ulnar, or radial nerves and may affect any or all three of these. Typically, there is no associated appearance of ischemia of the other tissues of the hand. The hand appears warm and well perfused, and the pulses are normal or at least comparable to the opposite side. When this is recognized, immediate treatment is indicated.

Vascular Steal Syndrome

Vascular steal syndrome occurs when blood derived from the ulnar artery is shunted through the palmar arch to the graft, depriving the hand of perfusion. This is due to the marked difference in resistance to flow presented by the arteriovenous shunt and the microcirculation of the hand. Diabetics, elderly individuals, patients with severe peripheral vascular disease, and those who have had multiple access attempts are at high risk for this complication. Ischemia is seen most often early after access construction, but it can occur anytime. It may first appear after the treatment of a venous stenotic lesion associated with a graft. Such treatment reduces the resistance within the vascular access circuit and promotes shunting from the higher resistance circuit of the hand.

Physical findings in patients with vascular steal syndrome are somewhat variable, depending on the severity of the problem and the preexisting status of the peripheral circulation. In most instances, it is helpful to compare the affected side to the opposite normal or relatively normal side. In the mildest cases, the affected hand is pale or cyanotic in appearance, it feels cold and has a diminished or absent radial pulse. It is helpful to know whether a radial pulse was present before surgery. Occlusion of the graft may be found to either increase the strength of a previously weak radial pulse or may result in the appearance of a previously absent pulse.

In more severe cases, evidence of ischemic changes in the skin, especially at the fingertips, may be present. At this time, the patient generally has significant pain and neuropathic changes. Signs and symptoms of ischemia are generally more prominent during dialysis.

Pseudoaneurysm Associated with an Arteriovenous Graft

Dialysis needles are unique; they are extremely sharp and have very thin walls. Because of this, they act like a cookie cutter. When the graft as cannulated, the needle either cuts

a core or creates a flap. In either instance, the graft is left with a defect. If cannulation sites are too close together, these defects become confluent. On physical examination, these confluent cannulation sites can be felt as a defect in the graft; that is, the roof of the graft is missing. Significant scarring of the skin overlying the defect is generally apparent as well. It is important to recognize the sites before performing endovascular procedures on an AVG. High-pressure dilatation of an angioplasty balloon within such an area can cause it to extend.

In patients with an associated venous stenosis, the increased pressure within the graft results in the formation of an area of dilatation at the site of the graft defect and the formation of a pseudoaneurysm (Fig. 18.8). This differs from the aneurysm seen in association with the AVF in that here there is no vessel present in the wall of the dilatation, nor is there any graft. There is only skin and a thin layer of fibrosed subcutaneous tissue.

Physical examination of the pseudoaneurysm is important. First, its presence should raise the concern for the associated venous stenosis that is present in most cases. Second, the overlying skin should be closely evaluated. With progressive enlargement, a pseudoaneurysm eventually can compromise circulation to the skin covering the AVG and ultimately may lead to rupture and severe hemorrhage. Any evidence of thinning of the skin, scarring, ulceration, or spontaneous bleeding should be noted.

Third, its size relative to the diameter of the graft should be determined. Large pseudoaneurysms can prevent access to the adjacent areas of the graft for needle placement, thereby limiting potential puncture sites. If the pseudoa-

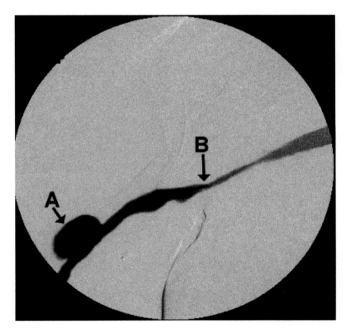

FIGURE 18.8. Pseudoaneurysm affecting upper arm arateriovenous graft. *A,* pseudoaneurysm; *B,* venous stenosis at the anastomosis.

neurysm exceeds twice the diameter of the adjacent normal graft, it should be referred to surgery for revision (19). Fourth, the pseudoaneurysm should be palpated for firmness, especially if the graft is thrombosed. A hard pseudoaneurysm in a thrombosed graft is indicative of the presence of retained thrombus. Frequently, this is represented by chronic, layered blood clot that is very resistant to removal by using endovascular techniques. This appearance, associated with the fact that the pseudoaneurysm is present, is justification for referring the patient to surgery for a declot–revision combination therapy.

CONCLUSION

Hemodialysis vascular access and its associated problems represent an extremely important part of the management of the chronic dialysis patient. A great deal of useful information can be gained through a simple but thorough physical examination of the dialysis vascular access. This is where access evaluation should start, and it should be done on a regular basis. Unfortunately, in this time of concern over medical costs and debate over the best method to screen for venous stenosis, we often ignore an effective technique that is literally at the tip of our fingers. The patient's access has a lot to say if we will but listen.

More mistakes are made from want of a proper examination than for any other reason.
Russel John Howard (1875–1942)

REFERENCES

1. Beathard GA. Physical examination of AV grafts. *Semin Dial* 1992;5:74.
2. Trerotola SO, Scheel PJ, Powe NR, et al. Screening for access graft malfunction: comparison of physical examination with ultrasound. *J Vasc Interv Radiol* 1996;7:15–20.
3. Safa AA, Valji K, Roberts AC, et al. Detection and treatment of dysfunctional hemodialysis access grafts: effect of a surveillance program on graft patency and incidence of thrombosis. *Radiology* 1996;199:653–657.
4. Migliacci R, Selli ML, Falcinelli F, et al. Assessment of occlusion of the vascular access in patients on chronic hemodialysis: comparison of physical examination with continuous-wave Doppler ultrasound. *Nephron* 1999;82:7–11.
5. NKF-DOQI Clinical Practice Guidelines For Vascular Access. Guideline 1: patient evaluation prior to access placement. *Am J Kidney Dis* 1997;30(Suppl 3):S154.
6. Beathard GA. Percutaneous transvenous angioplasty in the treatment of vascular access stenosis. *Kidney Int* 1992;42:1390–1397.
7. Silva MB Jr, Hobson RW 2nd, Pappas PJ, et al. A strategy for increasing use of autogenous hemodialysis access procedures: impact of preoperative noninvasive evaluation. *J Vasc Surg* 1998;27:302–307.
8. Kamienski RW, Barnes RW. Critique of the Allen test for continuity of the palmar arch assessed by Doppler ultrasound. *Surg Gynecol Obstet* 1976;142:861–864.
9. Beathard GA, Settle SM, Shields MW. Salvage of the nonfunctioning arteriovenous fistula. *Am J Kidney Dis* 1999;33:910–916.
10. Romero A, Polo JR, Morato EG, et al. Salvage of angioaccess after late thrombosis of radiocephalic fistulas for hemodialysis. *Int Surg* 1986;71:122–124.
11. Beathard GA. Physical examination of the dialysis vascular access. *Semin Dial* 1998;11:231–236.
12. Beathard GA, Settle SM, Shields MW. Salvage of the nonfunctioning arteriovenous fistula. *Am J Kidney Dis* 1999;33:910–916.
13. Morsy AH, Kulbaski M, Chen C, et al. Incidence and characteristics of patients with hand ischemia after a hemodialysis access procedure. *J Surg Res* 1998;74:8–10.
14. Albers F. Causes of hemodialysis access failure. *Adv Ren Replace Ther* 1994;1:107–118.
15. Depner TA. Techniques for prospective detection of venous stenosis. *Adv Ren Replace Ther* 1994;1:119–130.
16. Butterly DW. A quality improvement program for hemodialysis vascular access. *Adv Renal Replace Ther* 1994;1:163–166.
17. Miles AM. Upper limb ischemia after vascular access surgery: differential diagnosis and management. *Semin Dial* 2000;13:312–315.
18. Hye RJ, Wolf YG. Ischemic monomelic neuropathy: an under-recognized complication of hemodialysis access. *Ann Vasc Surg* 1994;8:578–582.
19. NKF-DOQI Clinical practice guidelines for vascular access. Guideline 27: treatment of pseudoaneurysm of dialysis AV grafts. *Am J Kidney Dis* 1997;30 (Suppl 3):S177.

tracorporeal circuit must be reversed, such that the arterial needle is now downstream from the venous return needle (Fig. 19.1). The indicator is injected into the venous return line, and if a single dilution detector is used, it is positioned at the arterial line. Use of a single detector requires knowledge of the precise amount of indicator injected and requires periodic calibration of the system to ensure accuracy. Adding a second matched detector on the venous line downstream from the injection site simplifies the process (Fig. 19.1) because neither the amount of injectant nor a separate calibration injection is required. The following descriptions outline the mathematical calculations of access flow when using either one or two detectors.

Because the lines are reversed, the blood flow between the two needles (Q_{mix}) is the sum of the access flow (Q_{acc}) and the blood flow in the extracorporeal circuit (Q_b) (Fig. 19.1). In the absence of ultrafiltration,

$$Q_{mix} = Q_{acc} + Q_b \qquad [Eq\ 2]$$

Rearranging Eq. 2 and combining with Eq. 1, Q_{acc} in the case of a single detector is simply

$$Q_{acc} = Q_{mix} - Q_b = \frac{\text{Amount injected}}{AUC_{mix}} - Q_b \quad [Eq\ 3]$$

where AUC_{mix} is the area under the concentration-versus-time curve at the arterial detector. When two detectors are used, rearranging Eq. 2 and combining it with Eq. 1 yields

$$Q_{acc} = Q_{mix} - Q_b = \frac{Q_b\,Q_{mix}}{Q_b} - Q_b$$

$$= Q_b \left(\frac{Q_{mix}}{Q_b} - 1 \right) \qquad [Eq\ 4]$$

$$Q_{acc} = Q_b \left(\frac{\text{Amount injected}/AUC_{mix}}{\text{Amount injected}/AUC_{inj}} - 1 \right) \qquad [Eq\ 5]$$

where AUC_{inj} is the area under the concentration versus time curve at the venous line detector downstream from its injection site. Because the amount of indicator injected is identical,

$$Q_{acc} = Q_b \left(\frac{AUC_{inj}}{AUC_{mix}} - 1 \right) \qquad [Eq\ 6]$$

When two sensors are used, recirculation in the vascular access between the needle tips can be determined easily using the indicator dilution technique:

$$\text{Fraction of } Q_b \text{ that recirculates} = \frac{AUC_{mix}}{AUC_{inj}} = R \qquad [Eq\ 7]$$

With the lines in the normal configuration, when there is no recirculation, indicator injected into the venous line (which is downstream from the arterial line) will not appear in the arterial line, and AUC_{mix} will be zero. When the lines are reversed, recirculation always occurs, and its magnitude is an inverse function of access blood flow. Substitution from Eq. 7 yields an alternative form of Eq. 6, allowing the calculation of access flow whenever the recirculation ratio (R) is known:

$$Q_{acc} = Q_b \left(\frac{1}{R} - 1 \right) \qquad [Eq\ 8]$$

PITFALLS OF THE INDICATOR DILUTION METHOD

Several pitfalls of the indicator dilution method have been identified by Krivitski and colleagues and by others (11–16) and recently were reviewed by Depner and Krivitski (8,17) (Table 19.1).

TABLE 19.1. FACTORS THAT AFFECT THE ACCURACY OF VASCULAR ACCESS FLOW (Q_{acc}) MEASUREMENTS AND PRACTICAL CLINICAL SOLUTIONS TO ELIMINATE OR MINIMIZE THE RESULTING ERRORS[a]

Factors Affecting Accurate Q_{acc} Measurement	Maneuvers to Eliminate or Minimize Errors
Errors in measuring Q_b	Turn off ultrafiltration
	Measure Q_b independently
Presence of cardiopulmonary recirculation	Inject indicator before the venous trap
	Inject indicator rapidly
Incomplete mixing of indicator with blood	Use a rapidly responding detector
	Insert arterial needle opposite to the direction of access flow
	Place needles ≥3 cm apart
	Keep Q_b ≥200 mL/min during measurement
Falling blood pressure during dialysis	Place needles in the same fistula branch
	Peform measurements during the first 90 min of dialysis

Q_b, blood flow through the dialyzer and blood tubing.
[a]For an explanation of these factors, please see text.

Accuracy of Blood Flow

As shown by Eq. 6 and Fig. 19.1, the accuracy of Q_{acc} depends on the accuracy of Q_b. Several factors can affect Q_b. During initial validation of the method, Krivitski (11) reported that ultrafiltration must be turned off when reversing the lines to start the access flow measurement and must be kept off until the measurement is complete. This maneuver will ensure that Q_b is identical at both the venous and arterial sensors. Additional experience with the technique has allowed modifications to the computer program that generates the area under the concentration versus time curve from the sensors to account for the ultrafiltration.

Accurate measurement of Q_b itself is also essential. Unfortunately, blood pump meters are notoriously inaccurate because they report Q_b as a simple function of the pump ro-

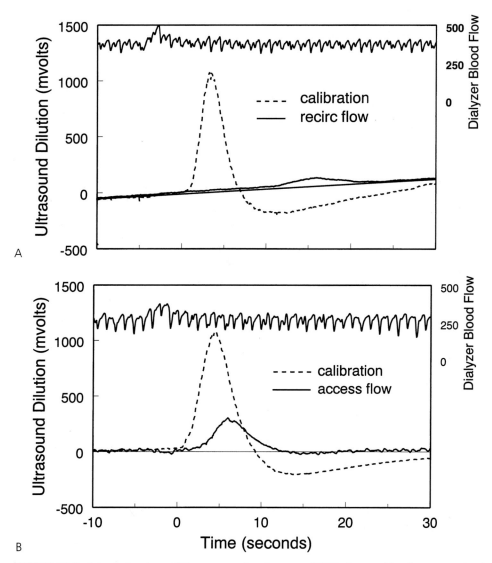

FIGURE 19.2. Sample tracings of the area under the curve (AUC) detected by the meter. Again, dual sensors are used and the curves are typical of those for the ultrasound dilution technique but are generally applicable to other indicators. **A**: Typical AUC tracing with the bloodlines in normal configuration. The first or venous sensor detected the bolus of saline immediately after injection, translated as the initial positive deflection in the calibration curve (*dashed line*). Because no spontaneous recirculation is present, the recirculation flow curve (*solid line*) does not have an initial upward deflection. The small deflection seen at about 15 seconds is due to cardiopulmonary recirculation. **B**: Typical AUC tracing with the bloodlines reversed to create recirculation. As in A, the initial positive defection in the calibration curve (*dashed line*) is due to the bolus of saline immediately after injection. The smaller positive deflection that appears slightly later in the access flow curve (*solid line*) indicates the presence of recirculation and is a function of the access blood flow. Significant cardiopulmonary recirculation is absent in this patient, as demonstrated by the absence of a second positive deflection in the access flow curve at about 15 to 20 seconds. The terminal negative deflection of the calibration curve in both figures results from using saline injections at ambient temperature.

tational speed (18–20). An independent accurate measure of Q_b helps to ensure the accuracy of access flow. Lastly, the speed and location of the injection itself can affect Q_b (12). To prevent errors in access flow from cardiopulmonary recirculation (see later), the injection must be relatively quick. Injection of 5 to 10 mL close to the vascular access caused Q_b to increase by 20% to 40% (12). Moving the injection to the venous bubble trap or just upstream from the trap decreased the error to 5% for most brands of tubing tested. This maneuver also has the advantage of eliminating the need for removing bubbles from the syringe before injection.

Effects of Cardiopulmonary Recirculation

Cardiopulmonary recirculation is another potential source of error (12). Soon after the technique was described, Depner and colleagues (17,21) found that the time required to complete the circuit from the vascular access through the heart and lungs and back to the vascular access (cardiopulmonary recirculation) is very short, about 5 to 20 seconds. After it passes through the heart and lungs the indicator appears as a second peak (Fig. 19.2). For access flow to be accurate, the two curves must be separable. Combining the two curves falsely decreases access flow by as much as 10% to 40%, proportional to the ratio of Q_{acc} to cardiac output. Separating the two curves requires a short, rapid injection of the indicator and a sensitive detector.

Importance of Mixing

Incomplete mixing of the indicator with the patient's blood is another potential source of error (11). The natural turbulence of flow in the vascular access helps to mix the indicator with blood rapidly and thoroughly. To guarantee rapid and complete mixing, the venous or return needle should be inserted in the direction opposite to access flow. Placing the two needles at least 3 cm apart and keeping Q_b above 200 mL per minute facilitates mixing, reducing the measurement error to less than 3%. The location of the tips of the venous and arterial needles with respect to each other and the vascular access wall (on the same side or on opposite sides) is a minor source of error (about 0%–5%) when Q_b is greater than 200 mL per minute. As the vascular access diameter increases from 6.6 to 10 mm (approximately the diameters of a synthetic graft and a native fistula), the error in access flow increases, probably because flow velocity decreases. Again, above a Q_b of 200 mL per minute, the error decreases to about 3% and the disparity disappears. If one mistakenly places the needles in separate branches of a fistula when measuring access flow, the results are unpredictable, and Q_{acc} values may be spuriously high from the lack of recirculation when the lines are reversed (8,22).

Effect of Blood Pressure

Because flow is determined by pressure and resistance (Flow $\cong$ Pressure $\div$ Resistance), the timing for measuring access flow during hemodialysis may be important as blood pressures usually fall during hemodialysis. Three studies reported that access flow decreased 7% to 8% during hemodialysis (14–16), although only the largest of the studies (16) found this difference to be statistically significant. The decrease in access flow was associated with a decrease in blood pressure (14,16) and cardiac output (14,15). The estimated magnitude of the reduction in access flow was modest during the first 90 minutes of dialysis (< 8% even with >25% decrease in mean arterial pressure) and more severe thereafter (14% with >10% decrease in mean arterial pressure and 28% to 50% with >15% to 25% drop in mean arterial pressure, respectively) (16). For most patients, it appears that the modest decrease in access flow during hemodialysis will not affect clinical decision making unless it is near or below the 600 to 800 mL per minute threshold for intervention (see later). For patients in whom a significant lowering of blood pressure (>10–15%) is anticipated, however, access flow is best measured during the first 90 minutes of dialysis.

Effect of Temperature

Some errors are more specific to the ultrasound dilution technique. The temperature of the injectant may have a minor effect on access flow measurements (13). When the indicator solution is at room temperature, it has a cooling effect on the extracorporeal circuit, which decreases the sound velocity of blood but increases the sound velocity of the tubing. These disparate effects alter the appearance of the dilution curves such that the curves become narrower and consist of a positive deflection followed by a negative deflection. Using only the positive deflection to calculate access flow yields an error of 5% to 6%. Because this error is relatively small and the ultrasound dilution software includes a correction for temperature, in clinical practice, indicator solutions can be injected at room temperature.

CLINICAL MEASUREMENT OF ACCESS BLOOD FLOW

As discussed, access flow may be measured using Doppler ultrasound, MRA, or the indicator dilution method. Doppler ultrasound and MRA are too expensive and inconvenient to use for frequent screening and require a radiology technician to perform the test. This section focuses on the various indicator dilution methods done in the dialysis unit by a trained dialysis technician or nurse.

Ultrasound Dilution Method

Transporting the theory behind indicator dilution techniques to clinical practice requires a suitable indicator, a sensitive detector for the indicator, a method of recording the indicator dilution curve, and an awareness of the assumptions made in applying the theory. The indicator dilution method with the most widespread use, the most extensive validation, and the most precise standardization is the ultrasound dilution technique. The indicator is a bolus of normal saline, and the detector is an ultrasound probe attached to the patient's bloodline. The detector simultaneously measures blood flow in the tubing using an established transit-time method (yielding an independent continuous measure of Q_b) while it detects the transient change in ultrasound velocity induced by saline dilution of the blood. Voltage signals from the detector are sent to the Transonic Hemodialysis Monitor (HD01 Monitor, Transonic Systems, Ithaca, NY, U.S.A.), which records the area under the voltage-time curve. The software in an attached computer then calculates access flow and access recirculation.

Initial measurements are taken with the bloodlines in the correct orientation to determine whether access recirculation is present (17). To accomplish this, the trained technician turns off ultrafiltration, places the ultrasound sensors on the bloodlines, and injects room-temperature saline into the venous drip chamber or into the bloodline before the venous drip chamber. If recirculation is not present, the technician turns off the blood pump and reverses the bloodlines to create artificial recirculation for measurement of access flow. While keeping the ultrafiltration off, the technician injects room-temperature saline as before. The test is repeated once or twice to ensure reproducibility. In clinical validation studies, the error of duplicate measurements in the same patient for recirculation is $3.9 \pm 2.8\%$ (21) and for access flow is $5.0 \pm 3.8\%$ (9).

Beginning the test with a measurement of recirculation has several advantages. First, it allows detection of unintentional line reversal as may occur when the dialysis technician and the nurse do not know the direction of blood flow in the vascular access. In such a case, evidence for recirculation will appear during the initial measurement but will disappear when the bloodlines are reversed. In the "reversed" configuration, flow of blood in the extracorporeal circuit is actually returned to the normal configuration, and the expected recirculating bolus of saline may not appear at the arterial sensor, indicating that something is wrong. Second, lack of recirculation with the bloodlines in the normal configuration accompanied by a low access flow strongly indicates the presence of access stenosis between the arterial and venous needles. Third, if no access recirculation is present with normal line orientation, the small ultrasound dilution curve detected by the arterial sensor is due to cardiopulmonary recirculation (CPR). Knowing the time to appearance and the magnitude of the CPR allows the Transonic hemodialysis monitor to eliminate it from the measured area under the curve (AUC) used to calculate access flow, which improves the accuracy of the measurements. This refinement of the technology also allows release of the normal saline indicator from an intravenous bag (which is detected over a longer period

and thus overlaps the CPR peak) to replace the saline injection, further simplifying the procedure.

The accuracy of the vascular access measurements was validated in an *in vitro* system using in-line flow sensor readings as the gold standard (11,13), in a sheep model using a perivascular flow probe as the gold standard (12), and in humans using Doppler ultrasound (9) or MRA (23) for comparison. The difference between access flow measured with the ultrasound dilution technique and with Doppler ultrasound approaches 10% (9,24), with the Doppler ultrasound measurement consistently lower. This difference is more likely due to errors in the Doppler ultrasound technique, which has a higher variance. Access flow measured with the ultrasound dilution method and with MRA agree closely ($r = 0.91$) (23). Under optimal conditions (Table 19.1), access flow values measured with the ultrasound dilution technique and those from direct measurements differ by only 5% (11–13). Access recirculation measured by the ultrasound dilution technique agreed closely with that obtained from urea dilution using the low flow clamp method ($r = 0.92$) (21).

Magnetic Inductance or Differential Conductivity Method

The principles of indicator dilution have been applied using other indicators and detectors to measure access flow (Table 19.2). Lindsay and colleagues described a technique for determining access recirculation (25) and access flow (26) using a bolus injection of hypertonic saline as the indicator that was detected by measuring the resulting induced current with a magnetic sensor. This inductance technique yielded excellent reproducibility, with a standard deviation of 1.8% for recirculation measurements and 7.9% for access flow (26). Access recirculation measured by the inductance technique correlated highly with the urea method ($r = 0.94$) (26), whereas access flow measurements correlated highly with those obtained from the ultrasound dilution technique ($r = 0.98$) in 15 patients (27). The inductance technique, however, did not provide an independent measure of Q_b. The technique also suffers from the disadvantage of requiring specially made blood tubing for the magnetic sensors to work and the potential risk to the patient from the injection of 23.4% saline.

Urea Method

If recirculation can be quantified in the reversed line configuration, access flow can be calculated using Eq. 8. Because the urea concentration in the venous outflow line is significantly lower than the concentration in the arterial inflow line, recirculation can be quantified by urea dilution. This method and other continuous methods differ from the bolus technique because they are unable to separate local access recirculation from CPR; so R in Eq. 8 is overestimated, lead-

TABLE 19.2. METHODS AND DEVICES FOR MEASURING VASCULAR ACCESS BLOOD FLOW (Q_{acc}) USING THE INDICATOR DILUTION TECHNIQUE[a]

Method	Indicator	Detector	Principle
Ultrasound dilution	Normal saline	Ultrasound sensor	Normal saline decreases ultrasound velocity of blood
Magnetic inductance	Hypertonic saline	Conductivity sensor	Hypertonic saline increases ability of blood to conduct a current in a magnetic field
Urea dilution	Endogenous urea	Arterial, venous, systemic blood urea concentration	Recirculation lowers urea concentration in the arterial line
Thermodilution	Dialysate temperature	Temperature sensor	Change in dialysate temperature changes arterial blood temperature
Hemodilution	Hematocrit	Optical sensor	Injection of saline leads to hemodilution
Ultrafiltration	Hematocrit	Optical sensor	Abrupt increase in ultrafiltration leads to hemoconcentration
Conductivity dialysance	Dialysate sodium	Conductivity sensor in the disalysate lines	Change in dialysate sodium alters blood sodium concentration to different extent when blood lines are in normal or reversed position

[a] The best validated method and device is the ultrasound dilution technique.

ing to an underestimation of access blood flow. In support of this theoretical analysis, Q_{acc} calculated from induced urea recirculation (reversing the lines) was consistently lower than Q_{acc} measured by the inductance technique (28). During a subsequent 8-month follow-up period, Q_{acc} measured by the urea technique could not predict vascular access outcome.

Thermodilution Method

Schneditz and colleagues (29,30) changed the dialysate temperature for 3 minutes and used the resultant change in blood temperature as the indicator. Temperature-sensitive thermistors were placed on the outside surface of the arterial and venous blood lines, and temperature was monitored using the Fresenius Blood Temperature Monitor (Fresenius Medical Care, Bad Homburg, Germany). The coefficient of variation was 7% to 8% (29). The thermodilution technique underestimated access recirculation by 1% to 2% and access flow by 500 to 600 mL per minute when compared with the ultrasound dilution technique (30), albeit the latter difference was not significant. Although these differences may not be clinically significant, they result from the significant overlap of the cardiopulmonary recirculation curve and the access recirculation curve and may give rise to larger magnitudes of errors when conditions (Table 19.1) are not optimal.

Optical Hemodilution and Hemoconcentration (Ultrafiltration) Methods

A technology originally designed to monitor changes in central blood volume during dialysis by measuring hematocrit continuously during hemodialysis has been adapted to measure access recirculation and flow (27,31), using the principles of indicator dilution with optical detection. The indicator is either a bolus of normal saline to cause hemodilution (27) or an abrupt increase in ultrafiltration to induce hemoconcentration (31). Optical sensors inserted into the blood tubing detect the change in hematocrit. Compared with the ultrasound dilution technique, measurements using hemodilution (27) consistently overestimate access flow and underestimate access recirculation, likely because of poor separation of access recirculation from CPR as described already. In addition, access flow calculations using hemodilution still require an accurate measure of dialyzer blood flow (Q_b), but the hemodilution technique does not provide an independent measure of Q_b. In these respects, the hemoconcentration method (also called the *ultrafiltration* method) (31) may offer an advantage.

The hematocrit in the dialyzer inflow (arterial) line is measured after 4 minutes of minimal ultrafiltration (H_0) with the blood lines in the usual position. After the ultrafiltration rate is abruptly increased to ≥ 1.8 L per hour for 4 minutes, the arterial hematocrit is measured again. Then the bloodlines are reversed and the measurements are repeated. Access flow then can be calculated using the following equation:

$$Q_{acc} = \frac{Q_f \cdot H_0}{(\Delta H_r - \Delta H_n)} \qquad [Eq\ 9]$$

where Q_f is the ultrafiltration rate, H_0 is the arterial hematocrit with minimal ultrafiltration, ΔH_n is the change in arterial hematocrit with lines in the normal configuration, and ΔH_r is the change in arterial hematocrit with the lines reversed.

This equation takes into account CPR and blood volume depletion and does not require any direct knowledge of Q_b but requires an accurate measurement of Q_f. Despite these advantages, access flow measured by the ultrafiltration method still consistently overestimates Q_{acc} by 16% compared with the ultrasound dilution method (31).

Conductivity or Ionic Dialysance Method

Recently, both Fresenius, Inc. and Hospal Dasco SpA (22) added sensitive conductivity meters at the dialysate inflow and outflow ports to monitor small solute clearance during hemodialysis as a measure of adequacy. Gotch and colleagues (32) and Mercadal and co-workers (22) devised a method to measure access flow using these meters. Altering the proportioning ratio of dialysate concentrate to water during dialysis changes the dialysate sodium concentration as well as the blood sodium concentration. The sodium dilution and the resultant change in conductivity in the dialysate (called *conductivity* or *ionic dialysance*) serve as the indicator for measuring access flow. Measuring the dialysance with the blood lines in their usual position (D) and after reversal (D_{rev}) allows calculation of Q_{acc} (32):

$$Q_{acc} = \left(\frac{D \cdot D_{rev}}{D - D_{rev}}\right)\left(\frac{1}{Blood\ water\ fraction}\right) \qquad [Eq\ 10]$$

Like the other indicator dilution methods, the mathematical derivations by Gotch and colleagues (32) assume ultrafiltration is zero. In their mathematical derivation, Mercadal and colleagues (22) allowed continued ultrafiltration while measuring dialysance, eliminating the need for (1/blood–water fraction) from Eq. 10. The dialysance technique eliminates the need for an accurate measurement of Q_b. This technique assumes, however, that there is no recirculation when the blood lines are in the normal position (22). It also consistently underestimates access flow compared with the ultrasound dilution technique at access flows below 1000 mL per minute (22,33).

CLINICAL SIGNIFICANCE OF VASCULAR ACCESS BLOOD FLOW

Access flow in both native fistulae and synthetic grafts range from less than 100 to more than 2,000 mL per minute (8).

Many studies (2–5,26,34–40) have attempted to correlate access flow with vascular access thrombosis to find a threshold value for Q_{acc}. These studies are summarized in Tables 19.3 and 19.4.

Threshold Access Flow as Predictor of Graft Thrombosis

In several cross-sectional studies, access flow was measured at a single point in time and then the patients were followed to determine the rate of access thrombosis within the next few months. These studies attempted to define a threshold value for Q_{acc} below which the incidence of access thrombosis accelerates. For access flow measured by Doppler ultrasound, investigators (2,3,5,34) found that the incidence of graft thrombosis increased markedly from 10% to 20% up to 63% to 93% at a threshold Q_{acc} below 300 to 800 mL per minute (Table 19.3). The length of follow-up in these studies ranged from 1 to 6 months. The largest study, involving 2,792 hemodialysis patients, showed that, compared with the reference Q_{acc} group of 700 to 1,000 mL per minute, the risk of access thrombosis increased by 40% for Q_{acc} between 300 and 500 mL per minute ($p = 0.01$) and doubled for Q_{acc} less than 300 mL per minute ($p = 0.0001$) (Table 19.3). Given the inherent problems of Doppler ultrasound measurements of access flow (see preceding in "Access Flow Measurement"), the threshold Q_{acc} values derived from this method may not apply to that derived using other methods. Of particular note is that average access flow values obtained from Doppler ultrasound range from 600 to 900 mL per minute (2–5,34) compared with the average of 1,100 mL per minute from the magnetic inductance method (26) and 900 to 1,200 mL per minute from ultrasound dilution (35–41). These discrepancies may be due to the tendency for Doppler ultrasound to underestimate access flow or to some other differences in the study population, but they highlight the importance of not applying the threshold Q_{acc} values derived from Doppler ultrasound to other methods of measuring access flow.

Using the magnetic inductance method to measure access flow, Lindsay and colleagues (26) reported thrombosis rates in polytetrafluoroethylene (PTFE) grafts and fistulae of 71% with Q_{acc} below 500 mL per minute and 50% with Q_{acc} below 750 mL per minute (Table 19.3). The thrombosis rate was 12% with Q_{acc} greater than or equal to 500 mL per minute and 7% with Q_{acc} greater than 750 mL per minute; however, only 41 patients were studied.

The first study (8,35) attempting to define a threshold Q_{acc} value using ultrasound dilution offered hope for a sensitive test in the battle against vascular access thrombosis. When access flow was below 800 mL per minute, the incidence of synthetic graft and native fistula thrombosis increased from 3% to 54% during the following 6 or more months (Table 19.3). Data from Besarab and colleagues (36) also suggested that access flow is an excellent discrim-

TABLE 19.3. SUMMARY OF OBSERVATIONAL STUDIES THAT EVALUATED THE IMPACT OF A SINGLE MEASUREMENT OF VASCULAR ACCESS BLOOD FLOW ON VASCULAR ACCESS THROMBOSIS

Study (Ref. No.)	Access No.	Grafts (%)	Method	Follow-up (mo)	Q_{acc} (mL/min)	N	Thrombosis (%)	Relative Risk	
Sands et al. (34)	177	100	Doppler US	6	≤801	14	93		
					≤1,300	69	42		
					≥1,603	38	26		
Strauch et al. (3)	57	100	Doppler US	6	<400	11	64		
					≥400	46	13		
					<500	18	50		
					≥500	39	11		
Bay et al. (4)	2,792	69	Doppler US	≥6	≤300			2.0[a]	
					300–500			1.4[a]	
					500–700			1.2	
					700–1000			1.0	
					>1,000			0.8	
Shackleton et al. (2)	18	100	Doppler US	2	≤450	8	63		
					>450	10	10		
Wang et al. (5)	39	100	Doppler US	1	<300		77		
					300–500		8		
					500–800		4		
					>800		0		
Lindsay et al. (26)	41	39	Magnetic inductance	8	<500	7	71		
					≥500	34	12		
					≤750	14	50		
					>750	27	7		
Depner (8) and Depner et al. (35)	68	57	US dilution	≥6	<800	35	54		
					≥800	33	3		
Besarab et al. (36)	114	100	US dilution	3	See text for discussion				
May et al. (37)	172	100	US dilution	3	<710	44	25	300[b]	2.39
					710–1,010		19	650[b]	1.67
					1,010–1,395		19	900[b]	1.29
					>1,395	43	9	1,150[b]	1.00
Bosman et al. (38)	41	100	US dilution	2	≤600	9	67		
					>600	32	6		
Wang et al. (39)	68	100	US dilution	2	<500		42	3.12	
					500–800		20	1.52	
					800–1,100		17	1.25	
					1,100–1,400		13	1.0	
					>1400		12	0.89	
Paulson et al. (40)	80	100	US dilution	3	See text for discussion				

US, ultrasound.
[a] $p < 0.05$.
[b] Relative risk for thrombosis at these Q_{acc}.

TABLE 19.4. SUMMARY OF OBSERVATIONAL STUDIES THAT EVALUATED THE IMPACT OF THE CHANGE IN VASCULAR ACCESS BLOOD FLOW ON VASCULAR ACCESS THROMBOSIS

Study (Ref. No.)	No. Access	Grafts (%)	Method	Frequency of Q_{acc} (mo)	Period of Follow-up	Change in Q_{acc} %	
						Thrombosed Grafts	Patent Grafts
Wang et al. (5)	39	100	Doppler US	1	1st to 2nd	−26	−13
					2nd to 3rd	−36	+16
Wang et al. (39)	68	100	US dilution	2	1st to 2nd	−25	−10
					2nd to 3rd	−21	+6
Neyra et al. (41)	95	76	US dilution	6	1st to 2nd	−22	−4
					2nd to 3rd	−41	+15
Paulson et al. (42)	83	100	US dilution	1	12 mo	See text for discussion	

inator of thrombosis-prone PTFE grafts. Grafts that remained patent at 3 months had a Q_{acc} of 1,121 ± 26 [standard error of the mean (SEM)] mL per minute, comparable to grafts that clotted in the absence of an anatomic lesion (1,209 ± 202 mL per minute). Grafts that clotted or required intervention and were found to have an anatomic lesion had a much lower access flow (656 ± 84 and 605 ± 45 mL per minute, respectively). Grafts that clotted with preceding evidence for access recirculation had an even lower access flow (270 ± 9 mL per minute). Subsequent experience suggested a threshold Q_{acc} of 500 to 700 mL per minute (37–39), below which the incidence of PTFE graft thrombosis during the subsequent 2 to 3 months varied from 25% to 67%. Above this threshold, the incidence of thrombosis may be as high as 20% (Table 19.3), making the threshold Q_{acc} a somewhat insensitive indicator of future thrombosis. This issue was illustrated further by May and colleagues (37), who found a 25% access thrombosis rate over 3 months in patients with access flow in the lowest quartile (< 710 mL per minute), decreasing only slightly to 19% in the next two quartiles (710–1,010 mL per minute and 1,010–1,395 mL per minute) (Table 19.3). Even with access flow in the highest quartile (>1,395 mL per minute), 9% of the PTFE grafts thrombosed. In multivariate analysis, after adjusting for potential confounding factors and assigning Q_{acc} of 1,150 mL per minute as the reference, the relative risk of graft thrombosis increased progressively with declining access flows: 1.29 for Q_{acc} 900 mL per minute, 1.43 for Q_{acc} 800 mL per minute, 1.67 for Q_{acc} 650 mL per minute, and 2.39 for Q_{acc} 300 mL per minute (Table 19.3). Wang and associates (39) also reported significant access thrombosis rates in the higher access flow ranges: 20% for Q_{acc} 500 to 800 mL per minute, 17% for Q_{acc} 800 to 1,100 mL per minute, 13% for Q_{acc} of 1,100 to 1,400 mL per minute, and 13% for Q_{acc} > 1,400 mL per minute. In this study, the relative risk for access thrombosis was 0.89 for Q_{acc} > 1,400 mL per minute, 1.25 for Q_{acc} 800 to 1,100 mL per minute, 1.52 for Q_{acc} 500 to 800 mL per minute, and 3.12 for Q_{acc} less than 500 mL per minute, compared with the reference Q_{acc} of 1,100 to 1,400 mL per minute. Differences in design of the various studies and in patient populations may account for the variable usefulness of access flow in predicting access failure or thrombosis. In particular, the longer the follow-up, the more sensitive access flow is as a predictor of access failure. Nevertheless, the data from these two studies raise the possibility that declining access flow may behave as a continuous risk factor for access thrombosis. It may not be possible to define a threshold value.

To address the issue of the value of access flow as a screening tool for impending access thrombosis, Paulson and colleagues (40) performed a meta-analysis using their data and published data to compute receiver operating characteristic (ROC) curves. ROC curves are generated by plotting the false-positive rate on the x-axis against sensitivity on the y-axis. A perfect screening test will have an AUC of 1.0; that is, the curve rises steeply to yield simultaneously a high sensitivity and a low-false positive rate. A screening test with no discriminative ability has an AUC of 0.5, that is, a 45° line that bisects the x-y plot. Whereas four of the studies yielded reasonable AUC values ranging from 0.84 to 0.90 (3,26,35,36), the other six studies had AUC values of 0.61 to 0.71 (40). Overall, the AUC was in the 0.7 range for all studies combined. These investigators argue that an optimal screening test should have an AUC of 0.90, yielding a sensitivity of 80% and a false-positive rate of 20% (42).

Current recommendations for clinical practice include intervention to prevent graft thrombosis when access flow falls below 600 to 800 mL per minute (8,43–45). The main objection to these recommendations comes from the analysis by Paulson and colleagues (40), whose study suggests that a single access flow value may not be a good screening test to select patients for intervention because of its insufficiently high sensitivity and specificity. Even in the studies with good sensitivity (only a small percentage of patients with access flow above threshold had an adverse graft event), a third to a half of the patients with flows below threshold did not progress to access thrombosis during at least 6 months of follow-up (3,26,35) (Table 19.3). Should these patients also be subjected to vascular access angiograms? What about the patient whose flow exceeds 800 mL per minute? In some studies, a fifth of these patients will develop thrombosis in their access within the next 2 to 3 months.

Progressive Fall in Access Flow as Predictor of Graft Thrombosis

To improve the sensitivity and specificity of blood flow as an indicator of access thrombosis, several investigators have evaluated the association of thrombosis with changes in access flow. Wang and colleagues reported that a 21% to 36% decline in access flow usually preceded graft failure in patients with a Q_{acc} above threshold [>300 mL per minute by Doppler ultrasound (5) or greater than 500 mL per minute by ultrasound dilution (39)] (Table 19.4). In contrast, patients with patent grafts had a nonsignificant decrease (10%–13%) or even an increase in access flow (6%–16%) during follow-up. In studies that measured access flow every 1 to 2 months, the threshold flow to predict graft failure appears to be lower (Table 19.3). This finding may be explained by the previous observation. Patients with apparent high access flow and access failure actually may have developed progressive vascular access stenosis, and flow may have fallen before the graft failed. Infrequent access flow measurements would not have detected this fall and the graft failure would then be associated with an apparently higher value.

Neyra and colleagues (41) expanded these observations by prospectively following 91 patients (95 accesses) for 18 months, measuring access flow using the ultrasound dilution method every 6 months. Flow declined progressively in accesses that developed thrombosis during follow-up [from 1,205 ± 277 mL per minute at baseline to 910 ± 381 (−22%) during the second period to 661 ± 276 (−41%) during the third period] but was unchanged in accesses that remained patent [1,579 ± 703, 1,301 ± 811 (−4%), 1,287 ± 638 (+15%) mL per minute, respectively] (Table 19.4). Defining vascular accesses with stable access flow as the reference group, a greater than 20% decrease in Q_{acc} conferred a 5.5-fold risk of access thrombosis in the following 12 weeks. For larger decreases in Q_{acc}, the risk of access thrombosis rose exponentially (a decrease in Q_{acc} greater than 35% conferred a relative risk of 13.6 and a decrease greater than 50% a relative risk of 34.7). Thrombosis-free survival analysis revealed that the probability of having a patent access at 90 days was 92% when access flow remained stable, 74% when Q_{acc} decreased by 25%, and 33% when Q_{acc} decreased by 40%. Studies like these have prompted recommendations to intervene to prevent access thrombosis when flow decreases by 20% to 30% (8,44), in addition to the previous recommendation of intervention when Q_{acc} is below 600 to 800 mL per minute.

Paulson and colleagues (42) attempted to quantify the ability of changes in flow to predict vascular access thrombosis through using ROC curves. Access flow was measured monthly for 3 months in 80 patients (83 PTFE grafts) using the ultrasound dilution method. Patients were monitored for the next 3 months to determine the incidence of access thrombosis. Of the patients with a clotted access, 53% had a Q_{acc} less than 600 mL per minute, 52% had a 20% or greater decrease in Q_{acc} over 3 months, and 72% had a 20% or greater decrease in Q_{acc} from month to month. Using these Q_{acc} and changes in Q_{acc} as threshold values, 3%, 17%, and 23%, respectively, of patients with patent accesses in the subsequent 3 months would have been selected for access intervention. Overall, the AUC for using a decrease in flow to predict graft thrombosis is 0.74 to 0.82, similar to the AUC values reported for using a single Q_{acc} measurement in this study (0.79–0.84), and the meta-analysis by the same group (40) (see preceding). In other words, taking into account the decline in flow did not improve the sensitivity or specificity of the test compared with a single flow measurement in this study. What if one were to combine the two parameters and use the criteria of either a Q_{acc} below 600 mL per minute or a decrease in Q_{acc} of 20% or greater over 3 months, as suggested by recent reviews (8,44,45)? This strategy would have detected 77% of patients who went on to develop access thrombosis while subjecting 23% of patients whose accesses remained patent after 3 months to an intervention (42).

How do we resolve the controversy generated by the Paulson study? Neyra and colleagues (41) clearly showed that decreasing access flow over 6 months is associated with an ex-

ponential increase in the risk of access thrombosis over the next 3 months. Paulson and associates (42) suggested that decreasing flow over 1 to 2 months is not a very sensitive or specific indicator of access thrombosis over the subsequent 3 months. The variable interval between flow measurements in the two studies may have contributed significantly to the difference in outcome. The patients in the study by Neyra and colleagues may have had the lower flow for a longer period before it was detected, making the "follow-up" time longer than the stated 3 months. If follow-up had been longer in the study by Paulson's group, more accesses with decreasing flow may have clotted. Because the main concern raised by Paulson and co-workers is subjecting patients with normal accesses to unnecessary interventions, we need to know whether the patients whose accesses did not clot were indeed normal and free of venous or arterial stenosis. Subsequent intervention studies will shed more light on this issue (see later section on the "Benefits of Monitoring Vascular Access Flow").

Flow as Predictor of Native Fistula Thrombosis

Most studies evaluating the predictive value of a single measurement of flow on access thrombosis included native fistulae but were unable to draw any conclusion about the relationship between flow and access thrombosis because of the much lower thrombosis rate (3,4,37). Other studies concluded that access flow did not predict thrombosis in native fistulas (4,39), but these studies may be confounded by the small number of patients (39), the low incidence of access thrombosis (4,39), and the less accurate flow measurements in native fistulas because of the problem of multiple draining veins (4,39). Two studies found that low access flow was associated with a higher incidence of access thrombosis in native fistulas (26,35), although the risk of thrombosis occurred at a lower flow (< 400 mL per minute) than in synthetic grafts. The relative risks for fistula thrombosis associated with progressive decreases in access flow are comparable to that for grafts (41).

Access Recirculation as Predictor of Thrombosis

Although all indicator dilution methods for measuring access flow also provide a measurement of access recirculation, recirculation should not be used to screen for access dysfunction because it occurs late in the course of access failure. As a stenosis develops in the vascular access, access flow will fall progressively, but access recirculation does not occur until Q_b exceeds Q_{acc} (36,46).

BENEFITS OF MONITORING VASCULAR ACCESS BLOOD FLOW

The goal of a successful vascular access surveillance program is to identify failing grafts and fistulas before they clot, thus permitting elective intervention without interrupting the patient's dialysis schedule (see Chapter 22). Even if intervention does not prolong the life of the access, it can prevent underdialysis from unrecognized access recirculation, reduce hospitalization, minimize the use of temporary dialysis catheters, and improve the quality of life. Several retrospective studies using historical controls suggest that an intensive vascular access surveillance program reduces the incidence of access thrombosis (47–53). Most of these studies used venous pressure measurements alone (47–49) or in combination with physical examination of the access, reports of difficulty in cannulation, prolonged bleeding from puncture sites, edema in the access extremity, decreased dialysis adequacy, and recirculation (50–52) to screen for vascular accesses at risk. Angiography and angioplasty of any stenosis greater than 50% followed.

A basic premise of all vascular access surveillance programs is that prophylactic or preemptive angioplasty will prevent or decrease graft thrombosis, even if it does not prolong graft function. Data from Lumsden and colleagues (54) initially refuted this premise. Color duplex ultrasound identified patients with a greater than 50% stenosis in their vascular access graft, confirmed by angiography. The 32 patients randomized to angioplasty had a 6-month graft patency of 69% and a 12-month patency of 51%, comparable to the patency rates of 70% and 47%, respectively, for the 32 patients randomized to observation. Time to access thrombosis from diagnosis (8.2 and 7.8 months, respectively) was also comparable. Potential confounding issues were a higher percentage of previous access interventions, a higher proportion of older accesses in the angioplasty patients, and patency measured from the time of diagnosis of the stenosis and not from the time of graft placement. All these factors may have increased the risk of thrombosis in the angioplasty patients. These researchers attempted to eliminate these confounders by performing a subgroup analysis of the 21 patients with a "virgin" vascular access (55), that is, an access that has not clotted or required angioplasty or surgical revision. The eight patients randomized to angioplasty had a graft thrombosis rate of 0.10 episodes per patient-year, compared with the thrombosis rate of 0.44 per patient-year in the 13 untreated patients with virgin grafts and 0.91 per patient-year in the nonvirgin grafts treated with angioplasty. That the thrombosis rate was lower after angioplasty despite the small number of patients, more diabetics, more smokers, and older grafts in the angioplasty group suggests a real effect.

Vascular Access Flow Monitoring Decreases Thrombosis

Two studies used access flow by ultrasound dilution as the vascular access monitor. Schwab and colleagues (53) measured access flow monthly with the ultrasound dilution method in 42 hemodialysis patients, one third of whom had native fistulas. Thirty-seven patients had a Q_{acc} less than 600 mL per minute or a 20% decrease in flow when Q_{acc} was less than 1,000 mL per minute. Thirty-five underwent angiography. All had at least one significant stenosis (> 50%), which was treated first with angioplasty and then with surgical revision if angioplasty was unsuccessful. Two patients declined angiography and developed access thrombosis. The average follow-up was 1.8 years. The average interval between angioplasties was 5.8 months for grafts and longer than 11.4 months for fistulas (only 1/24 fistulas required repeat intervention). The overall thrombosis rate of 0.16 episodes per patient-year compares favorably with the 0.25 per patient-year observed in historical controls monitored with dynamic venous pressures ($p < 0.05$). Arteriovenous fistulas thrombosis rate decreased from 0.16 to 0.07 episodes per patient-year ($p < 0.05$), whereas that of grafts decreased from 0.30 to 0.22, albeit the difference was not statistically significant.

Sands and associates (56) randomized 103 patients to monthly measurement of access flow using ultrasound dilution, monthly measurement of static venous pressure, or no additional access monitoring. If flow was less than 750 mL per minute or static venous pressure 0.5 or greater, the patient underwent angiography followed by angioplasty if a lesion with at least 50% stenosis was found. All groups also had a color flow Doppler ultrasound every 6 months. If Doppler ultrasound detected a flow of less than 800 mL per minute for a graft or 600 mL per minute for a fistula, a 50% or greater stenosis, or a 20% or greater decease in flow compared with prior studies, the patient also underwent angiography and possible angioplasty. During an average follow-up of 6.5 months, 9.7% of patients monitored monthly developed an access thrombosis, compared with 22% of the control patients. When all episodes of thromboses were analyzed, the two groups monitored monthly had 19 episodes of thrombosis per 100 patient-years compared with the 125 episodes per 100 patient-years in the control group. The access flow group had the lowest incidence of thrombosis (5.9 episodes per 100 patient-years), and the venous pressure group was intermediate (30.3 per 100 patient-years). Monthly monitoring reduced episodes of thrombosis from 27.1 to 16.8 episodes per 100 patient-years in the two thirds of patients with native fistulae and from 246.7 to 23.2 episodes per 100 patient-years in the remaining third of patients with grafts. Although access thrombosis episodes were lower in patients monitored with flow compared with venous pressure for both fistulae and grafts, the differences were not statistically significant. A potential confounder of the study is that accesses in the control group were older (2.3 years) than those in the other two groups (1.5 years). This confounder should actually lower and not increase the thrombosis rate in the control group, however, because older accesses thrombose less.

Recommendations for Vascular Access Blood Flow Monitoring

Although many studies have shown that access flow and fall in flow is an excellent tool to identify vascular accesses at risk of thrombosis (Table 19.3), Paulson and colleagues (40,42) questioned whether it has sufficient sensitivity and specificity to serve as a screening tool (see preceding). The fact that all patients with a low or declining flow were found to have one or more lesions with 50 % or greater stenosis refutes the argument that it does not have sufficient specificity. The patients with low or declining flow whose access did not clot may not have been followed long enough ($\leq$ 3 months). Further, the fact that using flow in a vascular access surveillance and intervention program significantly lowered the access thrombosis rate lends further support for its use as a screening tool. It is difficult to imagine that a stenosis that is causing a significant decline in access blood flow will not progress. One might ask, however, whether early angioplasty of a developing stenosis interrupts a healing process and predispose to future thrombosis and stenosis. Although Lumsden and colleagues (54) attempted to answer this question with a randomized control study, the significant differences in baseline characteristics between the observation and the angioplasty group rendered suspect the conclusion that angioplasty did not prevent thrombosis (see preceding). The definitive answer requires a well-designed controlled study. Another question that remains to be settled is whether the improved quality of life, less frequent missed dialysis, less hospitalization, less use of temporary vascular access offset the increased cost of access monitoring and more frequent angiography and angioplasty.

At present, a vascular access surveillance program using access flow as a guide to identify patients who may benefit from angiography and angioplasty appears to offer the most benefit and the lowest rate of access thrombosis. Doppler ultrasound and magnetic resonance imaging are cumbersome methods of measuring access flow given the expense and the difficulty, if not impossibility, of performing the test during dialysis. The indicator dilution techniques appear most promising for routine access flow monitoring, especially the ultrasound dilution technique for which the most experience has accumulated and is the best validated. In addition, it offers the added advantage of a direct measure of Q_b, which is not available with the other indicator dilution techniques. The authors of the Dialysis Outcomes Quality Initiative (43,45) recommended measurement of access flow as the preferred method for monitoring both arteriovenous fistulas and grafts. The ideal frequency of monitoring is not clear, but preferably at least once a month if funding will allow. If flow falls below 600 mL per minute in grafts or below 400 mL per minute in fistulas, or if flow decreases by 20% to 25%, then intervention consisting of angiography followed by angioplasty for lesions causing greater than 50% stenosis or surgical revision is appropriate.

REFERENCES

1. Basseau F, Grenier N, Trillaud H, et al. Volume flow measurement in hemodialysis shunts using time-domain correlation. *J Ultrasound Med* 1999;18:177–183.
2. Shackleton CR, Taylor DC, Buckley AR, et al. Predicting failure in polytetrafluoroethylene vascular access grafts for hemodialysis: a pilot study. *Can J Surg* 1987;30:442–444.
3. Strauch BS, O'Connell RS, Geoly KL, et al. Forecasting thrombosis of vascular access with Doppler color flow imaging. *Am J Kidney Dis* 1992;19:554–557.
4. Bay WH, Henry ML, Lazarus JM, et al. Predicting hemodialysis access failure with color flow Doppler ultrasound. *Am J Nephrol* 1998;18:296–304.
5. Wang E, Schneditz D, Levin NW. Predictive value of access blood flow and stenosis in detection of graft failure. *Clin Nephrol* 2000;54:393–399.
6. Oudenhoven LF, Pattynama PM, de Roos A, et al. Magnetic resonance, a new method for measuring blood flow in hemodialysis fistulae. *Kidney Int* 1994;45:884–889.
7. Bakker CJ, Bosman PJ, Boereboom FT, et al. Measuring flow in hemodialysis grafts by non-triggered 2DPC magnetic resonance angiography. *Kidney Int* 1996;49:903–905.
8. Depner TA. Analysis of new methods for access monitoring. *Semin Dial* 1999;12:376–381.
9. Depner TA, Krivitski NM. Clinical measurement of blood flow in hemodialysis access fistulae and grafts by ultrasound dilution. *ASAIO J* 1995;41:M745–M749.
10. Weitzel WF, Rubin JM, Swartz RD, et al. Variable flow Doppler for hemodialysis access evaluation: theory and clinical feasibility. *ASAIO J* 2000;46:65–69.
11. Krivitski NM. Theory and validation of access flow measurement by dilution technique during hemodialysis. *Kidney Int* 1995;48:244–250.
12. Krivitski NM, MacGibbon D, Gleed RD, Dobson A. Accuracy of dilution techniques for access flow measurement during hemodialysis. *Am J Kidney Dis* 1998;31:502–508.
13. Krivitski NM. Novel method to measure access flow during hemodialysis by ultrasound velocity dilution technique. *ASAIO J* 1995;41:M741–M745.
14. Sands J, Glidden D, Miranda C. Access flow measured during hemodialysis. *ASAIO J* 1996;42:M530–M532.
15. Pandeya S, Lindsay RM. The relationship between cardiac output and access flow during hemodialysis. *ASAIO J* 1999;45:135–138.
16. Rehman SU, Pupim LB, Shyr Y, et al. Intradialytic serial vascular access flow measurements. *Am J Kidney Dis* 1999;34:471–477.
17. Krivitski NM, Depner TA. Development of a method for measuring hemodialysis access flow: From idea to robust technology. *Semin Dial* 1998;11:124–130.
18. Depner TA, Rizwan S, Stasi TA. Pressure effects on roller pump blood flow during hemodialysis. *ASAIO Trans* 1990;36:M456–M459.
19. Schmidt DF, Schniepp BJ, Kurtz SB, et al. Inaccurate blood flow rate during rapid hemodialysis. *Am J Kidney Dis* 1991;17:34–37.
20. Sands J, Glidden D, Jacavage W, et al. Difference between delivered and prescribed blood flow in hemodialysis. *ASAIO J* 1996;42:M717–M719.
21. Depner TA, Krivitski NM, MacGibbon D. Hemodialysis access recirculation measured by ultrasound dilution. *ASAIO J* 1995;41:M749–M753.
22. Mercadal L, Hamani A, Bene B, et al. Determination of access blood flow from ionic dialysance: theory and validation. *Kidney Int* 1999;56:1560–1565.

23. Bosman PJ, Boereboom FT, Bakker CJ, et al. Access flow measurements in hemodialysis patients: *in vivo* validation of an ultrasound dilution technique. *J Am Soc Nephrol* 1996;7:966–969.

24. Sands J, Glidden D, Miranda C. Hemodialysis access flow measurement: comparison of ultrasound dilution and duplex ultrasonography. *ASAIO J* 1996;42:M899–M901.

25. Lindsay RM, Blake PG, Malek P, et al. Accuracy and precision of access recirculation measurements by the hemodynamic recirculation monitor. *Am J Kidney Dis* 1998;31:242–249.

26. Lindsay RM, Blake PG, Malek P, et al. Hemodialysis access blood flow rates can be measured by a differential conductivity technique and are predictive of access clotting. *Am J Kidney Dis* 1997; 30:475–482.

27. Lindsay RM, Bradfield E, Rothera C, et al. A comparison of methods for the measurement of hemodialysis access recirculation and access blood flow rate. *ASAIO J* 1998;44:62–67.

28. Lindsay RM, Blake PG, Bradfield E. Estimation of hemodialysis access blood flow rates by a urea method is a poor predictor of access outcome. *ASAIO J* 1998;44:818–822.

29. Schneditz D, Fan Z, Kaufman A, et al. Measurement of access flow during hemodialysis using the constant infusion approach. *ASAIO J* 1998;44:74–81.

30. Schneditz D, Wang E, Levin NW. Validation of haemodialysis recirculation and access blood flow measured by thermodilution. *Nephrol Dial Transplant* 1999;14:376–383.

31. Yarar D, Cheung AK, Sakiewicz P, et al. Ultrafiltration method for measuring vascular access flow rates during hemodialysis. *Kidney Int* 1999;56:1129–1135.

32. Gotch FA, Buyaki R, Panlilio F, et al. Measurement of blood access flow rate during hemodialysis from conductivity dialysance. *ASAIO J* 1999;45:139–146.

33. Gotch F, Panlilio F, Buyaki R, et al. A comparative study of ultrasound and conductivity dialysance methods to measure blood access flow rate. *J Am Soc Nephrol* 1998;9:171(abst).

34. Sands J, Young S, Miranda C. The effect of Doppler flow screening studies and elective revisions on dialysis access failure. *ASAIO J* 1992;38:M524–M527.

35. Depner TA, Reasons AM. Longevity of peripheral A-V grafts and fistulas is related to access blood flow. *J Am Soc Nephrol* 1996;7: 1405(abst).

36. Besarab A, Lubkowski T, Frinak S, et al. Detecting vascular access dysfunction. *ASAIO J* 1997;43:M539–M543.

37. May RE, Himmelfarb J, Yenicesu M, et al. Predictive measures of vascular access thrombosis: a prospective study. *Kidney Int* 1997; 52:1656–1662.

38. Bosman PJ, Boereboom FT, Eikelboom BC, et al. Graft flow as a predictor of thrombosis in hemodialysis grafts. *Kidney Int* 1998; 54:1726–1730.

39. Wang E, Schneditz D, Nepomuceno C, et al. Predictive value of access blood flow in detecting access thrombosis. *ASAIO J* 1998; 44:M555–M558.

40. Paulson WD, Ram SJ, Birk CG, et al. Does blood flow accurately predict thrombosis or failure of hemodialysis synthetic grafts? A meta-analysis. *Am J Kidney Dis* 1999;34:478–485.

41. Neyra NR, Ikizler TA, May RE, et al. Change in access blood flow over time predicts vascular access thrombosis. *Kidney Int* 1998;54:1714–1719.

42. Paulson WD, Ram SJ, Birk CG, et al. Accuracy of decrease in blood flow in predicting hemodialysis graft thrombosis. *Am J Kidney Dis* 2000;35:1089–1095.

43. National Kidney Foundation-Dialysis Outcomes Quality Initiative. NKF-DOQI clinical practice guidelines for vascular access. *Am J Kidney Dis* 1997;30:S150–S191.

44. Hakim R, Himmelfarb J. Hemodialysis access failure: a call to action. *Kidney Int* 1998;54:1029–1040.

45. National Kidney Foundation-Dialysis Outcomes Quality Initiative. NKF-K/DOQI clinical practice guidelines for vascular access: update 2000. *Am J Kidney Dis* 2001;37:S137–S181.

46. Besarab A, Sherman R. The relationship of recirculation to access blood flow. *Am J Kidney Dis* 1997;29:223–229.

47. Schwab SJ, Raymond JR, Saeed M, et al. Prevention of hemodialysis fistula thrombosis: early detection of venous stenoses. *Kidney Int* 1989;36:707–711.

48. Besarab A, Sullivan KL, Ross RP, et al. Utility of intra-access pressure monitoring in detecting and correcting venous outlet stenoses prior to thrombosis. *Kidney Int* 1995;47:1364–1373.

49. Roberts AB, Kahn MB, Bradford S, et al. Graft surveillance and angioplasty prolongs dialysis graft patency. *J Am Coll Surg* 1996; 183:486–492.

50. Safa AA, Valji K, Roberts AC, et al. Detection and treatment of dysfunctional hemodialysis access grafts: effect of a surveillance program on graft patency and the incidence of thrombosis. *Radiology* 1996;199:653–657.

51. Cayco AV, Abu-Alfa AK, Mahnensmith RL, et al. Reduction in arteriovenous graft impairment: results of a vascular access surveillance protocol. *Am J Kidney Dis* 1998;32:302–308.

52. Gallego Beuter JJ, Hernandez LA, Herrero CJ, et al. Early detection and treatment of hemodialysis access dysfunction. *Cardiovasc Intervent Radiol* 2000;23:40–46.

53. Schwab SJ, Oliver MJ, Suhocki P, et al. Hemodialysis arteriovenous access: detection of stenosis and response to treatment by vascular access blood flow. *Kidney Int* 2001;59:358–362.

54. Lumsden AB, MacDonald MJ, Kikeri D, et al. Prophylactic balloon angioplasty fails to prolong the patency of expanded polytetrafluoroethylene arteriovenous grafts: results of a prospective randomized study. *J Vasc Surg* 1997;26:382–390.

55. Martin LG, MacDonald MJ, Kikeri D, et al. Prophylactic angioplasty reduces thrombosis in virgin ePTFE arteriovenous dialysis grafts with greater than 50% stenosis: subset analysis of a prospectively randomized study. *J Vasc Interv Radiol* 1999;10:389–396.

56. Sands JJ, Jabyac PA, Miranda CL, et al. Intervention based on monthly monitoring decreases hemodialysis access thrombosis. *ASAIO J* 1999;45:147–150.

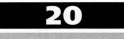

DOPPLER ULTRASOUND AND HEMODIALYSIS ACCESS MANAGEMENT

JEFFREY J. SANDS

Color-flow Doppler ultrasound provides a noninvasive image of the dialysis access, a measurement of the velocities of blood flowing through the access, and a measurement of the hemodialysis access blood flow. It is mobile, noninvasive, and can be performed serially. It is the only noninvasive mobile technique that can provide both anatomic and physiologic (hemodynamic) information about the function of the dialysis access. Although magnetic resonance imaging (MRI) and magnetic resonance and magnetic resonance angiography (MRA) can provide comparable information, their lack of mobility, limited availability, and high cost have limited their current role to that of a research tool. Angiography has been considered the gold standard in the evaluation of the hemodialysis access abnormalities. In reality, however, duplex ultrasound provides more information without the potential risks associated with the use of contrast agents. This ability to evaluate hemodialysis access anatomy and physiology noninvasively makes Doppler ultrasound an attractive modality for evaluating and following a patient's vascular access function.

DOPPLER ULTRASOUND PROTOCOLS AND TECHNIQUE

A dialysis access Duplex ultrasound includes gray scale and color-flow images of the entire access with transverse and longitudinal views of the arterial anastomosis, the length and body of the access, the venous anastomosis and venous runoff, including the subclavian vein to the level of the clavicle. A Doppler evaluation of the velocity of blood flow is performed throughout the access and access flow is measured. Often an image of the native inflow artery and a calculation of volume flow in the inflow artery also are performed (1).

The adequacy of Doppler Ultrasound is dependent on the ability and experience of the operator, the anatomy of the access, and the capability and the characteristics of the ultrasound machine used. Potential sources of variance include difficulty in measuring the cross-sectional area of the vessel, difficulties in obtaining an adequate Doppler angle,

and an inability to obtain an adequate Doppler signal. In particular, measurement of access flow can be affected by these parameters. Access flow is generally measured in an area of laminar flow, avoiding areas of turbulence. Volume flow is calculated by multiplying the cross-sectional area of the access by the measured velocity of blood integrated across the cross section. Different machines use different algorithms to compute the velocity used for the calculation of access flow (based on, e.g., mean velocity, peak velocity, both, time domain correlation). For this reason, flow volume measurements may vary with the brand of ultrasound machine being used.

Winker and colleagues (2) compared volume flow measurements in five commercially available duplex machines with a phantom model at flow rates between 150 to 823 mL per minute. Variation in the measured flow volumes ranged from an underestimation of 10.8% to 33.6% (Siemens-Quantum QAD1) (*mean velocity method*) to overestimates of 9.2% to 39.1% (H.P. Sonos 1000) (*peak velocity method*), 6.0% to 77.9% (ATL Ultramark 9), and 2.3% to 37.5% (Acuson128XP/10) (*both peak and mean velocity methods*). The most accurate measurements (within -3.1%–$+0.5\%$ of flow settings) were obtained by time domain correlation (Phillips CVI). These systemic differences must be considered when comparing measurements using different machines or techniques. Access flow measured by Doppler ultrasound correlates with measurements obtained by other methods. Sands and colleagues (3) compared access flow measurement by Doppler ultrasound with time domain correlation to online measurement of access flow by ultrasound dilution (Transonic HDO1 monitor, Transonic Systems, Ithaca, N.Y., U.S.A.). Results were comparable by both methods with a correlation coefficient of 0.83.

USES OF COLOR-FLOW DOPPLER ULTRASOUND IN VASCULAR ACCESS

Color-flow Doppler ultrasound has multiple uses in vascular access management. These include preaccess vascular imaging to determine the best potential sites for AV fistula placement, prediction of access failure by detection of stenosis and other pathology and monitoring flow volume, helping to determine the most appropriate access intervention (e.g., surgical revision, angioplasty, elective creation of a secondary AV fistula), and evaluation of the success of interventional procedures.

Preoperative Imaging

Several groups have reported the ability to use Doppler ultrasound to select appropriate vessels for access creation (See Chapters 10, 11, and 14). Koksoy and colleagues (4) compared the effect of preoperative Doppler evaluation on the initial and long-term patency rate of straight brachial polytetrafluoroethylene (PTFE) grafts placed in patients with failed arteriovenous (AV) fistulas. Doppler studies identified problems in the proposed access arm in 5 of 17 patients (two with decreased brachial artery flow, three with subclavian vein stenosis) that resulted in use of the other arm for access placement. After 1 month, all 17 patients in the Doppler group had functioning grafts; however, 3 of 21 controls developed thrombosis. At 6 months, only 2 of 17 Doppler patients compared with 8 of 21 control patients had developed thrombosis ($p = 0.06$). After 1 year, 5 of 17 patients in the Doppler group had developed thrombosis; all five had preoperative brachial artery flow rates below 70 mL per minute. The nine patients with brachial artery flow rates greater than 70 mL per minute remained patent.

Silva and colleagues (5) increased successful AV fistula placement through the use of preoperative Doppler ultrasound to identify the appropriate sites for AV fistula placement. Their criteria include having an arterial diameter of 2 mm or greater, no pressure differential between the patients' two arms, and having a patent palmar arch. Veins are required to be 2.5 mm or larger for AV fistulas and 4 mm or larger for PTFE grafts. Veins had to be patent, without segmental stenosis or occluded segments, have continuity with the upper-arm deep venous system, and have no evidence of ipsilateral central vein stenosis. Using these criteria, early AV fistula failure decreased from 38% to 8.3%, and AV fistula prevalence increased from 14% to 63% over a 2.5-year period. In subsequent work, Silva and colleagues used Doppler ultrasound mapping to select deep forearm veins for transposition to the surface for the use in AV fistula creation (6). Ascher and colleagues (7) also reported increasing AV fistula prevalence through a program emphasizing preoperative ultrasound to select appropriate vasculature for AV fistula creation. Using criteria requiring a vein measuring larger than 2 mm at the wrist or larger than 3 mm in the upper arm, they were able to increase fistula placement from 5% to 68% from 1996 through 1999. In the last year of their program, more than 95% of patients underwent AV fistula creation. Successful 6-week maturation ranged from 75% to 91% (75% radial–cephalic, 91% brachial–cephalic, 87% brachial–basilic).

Stenosis Detection

Ultrasound accurately detects stenosis. Tordoir and colleagues (8) compared stenosis determination in 64 accesses by using Doppler ultrasound and arteriography. Ultrasound successfully identified greater than 50% stenotic lesions in AV fistulas with a sensitivity of 79% and a specificity of 84% and greater than 50% stenoses in PTFE grafts (all sites) with sensitivity of 92%. Stenosis at the venous anastomosis was identified with 95% sensitivity and 97% specificity. Gadallah and co-workers (9) found that of 38 patients prospectively evaluated by both techniques, all 19 patients with greater than 50% stenosis by angiography had greater than 40% stenosis by ultrasound. The other 19 patients had no significant stenosis by either technique. The differences in the estimation of the extent of stenosis between angiography and ultrasound are related to the differences in the techniques themselves. Ultrasound images both the inside and outside vessel wall and clearly defines the area where blood is flowing. Angiography shows only the column of moving contrast (blood). This results in somewhat different information. Miranda and Sands (10) reviewed 71 accesses referred for angiographic evaluation because of significant stenosis (>50%) found on ultrasound evaluation. Angiography confirmed lesions in 60 accesses (85%). Of the 11 remaining cases, ten angiograms were subsequently reviewed by a second radiologist (one was lost), and five of these ten angiograms were misread initially and had significant abnormalities, which correlated with the ultrasound findings. Four others disagreed only about the degree of stenosis present. The final correlation rate was 97%.

Access Monitoring

Doppler ultrasound has been used successfully to predict accesses at risk of failure. Strauch and associates (11) reported that PTFE grafts with a greater than 50% stenosis had a 57.1% thrombosis rate within 6 months compared with a 9.5% to 11.4 % grafts with less than 50% stenosis. Patients who developed thrombosis had lower access flow rates (357 versus 638.5 mL per minute)(Siemens-Quantum) than grafts that remained patent.

May and colleagues (12) also showed with significant correlation of stenosis with subsequent access thrombosis. In their study, 57% of PTFE grafts with a greater than 70% stenosis thrombosed over the subsequent 6 months, compared with a less than 8% thrombosis rate in PTFE grafts with lower grade of stenosis. Sands and colleagues evaluated 253 patients with duplex ultrasonography (13). Patients with PTFE grafts with flow rates less than 800 mL per minute by Doppler ultrasound (Hewlett Packard Sonos 100) had a 92.9% incidence of thrombosis over 6 months compared with a 25% to 28% thrombosis rate in those with higher flows. In a later study, Miranda and Sands (14) reviewed 1,308 ultrasound-derived flow volume measurements (Hewlett Packard Sonos 100) performed on 831 PTFE grafts and 477 AV fistulas. Six-month patency without intervention was 5% for PTFE grafts with flow less than 400 mL per minute and 18% with flow of 401 to 800 mL per minute compared with a 44% to 66% patency in grafts with flow greater than 800 mL per minute ($p < 0.0001$). In AV fistulas, 26% with flow less than 400 mL per minute remained patent without intervention for 6 months, compared with 57% to 85% in fistulas with flow volumes greater than 400 mL per minute ($p < 0.0001$).

It is important to note that ultrasound-based programs, including monitoring coupled with elective repair of stenotic lesions, effectively decrease access thrombosis. In the previous study by Miranda and Sands (14), 22% of nonrevised PTFE grafts, with flow less than 800 mL per minute, accesses remained patent after 6 months, compared with 47% of those who underwent revision. This improved 6-month patency was noted even at higher flow rates. Of grafts with flows greater than 800 mL per minute who underwent correction of a greater than 50% stenosis, 80% remained patent, compared with 65% that were not revised. Similarly, in AV fistulas, those with flows less than 800 mL per minute who underwent revision had a 77% versus a 59% patency at 6 months in those that were not revised (14).

Other groups have shown similar results. Mayer and colleagues (15) prospectively randomized 70 new PTFE grafts from initial placement to either clinical evaluation or monitoring by Doppler ultrasound. Patients with greater than 50% stenosis by Doppler ultrasound were referred for surgical revision. Patients in the ultrasound group required less surgery (0.7 procedures versus 1.6, $p < 0.05$) and had fewer episodes of thrombosis. Life-table analysis revealed significantly improved patency at 6, 12, 24, and 36 months. Altman and colleagues (16) decreased thrombosis rates from 94.6 per 100 patient-years to 41.1 per 100 patient-years using a program of 2- to 3-month ultrasounds, coupled with angioplasty of greater than 50% stenotic lesions. In another study, 55 patients with PTFE grafts were randomized to a program of ultrasound followed by angioplasty of 50% stenosis or a control group. In the intervention group, thrombosis rates were 19 per 100 patient-years versus 126 per 100 patient-years in controls. The total number of interventions (21.9 per 100 patient-years in the ultrasound group versus 138.8 in the control group), access-related hospital admissions [7 admissions per 100 patient-years (U.S.) versus 92 controls] and hospitalized days [73 days per 100 patient-years (U.S.) versus 210 controls) were significantly lower in the ultrasound group (17).

In 1997, the effectiveness of an ultrasound–angioplasty program was called to question in a study by Lumsden and co-workers (18). Life-table analysis comparing PTFE grafts with 50% stenosis (by ultrasound and confirmed with angiography) randomized to angioplasty or observation revealed no difference in outcomes between the two groups. Despite randomization, however, this study was limited by

demographic differences between the two groups. The intervention group had more central stenosis and more prior thrombosis than the control group. Subsequently, a subgroup analysis was performed on the 21 patients with PTFE grafts with no prior access interventions (19). Fewer patients who underwent elective angioplasty developed thrombosis (25% versus 69%), thrombosis rates were significantly lower (0.1 thrombosis per patient-year versus 44 thromboses per patient-year) after elective angioplasty, and life-table analysis showed improved survival for the PTFE grafts in the elective angioplasty group compared with controls. These studies confirm the usefulness of ultrasound monitoring with elective correction of stenosis to decrease thrombosis rates.

Access flow measurement was recommended by the Dialysis Outcome Quality Improvement (DOQI) (20) as the best method for monitoring; however, the sensitivity and specificity of access flow measurement alone to predict thrombosis has been questioned. Monitoring is effective only if one can identify and repair lesions that result in improved patient outcome. Sands and associates (21) evaluated measurements of access flow by Doppler ultrasound and measurement of access stenosis to determine the sensitivity and specificity of access flow alone to predict a 50%-diameter stenosis. Studies were performed on 1,604 AV fistulas and 1,364 PTFE grafts over a 7-month period. In AV fistulas, access flow of less than 400 mL per minute had a 42.9% sensitivity and a 79.5% specificity for identifying a 50%-diameter stenosis. Flow of less than 300 mL per minute had a 22.6% sensitivity and 88.4% specificity, and flows of less than 200 mL per minute had a 10.7% sensitivity and a 96% specificity for identifying a 50%-diameter stenosis. In PTFE grafts, access flow of less than 600 mL per minute had a 50.2% sensitivity, an 81.5% specificity, and a false-positive rate of 18.5% for identifying a 50%-diameter stenosis. Even at access flows of less than 500, there was only a 33.5% sensitivity and a 89.1% specificity with a false-positive rate of 10.9%. Referral for angiography based on the Kidney Disease Outcomes Quality Initiative (K/DOQI) criteria of access flow of less than 600mL per minute might result in a significant number of negative angiograms.

Currently, both the K/DOQI and SCVIR recommend angioplasty of greater than 50% stenotic lesions only if they are hemodynamically significant (determined by elevated dynamic or static venous pressure or decreased access flow). This approach hinges on the adequacy, efficacy, and frequency of the "hemodynamic" monitoring. Access monitoring (see Chapters 19 and 21) techniques differ greatly and may vary significantly during and between treatments. Often they are not readily available or performed infrequently if at all. There is no evidence that shows that correction of only "hemodynamically" significant stenosis is a superior strategy than to correct all greater than 50% stenosis. In fact, the best strategy may be determined by the details of the particular monitoring program and the ability to obtain prompt intervention when indicated. Further studies are necessary to clarify this issue.

REIMBURSEMENT ISSUES

Reimbursement issues play a significant role in the clinical decisions on access management. Currently, there is no reimbursement in the United States for access flow measurement (22), and the stringent criteria for reimbursement for Doppler ultrasound have limited its utility. It remains unclear whether reimbursement will allow the effective use of Doppler ultrasound as part of coordinated access management programs. These policies are short sighted and complicate patient care.

CONCLUSION

In conclusion, ultrasound provides reliable anatomic and physiologic data that correlate closely with angiographic evaluation of dialysis accesses. Color-flow Doppler can reliably predict the subset of patients at increased risks of access failure. Prospectively, trials show that ultrasound-based programs can decrease thrombosis rates, prolong access longevity, and decrease the cost of hemodialysis access management. Color-flow Doppler ultrasound should be included as a part of an integrated approach to dialysis access management.

REFERENCES

1. Sands J, Kapsick B. Assessment of hemodialysis access performance by color-flow Doppler ultrasound. *J Biomater Appl* 1999; 13:224–237.
2. Winkler AJ, WuJ, Case T, Ricci MA. An experimental study of the accuracy of volume flow measurements using commercial ultrasound systems. *J Vasc Technol* 1995;19:175–180.
3. Sands J, Glidden D, Miranda C. Hemodialysis access flow measurement comparison of ultrasound dilution and duplex ultrasonography. *ASAIO J* 1996;Sept–Oct:M899–M901.
4. Koksoy C, Kuzu A, Erden I, et al. Predictive value of color Doppler ultrasonography in detecting failure of vascular access grafts. *Br J Surg* 1995;82:50–52.
5. Silva MB, Hobson II RW, Pappas PJ, et al. A strategy for incasing use of autogenous hemodialysis access procedures: impact of preoperative noninvasive evaluation. J Vasc Surg 1998;27:302–308.
6. Silva MB, Hobson RW, Pappas PJ, et al. Vein transposition in the forearm for autogenous hemodialysis access. *J Vasc Surg* 1997; 26:981–988.
7. Ascher E, Gade P, Hingorani A, et al. Changes in the practice of angioaccess surgery: impact of dialysis outcome and quality initiative recommendations. *J Vasc Surg* 2000;31:84–92.
8. Tordoir JH, de Bruin HG, Hoeneveld H, et al. Duplex ultrasound scanning in the assessment of arteriovenous fistulas created for hemodialysis access. *J Vasc Surg* 1989;10:122–128.
9. Gadallah MF, Paulson WD, Vickers B, et al. Accuracy of Doppler ultrasound in diagnosing anatomic stenosis of hemodialysis arteriovenous access as compared with fistulography. *Am J Kidney Dis* 1998;32:273–277.
10. Miranda CL, Sands JJ. Duplex referral of hemodialysis access for percutaneous balloon angioplasty. *J Vasc Technol* 1996;20:99–103.
11. Strauch BS, O'Connell RS, Geoly KL. Forecasting thrombosis of vascular access with Doppler color flow imaging. *Am J Kidney Dis* 1992;19:554–557.
12. May RE, Himmelfarb J, Yenicesu M, et al. Predictive measures of vascular access thrombosis: a prospective study. *Kidney Int* 1997; 52:1656–1662.
13. Sands JJ, Young SF, Miranda CL. The effect of Doppler flow screening studies and elective revisions on dialysis access failure. *Trans Am Soc Artif Intern Organs* 1992;38:524–527.
14. Miranda CL, Sands JJ. Flow volumes as a predictor of hemodialysis access failure. *J Vasc Technol* 1998;22:73–76.
15. Mayer DA, Zingale RG, Tsapogas MJ. Duplex scanning of expanded polytetrafluoroethylene dialysis shunts: impact on patient management and graft survival. *Vasc Surg* 1993;27:647–658.
16. Altman SD, Arthur TS, Altman NR, et al. Maintenance angioplasty of hemodialysis access stenoses in a mobile setting. In: Henry MG, Ferguson RM, eds. *Vascular access for hemodialysis*. Chicago: W.L. Gore & Associates and Precept Press, 1997: 178–185.
17. Sands J, Gandy D, Finn M, et al. Ultrasound-angioplasty program decreases thrombosis rate and cost of PTFE graft maintenance. *J Am Soc Nephrol* 1997;8:171(abst).
18. Lumsden A, MacDonald J, Kikeri D, et al. Prophylactic balloon angioplasty fails to prolong the patency of expanded polytetrafluoroethylene arteriovenous grafts: results of a prospective randomized trial. *J Vasc Surg* 1997;26:382–392.
19. Martin LG, MacDonald MJ, Kikeri D, et al. Prophylactic angioplasty reduces a thrombosis in virgin ePTFE arteriovenous dialysis grafts with greater than 50% stenosis: subset analysis of a prospectively randomized study. *J Vasc Interv Radiol* 1999;10: 389–396.
20. National Kidney Foundation K/DOQI clinical practice guidelines for vascular access 2000. *Am J Kidney Dis* 2001;37(Suppl 1):S137–S181.
21. Sands J, Uddin L, Espada C, et al. Access flow measurement poorly predicts a 50% stenosis. *J Am Soc Nephrol* 2000;11: A1553(abst).
22. HCFA Program Memorandum Transmittal AB-00-55 June 2000.

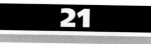

PRESSURE MEASUREMENTS IN THE SURVEILLANCE OF VASCULAR ACCESSES

ANATOLE BESARAB
STANLEY FRINAK
MOHAMMAD A. ASLAM

Recognizing and treating a failed vascular access remain major issues for nephrologists and their hemodialysis patients. Failure of access function, defined as the delivery of less than 400 mL per minute of blood flow to the dialyzer, can limit the delivered dose of dialysis and affect patient survival (1).

Tests to assess hemodynamics within the access, access pressure, or flow, can detect vascular accesses at risk for thrombosis. Available tests have different utility in detecting lesions within an arteriovenous (AV) fistula compared with a synthetic graft (2). Anatomic features and location of lesions produce differences in the flow-pressure characteristics (2). Access type, that is, autologous native fistula versus prosthetic bridge graft, also may influence the risk for thrombosis at a given flow (3,4).

A firm understanding of access hemodynamics as well as what pressures are being measured is required to use pressure measurements as a surveillance method for detecting access dysfunction. Different lesions and anatomic locations produce different changes in the flow-pressure characteristics within the access (5).

DIALYSIS CIRCUIT AND SITES OF PRESSURE MEASUREMENT

A typical dialysis circuit is shown in Figure 21.1. A loop prosthetic graft access is shown cannulated with fistula needles in the arterial and venous segments. The arterial segment of a vascular access is defined as that portion of the access in which the "arterial" needles are placed that permit withdrawal of blood into the extracorporeal dialysis circuit. The venous segment is that portion of the access that is cannulated with "venous needles" to return blood from the extracorporeal circuit and back into the vascular system.

The blood pump generates a negative pressure, inducing blood flow into the arterial segment of the dialyzer tubing (6). Because the pump is occlusive, pressure becomes positive after the pumping, and it is this pressure that drives blood through the dialyzer, venous tubing, and needle and then back into the vascular access. On many delivery systems (Cobe/Gambro, Althin, Lakewood, CO, U.S.A.; Fresinius, Lexington, MA, U.S.A.) prepump (negative pressures) can be measured. On other systems (Baxter, McGraw Park, IL, U.S.A.) only postpump (positive pressure) can be measured. Dynamic pressure measurements are conducted with the blood pump running and typically are measured from the venous drip chamber. Static pressures are measured with the blood pump shut off and more directly reflect the pressures in the access. To detect all access lesions maximally, static pressure measurements should be recorded from both the arterial and venous segments (See below).

Measurements of pressure from the dialysis circuit were not designed originally to measure access function either directly or indirectly. They were used to determine the mean pressure needed to obtain a given hydraulic ultrafiltration rate so that fluid could be removed from patients. The desired ultrafiltration rate was calculated as the weight gained divided by the total treatment time. Each dialyzer was capable of delivering a different rate when a given transmembrane pressure gradient was applied. Thus, it was necessary to calculate the transmembrane pressure needed from the desired ultrafiltration rate and the membrane ultrafiltration coefficient (typically provided by the manufacturers of the membranes). The mean transmembrane pressure in the dialyzer was equated to the average of the postpump predialyzer drip chamber pressure and the venous return drip chamber pressure. Thus, it is necessary to know both pressures on either side of the dialyzer. The development of volumetric control systems made measurement of these pressures obsolete. Pressure measurements were retained because of safety issues.

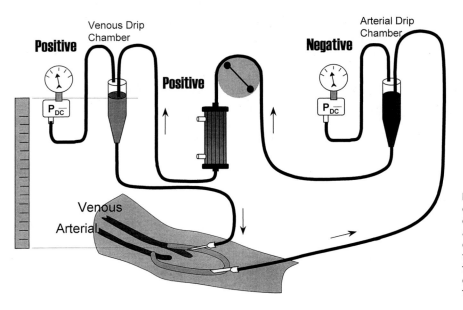

FIGURE 21.1. Diagram of a typical dialysis circuit. A loop prosthetic graft access is shown cannulated with fistula needles in the arterial and venous segments. The blood pump generates a negative pressure, inducing blood flow into the tubing. Pressure becomes positive post pump, and it is this pressure that drives blood through the dialyzer and venous tubing and back into the vascular access.

Prepump arterial segment pressures are now chiefly used to determine whether the access can deliver the prescribed flow without generating excessively negative pressures (7). A common sign of inadequate access inflow is excessive negative pressures at the arterial needle. At high negative pressures, collapse of the pump segments reduces the delivered (true dialyzer) blood flow compared with the set blood flow (8,9). This can produce underdialysis. Excessively negative pressures also can lead to cavitation and hemolysis (10). This is particularly dangerous in systems that only use a "pillow" to detect these excessively negative pressures.

The venous drip chamber pressure is sensitive to changes in venous needle outflow obstruction. The pressure at the venous drip chamber was used to detect infiltration or malposition of the needle because infiltration into the soft tissue or flow through a partially occluded orifice would quickly produce pressures greater than 300 mm Hg and either alarm the system or shut the blood pump off. Because there was no algorithm to detect low pressures, dislodgement of the venous needle could lead to exsanguination (11).

FLOW CHANGES IN ACCESSES WITH MATURATION AND DISEASE

Blood flow in an AV fistula increases progressively over the first 3 to 6 months after construction while the access undergoes maturation. Once developed, a matured native fistula maintains its flow for years. By contrast, blood flow in an AV graft is maximal within 2 to 5 weeks of its construction (12) and then decreases variably over time. In some patients, flow is maintained for years and in others only for 3 to 4 months. Despite the differences in pressure profiles along the access between native AV fistulae and prosthetic AV grafts (see later discussion), access flow rates tend to be

quite similar when compared at similar anatomic locations. This results from the similar overall resistances for the two access types. In general, well-functioning grafts and native fistulas provide the same flow when the same artery is used for construction. The major determinant of the initial access flow is the artery used for the arterial anastomosis: axillary > brachial > radial. Well-functioning forearm straight grafts from the radial artery average 600 to 800 mL per minute, forearm loop grafts from the brachial artery about 1,000 mL per minute. Upper-arm graft flow is somewhat higher and may range up to 3 L per minute (4,13,14).

A body of evidence suggests that an access flow rate less than 600 mL per minute in a graft predicts failure of the access (15–22). Most grafts cannot sustain patency for more than 6 weeks at flows less than 350 mL per minute. Native fistulas can maintain long-term patency at flows lower than those in grafts. Because access flow determines patency, a strong impetus for measurement of access flow has evolved in the last 5 years to predict the likelihood of access dysfunction; however, pressure measurements, the mainstay of access surveillance in the last few years, will continue to be used.

PRESSURE–FLOW RELATIONSHIPS IN NORMAL VASCULAR ACCESSES

Pressure is a surrogate for flow. Access flow, intra-access pressure, and flow resistance are mathematically related (23,24). The intra-access pressure (P_{IA}) profiles of grafts and native fistulas differ significantly when measured as pullback pressures starting in the artery, proceeding longitudinally along the length of the access, and concluding with measurements from the draining and central veins (3,25). This is illustrated in Figure 21.2. Because systemic blood pressure influences intra-access pressure, the ordinate in Figure 21.2 expresses the pressure at any point along the access as a percentage of mean arterial pressure (MAP) in the artery supplying the access (P_{IA}/MAP). Blood entering an AV graft can exit only through the venous outlet and its draining veins. In a normal AV graft, most of the arterial pressure is dissipated across the two anastomoses (35%–50% arterial and 20%–25% venous) as shown in Figure 21.2. These gradients at the two anastomoses develop in the absence of any anatomic lesions and are believed to represent loss of energy resulting from compliance mismatch (26) and tissue vibration from turbulent flow (27). The pressure gradient along the graft itself from arterial to venous cannulation sites (usually <30 mm Hg) is only 20% to 25% of the arterial pressure head. As newer configurations are developed that modify the venous anastomotic outlet (hooded grafts), the intra-access pressure profile is likely to change somewhat.

In AV fistulae, blood entering the venous system can return to the heart via multiple collateral veins unless the main trunk has been "pruned" to force blood to go through the main cephalic vein as part of a maturation procedure (28). The intra-access pressure falls to about 20% of the arterial pressure in the *earliest* segment of the fistula used for arterial needle insertion. A pressure gradient of less than 10 mm Hg (29) is sufficient to maintain flows of 1 L per minute or more through the fistula system. Vascular resistance of native AV fistulae is lower than in grafts, in part because of the multiple parallel venous pathways returning blood to the central venous system, and in part because of vasoactive properties associated with an intact endothelium. In humans, grafts are endothelialized for only a few centimeters at either of the two anastomoses (30). Patency of grafts depends on a high flow rate; by contrast, the endothelium of autologous fistula releases anticoagulant factors, which inhibit thrombosis.

EFFECT OF STENOSIS ON PRESSURE PROFILES IN ARTERIOVENOUS ACCESSES

The location of the stenosis within the vascular access affects the longitudinal pressure patterns in both native (Fig. 21.3) and prosthetic grafts (Fig. 21.4). Typically, stenoses are described as being inflow (at the arterial anastomoses or early arterial cannulation segment), within the body of the access, or in the outflow tract. In grafts, the outflow tract consists of the venous–graft anastomoses, the draining vein(s), and the central vein.

When outflow stenosis develops in a graft (sometimes within a month of construction), a pressure gradient develops, increasing the intra-access pressure proximally (Fig. 21.3). Stenosis before the graft–vein anastomosis (venous outlet) is usually the result of neointimal hyperplasia. The magnitude of pressure increase within the access upstream to the stenosis is proportional to the degree of stenosis. When venous outlet systolic pressure rises above 50% of the MAP, a 50% diameter stenosis is likely (29,31). If a stenosis develops in the body of the graft between the areas used for arterial and venous limb cannulation, venous outlet pressures (measured at the venous needle) will remain normal. Detection of such lesions requires measurement of the upstream arterial segment pressure as well.

Typical profiles for native AV fistulae are shown in Figure 21.4. The solid line depicts the normal profile. An arterial lesion produces a lower than expected intra-access pressure in the arterial segment. Because venous pressures are low to begin with it, it is difficult to detect. An inflow lesion on the first 5 cm of a fistula may develop before the actual use of a fistula and impair maturation of the fistula. Lesions within the body of the fistula are often clinically silent. A major increase in intra-access pressure may be prevented by collateral flow through deeper veins. The difficulty becomes

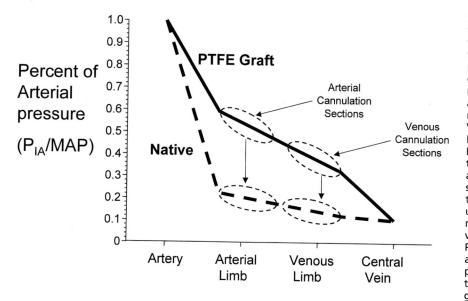

Percent of Arterial pressure (P_{IA}/MAP)

FIGURE 21.2. Pressure profiles within prosthetic graft (*solid line*) and autologous or native (*dashed line*) vascular accesses. In a well-functioning normal graft access, systolic pressure in the early arterial segment decreases to about one half to two thirds of the mean arterial pressure within the feeding artery and to one quarter to one third of mean arterial pressure at the venous segment. Variations in intra-access pressure of 10 mm Hg occur from needle-site rotation in grafts. By contrast, the pressure in the segment of the fistula within 5 cm of the arteriovenous anastomosis is one fifth of the arterial pressure. Because of the low resistance to flow, the pressure gradient between the section used for arterial needle cannulation and the more distal segments of the fistula used for venous cannulation is less than 10 mm Hg. Pressures in the more central draining veins are equal in the two access types. Variations in pressure resulting from rotation of cannulation sites are smaller in native fistulae than grafts.

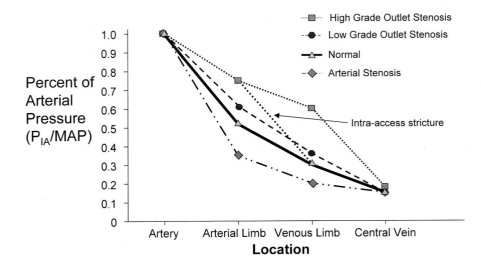

FIGURE 21.3. Effect of stenosis location on intra-access pressures in prosthetic grafts. The *solid line* indicates the normal profile. A venous outlet stenosis increases all pressures proximal to the lesion; the degree of elevation is proportional to severity of stenosis (*dashed lines* connecting circles and squares, respectively). Thus, both the venous segment and arterial segment pressures increase. A stenosis in the body of the graft (intra-access stricture) between the needles elevates the pressure only in the arterial limb, leaving pressures in the venous segment at normal levels (*dashed line* connecting the *squares* and *triangle*). An arterial segment stenosis lowers all pressures in the graft (*dashed dotted line*).

one of being able to cannulate the superficial veins that are now relatively collapsed. If the stenosis is very central in the axillary or central veins, collateral flow is largely precluded, and pressure will increase in all parts of the fistula. In this case, the pressure profile then resembles that in a graft; access flow is compromised, and prolonged bleeding following needle withdrawal is frequently observed. In my experience, upper-arm native fistulae are more likely to develop pressures comparable to those seen in grafts because the opportunity for collateral vein development is less.

As stated earlier, access pressure is a surrogate for access flow. The effect of stenosis on the pressure flow characteristics of native and graft fistulae differs. In grafts, stenoses within the body of the access or in the outflow tract increase resistance to flow. Consequently, flow decreases and the pressure within the access upstream to the stenosis increases. This is schematically illustrated in Fig. 21.5 for a venous outlet lesion, although hemodynamically, it does not matter whether the lesion is in the body of the graft or in the outflow tract because similar degrees of flow reduction are produced by the two differing sites of stenosis (29,32). Three

areas are depicted in Fig. 21.5. The area enclosed by the oval is the area of good graft function with flows of 1 to 2 L per minute. The crosshatched shaded area is the region of increased risk for thrombosis, and the lightly shaded area the region in which access recirculation could occur, depending on whether access flow and blood pump flow setting were mismatched.

Note in Figure 21.5 that the region of increased thrombosis risk (flow <800 mL per minute) with venous outlet lesions is entered when the venous outlet systolic pressure exceeds 50% of the arterial pressure. As pressure increases further, flow decreases even more. Thrombosis rates increase with the degree of stenoses (21). Different investigators have used different absolute values of access flow to predict the likelihood of thrombosis in grafts (16–22). This reflects the differing observation periods among the studies. In general, the shorter the period of observation, the lower the flow that predicts the probability of access thrombosis within the observation period. The likelihood of thrombosis within 6 months increases fourfold when access flow decreases below 600 to 700 mL per minute (17,19,33). The

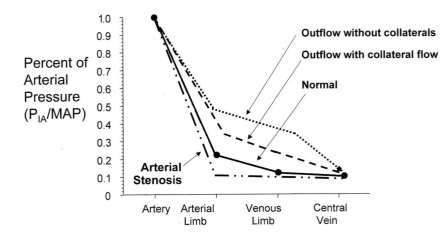

FIGURE 21.4. Effect of stenosis location on intra-access pressures in autologous fistula. The profile of an access without lesions is depicted by the *solid line* connecting the *circles*. The effect of outflow stenosis on pressures in the absence of collaterals (*top curve, dotted line*) and in the presence of collaterals (*dashed line*) is shown. An inflow lesion proximal to the usual "arterial cannulation" area lowers all pressures in the access.

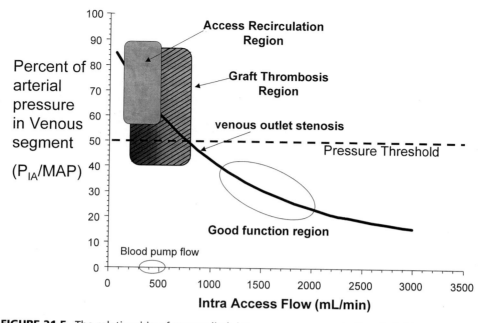

FIGURE 21.5. The relationship of venous limb intra-access pressure to flow in bridge grafts. Venous segment pressure in the access (P_{IA}) is normalized by the mean arterial pressure (*MAP*). The *dark-shaded cross-hatched area* shows the risk of thrombosis in grafts, which begins at about 800 mL per minute. Intra-access pressure increases proximal to the recording venous needle in both loop and straight arteriovenous grafts as stenosis develops. A P_{IA}/ MAP ratio of 0.5 predicts stenosis. Such values are reached before entering the area of increasing risk for thrombosis. Note that for grafts, the risk for thrombosis begins at flows greater than those typically prescribed for dialysis (i.e., pump blood flow rates of 300–500 mL per minute). (Adapted from data in Besarab A, Ross R, Al-Ajel F, et al. The relation of intra-access pressure to flow. *J Am Soc Nephrol* 1995;7:483, with permission, in which longitudinal measurements of pressures and ultrasound measured flow were made at 6 month intervals for 1 year.)

risk increases twofold over 2 months at a blood flow of 500 mL per minute (22). Over a still shorter 6-week observation period, the threshold access flow value indicating impending thrombosis is even lower at 400 mL per minute (20). Such observations are expected because the stenotic lesion is dynamic and progressive over time. In our studies, we also noted that the odds ratio of an access event (i.e., the need for intervention to prevent an access thrombosis) in newly constructed accesses within 6 months is a function of both the initial flow and its rate of change, but it differs for grafts and native AV fistulae (4). Native fistulae can maintain patency at lower flows than grafts, but changes in flow increase the likelihood of intervention because the adequacy of dialysis is compromised.

Note also in Figure 21.5 that the time-honored method to evaluate access adequacy, access recirculation, is a very late indicator of access dysfunction in grafts. Fewer than 20% of grafts can maintain patency at the low flows needed to induce access recirculation (29,32). Access recirculation should not be used in grafts as a surveillance method. In contrast, access recirculation develops in half of the native accesses that require intervention because of inadequate flow.

Unlike the progressive increase in pressure with decreasing access flow seen in two thirds of grafts, the ratio of venous limb intra-access pressure at the venous cannulation segment to arterial pressure usually does not change in autologous AV fistulae, as blood flow progressively decreases (14). This represents the effect of several processes in native fistulae. First, collateral flow permits the exit of the inflowing blood and thus preservation of flow without an increase in pressure (shunt pathways). In fact, accessory side or deep veins sometimes prevent adequate maturation of native cephalic vein fistulae. For pressure to rise in a native vein fistula, the stenosis must be more central in the axillary, subclavian, or innominate system (Fig. 21.4). Second, many lesions are in the arterial inflow tract or body of the fistula within 5 cm of the anastomosis. Resistance to flow and the pressure gradient are proximal to the venous cannulation sites. As a result, measurement of venous pressures alone is not sufficient to detect most stenosis.

PRESSURE MEASUREMENTS: DYNAMIC AND STATIC

Data indicate that flow is the best predictor of the risk for thrombosis in grafts. We found that both the absolute flows as well as the change in flow were important determinants of the probability of clotting (4). Flow measurements, however, are the most time consuming and require a significant amount of staff time. Pressure measurements, however, are fast, easy, and less expensive.

I believe the greatest efficiency derives from a method that can be done quickly, repeatedly, and cheaply to detect the presence of a lesion (pressure measurements) combined with a method that helps to refine the timing for intervention (flow). It is important that the lesion be detected when its severity is moderate (i.e., degree of luminal reduction that is between 50% and 70%) so that there is adequate time to plan nonurgent intervention. The rate of change in access flow among patients varies from less than 50 mL per minute per year to more than 200 mL per minute per month (4). Patients with the latter type of access behavior invariably thrombose their grafts if the interval between measurements is more than several months.

Pressure measurements under certain circumstances can be obtained using the pressure transducers built into the dialysis system. The following considerations must be kept in mind when considering the use of pressure monitoring. First, the method used should be able to detect functionally flow-limiting stenosis. Second, the test must be reproducible and accurate. Because the development of stenosis is common in grafts, tests that do not achieve a sensitivity and specificity of 75% or better in grafts are not useful. No test, including access flow measurement, has perfect accuracy or predictive power (33). The accuracy of some techniques also depends on the location of the lesion(s) within the access or its outflow tract (32).

Dynamic Pressure Measurements

The finding of a persistently elevated venous drip chamber pressure (P_{DC}) is a well-accepted means of screening for the presence of a functionally significant venous outlet stenosis (34). As shown in Figure 21.1, the pressure measured by the transducer at the venous drip chamber is far upstream of the pressure in the venous segment of the vascular access. In addition, the pressure measured at the drip chamber differs

from that in the access by the magnitude of the height difference between the drip chamber and the access. Aside from these considerations, pressure measured at the drip chamber is a function of three additional factors: blood flow rate, needle gauge, and hematocrit, as shown in Figure 21.6. The blood pump setting determines the blood flow through the venous tubing and needles. The pressure drop through tubing and needle is a function of their diameter. The venous needle, having a much smaller diameter than the tubing, is the major site of pressure gradient dissipation. The magnitude of pressure drop for equivalent length needles varies with the needle gauge used. These vary from large-bore 14-gauge needles (used to attain very high flows of >600 mL per minute) to 16-gauge needles used to deliver flows up to 350 mL per minute. In children, even smaller-gauge needles are used. Figure 21.6 clearly shows that at any flow rate, pressure increases as needle gauge increases (and needle diameter decreases). The hematocrit of blood determines viscosity; more viscous fluids require a larger pressure gradient to achieve the same flow in identical circuits. The effect of varying hematocrit from 22% to 38% as might be found in the clinic setting is shown by the dotted lines on either side of the 16-gauge needle pressure–flow curve in Figure 21.6. For a 16-gauge needle, at 200 mL per minute blood flow, the pressure gradient attributable to hematocrit effects is 28 to 30 mm Hg.

As shown in Figure 21.6, the pressure measured at the drip chamber under conditions of flow is actually the sum of the pressure within the access (at the site of needle insertion), and the pressure drops through the needle and tubing. For simplicity, the drip chamber and vascular access are assumed to be at the same level to obviate the need for any hydrostatic pressure difference correction. As illustrated, at a blood flow of 200 mL per minute, the most commonly used flow, and using a 16-gauge needle, the pressure measured at the drip chamber (P_{DC}) is 150 mm Hg compared with an intra-access pressure (P_{IA}) of only 30 mm Hg. The P_{DC} thresholds using 15- and 14-gauge needles decrease to 115 and 88 mm Hg, respectively, whereas P_{IA} remains un-

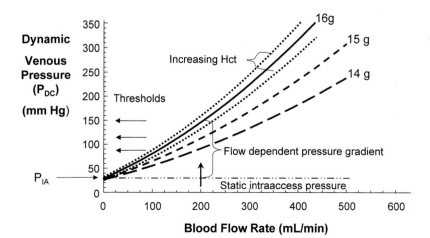

FIGURE 21.6. The relationship of venous drip chamber pressure to blood pump flow as a function of hematocrit and needle gauge. Needle gauge is a strong determinant of pressure. At a blood flow of 200 mL per minute (*vertical arrow*), which is commonly used for dynamic pressure monitoring, the critical pressure (*horizontal arrows*) varies from 90 mm Hg for a 14-gauge needle to 150 mm Hg for a 16-gauge needle when hematocrits are 30%. A variation in hematocrits of 8 points around the mean value of 30% produces changes of 8 to 15 mm Hg. Note that at zero pump flow (static), these influences disappear. For a 16-gauge needle, 120 of the 150 mm Hg is due to pressure gradients in the tubing and needle.

changed. Thus, the threshold pressure (left pointing horizontal arrows) that triggers further access evaluation varies significantly with needle gauge being greater than 150 mm Hg for 16-gauge, 110 to 120 mm Hg for 15-gauge, and 80 to 90 mm Hg for 14-gauge fistula needles. These guidelines are for grafts that normally carry 15 to 20 mm Hg higher pressures in the venous segment than do autologous fistula. Thus, the thresholds in native fistula should be set lower than those for grafts.

Schwab and co-workers (34) originally recommended that dynamic pressure measurement be made at low pump blood flow rate (150–200 mL/min) to minimize the contribution to pressure from the resistance in the blood lines and venous needle at higher blood flow rates. Others have recommended pressure measurements at higher flows. I disagree with the latter because I believe the signal-to-noise ratio diminishes at higher blood flows. Even at the recommended lower blood flow rates of 150 to 200 mL per minute, however, the measured drip chamber venous pressure, resulting largely from needle resistance, is still threefold to fivefold higher than the actual intra-access pressure (Fig. 21.6) (31,35). Variations in hematocrit between 22% and 38% produce 10 to 30 mm Hg variations in dynamic pressure at the same blood flow. These factors mandate that trend analysis as well as multiple occasions of exceeding the threshold be used when evaluating dynamic pressure measurements. Trend analysis is *much* more important than any single value.

Optimum use of dynamic pressure measurements thus requires frequent sequential measurements. Ideally, a baseline value should be established when the access is first used (new) and unlikely to have any stenoses. Although neointimal hyperplasia can develop quickly in some patients, it is rare to have a hemodynamically significant lesion develop within the 2- to 4-week period needed to mature and begin using a graft. The dynamic pressure should be measured within the first 2 to 5 minutes into each dialysis, and the venous needles must be within the lumen and not partially occluded by the vessel wall. Dynamic pressure measurements

are very sensitive to partial occlusion of the venous needle orifice that can produce high values of P_{DC}, even at low blood pump flows. Stenosis at the venous anastomotic site is suggested by progressive increase in P_{DC}. The threshold should be exceeded on three consecutive dialysis treatments to be meaningful. A lesion within the body of the access or in the inflow will be missed because the lesion and the site of pressure dissipation are proximal to the venous needle. This lowers the sensitivity and specificity of the method.

Other approaches to dynamic pressure measurements have examined the possibility of extracting the intra-access pressure (P_{IA}) from measurements conducted at any blood flow during the dialysis session. In principle, because pressure measurements are recorded six to eight times in any dialysis session, one could "back calculate" P_{IA} from P_{DC} if one knows the relationship between flow (Qb) and pressure, the effect of hematocrit on the pressure, and the magnitude of the hydrostatic pressure between drip chamber and venous needle. One then could determine the average venous segment pressure during the session. Any noise in the signal would be reduced by "regression to the mean" when multiple measurements are made. Such an approach is illustrated in Figure 21.7. The relationship between blood flow and pressure drop in the venous return portion of the dialysis circuit can be determined *in vitro* (for a given needle gauge and length) by diluting blood with albumin (31) or type-specific plasma (35) and placing the venous return needle over a container a suitable distance below the drip chamber (to mimic the usual difference in height between drip chamber and access). The relationship between pressure and flow is quadratic (31,35). Hematocrit in turn has a quadratic effect on Qb. For a given Qb and hematocrit, one can calculate the dynamic pressure resulting from flow through the system as if the access was not there. The differences in pressure between the displayed pressure and the calculated pressure reflect the pressure in the access. This then permits calculation of the P_{IA}/MAP ratio in the venous segment as though one had measured it directly.

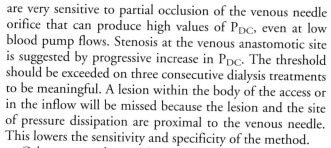

$$P_{IA} = P_{DC@Qb} - P_{DC@Qb=0}$$

$$P_{DC@Qb=0} = 0.00042 \cdot Qb^2$$
$$+ (0.62116 \cdot Hct^2 + 0.01203 \cdot Hct + 0.12754) \cdot Qb$$
$$-17.32 = 153 \text{ mm Hg} \quad \text{(for 15 gauge needle)}$$

$$P_{IA} = 220 \text{ mmHg} - 153 \text{ mmHg} = 67 \text{ mmHg}$$

MAP = 100 mmHg; Hct = 30 %

P_{DC} = 220 mmHg

Qb = 450 ml/min

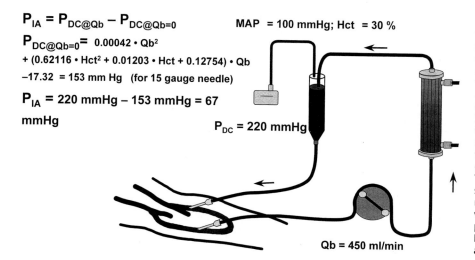

FIGURE 21.7. Extracting intra-access pressure (P_{IA}) from the venous drip chamber pressure (P_{DC}). In the illustration, a 15-gauge fistula needle is used, the mean arterial pressure (*MAP*) is 100 mm Hg, the blood hematocrit is 30%, and the blood pump flow is 450 mL per minute. The hydrostatic pressure difference between access and drip chamber is assumed to be 17 mm Hg. The venous drip chamber is 220 mm Hg. At a hematocrit of 30% and a blood flow of 450 mL per minute, the calculated pressure drop through the needle and tubing as well as the correction for the hydrostatic pressure difference is calculated from the equation as 153 mm Hg. The difference between the dynamic pressure measured and the calculated pressure reflects the pressure within the access at the venous needle site, 67 mm Hg. At a mean pressure of 100 mm Hg, this indicates a P_{IA}/MAP ratio of 0.67, which is indicative of an outlet stenosis.

One should be cognizant of several sources of error in the above technique. One cannot use one equation for all needle gauges (Fig. 21.6). Needle length also influences the pressure drop. Furthermore, hematocrit is not constant and changes over time. Thus, it is important to have weekly measurements of hematocrit to have accurate measurements. Hematocrit also changes during the course of dialysis. At a hematocrit of 33%, fluid removal equivalent to 3% to 5% of body weight induces changes in hematocrit of 4 to 6 points during the course of treatment. In addition, the hydrostatic pressure from the relative positions of the drip chamber and the access will vary among patients. Finally, one must be cognizant that the blood pump flow measured during *in vitro* experiments to determine the pressure–flow relationship may differ *in vivo* (36).

Alternative methods of determining P_{IA} at pump flows that are not zero have been attempted. In one iteration of the theme, measurements of P_{DC} at several different blood flows are made, and a computer curve fits the data so that P_{IA} is calculated at zero pump blood flow. This method suffers from the need for multiple measurements and data input. Another method makes measurements at a flow of 50 to 60 mL per minute that is enough flow to generate a pressure equal to the hydrostatic offset in "most" patients.

Static Intra-Access Pressures

The preceding attempts clearly emphasize the need for direct measurement of intra-access pressure. It is logical that the sensitivity and specificity of pressure measurements in detecting lesions would be improved if intra-access pressures were measured directly and used to screen for access stenosis rather than going through complicated procedures that attempt to "estimate" P_{IA} from the venous drip chamber pressures under conditions of flow. Direct measurement of P_{IA} eliminates flow effects and the effects of partial occlusion of the needle orifice. Because systemic blood pressure influences intra-access pressure, the utility of intra-access pressure measurements in detecting lesions is refined by using a ratio of intra-access pressure to systemic pressure rather than the intra-access pressure alone (25,31). Measurements of systolic P_{IA}/ MAP are superior to drip-chamber venous pressures as a screening modality to detect stenoses in AV grafts (37,38). In the latter study, dynamic pressures, static pressure ratios, and access flow measurements were determined in grafts in an attempt to determine which tests best predicted access dysfunction. Static pressure measurements (every 2 weeks) were as good as access flows (measured every 2 months) in detecting lesions that required radiologic intervention or surgical correction. Static pressure thresholds were reached before dynamic thresholds, even though the latter were conducted at every dialysis session. This study clearly showed that dynamic pressures (pressures from the venous needle under conditions of low blood flow, 150–200 mL per minute) should be replaced by measurement of static intra-access pressure, P_{IA}, under conditions of no pump flow.

A reproducible observation is that venous outlet stenotic lesions are more likely to manifest increased intra-access pressures in PTFE grafts. Because access lesions can develop in other segments of the access, however, sensitivity is reduced in direct proportion to the frequency of nonoutlet stenoses. If a stenosis develops in the body of the graft between the arterial and venous limb cannulation sites, intra-access pressure at the venous needle remains normal, but flow still decreases (29,32). Detection of such a lesion requires measurement of the upstream arterial segment pressure as well (Figs. 21.3 and 21.4). In our experience (29,32), such lesions account for about a third of all graft lesions and more than half of lesions in native fistulae. Other researchers have found that nonoutlet lesions can account for up to half of all stenosis (39,40).

It is impractical to measure intra-access pressures directly by using separate transducer and recorder systems as originally described (31). The technique for measuring P_{IA} has evolved to use regular available dialysis equipment (41) rather than a specialized external transducer. When there is no flow in the dialysis circuit, the only difference in pressure, ΔP_H, between an external transducer (P_T) and the drip chamber transducer (P_{DC}) arises from the difference in height (ΔH) of the drip chamber relative to the fistula (41), a quantity easily measured and converted to millimeters of mercury. Thus, the simplified technique for determining venous segment intra-access pressure ratio ($_{EQ}P_{IA}$/MAP) uses the pressures from the venous drip chamber measured with the blood pump turned off, a "cuff" blood pressure, and ΔH to determine $_{EQ}P_{IA}$. After the blood pump is stopped, a clamp is placed upstream to the venous drip chamber. After 30 to 40 seconds, the pressure in the venous drip chamber stabilizes and is read. If the transducer is properly calibrated, this "static" pressure accurately reflects intra-access pressure. After measuring ΔH in centimeters, offset pressure ΔP_H in millimeters of mercury can be calculated by multiplying the height by 0.76 (the theoretic value for blood) (Fig. 21.8). Correcting for ΔP_H permits the sequential measurement of an equivalent intra-access pressure ($_{EQ}P_{IA} = P_{DC}$ static $+ \Delta P_H$) in a prospective way without any special equipment or cost. A value of $_{EQ}P_{IA}$/MAP greater than 0.5 is highly specific for a 50% luminal outlet stenosis in an AV graft (39). The height offset varies significantly from patient to patient (Fig. 21.9). For example, values of 10.0 to 12.5 mm Hg are found in patients with arm accesses and up to 30 mm in those with thigh grafts when measured in the sitting position. It is therefore important to measure the height offset in individual patients. This permits the use of an absolute limit (e.g., P_{IA}/MAP > 0.5) as the criteria for further imaging or intervention (Table 21.1).

On the other hand, if an increase above baseline is used as an action threshold (Table 21.1), the exact value for the offset is not as critical. We have found that the mean value

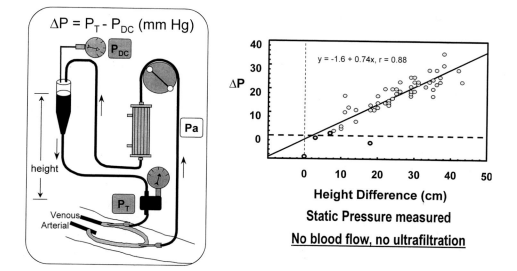

FIGURE 21.8. Influence of the height difference measurement on intra-access pressure (P_{IA}). A dialysis circuit is shown on the left. The pressure can be measured at the drip chamber (P_{DC}) or by a separate transducer introduced between the tubing and fistula needle (P_T). The separate transducer can be leveled at the same height as the venous needle so there is no height offset. With the blood pump shut off and the line to the venous drip chamber clamped to prevent ultrafiltration (dialysate side flow and pressures are not interrupted), the difference between the two pressures, $\Delta P = P_T - P_{DC}$, is a linear function of the height offset between the two transducers as shown by the right side of this figure. Note that the slope of 0.74 is statistically indistinguishable from the theoretical value of 0.76 based on the specific gravity of blood relative to mercury.

for the offset at a given treatment center is directly related to the height difference between the arm of the chair and the drip chamber (41). This value can be used rather than having to measure the offset for each and every patient (41). Using this method, it is crucial to measure access pressure when the access is functioning well (usually within a month of construction) because this establishes the baseline.

As previously emphasized, the use of both static prepump arterial and venous drip chamber pressures can detect both intra-access and venous outlet stenoses (29,32). Reproducible arterial segment pressure ratios greater than 0.8 or venous segment ratios greater than 0.5 in grafts are highly suggestive of hemodynamically significant stenosis greater than 50% by diameter (Table 21.1). Although the pressure ratios are lower in autologous native fistulae for the same kind of lesions, criteria for action can be developed.

The use of the venous segment pressures alone would fail to detect lesions between the needles. If prepump pressures are not available, lesions between the needles can be detected by palpation and auscultation. Physical examination is a valuable part of the armamentarium although uncommonly performed (see Chapter 18).

Although the method for measuring static pressures from the prepump and venous drip chambers is straightforward (Fig. 21.10), it is also very tedious and requires that 12 separate steps be carefully and accurately performed, including verification that the built-in transducers are appropriately zero calibrated. The multiple steps that ensure accuracy make the procedure "user unfriendly," and staffs frequently rush through the procedure. Poor zero calibration of the transducers can lead to large variations between sessions, particularly if patients are rotated among machines. In some centers,

TABLE 21.1. INTRA-ACCESS PRESSURE RATIOS FOR DETECTING STENOSIS

Degree of Stenosis	Graft: Arterial Segment		Graft: Venous Segment	Native: Arterial Segment		Native: Venous Segment
<50% Diameter	0.35–0.74		0.15–0.49	0.13–0.43		0.08–0.34
>50% Diameter						
Venous outlet	>0.75	or	>0.5	>0.43	or	>0.35
Intraaccess	>0.65	and	<0.5	>0.43	and	<0.35
Arterial Inflow	<0.3		Clinical findings	<.13 + Clinical findings		Clinical findings

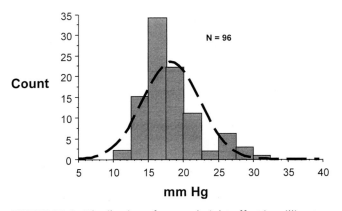

FIGURE 21.9. Distribution of venous height offset in millimeters of mercury in 96 patients with vascular accesses. Note that the mode is 15 to 17.5 mm Hg. The mean is 17.7 mm Hg; the range is 10 to 32.5 mm Hg. The distribution is skewed to the left compared with a normal distribution (*dashed line*). Lower offsets are found in those with upper-arm locations, intermediate in those with forearm accesses, and highest in those with thigh grafts.

prepump drip chambers and transducers are not used at all; so arterial segment measurements are not possible.

A device, Access Alert (Medisystems), consisting of a sterile hydrophobic luer connector, simplifies the entire procedure because it can join a generic sterile fistula needle to a manometer via a short tubing set (Fig. 21.11). Intra-access pressures are measured at the time of access cannulation (predialysis) and therefore do not produce any interruption of the dialysis treatment. Because the measurements are made at the level of the access, there is no need for any height corrections, and the aneroid displays zero directly so that incorrect calibration is easily detected. Recent studies have validated that this technique is able to detect access stenosis and correlates with access flow (Fig. 21.12) (42). The device performs as well if not better than the standard method using static pressures derived from the drip chambers. The system detects the majority of graft accesses at risk (inflow, midgraft, and outflow stenoses), and preemptive correction based on pressure measurements by the Access Alert Device prevents thrombosis and improves flow within accesses (Fig. 21.13) (42).

RECOMMENDATIONS FOR PRESSURES IN A MONITORING PROGRAM

In a successful monitoring program, more than half of all graft access stenoses should be detected before thrombosis. Successful angioplasty or surgical revision should be accompanied by a decrease in either dynamic (blood pump running) or static (blood pump off) access pressures into the "normal" range. In our experience, flow usually doubles

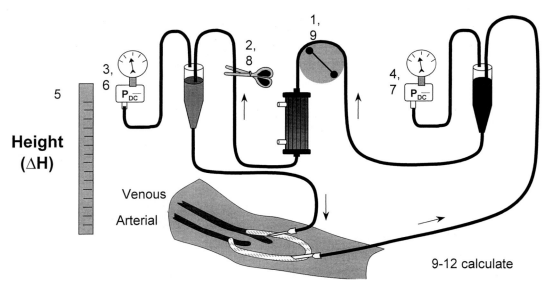

FIGURE 21.10. Graphic representation of the dialysis circuit and the steps needed to make accurate measurements of static pressures from both the arterial and venous segments of the access. The steps necessary for accurate measurement are the following: *1.* Shut off the blood pump; *2.* Clamp the prevenous drip chamber tubing (or shut off ultrafiltration); *3.* Record the venous drip chamber pressure at 30 to 45 seconds ($P_{DC,V}$); *4.* Record the arterial drip chamber pressure at 30 to 45 seconds ($P_{DC,A}$); *5.* Measure the height offset (can be done once during the life of the access) and convert to mm Hg (ΔP_H); *6.* Clamp the line to the venous drip chamber transducer, pull off the line, and record zero pressure value ($P_{V,0}$); *7.* Clamp the line to the arterial drip chamber transducer, pull off the line, and record zero pressure value ($P_{A,0}$); *8.* Release the clamp from the tubing to the venous drip chamber; *9.* Turn the blood pump to the prescribed blood flow; *10.* Calculate the venous segment intra-access pressure, $P_{IA,V} = P_{DC,V} + \Delta P_H + P_{V,0}$; *11.* Calculate the arterial segment intra-access pressure, $P_{IA,A} = P_{DC,A} + \Delta P_H + P_{A,0}$; and *12.* Measure the arterial blood pressure in the contralateral arm and calculate the arterial and venous segment ratios.

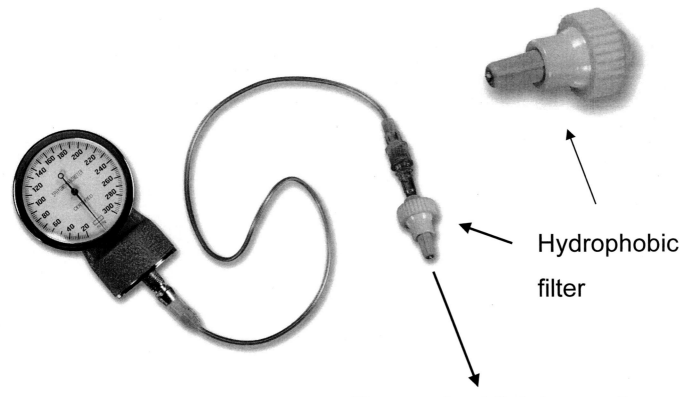

FIGURE 21.11. AccessAlert Device for measuring static pressures. A hydrophobic luer connector (orange/yellow) connects to a standard dialysis needle. Pressure is read on the aneroid display.

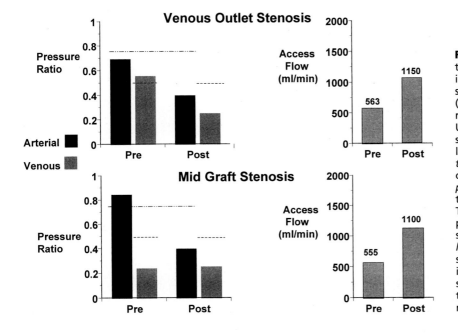

FIGURE 21.12. Illustrative cases detected by intra-access pressure measurements before initiating dialysis using AccessAlert. The *left panels* show the static arterial (*black bars*) and venous (*gray bars*) segment pressures; the *right panels* reflect the access flows (Transonics, Ithaca, NY, U.S.A.) during the same dialysis session. Data are shown for before and after percutaneous transluminal angioplasty (PTA). The *dashed horizontal lines* reflect the upper limits for the absence of a 50% stenosis in the outflow tract. In the *top panel*, a venous outlet stenosis raises pressure so that the venous segment ratio of 0.5 is exceeded. The stenosis is associated with a flow of 563 mL per minute. Following PTA, arterial and venous segment ratios decrease and flow doubles. In the *lower panels*, the effect of a midgraft stenosis is shown. Only the arterial segment pressure ratio is elevated, whereas the venous segment pressure is normal. Flow, however, is decreased to the same extent as in the top panel. Angioplasty reduces the pressure and again doubles the flow.

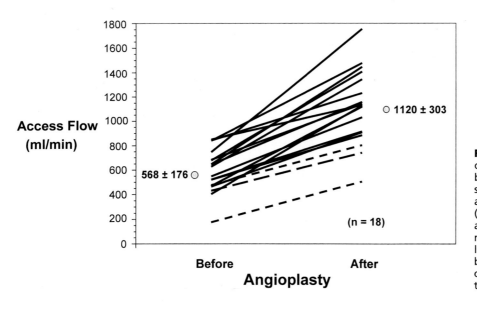

FIGURE 21.13. The effect of intervention on access flow. All lesions were detected by prospective surveillance of the venous segment of the accesses. Grafts (n = 15) are shown as *solid lines* and native fistula (n = 3) as *dashed lines*. All graft accesses achieved a flow greater than 750 mL per minute following angioplasty. Native fistulas did not respond to PTA as well as grafts because of lower flows (in part because of concomitant arterial inflow problems) and the presence of multiple stenoses.

(Fig. 21.13). Static pressure monitoring prompted all the interventions in Figure 21.12. Restenosis over a period of 3 to 12 months is a frequent event, and thus ongoing monitoring is needed.

Static prepump arterial and venous drip chamber pressures can detect both intra-access and venous outlet stenoses. In grafts, reproducible arterial segment pressure ratios greater than 0.8 (Table 21.1) or venous segment ratios greater than 0.5 are highly suggestive of greater than 50% stenosis. Lower ratios are used in native fistulae, as shown in Table 21.1. We believe that use of the venous segment pressures alone may fail to detect lesions between the needles. If only one pressure is measured, the arterial segment provides more information. The policy of using

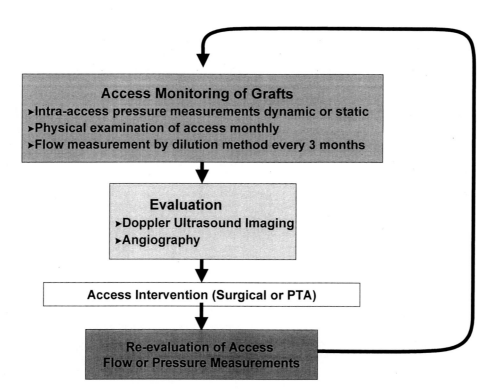

FIGURE 21.14. Schematic outlining the procedure for prospective graft monitoring and intervention (see text for details). The key component is the improvement in graft hemodynamics as revealed by flow, pressure, or physical examination following intervention. *PTA,* percutaneous transluminal angioplasty.

arterial tubing sets containing a prepump pillow without any means of measuring pressure prepump should be abandoned. Units choosing to continue the use of dynamic pressures need to validate the pressure thresholds they use at the chosen blood-pump flow rate and for the appropriate needle gauge and length.

We recommend the algorithm illustrated in Figure 21.14 for access monitoring of grafts. All grafts should be examined monthly by physical examinations. Static arterial and venous segment pressures are measured every 2 weeks. If dynamic measurements are made in place of statics, then measurements are conducted at every treatment. Flow measurements are conducted every 3 months but are advanced if the pressure measurements indicate rapid evolution of a stenosis. A steady progressive increase in venous static pressures and decrease in flow is an indication for *direct referral* to angiography. Doppler evaluation is usually limited to those cases in which the data are not clear; for example, a palpable stricture is believed to be present by examination, but flow measurements are erratic. Autologous fistulas and grafts with Doppler ultrasound flows greater than 800 mL per minute are observed, and those with less than 600 mL per minute are sent directly for surgical or radiologic correction, depending on the length of stenosis and other characteristics. Following any procedure, pressures and flows are repeated at the next dialysis session and within 2 weeks to ensure that hemodynamics have improved. Rapid recurrence of abnormality indicates an elastic lesion or technically unsuccessful intervention.

REFERENCES

1. Held PJ,.Port FK, Wolfe RA, et al. The dose of hemodialysis and patient mortality. *Kidney Int* 1996;50:550–556.
2. Sherman R, Besarab A, Schwab SJ, et al. Recognition of the failing vascular access: a current perspective. *Seminars in Dialysis* 1997;10:1–5.
3. Sullivan KL, Besarab A, Bonn J, et al. Hemo-dynamics of failing dialysis grafts. *Radiology* 1993;186:867–872.
4. Besarab A, Lubkowski T, Ahsan M, et al. Access flow (Q$_A$) as a predictor of access dysfunction. *J Am Soc Nephrol* 1999;11:202A (abst).
5. Sullivan KL, Besarab A. Hemodynamic screening and early percutaneous intervention reduce hemodialysis access thrombosis and increase graft longevity. *J Vasc Interv Radiol* 1997;8:163–170.
6. Polaschegg HD. The extracorporeal circuit. *Seminars in Dialysis* 1995;8:299–304.
7. Polaschegg HD. Access physics. *Seminars in Dialysis* 1999;12 (Suppl 1):S33–S40.
8. Depner TA, Rizwan S, Sasi TA. Pressure effects on roller pump flow during hemodialysis. *ASAIO Trans* 1990;31:M456–M459.
9. Sands J, Glidden D, Jacavage W, Jones B. Difference between delivered and pre-scribed blood flow in hemodialysis. *ASAIO J* 41996;42:M717–M719.
10. Francos GC, Burke JF, Besarab A, et al. An unsuspected cause of acute hemolysis during hemodialysis. *ASAIO Trans* 1983;29:140–146.
11. Besarab A, Frinak S. Effect of dislodgement of venous needle on venous pressure. *Seminars in Dialysis* 1996;9:289–290.
12. Johnson CP, Yong-ran Z, Matt C, et al. Prognostic value of intraoperative blood flow measurements in vascular access surgery. *Surgery* 1998;124:729–738.
13. Besarab A, Hall B, Al-Ajel F, et al. The relation of brachial artery flow to access flow. *J Am Soc Nephrol*1995;7:483(abst).
14. Besarab A, Ross R, Al-Ajel F, et al. The relation of intra-access pressure to flow. *J Am Soc Nephrol* 1995;7:483(abst).
15. Bay WH, Henry ML, Lazarus JM, et al. Predicting hemodialysis access failure with color flow Doppler ultrasound. *Am J Nephrol* 1998;18:296–304.
16. Bosman PJ, Boereboorn FTJ, Eikelboom BC, et al. Graft flow as a predictor of thrombosis in hemodialysis grafts. *Kidney Int* 1998;54:1726–1730.
17. Depner TA, Reason AM. Longevity of peripheral A-V grafts and fistulas for hemodialysis is related to access blood flow. *J Am Soc Nephrol* 1996;7:1405(abst).
18. Lindsay RM, Blake PG, Malek P, et al. Hemodialysis access flow rates can be measured by a differential conductivity technique and are predictive of access clotting. *Am J Kidney Dis* 1997;30:475–482.
19. May RE, Himmelfarb J, Yenicesu M, et al. Predictive measures of vascular access thrombosis—a prospective study. *Kidney Int* 1997;52:1656–1662.
20. Schackelton CR, Taylor DC, Buckley AR, et al. Predicting failure in polytetrafluoroethylene vascular access grafts for hemodialysis: a pilot study. *Can J Surg* 1987;30:442–444.
21. Strauch BS, O'Connell RS, Geoly KL. Forecasting thromboses of vascular access with Doppler color flow imaging. *Am J Kidney Dis* 1992;19:554–557.
22. Wang E, Schneditz D, Nepomuceno C, et al. Predictive value of access blood flow in detecting failure of vascular access. *ASAIO J* 1998;44:M555–M558.
23. Guyton AC, Hall JE. Interrelationships among pressure, flow, and resistance. In: Guyton AC, Hall JE, eds. *Textbook of medical physiology*, 9th ed. Philadelphia: WB Saunders, 1996:163–169.
24. van stone JC, Jones MJ, Van Stone J. Detection of hemodialysis access stenosis by measuring outlet resistance. *Am J Kidney Dis* 1994;23:562–568.
25. Sullivan KL, Besarab A, Dorrell S, et al. The relationship between dialysis graft pressure and stenosis. *Invest Radiol* 1992;27:352–355.
26. Kim YH, Chandran KB, Bower TJ, et al. Flow dynamics across end-to end vascular bypass anastomoses. *Ann Biomed Eng* 1993;21:311–320.
27. Bassiouny HS, White S, Glasgov S, et al. Anastomotic intimal hyperplasia: mechanical injury or flow induced? *J Vasc Surg* 1992;15:708–715.
28. Beathard GA, Settle SM, Shields MW. Salvage of the nonfunctioning arteriovenous fistula. *Am K Kidney Dis* 1999;33:910–916.
29. Besarab A, Lubkowski T, Frinak S, Ramanathan S, Escobar F. Detecting vascular access dysfunction. *ASAIO J* 1997;43:M539–M543.
30. Clowes AW, Zacharias RK, Kirkman TR. Early endothelial coverage of synthetic arterial grafts: porosity revisited. *Am J Surg* 1987;153:501–504.
31. Besarab A, Sullivan KL, Ross R, et al. The utility of intra-access monitoring in detecting and correcting venous outlet stenoses prior to thrombosis. *Kidney Int* 1995;47:1364–1373.
32. Besarab A, Lubkowski T, Frinak S, et al. Detection of strictures and vascular outlet stenoses in vascular accesses: which test is best?. *ASAIO J* 1997;43:M543–M547.
33. Paulson WD, Ram SJ, Work J. Does blood flow accurately predict thrombosis or failure of hemodialysis synthetic grafts? A meta-analysis. *Am J Kidney Dis* 1999;34:478–445.

34. Schwab SJ, Raymond FR, Saeed M, et al. Prevention of hemodialysis fistula thrombosis: early detection of venous stenosis. *Kidney Int* 1989;36:707–711.

35. Frinak S, Zasuwa G, Dunfee T, et al. Computerized vascular access monitoring for hemodialysis. *J Am Soc Nephrol* 2000;12:184A(abst).

36. Sands J, Glidden D, Jacavage W, et al. Difference between delivered and prescribed blood flow in hemodialysis. *ASAIO J* 1996;42:M717–M719.

37. Dinwiddie LC, Frauman AC, Jaques PF, et al. Comparison of measures for prospective identification of venous stenosis. *Am Nephrol Nurse Assoc J* 1996;23:593–600.

38. Smits JHM, van der Linden J, van den Dorpel MA, et al. Graft surveillance: venous pressure, access flow or the combination. *J Am Soc Nephrol* 1999;10:218A(abst).

39. Strauch BS, O'Connell RS. Permanent vascular access for hemodialysis: the role of color Doppler flow imagining in the assessment of the hemodialysis vascular access. *Seminars in Dialysis* 1995;8: 142–146.

40. Kanterman RY, Vesely TM, Pilgram TK, et al. Dialysis access grafts: anatomic location of venous stenoses and results of angioplasty. *Radiology* 1995;195:135–139.

41. Besarab A, Frinak S, Sherman RA, et al. Simplified measurement of intra-access pressure. *J Am Soc Nephrol* 1998;9:284–289.

42. Besarab A, Lubkowski T, Frinak S. A simpler method for measuring intra-access pressure. *J Am Soc Nephrol* 1999;11: 202A(abst).

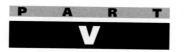

TREATMENT FOR ACCESS DYSFUNCTION

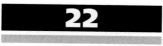

PROPHYLACTIC ANGIOPLASTY: IS IT WORTHWHILE?

22A

PRO VIEWPOINT

KARIM VALJI

The maintenance of vascular access for chronic hemodialysis is a significant burden on patients with end stage renal disease (ESRD), health care systems, and society as a whole. A substantial portion of the Medicare budget for ESRD must be devoted to the initial placement and subsequent maintenance of arteriovenous (AV) fistulas, synthetic bridge grafts, and tunneled catheters. The problem is particularly great in the United States, where there is undue reliance on synthetic grafts, which are notoriously difficult to maintain because of the high rates of infection and thrombosis. For example, the 1-year primary patency of polytetrafluoroethylene (PTFE) dialysis grafts is about 60% to 80% (1,2). After the first episode of thrombosis, patency rates with percutaneous treatment or surgical revision are usually less than 50% at 3 and 6 months (3). AV fistulas, although more durable than synthetic grafts, also have a limited life span, particularly after the first episode of thrombosis.

The primary reason for graft failure and the need for subsequent graft revision or replacement is thrombosis, most often due to intimal hyperplasia at the venous anastomosis. Neither operative nor endovascular techniques are able to provide durable graft function after thrombosis occurs. For this reason, there has been a growing interest over the last decade in the early detection of dialysis graft dysfunction through routine surveillance and subsequent prophylactic treatment before complete graft failure. Although this algorithm has been advocated by the National Kidney Foundation through the Kidney Disease Outcomes Quality Initiative (K/DOQI), the approach has not been universally accepted or adopted (4).

There are two options for managing hemodialysis access: (a) prophylactic treatment of failing grafts (either by percutaneous or surgical means) or (b) treatment of clotted accesses (by endovascular means, surgical revision, or replacement) when they fail completely. Boiled down to a simple question, we must ask whether this approach to hemodialysis access provides a cost-effective alternative to conventional management of clotted grafts. That is, do the benefits to patients and society in terms of less frequent graft thrombosis, increased graft patency, and improved quality and length of life outweigh the costs (to the patient, health care system, and society as a whole) of a program of routine surveillance followed by prophylactic and often repeated angioplasty?

PROLONGATION OF DIALYSIS ACCESS PATENCY

The key potential benefit of the screening/angioplasty algorithm is prolonged graft longevity and preservation of vein. Patients on chronic hemodialysis have limited sites for graft placement. Each graft revision or replacement exhausts precious venous "real estate" on which the patient is dependent for life. Thrombosed AV fistulas usually are managed operatively by abandoning the fistula and placing a graft. Thrombosed synthetic grafts can be treated by patch revision. In reality, however, many surgeons prefer to extend the graft up the arm, thus using up more valuable vein.

Schwab and colleagues were among the earliest proponents of prophylactic balloon angioplasty to reduce the incidence of dialysis graft thrombosis (5). In their seminal report published in 1989, venous pressures were routinely measured in a population of 168 patients, most of whom had PTFE bridge grafts. Angiography (followed by angioplasty as indicated) was performed in patients with serial venous pressure levels above 150 mm Hg. Venous stenoses were documented by venography in 86% of such cases. The graft thrombosis rates in the subpopulations with venous pressures lower than 150 mm Hg, elevated pressures who subsequently underwent angiography and angioplasty, and elevated pressures but no treatment were 0.13, 0.15, and 1.4 episodes per patient-year, respectively.

Since the time of that report, numerous studies have confirmed the value of surveillance programs, with early treatment of dysfunctional grafts by angioplasty in lowering the

TABLE 22A.1. EFFECT OF PROPHYLACTIC ANGIOPLASTY ON DIALYSIS GRAFT FUNCTION

Study (yr) (Ref No.)	No. of Patients	Reduction in Thrombosis Rate	Increase in Mean Graft Survival
Schwab et al. (1989) (5)	168	1.4 vs. 0.15/patient-yr	26 → 7% replace/patient-yr
Besarab et al. (1995) (6)	107	0.58 → 0.19/patient-yr	2.0 → 3.0 yr
Roberts et al. (1996) (7)	121	1.0 → 0.5/patient-yr	6.3 → 15.8 mo
Safa et al. (1996) (8)	57	48% → 17%	
Lumsden et al. (1997) (9)	64		51% vs. 47% at 1 yr
Martin et al. (1999) (10)	21	0.10 vs. 0.44/patient-yr (virgin grafts only)	

incidence of dialysis graft thrombosis (Table 22A.1) (5–10). Almost all these studies have shown a significant reduction in the frequency of graft thrombosis or significant improvement in graft patency through routine graft surveillance followed by angioplasty or operative revision of significant stenoses. For example, an aggressive surveillance program conducted at the University of California, San Diego, by a single nephrologist and based primarily on careful graft examination reduced the frequency of graft clotting from 48% to 17% compared with a historical control group (8). The program also allowed 1-year primary assisted patencies rates of 67% and 68% for AV fistulas (AVFs) and synthetic grafts, respectively. The design of the monitoring programs differed among the various institutions, but most studies used the commonly accepted parameters of venous pressure (static or dynamic), physical examination of the grafts, and duplex sonography, alone or in combinations (11–17).

Whereas most of these reports involved synthetic bridge grafts, comparable results have been achieved when close hemodynamic monitoring of native AVFs is followed by repeated balloon angioplasty (and occasionally stent placement). In the study by Turmel-Rodrigues and colleagues, 32 Brescia–Cimino fistulas were identified with hemodynamically significant stenoses and underwent prophylactic angioplasty, sometimes with repeated procedures (18). Primary and secondary patencies at 1 year for AVFs were 62% and 82%, respectively. Similarly, Gallego Beuter and co-workers achieved one-year primary and primary assisted patency rates of 71% and 89%, respectively, for 110 Brescia–Cimino fistulas treated with angioplasty when routine monitoring suggested a hemodynamic problem (19).

Comparable results have been found with elective surgical revision of failing dialysis grafts. In a study by Sands and colleagues, 56 AV fistulas and 97 PTFE grafts were followed and categorized into two groups: one subset with elective repair (endovascular or operative) and another subset in which the first intervention was graft thrombectomy (20). Both the total number of clotting episodes and the number of subsequent interventions were reduced significantly in the former group.

Despite the strong evidence in support of the dialysis access surveillance/angioplasty algorithm, there are some skeptics who refute these studies. Lumsden and his colleagues reported the results of prospective study in which a population of patients with PTFE bridge grafts underwent duplex sonography (9). Patients with a suspected greater than 50% stenoses confirmed at angiography were studied every 3 months thereafter with duplex sonography. The 65 patients were randomized to either prophylactic angioplasty (repeated as needed) or observation. No significant difference in 12-month primary patency was noted (47% ± 4% in the untreated subgroup and 51% ± 6% in treatment group). Most of these anatomic lesions were not confirmed, however, by a validated test to be clinically or hemodynamically significant. In addition, the two populations were not comparably matched with regard to the number of prior interventions or coexistent central venous stenoses (greater for both in the treatment group). Later analysis of the subgroup of patients in this cohort with "virgin" grafts with no prior intervention to maintain patency (albeit a smaller population) demonstrated a significant prolongation of graft patency and reduction in graft thrombosis rate with prophylactic angioplasty (10).

COST-EFFECTIVENESS ANALYSIS

Although proving the benefits of screening and prophylactic treatment of dialysis access in reducing the rate of graft thrombosis and prolonging graft life is relatively straightforward, evaluating true long-term cost-effectiveness is a far more complex problem. The bottom line is that properly conducted studies to answer this important question do not exist. Hunink provided a framework for medical decision making with respect to interventional radiology procedures (21). Rigorous evaluation requires investigators to pose the question properly, frame the issues using multiple perspectives, consider all alternative approaches (including nontreatment), assess the consequences of each alternative appropriately (via trials or decision models), consider tradeoffs in costs (to patients and all parties) and effectiveness (quantified by life years and by accepted measures of quality of life), and then integrate the values and evidence.

Lumsden and co-workers recently published one of the few studies of cost-efficacy using the population of patients described in his previously mentioned study (9,22). The investigators refuted the value of such a screening program because of the comparable rates of graft patency in the treated and observed groups and because of the excess costs incurred through routine graft monitoring (estimated at $440,835 for 32 patients). This report has several major weaknesses, however. It fails to have many of the components of a sophisticated analysis as suggested by Hunink and others. Second, the cost analysis was based primarily on hospital charges, which often have little bearing on Medicare reimbursements or actual costs to the patient, the health care system, or society. Other important cost considerations, such as production losses, resource costs, and costs of patient and dialysis unit time were not considered.

Finally, the surveillance program designed by Lumsden's group relied on periodic sonography for graft monitoring. Duplex sonography is quite accurate in detecting peripheral dialysis graft-related venous stenoses; however, the role of duplex ultrasound in this setting has diminished significantly with the availability of other much cheaper and equally accurate screening tests that evaluate for clinical or hemodynamic abnormalities. Direct inline measurement of dialysis graft flow and sustained elevations in venous pressure are probably the best methods for detecting dialysis graft dysfunction and impending graft failure (23). Even simple graft examination is an excellent screening test for dialysis graft dysfunction. (8,24). Trerotola and colleagues found that physical examination had a negative predictive value of 96% when studied in reference to sonographically obtained volume flow measurements (24). These other screening parameters can be obtained at every dialysis session without the need for a separate procedure or the costs entailed with it.

Despite the lack of convincing proof of the cost-effectiveness of the screening/angioplasty model, there are numerous reasons to advocate this approach. Routine dialysis graft surveillance and elective angioplasty allow for efficient, continuous, uninterrupted dialysis. Dialysis sessions can be completed more quickly, which is a benefit in terms of patients' time, productivity, and dialysis unit efficiency. When a dialysis graft clots, the dialysis unit (and often the interventional radiology) schedule is upset; there is added inconvenience for the patient. Because of room and staffing constraints, placement of a temporary catheter for immediate dialysis may be necessary. This procedure entails added cost, immediate risk (albeit slight), and the possibility of deleterious effects on central veins (even when the internal jugular or femoral vein is used). Hospitalization is much more likely due to the patient's medical condition or the use of general anesthesia for surgical revision (25).

Well-designed cost-effectiveness analyses are needed to establish the benefit of routine and universal dialysis graft surveillance/angioplasty scheme for patients on chronic hemodialysis. As the Medicare program moves rapidly toward capitation of patients with ESRD, the burden of proof will lie with the health care providers who will bear the added costs of an inefficient approach to dialysis access management.

KIDNEY DISEASE OUTCOMES QUALITY INITIATIVE GUIDELINES

Perhaps the most convincing support for widespread adoption of these programs is the strong endorsement by the Vascular Access Work Group of the National Kidney Foundation (4). This multidisciplinary group is composed of nephrologists, vascular surgeons, and interventional radiologists and has performed the most thorough and least biased analysis of the question of dialysis graft monitoring and prophylactic repair. The K/DOQI guidelines support all measures necessary to preserve veins of patients on chronic hemodialysis. They provide direct evidence that prospective surveillance of dialysis grafts and fistulas followed by early treatment will reduce the frequency of graft thrombosis and prolong access patency. The guidelines recommend weekly graft examination and frequent measurement of intragraft flow and static venous pressure, all of which incur almost no marginal cost. Recirculation percentage may be of greater value to patients with AV fistulas. Routine Doppler ultrasound studies are also considered of value; the group hesitated to endorse this approach given the additional costs for such a program in the absence of substantial evidence of its cost-efficacy.

The K/DOQI guidelines advocate prophylactic treatment of all hemodynamically significant stenoses (defined as >50% diameter stenosis along with functional, hemodynamic, or clinical evidence for graft dysfunction). Patent but significantly stenotic grafts are less efficient for providing dialysis. Lesions treated by angioplasty prior to graft thrombosis respond better and remain patent longer than lesions treated in the setting of graft thrombosis. For example, the 3-month primary patency rates for stenotic grafts treated before or after graft thrombosis were 79% and 40%, respectively (26). Inefficient dialysis is an even greater problem with native AVFs. For this reason, among others, prophylactic treatment of detected stenoses is warranted.

With regard to the mode of treatment, K/DOQI supports either balloon angioplasty or surgical revision, depending on procedure availability and local expertise. Angioplasty should produce less than a 30% residual stenosis, return of normal or near normal graft function, and primary unassisted patency at 6 months of at least 50%. Operative revision should have an expected primary unassisted patency of 50% at 1 year. Stents should be reserved for failures of angioplasty in selected cases. Aggressive restenoses (i.e., more than two angioplasty treatments over a 3-month period) should prompt surgical intervention.

REFERENCES

1. Munda R, First MR, Alexander JW, et al. Polytetrafluoroethylene graft survival in hemodialysis. *JAMA* 1983;249:219–222.
2. Palder SB, Kirkman RL, Whittemore AD, et al. Vascular access for hemodialysis: patency rates and results of revision. *Ann Surg* 1985;202:235–239.
3. Gray RJ. Percutaneous intervention for permanent hemodialysis access: a review. *J Vasc Interv Radiol* 1997;8:313–327.
4. National Kidney Foundation. K/DOQI clinical practice guidelines for vascular access, 2000. *Am J Kidney Dis* 2001;37(Suppl 1):S137–S181.
5. Schwab SJ, Raymond JR, Saeed M, et al. Prevention of hemodialysis fistula thrombosis: early detection of venous stenoses. *Kidney Int* 1989;36:707–711.
6. Besarab A, Sullivan KL, Ross RP, et al. The utility of intra-access pressure monitoring in detecting and correcting venous outlet stenoses prior to thrombosis. *Kidney Int* 1995;47:136–147.
7. Roberts AB, Kahn MB, Bradford S, et al. Graft surveillance and angioplasty prolongs dialysis graft patency. *J Am Coll Surg* 1996;183:486–492.
8. Safa AA, Valji K, Roberts AC, et al. Detection and treatment of dysfunctional hemodialysis access grafts: effect of a surveillance program on graft patency and the incidence of thrombosis. *Radiology* 1996;199:653–657.
9. Lumsden AB, MacDonald MJ, Kikeri D, et al. Prophylactic balloon angioplasty fails to prolong the patency of expanded polytetrafluoroethylene arteriovenous grafts: results of a prospective, randomized study. *J Vasc Surg* 1997;26:382–390.
10. Martin LG, MacDonald MJ, Kikeri D, et al. Prophylactic angioplasty reduces thrombosis in virgin ePTFE arteriovenous dialysis grafts with greater than 50% stenosis: subset analysis of a prospectively randomized study. *J Vasc Intervent Radiol* 1999;10:389–396.
11. Sullivan KL, Besarab A. Hemodynamic screening and early percutaneous intervention reduce hemodialysis access thrombosis and increase graft longevity. *J Vasc Interv Radiol* 1997;8:163–170.
12. Besarab A, Al-Saghir F, Al-Nabhan, et al. Simplified measurement of intra-access pressure. *ASAIO J* 1996;42::M682–M687.
13. Sullivan KL, Besarab A, Bonn J, et al. Hemodynamics of failing dialysis grafts. *Radiology* 1993;186:867–872.
14. Trerotola SO, Scheel PJ Jr, Powe NR, et al. Screening for dialysis access graft malfunction: comparison of physical examination with US. *J Vasc Interv Radiol* 1996;7:15–20.
15. Cinat ME, Hopkins J, Wilson SE. A prospective evaluation of PTFE graft potency and surveillance techniques in hemodialysis access. *Ann Vasc Surg* 1999;13:191–198.
16. Sands J, Young S, Miranda C. The effect of Doppler flow screening studies and elective revisions on dialysis access failure. *ASAIO J* 1992;M524–M527.
17. Dousset V, Grenier N, Douws C, et al. Hemodialysis grafts: color Doppler flow imaging correlated with digital subtraction angiography and functional status. *Radiology* 1991;181:89–94.
18. Turmel-Rodrigues L, Pengloan J, Blanchier D, et al. Insufficient dialysis shunts: improved long-term patency rates with close hemodynamic monitoring, repeated percutaneous balloon angioplasty, and stent placement. *Radiology* 1993;187:273–278.
19. Gallego Beuter JJ, Lezana AH, Calvo JH, et al. Early detection and treatment of hemodialysis access dysfunction. *Cardiovasc Intervent Radiol* 2000;23:40–46.
20. Sands JJ, Mirand CL. Prolongation of hemodialysis access survival with elective revision. *Clin Nephrol* 1995;44:329–333.
21. Hunink MG. Appraising decision and cost-effectiveness analyses. *J Vasc Interv Radiol* 2001;12:783–787.
22. Lumsden AB, MacDonald MJ, Kikeri D, et al. Cost efficacy of duplex surveillance and prophylactic angioplasty of arteriovenous ePTFE grafts. *Ann Vasc Surg* 1998;12:138–142.
23. Smits JH, van der Linden J, Hagen EC, et al. Graft surveillance: venous pressure, access flow, or the combination? *Kidney Int* 2001;59:1551–1558.
24. Trerotola SO, Scheel PJ Jr, Powe NR, et al. Screening for dialysis access graft malfunction: comparison of physical examination with US. *J Vasc Interv Radiol* 1996;7:15–20.
25. Marston WA, Criado E, Jacques PF, et al. Prospective randomized comparison of surgical versus endovascular management of thrombosed dialysis access grafts. *J Vasc Surg* 1997;26:373–381.
26. Beathard GA. Percutaneous angioplasty for the treatment of venous stenosis: a nephrologist's view. *Semin Dial* 1995;8:166–170.

22B

CON VIEWPOINT

ALAN B. LUMSDEN
PETER H. LIN

BACKGROUND

Is prophylactic angioplasty of the venous anastomosis of an arteriovenous (AV) graft worthwhile? In our opinion, this is a complex question to answer. The concept of prophylactic angioplasty was based on the observation in lower-extremity vein bypass grafts for peripheral arterial disease that Doppler ultrasound surveillance of a graft leads to the detection of preocclusive stenoses and that correction of stenoses before graft failure leads to prolongation of graft patency. This led to the development of several important concepts and terms:

Primary patency is uninterrupted patency from the time of graft insertion without any form of prophylactic intervention.

Assisted primary patency is continuous graft patency without any type of prophylactic intervention to assist continued patency.

Secondary patency is patency achieved after a graft has occluded and been reopened, measured from the time of graft insertion.

There is no argument that prophylactic intervention on lower-extremity venous bypass grafts leads to prolongation of graft patency. It is strongly believed that thrombosis of a vein alters the endothelium and vessel wall, perhaps because of ischemic damage, leading to frequent recurrent failure and a striking reduction in long-term patency. Whether these observations can be applied to AV fistulae is unknown. Furthermore, it never has been demonstrated conclusively that prophylactic intervention in any kind of prosthetic graft prolongs assisted primary patency.

TRAVESTY OF THE ARTERIOVENOUS GRAFT

Unfortunately, much of the treatment of AV grafts is dictated by a physician's "clinical experience," local practice patterns, and nihilism: "nothing works!" That there are huge numbers of these grafts being treated begs the question, Why don't we know the answers? This problem lends itself to multicenter large-volume prospective, randomized clinical trials. The DOQI authors are to be congratulated on trying to make sense from a confused publication environment. The next phase should be establishment of such trials with enrollment numbers that are close to those achievable in the interventional cardiology literature. The questions are as follows:

1. Percutaneous transluminal angioplasty (PTA) of a venous anastomosis is performed for a 70% lesion: How durable is this? Ultrasound post PTA days 3, 7, 14, and so on will provide us an answer easily. If it is not durable, is it justifiable?
2. Which intervention is most durable for an isolated venous stenosis: patch angioplasty versus balloon angioplasty?
3. When should prophylactic angioplasty be abandoned?
4. How do tandem central venous stenoses influence interventions on a venous anastomotic stenosis?

VENOUS ANASTOMOTIC LESION

Nowhere in the body is balloon angioplasty alone particularly effective for restenotic lesions. Venous lesions in general respond more poorly to balloon angioplasty than do arterial lesions. The venous anastomotic lesion is actively proliferative and contains a large amount of ground substance (1,2). It is rubbery and recoils following dilatation. Furthermore, it can be extraordinarily difficult to dilate. Indeed, high-pressure balloons are designed specifically to dilate this lesion because of this well-recognized difficulty. Despite using very high pressures even up to 20 atm, it may prove impossible to resolve the "waist" that is usually regarded as the determination of a successful outcome (Fig 22B.1).

It is very clear that all venous anastomotic lesions are not equal, varying from short-segment focal lesions to extensive stenoses with near total obliteration of the outflow venous segment over considerable lengths. Only Beathard (3) has attempted to classify the type of lesion detected based on the number of stenoses, anatomic location, severity, and length of stenosis or occlusion. He noted that a greater number of subclavian and brachiocephalic lesions were immediate technical failures compared with axillary or more peripheral lesions. The duration of efficacy (*clinical patency*) also was

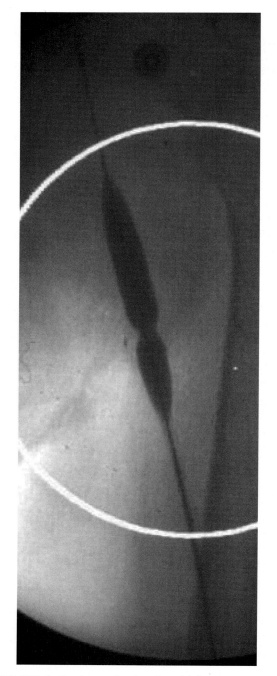

FIGURE 22B.1. Persistent "waist" in a high-pressure balloon, frequently observed during dilatation of venous anastomotic stenoses.

less for long venous lesions and subclavian lesions than for other venous stenoses. Perhaps surprisingly, Beathard noted no difference in outcome for total occlusions versus stenoses and no difference between the first and subsequent dilatations.

Schwab and colleagues (4) reported that in 27% of lesions, high-pressure balloons were required to dilate the stenoses. Even with high-pressure balloons, lesions resistant to dilatation are encountered. In our series, pres-

sures in excess of 10 atm were required in 20% of the cases (5).

The mechanism of action of PTA in hemodialysis-associated stenoses was examined by Davidson and colleagues (6) using intravascular ultrasound. Vessel dissection occurred in 16% of cases, stretching in 50%, but significant elastic recoil occurred in 50%. This is very different from the mechanism of action in arterial stenoses, where dissection of the plaque may be the primary mode of the therapeutic efficacy.

The benefit of balloon angioplasty in the treatment of the failing graft has not been validated in our experience, by both retrospective (5) and prospective randomized clinical trials (7). In a retrospective study of 40 patients with symptomatic or dysfunctional grafts, we reported the assisted primary patency at 1 month, 6 months, and 12 months to be 76%, 27%, and 10% (5). In a prospective randomized trial, color-flow duplex scanning was used to detect stenoses in functioning polytetrafluoroethylene (ePTFE) grafts of greater than 50% (7). Patients were subject to confirmatory angiography. Those with angiographic stenoses greater than 50% were randomized to balloon angioplasty versus observation. Patients were followed up with duplex scanning every 2 months. Statistical analysis was performed using the Kaplan—Meier technique. In the treatment and observation group, the 6-month patencies were 69% ± 7% and 70% ± 7%, respectively. Twelve-month patencies for the treatment and observation groups were 51% ± 6% and 47% ± 4%. There was no significant difference between these two groups ($p = 0.97$), with an 80% confidence limit for detection of a difference greater than 20% (Fig. 22B.2).

Our conclusion was that this study demonstrates that a generic approach of PTA to treat all ePTFE grafts with stenoses greater than 50% does not prolong patency and cannot be supported. This study was flawed by the lack of a synchronous functional evaluation. Nevertheless, with the selection criteria defined in this study, no benefit could be ascertained. In a subsequent report, we did note the efficacy of prophylactic angioplasty in "virgin" grafts, that is, those that had no prior intervention (7) (Fig 22B.3).

COSTS OF A PROPHYLACTIC INTERVENTIONAL REGIMEN

We analyzed the charges generated in the prospective randomized trial described already (8). Relevant charges were considered to be (a) initial duplex screening of the entire ePTFE dialysis group, (b) cost of transportation to the hospital for angiography, (c) professional and technical fees for angiography and angioplasty, (d) follow-up duplex scanning and repeat angioplasty, and (e) costs of lytic therapy for an intraprocedure lysis.

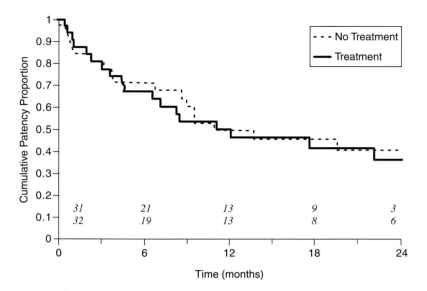

FIGURE 22B.2. Life-table analysis of prospective randomized trial evaluating the efficacy of prophylactic, maintenance angioplasty versus observation alone.

The charge for duplex screening of all patients in the dialysis unit with ePTFE grafts was $40,440 (at $337 each × 120 patients). Total charges for initial angiography were $178 (angioplasty costs were $143,040). Cost of the follow-up duplex ultrasound scanning in the treated group was $32,352. Cost of repeat angiograms in those with recurrent stenoses was $83,682 (professional fee $1,733 + $229 technical fee + $820 equipment charges × 32 × 0.94). One patient required urokinase therapy for an occlusion following PTA. The overall charge for treating the 32 patients in the treatment arm of this study was $440,834, with no net improvement in patency (9). A policy of generic graft surveillance and prophylactic is extremely expensive and in this study did not lead to improved patency. Until an effective inter-

vention is defined by prospective randomized trial, surveillance duplex scanning and intervention based on the criteria defined in this study cannot be recommended.

CONCLUSION

Is prophylactic angioplasty of the venous anastomosis of an AV graft worthwhile? My answer has to be yes. The reason: I do it. But the rationale is borne more out of having few better options and a desire to minimize surgical interventions, hospital time, and immediate costs, rather than convincing scientific data that it is the right thing to do. All of us who do angioplasty know of the high failure rate and re-

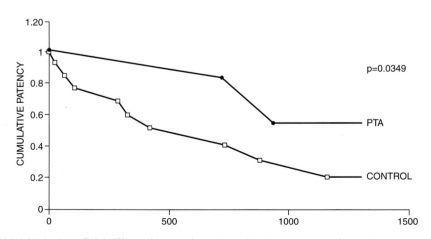

FIGURE 22B.3. Beneficial effect of angioplasty in prolonging patency of "virgin" arteriovenous grafts.

volving door approach to these patients. The DOQI guidelines set us on the right approach for evidence-based decision making; however, our somewhat skeptical use of maintenance angioplasty needs to be formally evaluated by prospective randomized trial: The patients are there, the lesion is frequent, and the questions are obvious. These kinds of hard data are what we need to formulate very costly national maintenance angioplasty policies.

REFERENCES

1. Lumsden AB, Chen C, Ku DN. Neovascularization in the venous neointimal hyperplastic lesions of arteriovenous grafts. *J Am Soc Nephrol* 1994;5:421.
2. MacDonald MJ, Martin LG, Hughes JD, et al. Distribution and severity of stenoses in functioning arteriovenous grafts: a duplex and angiographic study. *J Vasc Technol* 1996;20:131–136.
3. Beathard GA. Percutaneous transvenous angioplasty in the treatment of vascular access stenosis. *Kidney Int* 1992;42:1390–1397.
4. Schwab SJ, Raymond JR, Saeed M, et al. Prevention of hemodialysis fistula thrombosis: early detection of venous stenoses. *Kidney Int* 1989;36:707–711.
5. Lumsden AB, Macdonald MJ, Harker LA, et al. Hemodialysis access graft stenosis: percutaneous balloon angioplasty. *J Surg Res* 1997;68:181–185.
6. Davidson CJ, Newman GE, Sheikh KH, et al. Mechanisms of angioplasty in hemodialysis fistula. *Kidney Int* 1991;40:91–95.
7. Lumsden AB, Macdonald MJ, Kikeri D, et al. Prophylactic balloon angioplasty fails to prolong the patency of ePTFE Arteriovenous grafts: results of a prospective randomized trials. *J Vasc Surg* 1997;26:382–392.
8. Martin LG, Macdonald JM, Kikeri D, et al. Prophylactic angioplasty reduces thrombosis in virgin ePTFE arteriovenous dialysis grafts with greater than 50% stenosis: subset analysis of a prospectively randomized study. *J Vasc Interv Radiol* 1999;10:389–396.
9. Lumsden AB, Macdonald MJ, Kikeri D, et al. Cost efficacy of duplex surveillance and prophylactic angioplasty of Arteriovenous ePTFE grafts. *Ann Vasc Surg* 1997:12:138–142.

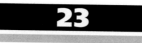

ENDOVASCULAR INTERVENTIONS: FISTULOGRAPHY, ANGIOPLASTY, AND STENTS

JOSHUA L. WEINTRAUB
JOHN H. RUNDBACK

More than 250,000 patients receive hemodialysis each year in the United States (1). Access failure is the leading cause for hospital admission and outpatient procedures. In 1997, the National Kidney Foundation published the Dialysis Outcomes Quality Initiative (NK-DOQI), which contained consensus guidelines intended to improve vascular access outcomes and survival (2). The implementation of the DOQI guidelines into clinical practice has been reported to have reduced access-related complications and thrombosis rates (3), largely attributable to aggressive screening and the early use of percutaneous techniques to maintain function in jeopardized grafts and fistulae (4,5). (See Chapter 22 for a discussion of prophylactic angioplasty.)

Since first described in 1982 (6,7), percutaneous transluminal balloon angioplasty (PTA) has become the mainstay of treatment for accesses failing because of underlying central or peripheral venous stenoses (8). When angioplasty alone fails, alternative treatment modalities, including atherectomy and stent placement, allow immediate salvage in most cases. This chapter discusses the methods, indications, and outcomes for percutaneous evaluation and treatment of the failing hemodialysis arteriovenous (AV) access.

DIAGNOSTIC ANGIOGRAPHY (FISTULOGRAPHY)

Indications and Screening

The DOQI vascular access guidelines strongly encourage regular assessment of the access conduit for signs of impending failure. At a minimum, weekly physical examination of the graft should be performed, with pulsatility or other change in the normal characteristic continuous thrill mandating fistulography (9). A monthly dialysis screening program also should be established using either direct measurements of intra-access flow (e.g., dilution techniques) or indirect measures (e.g., recirculation or venous pressures). Any abnormal values or changes over time in the study parameters should prompt fistulography, with the objective of definitively assessing and treating latent flow-limiting, access-related vascular stenoses.

Technique of Fistulography

Synthetic Grafts

Before fistulography, it is important to examine the patient's graft to establish the configuration, location, and direction of flow. Graft examination may help to determine the site of a stenosis by the presence of a transition from a pulse upstream to the lesion changing to a thrill downstream from the stenosis (see Chapter 18). In most synthetic grafts, stenosis occurs at the venous anastomosis or in the venous outflow, and the initial diagnostic puncture can therefore be placed within the graft and directed toward the vein. In uncertain cases, the venous end of a synthetic graft can be easily determined by brief manual compression of the graft to ascertain which side is pulsatile and, therefore, the arterial end.

Fistulography is performed by puncturing the graft with a small-gauge needle and injecting contrast through a needle cannula or subsequently introduced catheter. Usually, the venous limb of the graft and venous outflow are evaluated first. If the central veins (subclavian and innominate) are insufficiently visualized, a 4- or 5- French catheter may be advanced over a guidewire for directed angiography of this area. Any stenosis greater than 50%, particularly when producing venous collaterals, is considered hemodynamically significant (2), and endovascular intervention should be performed if the stenosis is consistent with the associated clinical or screening abnormality.

After examining the venous outflow, the arterial anastomosis and arterial limb must be evaluated by using a technique that enables reflux into the artery during contrast injection. We routinely compress the venous side of the graft using a surgical clamp, thereby decreasing hand exposure to the operator. Alternatively, inflating a blood pressure cuff above the graft to suprasystolic pressure will allow reflux of contrast across the arterial anastomosis. If a venous intervention has been performed or is anticipated, a thromboembolectomy or angioplasty balloon can be introduced and inflated within the graft, thus producing arterial reflux during injection through the sidearm of the sheath (Fig. 23.1). Any additional hemodynamically significant stenosis (>50%) uncovered in the arterial side of the graft may be treated using a second access puncture directed toward the lesion.

If initially both arterial and venous stenoses are suspected in a loop configuration graft, the apex technique (10) can be used, which allows access to both ends. For this technique, the initial puncture is made with a micropuncture set approximately 1 to 2 cm below the apex of the graft, making a short subcutaneous tunnel. It is preferable to enter the side of the graft and not the anterior surface. Evaluation of the venous side is performed initially, and any amenable venous stenosis is corrected. The arterial anastomosis is then studied using the reflux method previously described. If an additional lesion exists in the arterial limb of the access, the catheter can be redirected toward the arterial anastomosis and a second puncture site avoided.

After completing the diagnostic fistulogram and necessary endovascular interventions, several methods are available for facilitating hemostasis. By far the most common and simple method is manual compression performed by applying firm but nonocclusive pressure directly to the puncture. We routinely use compressive bandages (Tip-

Stop, Gambro Healthcare, Lakewood, NJ, U.S.A.) over the site while compressing manually for 5 to 10 minutes. Alternatively, a pursestring suture technique has been described (11). Using a 0-silk or smaller suture (some prefer monofilament sutures), two or three small superficial "in-and-out" bites are taken around the sheath and tightened on removal of the sheath. Manual pressure then is applied for several minutes to decrease the risk of pseudoaneurysm.

Arteriovenous Fistula

The venous outflow is usually punctured near the AV anastomosis. We routinely use a micropuncture set (Cook, Bloomington, IN, U.S.A.) to obtain initial access. An antegrade approach should be used if a venous outflow stenosis is suspected; a retrograde approach is appropriate for stenoses close to the anastomosis and upstream from the puncture site. The AV anastomotic site is a common location for vascular narrowing and must be evaluated carefully using refluxing methods. In our experience, the blood pressure cuff technique is most reliable for this purpose because the presence of multiple and variable venous anatomy frequently precludes point compression of all draining veins sufficient to cause arterial reflux (Fig. 23.2). Rarely, insertion of an intravenous-type cannula or small catheter into the brachial artery at the elbow is necessary to delineate stenoses located within the feeding artery or at the AV anastomosis. An entire fistulogram should be performed, including evaluation of the central venous system. If a stenosis is identified, endovascular intervention should be performed. As opposed to synthetic grafts, we routinely use manual compression to obtain hemostasis after the proce-

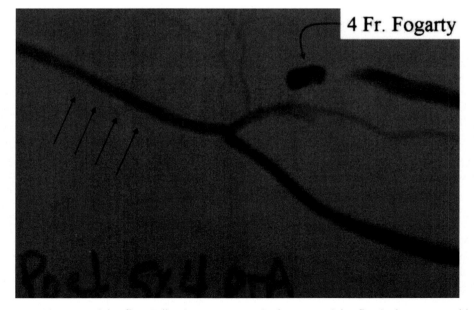

FIGURE 23.1. Arterial reflux. Following venous angioplasty, arterial reflux is demonstrated by inflating a Fogarty balloon (Baxter, Minneapolis, MN, U.S.A.) within the graft during contrast injection.

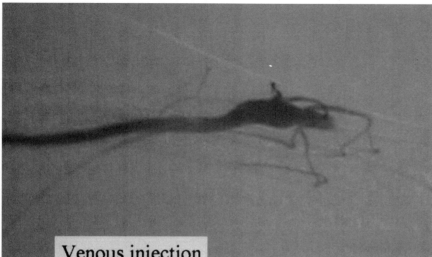

Venous injection

A

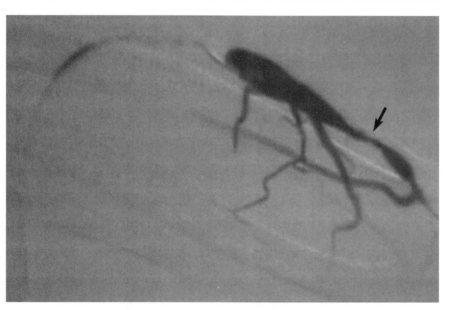

B

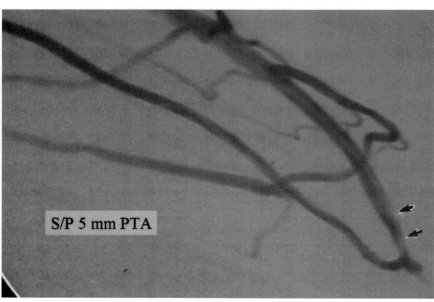

S/P 5 mm PTA

C

FIGURE 23.2. Autogenous arteriovenous fistula angioplasty. **A**: Contrast injection through an 18-gauge intravenous catheter fails to show the arterial anastomosis despite manual outflow compression. **B**: Following suprasystolic inflation of a blood pressure cuff, angiography demonstrates reflux across the arteriovenous anastomosis, revealing a short high-grade stenosis (*arrow*). **C**: Following 5-mm percutaneous transluminal angioplasty, there is no significant residual stenosis. Note that the guidewire has been left across the treated site.

dure. (See Chapter 24 for more on fistulography technique in autologous fistulas.)

Alternative Contrast Techniques

In patients with severe contrast hypersensitivity or residual renal function, fistulography may be performed using non-nephrotoxic carbon dioxide gas (CO_2) (12) or gadolinium chelates.

The technique of CO_2 fistulography is analogous to that already described, although digital subtraction is necessary and images should be acquired at a higher frame rate (six images per second) to allow sequential visualization or electronic "stacking" of all segments of the access anatomy. Because of its low viscosity, CO_2 freely refluxes across the arterial anastomosis even without occlusion of the venous outflow. For high-grade venous anastomotic lesions, care must be taken to avoid reflux into the vertebral and carotid arteries. CO_2 is drawn into a 50-mL syringe using a water-seal or closed bag technique to prevent contamination by insoluble room air and injected manually while visualizing the adequacy of vessel filling. Whereas too fast an injection of CO_2 is painful and causes patient movement, underfilling may be insufficient to visualize the central veins. If necessary, central venous evaluation can be augmented by injecting CO_2 through a centrally positioned catheter.

Gadolinium chelates also can be used as vascular contrast agents (13), providing approximately one third of the contrast resolution seen with iodinated contrast material. The k-edge of gadolinium is close to 90 KV, requiring recalibration of the angiography equipment or manual adjustment of the imaging technique to maximize image quality.

Results of Fistulography

The vast majority of stenoses in synthetic dialysis grafts occur at or within 10 cm of the venous anastomosis (Fig. 23.3) (14). One explanation for this finding is that the venous anastomosis has turbulent blood flow and is therefore subject to neointimal hyperplasia (see Chapter 8). Central venous stenoses related to prior catheterization are not uncommon; they are found in more than 50% of patients with prior or existing subclavian dialysis catheters (15). Hemodynamically significant lesions usually manifest numerous bridging collaterals, which often are noted to resolve after successful treatment.

It is widely believed that true arterial stenoses resulting from intimal hyperplasia account for fewer than 5% and possibly fewer than 1% of stenoses in dialysis grafts (14). There is recent evidence in the abstract literature that the incidence of arterial inflow lesions may be much higher, up to 39% in one abstract presentation. This is still controversial, and peer-reviewed studies are needed. In any event, most stenoses encountered at the arterial anastomosis are the result of the presence of a densely compacted fibrin and red blood cell "plug,"

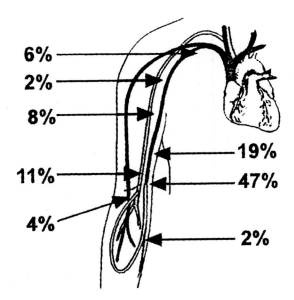

FIGURE 23.3. Location of vascular access stenosis.

especially if there has been a recent surgical or percutaneous thrombectomy. Any flow-compromising arterial plug must be removed completely. Although this may be attempted using balloon angioplasty to macerate the plug, resistant or adherent lesions should be resolved by using techniques directed at clot removal, such as a Fogarty balloon thrombectomy catheter (Baxter, Minneapolis, MN, U.S.A.), the Fogarty adherent clot catheter (Baxter), or a mechanical thrombolytic device. Although some institutions consider angioplasty of the arterial plug to be acceptable or even preferable, others suggest that this may be associated with a higher restenosis rate.

In autologous arteriovenous fistulae, stenosis is very frequent in the anastomotic area and proximal outflow vein, presumably secondary to the turbulent flow and neointimal hyperplasia. Repetitive vein punctures also may result in stenosis or pseudoaneurysms within the venous outflow.

ENDOVASCULAR INTERVENTIONS

Angioplasty and Stents

Techniques

Once a significant stenosis is identified, PTA almost always should be attempted. The initial diagnostic cannula or catheter is exchanged over a guidewire for a short vascular sheath of an appropriate caliber to accommodate the selected balloon catheter. The balloon diameter is selected by measuring the normal diameter of the vein proximal to the stenosis or distal to the poststenotic dilatation. For synthetic grafts, the balloon can be sized to 1 mm larger than the prosthetic portion of the graft, if that width is known. For most polytetrafluoroethylene (PTFE) grafts, a 7- or 8-mm-diameter balloon is usually appropriate for the venous anastomosis or adjacent outflow (Fig. 23.4). Some operators use 8-mm balloons for all 6-mm PTFE grafts and the adjacent venous anastomoses, unless the outflow vein is unusually small. Central venous stenoses generally require balloons ranging from 10 to 14 mm in diameter.

In forearm fistulae, a balloon at least 4-mm in diameter must be used to treat stenoses involving the feeding artery, with balloons of at least 5 mm needed in forearm veins to provide durable results. Dilatation of a stenosis close to the arterial anastomosis can create arterial spasm, and it is therefore recommended to leave a guidewire through the anastomosis during such dilatations to be able to reopen the artery rapidly if necessary (Fig. 23.2).

Once the lesion is crossed with the guidewire and the balloon, inflation generally is performed for at least 20 to 30 seconds to minimize elastic recoil. High-pressure balloons and inflation devices may be necessary to efface completely the fibrous lesions. During the balloon expansion, the patient usually will experience localized pain, which can be reduced by the use of intravenous analgesia immediately before inflation. Some have infiltrated the tissues around the lesion site with lidocaine for pain control. After PTA, the balloon is withdrawn, and a repeat angiogram is performed through the vascular sheath. Residual narrowing of more than 30% usually portends a poor outcome and should be treated by repeat PTA using a larger balloon (Fig. 23.4) or by stent deployment (Fig. 23.5). We successfully treated resistant lesions with repeat PTA using an intentionally undersized balloon capable of exerting greater radial force, followed by the use of balloons of serially increasing diameter. In synthetic grafts, a satisfactory PTA results in normalization of the thrill within the graft and disappearance of any initially noted venous collaterals. Direct pressure measurements also can be used as an endpoint for intervention in venous anastomotic or outflow lesions, although these are not reliable for central venous stenoses or in autologous fistulae. Hemodynamic success is conferred by a less than 10 mm Hg residual translesional gradient or a normalized pressure ratio (ratio of the systolic venous limb pressure to the cuffed arm systolic pressure) of less than 33% (16). (See Chapter 25 for a detailed discussion of stent deployment technique.)

Indications

The DOQI guidelines strongly support the judicious use of PTA and stents to preserve access function (Table 23.1). Furthermore, although not described in DOQI, stents may allow a treatment option in patients who have recurrent graft dysfunction despite repeated angioplasty.

Prophylactic Percutaneous Transluminal Angioplasty for the Failing Access

Guideline 10 of the DOQI supports the screening and early angiography of a failing hemodialysis access. Clinical or hemodynamic indicators of graft failure warranting angiography include arm swelling, prolonged bleeding after needle withdrawal, graft pulsatility, abnormal static or dynamic venous pressures, elevated recirculation, and reduced graft flow rates (<600 mL per minute). DOQI guidelines 17 (for dialysis grafts) and 18 (for primary AV fistulae) recommend prophylactic PTA for angiographically demonstrated stenoses exceeding 50% associated with an abnormal clinical or hemodynamic parameter. This approach has been documented to result in an approximately twofold to threefold decrease in the incidence of access thrombosis and surgical graft revision or replacement (17,18). The results of prophylactic PTA are shown in Table 23.2 (6,14,19–21). (See Chapter 22 for a discussion on prophylactic angioplasty.)

Guideline 19 of the DOQI defines technical success of balloon angioplasty as less than 30% residual stenosis and resolution of the abnormal clinical parameter. The threshold for long-term patency is established as 50% primary patency at 6 months. PTA *failure* is defined as a recurrent stenosis requiring angioplasty more than twice over a 3-month period and should be treated by a stent or surgical revision. Restenosis is more likely to occur with central venous stenoses, in lesions longer than 6 cm, in less mature grafts, in straight (compared with loop) grafts, and for PTA performed after thrombectomy compared with PTA performed (prophylactically) for nonthrombosed grafts.

Percutaneous Transluminal Angioplasty of Underlying Stenoses after Thrombolysis or Thrombectomy

Guideline 21 advocates complete angiography after successful thrombolysis or thrombectomy. In most radiologic series, venous anastomotic or outflow stenoses responsible for access failure are identified in about 90% of cases (compared with only 50% for intraoperative angiography) (22). PTA following declotting is successful 90% of the time and yields results equivalent to surgical revision with the advantages of preserving proximal veins, requiring less anesthesia and eliminating or reducing hospital stays (20,23). (See Chapter 29 for more on the relative merits of surgical and percutaneous thrombectomy.)

Atherectomy for Fibrous Lesions Resistant to Percutaneous Transluminal Angioplasty

Venous anastomotic and proximal venous outflow stenoses account for nearly 75% of all lesions threatening hemodialysis access function. These lesions tend to be fibrous and thus resistant to balloon dilatation, which requires the use of high-pressure balloons and inflation devices. Occasionally, the waist on the balloon cannot be effaced despite these techniques. In these instances, extirpative directional atherectomy successfully debulks the neointimal tissue and may allow successful adjunctive angioplasty (24). (Others have used multiple tiny-gauge needle punctures at the lesion site to allow complete balloon inflation subsequently.) Atherectomy also may be beneficial for the

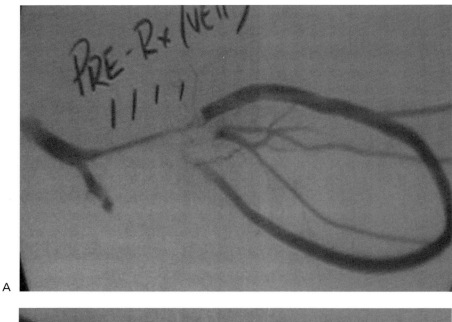

A

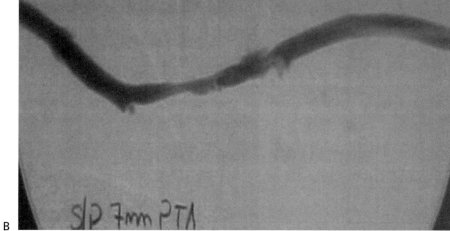

B

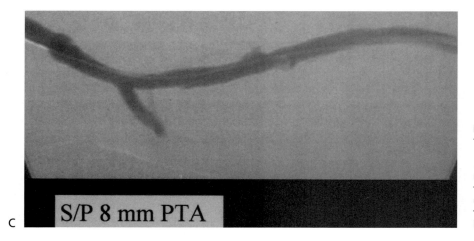

C

FIGURE 23.4. Fistulogram and percutaneous transluminal angiography (PTA) of a forearm loop graft. **A**: Fistulogram demonstrates a long-segment venous outflow and anastomotic stenosis. **B**: Following 7-mm PTA (sized to the known graft diameter), there is residual narrowing at the treated site. **C**: Completion fistulogram after 8-mm PTA shows resolution of the stenosis.

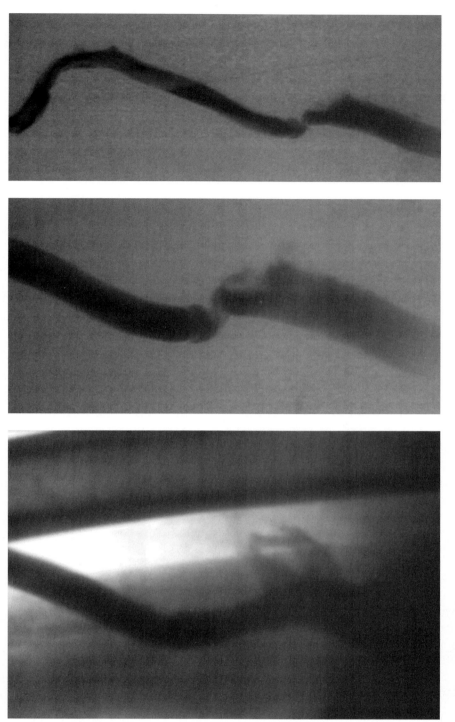

A

B

C

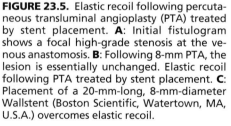

FIGURE 23.5. Elastic recoil following percutaneous transluminal angioplasty (PTA) treated by stent placement. **A**: Initial fistulogram shows a focal high-grade stenosis at the venous anastomosis. **B**: Following 8-mm PTA, the lesion is essentially unchanged. Elastic recoil following PTA treated by stent placement. **C**: Placement of a 20-mm-long, 8-mm-diameter Wallstent (Boston Scientific, Watertown, MA, U.S.A.) overcomes elastic recoil.

TABLE 23.1. INDICATIONS FOR PTA AND STENTS

Prophylactic PTA for failing access
PTA of underlying stenoses after thrombolysis or thrombectomy
Stents for central venous stenoses failing PTA
Stents for recurrent peripheral stenoses[a]
Stents for flow-limiting dissections occurring after PTA[a]
Stents for vein ruptures[a]

PTA, percutaneous transluminal angiography.
[a] See text for explanation.

treatment of intragraft stenoses or in-stent restenoses that do not respond to angioplasty alone. Unfortunately, the directional atherectomy device is currently unavailable, and its use is not addressed in the DOQI guidelines.

Stent Deployment for Central Venous Stenoses Failing Percutaneous Transluminal Angioplasty

Prior temporary subclavian venous catheters account for most central venous stenoses encountered in the dialysis

TABLE 23.2. RESULTS OF BALLOON ANGIOPLASTY

Author (Ref. No.)	No. of Patients	Primary Patency		Secondary Patency	
		6 Mo	12 Mo	6 Mo	12 Mo
Beathard (6)	285	62	38		
Turmel-Rodrigues et al. (19)[a]	63	51	43	72	63
Kanterman et al (14)	47	63	40		
Schwartz et al. (20)[b]	24	38	10	46	8
Safa et al. (21)	90	87	22	68	51

[a] Approximately half were autologous fistulae and half grafts; other studies in table were predominantly or exclusively grafts.
[b] Percutaneous transluminal angiography after surgical thrombectomy, other studies in table were for screened populations.

population. These lesions tend to be both fibrous and elastic and respond poorly to PTA. DOQI guideline 20 suggests PTA as the initial treatment of choice for central stenoses and supports the use of stents for restenoses developing within 3 months of balloon dilatation. An in-depth discussion of the results of central venous stent deployment is provided in Chapter 25.

Stents for Recurrent Peripheral Stenoses

Unlike central stenoses, stent placement for peripheral venous stenoses has not been shown to improve access patency rates when directly compared with PTA (25). Nevertheless, Turmel-Rodrigues et al. placed stents in 49 dialysis grafts for post-PTA elastic recoil (n = 13) or early (n = 33) or late (n = 3) restenosis. Primary patency was 47% at 6 months and 20% at 12 months. With repeated interventions, it was possible to maintain access function in 88% of patients at 1 year. In patients treated for early restenosis after prior PTA, the interval between subsequent reinterventions was doubled after stent placement (26). To date, others have not replicated these results. The DOQI guidelines recommend stents for peripheral lesions after PTA fails (or recurs more than twice in 3 months) only when surgery is not an option or limited residual access sites are available.

Stents for Flow-limiting Dissections Occurring after Percutaneous Transluminal Angioplasty

Although stents have not improved patency rates relative to PTA, stents still can be used as a "bailout" technique for PTA complicated by the development of a flow-limiting dissection. In this setting, percutaneous stent deployment may successfully preserve initial graft function, thereby avoiding the need for urgent surgical revision or the placement of a temporary hemodialysis catheter. Stents are especially useful for a flow-limiting dissection (or rupture; see later) that threatens immediate graft thrombosis in a graft that has not previously thrombosed. These particular situations are not addressed in the DOQI guidelines.

Stents for Vein Ruptures

A more recently recognized role for dialysis access stenting is in the management of post-PTA vein ruptures, a complication that occurs in 0.7% to 4.5% of cases. When observation (for limited extravasation) or prolonged balloon angioplasty at the site of vessel injury fails, stent placement often is effective in limiting further extravasation (27,28). Presumably, the stent creates a "path of least resistance" toward the central veins and may seal the site of vein rupture by apposing intact intima against the vessel defect.

CONCLUSION

Overall, the DOQI guidelines strongly support the role of carefully used fistulography, angioplasty, and stent placement for the evaluation and treatment of venous stenoses threatening vascular access function. Newer developments, including brachytherapy, radioactive and drug-incorporated stents, cutting angioplasty, and local drug delivery, in the future may improve the results of these techniques. When percutaneous methods fail, surgical revision or graft replacement remains the mainstay of therapy. In general, the credo is not "angioplasty *or* surgery"; rather, the credo is "angioplasty *and* surgery."

REFERENCES

1. 2001 United States Renal Data Systems (USRDS) Annual Report. Treatment Modalities. Available at: *www.usrds.org*. Accessed January 22, 2002.
2. Schwab S, Besarab A, Beathard G, et al. NKF-DOQI clinical practice guidelines for vascular access. *Am J Kidney Dis* 1997;30 (Suppl 3):S150–S191.
3. Allon M. Bailey R, Ballard, et al. A multidisciplinary approach to hemodialysis access: prospective evaluation. *Kidney Int* 1998; 53:473–479.
4. Sullivan KL, Besarab A. Hemodynamic screening and early percutaneous intervention reduce hemodialysis access thrombosis and increase graft longevity. *J Vasc Interv Radiol* 1997;8:163–170.
5. Schwab SJ, Oliver MJ, Suhocki P, et al. Hemodialysis arteriovenous access: detection of stenosis and response to treatment by vascular access blood flow. *Kidney Int* 2001;59:358–362.
6. Beathard GA. Percutaneous transvenous angioplasty in the treatment of vascular access stenosis. *Kidney Int* 1992;42:1390–1397.
7. Gordon DH, Glanz S, Butt KM, et al. Treatment of stenotic lesions in dialysis access fistulas and shunts by transluminal angioplasty. *Radiology* 1982;143:53–58.
8. Gray RJ. Percutaneous intervention for permanent hemodialysis access: a review. *J Vasc Interv Radiol* 1997;8:313–327.
9. Trerotola SO, Scheel PJ Jr, Powe NR, et al. Screening for dialysis access graft malfunction:comparison of physical examination with US. *J Vasc Interv Radiol* 1996;7:15–20.
10. Hathaway PB, Vesely TM. The apex-puncture technique for mechanical thrombolysis of loop hemodialysis grafts. *J Vasc Interv Radiol* 1999;10:775–779.
11. Vesely TM. Use of a purse string suture to close a percutaneous access site after hemodialysis graft interventions. *J Vasc Interv Radiol* 1998;9:447–450.

12. Ehrman KO, Taber TE, Gaylord GM, et al. Comparison of diagnostic accuracy with carbon dioxide versus iodinated contrast material in the imaging of hemodialysis access fistulas. *J Vasc Interv Radiol* 1994;5:771–775.

13. Spinosa DJ, Angle JF, Hagspiel KD, et al. CO_2 and gadopentetate dimeglumine as alternative contrast agents for malfunctioning dialysis grafts and fistulas. *Kidney Int* 1998;54: 945–950.

14. Kanterman RY, Vesely TM, Pilgram TK, et al. Dialysis access grafts: anatomic location of venous stenosis and results of angioplasty. *Radiology* 1995;195:135–139.

15. Surratt RS, Picus D, Hicks ME, et al. The importance of preoperative evaluation of the subclavian vein in dialysis access planning. *AJR Am J Roentgenol* 1991;156:623–625.

16. Sullivan KL, Besarab A. Strategies for maintaining dialysis access patency. In: Cope C, ed. *Current techniques in interventional radiology*, 2nd ed. Philadelphia: Current Medicine, 1995:125–131.

17. Schwab SJ, Raymond JR, Saeed M, et al. Prevention of hemodialysis fistula thrombosis: early detection of venous stenoses. *Kidney Int* 1989;36:707–711.

18. Roberts AB, Kahn MB, Bradford S, et al. Graft surveillance and angioplasty prolongs dialysis graft patency. *J Am Coll Surg* 1996;183:486–492.

19. Turmel-Rodrigues L, Pengloan J, Blanchier D, et al. Insufficient dialysis shunts: improved long-term patency rates with close hemodynamic monitoring, repeated percutaneous balloon angioplasty, and stent placement. *Radiology* 1993;187:273–278.

20. Schwartz CI, McBrayer CV, Sloan JH, et al. Thrombosed dialysis grafts: comparison of treatment with transluminal angioplasty and surgical revision. *Radiology* 1995;194:337–341.

21. Safa AA, Valji K, Roberts AC, et al. Detection and treatment of dysfunctional hemodialysis access grafts: effect of a surveillance program on graft patency and the incidence of thrombosis. *Radiology* 1996;199:653–657.

22. Valji K, Bookstein JJ, Roberts AC, et al. Pharmacomechanical thrombolysis and angioplasty in the management of clotted hemodialysis grafts: early and late clinical results. *Radiology* 1991;178:243–247.

23. Polak JF, Berger MF, Pagan-Marin H, et al. Comparative efficacy of pulse-spray thrombolysis and angioplasty versus surgical salvage procedures for treatment of recurrent occlusion of PTFE dialysis access grafts. *Cardiovasc Intervent Radiol* 1998;21:314–318.

24. Gray RJ, Dolmatch BL, Buick MK. Directional atherectomy treatment for hemodialysis access: early results. *J Vasc Interv Radiol* 1992;3:497–503.

25. Hoffer EK, Sultan S, Herskowitz MM, et al. Prospective randomized trial of a metallic intravascular stent in hemodialysis graft maintenance. *J Vasc Interv Radiol* 1997;8:965–973.

26. Turmel-Rodrigues LA, Blanchard D, Pengloan J, et al. Wallstents and Craggstents in hemodialysis grafts and fistulas: results for selective indications. *J Vasc Interv Radiol* 1997;8:975–982.

27. Funaki B, Szymski GX, Leef JA, et al. Wallstent deployment to salvage dialysis graft thrombolysis complicated by venous rupture: early and intermediate results. *AJR Am J Roentgenol* 1997;169:1435–1438.

28. Rundback JH, Leonardo R, Rozenblit G, et al. Vein rupture complicating hemodialysis access angioplasty: percutaneous treatment and outcomes in seven patients. *AJR Am J Roentgenol* 1998;171:1081–1084.

DIAGNOSIS AND ENDOVASCULAR TREATMENT FOR AUTOLOGOUS FISTULAE-RELATED STENOSES

LUC TURMEL-RODRIGUES

All the reports in the literature show that the incidence of stenosis and the risk of thrombosis are smaller in native fistulae than in prosthetic grafts. For this reason, the creation of any type of native fistula is preferable to placement of any type of graft (1–3). Some centers even achieve 100% primary native fistulae in their hemodialyzed patients, including diabetic patients (4). Nevertheless, stenosis and subsequent thrombosis remain the most frequent complications (1,2).

DETECTION OF STENOSIS

Flow-Rate Monitoring

Sands and Schwab and their colleagues demonstrated the value of monthly monitoring by access flow measurement with the Transonic machine (Transonic Systems Inc., Ithaca, NY, U.S.A.) to detect stenosis and indicate treatment in native fistulae (5,6), although venous collaterals can bias the measurements. It is likely that a reduction of flow at 1-month intervals is a more significant harbinger of thrombosis than a raw low-flow rate [Dialysis Outcomes Quality Improvement (DOQI) guideline 10], whose threshold is still debatable and not determined in native fistulae (see Chapter 19).

Clinical Examination

Clinical examination should remain the key detection method, although it is unfortunately operator dependent, and there is a learning curve. A *thrill* is the systolic turbulence resulting from the passage of blood from the high-pressure arterial system to the low-resistance venous system. It can be palpated with the fingers (*thrill*) or heard with a stethoscope (*bruit*). In a normal fistula, the thrill is best palpated or heard at the (arterial) anastomosis and then is lost relatively more rapidly (but never suddenly) than in grafts. In typical cases, the thrill is reinforced at the level of a stenosis and disappears downstream from the stenosis.

Many stenoses lie just under the skin and can be palpated as a tough cord with a firm dilated pulsatile vein upstream and a flat vein downstream. A tourniquet can help sensitize the location of the stenosis because the soft normal vein swells, whereas the tough stenotic segment does not.

Stenoses of the arterial inflow are responsible for an overall flat fistula, which is difficult to cannulate without the help of a tourniquet, and can cause a vacuum phenomenon during dialysis. Because most forearm fistula stenoses are located near the anastomosis, it is a common situation to be able to palpate the fistula easily only in the area of the anastomotic scar.

Stenoses of the venous outflow are typically responsible for a "too convenient fistula," which is much too visible and easy to puncture, but result in increased compression times after dialysis and formation of venous aneurysms, which can become painful and lead to skin necrosis. Pressure upstream to a venous outflow stenosis can, however, be reduced by alternative flow into collaterals, which are therefore also a sign of dysfunction and it it essential to look for them. Edema can occur when collaterals are insufficiently developed to compensate for a stenosis or when they run in the retrograde fashion down to the hand, involving the whole limb in cases of central vein stenosis but sometimes limited to the hand in cases of more peripheral stenoses. This is the main reason why side-to-side surgical anastomoses must be prohibited.

The aneurysms that are common in cannulation sites after some months of dialysis are ideal examination points because the skin is even thinner at their level: An aneurysm under tension indicates an outflow stenosis, whereas an abnormally flat and depressible aneurysm indicates an inflow problem. In cases of stenosis developing between the two cannulation sites, the "arterial" aneurysm is tough, whereas the "venous" aneurysm is soft. Stenoses in cannulation areas also can make routine needling impossible.

Placing the limb in the upright position can help sensitize the examination. Stenosis of the venous outflow can be ruled out if the fistula collapses, but stenosis of the arterial inflow can be suspected. If the fistula remains unchanged, venous outflow stenosis from the elbow or excessively high fistula flow can be suspected.

Palpation can be misleading, however. When stenosis of the venous outflow is associated with stenosis of the arterial inflow, the fistula appears clinically normal. Venous stenosis does not cause any upstream distension because the arterial inflow is poor and the arterial stenosis does not result in a flat fistula because the venous stenosis acts as a dam. Auscultation is particularly helpful in such cases because the systolic bruit is abnormally reinforced at the level of the "arterial" stenosis.

Examination of the hand is a mandatory stage of the clinical examination of any upper-arm fistula. Arterial ischemia by *steal syndrome* (i.e., painful, pale, cold, numb fingers, sometimes with ulcers) is often underestimated by nephrologists and nurses in older patients who are fatalistic and less demanding about physical limitations of their hands. Venous ischemia attributable to hand edema is the consequence of abnormal reflux of blood from the fistula down to the hand as a result of obstruction of the most direct venous outflow. Finally, a generally large fistula is highly suggestive of excessive high flow, with potential cardiac consequences. (For more on physical examination, see Chapter 18.)

Duplex Ultrasound

In experienced hands, duplex ultrasound can reliably detect stenoses and also can measure fistula flow rate (7,8). It can play a role in preselection of patients who can be directly referred to the surgeon (e.g., stenoses in the anastomotic area of wrist fistulae) and determine which patients require angiographic evaluation (see Chapter 20).

Recirculation is a very late sign of stenosis and should no longer be used in this setting.

DIAGNOSTIC ANGIOGRAPHY

Diagnostic angiography is performed within a scheme of a concomitant interventional procedure, and normal angiograms should be rare. Gadolinium can be used as the contrast agent in cases of absolute contraindication for iodine injection, but the cost is much higher (9). We recommend the cautious use of carbon dioxide gas only for treatment of venous outflow stenoses located far from the anastomosis because we experienced a casualty as a result of arterial reflux into the cerebral arteries (10,11).

The angiography technique depends on the clinical situation. In cases of *poor inflow* (the most frequent situation in forearm fistulae), retrograde puncture of the brachial artery at the elbow with an 18- to 20-gauge needle is the most physiologically appropriate approach to visualize the arteriovenous anastomosis and to avoid misinterpretation of the quality of arterial feed to the fistula (Figs. 24.1 and 24.2). This approach is the one most commonly used for the exploration of delayed maturation, a specific case where inflow and venous cannulation problems predominate. One hour's bedrest and armrest are required after brachial artery needle removal before discharging outpatients.

In cases of *outflow obstruction*, antegrade puncture of the vein is performed just after the anastomosis. This is usually easy to do becasue this venous segment is under tension (Fig 24.3–24.7).

In cases of *high outflow or hand ischemia*, complete visualization of the arteries of the limb is required to evaluate the possibility of fistula flow reduction or peripheral flow improvement. Retrograde puncture of the brachial artery is usually sufficient, and the femoral route is rarely necessary. In cases of distal ischemia, acquisitions centered on the forearm and hand must be performed before and during compression of the fistula to evaluate the respective roles of steal and intrinsic arterial lesions in the process.

Location of Stenoses

Stenoses can occur anywhere from the feeding artery to the superior vena cava, but they predominate in the anastomotic area for forearm fistulae and in the venous outflow for upper-arm fistulae (12).

Stenosis Grading

Stenosis in the arterial system is graded according to the narrowing of the diameter in the most pejorative incidence, the reference being the diameter of the immediately upstream or downstream normal vessel. Stenosis of more than 50% or 70% is considered significant, depending on the researcher and the location of the stenosis. The reference diameter can be difficult to determine in irregular and aneurysmal veins or at the confluence of two vessels. Symptomatic stenoses are mostly extremely tight, however, and there is rarely uncertainty.

In doubtful cases, pull-back pressure measurement can be performed, and this is not operator dependent (Fig. 24.3). We suggest grading according to the percentage of drop in systolic pressure through the presumed stenosis; significant stenosis induce a greater than 50% loss. It is, however, still not the perfect tool. This pressure gradient is fully reliable when no collaterals are visible upstream from the stenosis, but it underestimates the obstruction if there are collaterals leaving the fistula before the stenosis that reduce the upstream pressure. On the other hand, upstream pressure is abnormally high and leads to overestimation of the stenosis in excessively high-flow fistulae (<1.5 L per minute) (Fig. 24.4).

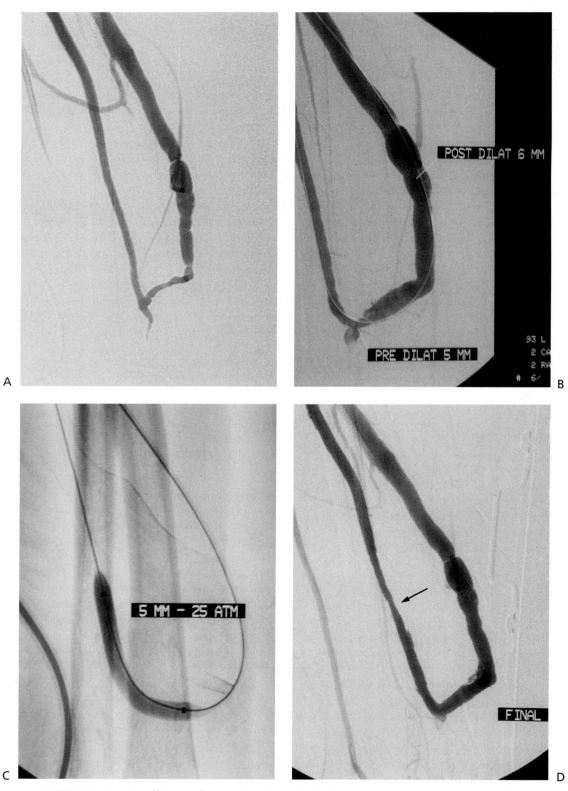

FIGURE 24.1. A: Insufficient inflow in this radio-cephalic fistula of 5 months' duration was mainly explained by a 3-cm-long stenosis starting from the anastomosis. **B**: Dilatation to 6 mm was performed to match the diameter of the cephalic vein in the upper part of the forearm. The balloon could not be placed across the anastomosis, however, because the radial artery had only a 4-mm caliber. The result was a greater than 50% residual stenosis of the immediately postanastomotic venous segment. **C:** Dilatation across the anastomosis was presumed feasible with a 5-mm balloon that had to be inflated to 25 atm to abolish any residual waisting. **D:** The final result is as satisfactory as possible given the anatomic constraints. Residual stenosis is about 30% in the immediately postanastomotic venous segment, and there is minor residual spasm on the radial artery (*arrow*) where overdilatation induced transient minor rupture.

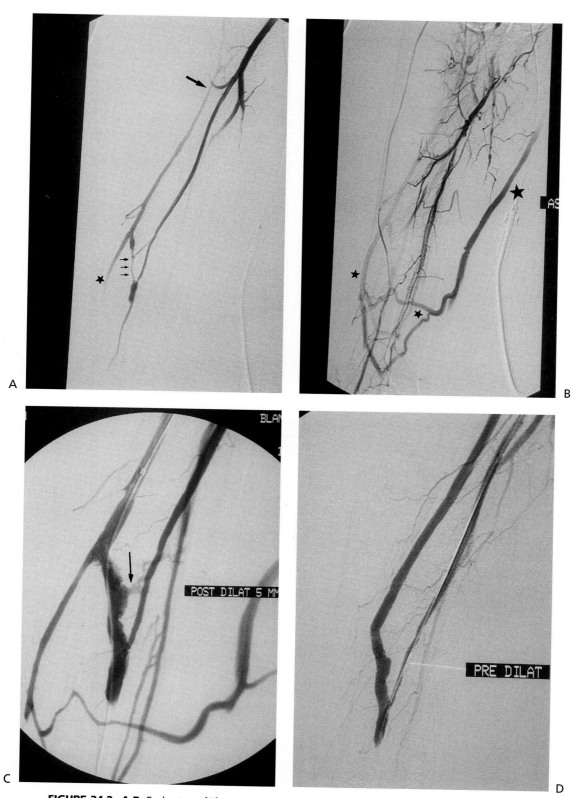

FIGURE 24.2. A,B: Early-stage **(A)** and late-stage angiography **(B)**. This radiocephalic fistula was created 7 weeks earlier in this 40-year-old diabetic patient. Delayed maturation was explained by stenoses on the distal feeding artery and on the vein at the postanastomotic level (*small arrows*) as well as at the elbow level (*larger arrow*). The elbow stenoses explain why the contrast medium re-fluxed through side branches (*small stars*) down to the wrist before reaching the basilic vein (*large star*). **C**: Dilatation of the postanastomotic venous stenosis to 5 mm caused transient rupture (*arrow*), which then was controlled by simple 5 minutes' low-pressure balloon tamponade. **D**: Flow through collaterals disappeared after dilatation of all the venous stenoses to 5 mm, but the thrill in the fistula remained insufficient because of the poor arterial inflow. Dilatation of the distal radial artery was performed after antegrade catheterization of the brachial artery at the elbow.

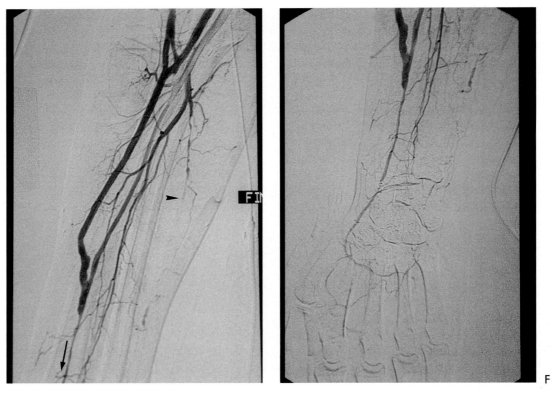

FIGURE 24.2. *(Continued.)* **E**: The final result was angiographically and clinically satisfactory after dilatation of the artery to 4 mm. It is important to take note of the persistence of antegrade flow in the radial artery beyond the anastomosis (*arrow*). The ulnar artery is virtually occluded (*arrowhead*). **F**: Vascularization of the hand depends only on the radial and interosseous arteries.

DILATATION

Indications

Stenosis should be treated only if it explains clinical impairment or if it threatens access patency because of low flow (DOQI guideline 18) (2). For example, apparent stenoses of the anastomosis of native fistulae must be dilated only in cases of insufficient flow because dilatation of a well-functioning fistula could lead to secondary high flow or steal phenomenon or because it could "awaken" the stenosing process and lead to early restenosis that could be more severe and lead to thrombosis. Similarly, subclavian and brachiocephalic stenoses are never responsible for native fistula thrombosis and must be dilated only in cases of clinically impairing upper-limb edema.

Regular Dilatation Technique

Dilatation is an outpatient procedure (13). Mature hemodialysis fistulae are made to be punctured and must be used for introduction of dilatation catheters. Clinical examination is essential to choose the best cannulation site. Puncture of the fistula for dilatation must be performed with the patient under local anesthesia in the direction of, but far enough away from (3 cm), the presumed stenosis. Aneurysms should not be punctured.

An antegrade approach should be used for stenoses located far enough from the anastomosis, and a retrograde approach should be used for stenoses close to the anastomosis. A tourniquet often helps this initial catheterization stage.

A 16- to 18-gauge needle and a 0.035-inch guidewire offer good support for placement of a 6 to 9 French introducer sheath. A small subcutaneous tunnel between the skin entry point and the vein entry point will facilitate the final compression and decrease the risk of pseudoaneurysm.

A soft-tipped Bentson-type guidewire is preferred to traverse stenoses. Angled catheters are helpful for selective catheterization of branches. Hydrophilic guidewires are very effective but must be used carefully because of their propensity to dissect vessel walls in stenosed areas. Heparin may be injected (2,000–3,000 U) once a guidewire has passed through the stenosis, but our experience indicates that it is only necessary in small-diameter or low-flow fistulae.

The diameter of the dilatation balloon should be equal to or 1 mm greater than the diameter of the immediately upstream or downstream normal vessel (take the smaller one first in cases of discrepancy). Angiography of the stenosed area must therefore be performed with the superimposition of a lead millimeter ruler (Fig. 24.4). A fistula of less than 3 months must be dilated at least to 5 mm (Fig. 24.2); a fistula of more than 1 year must be dilated at least to 7 mm (Fig. 24.5).

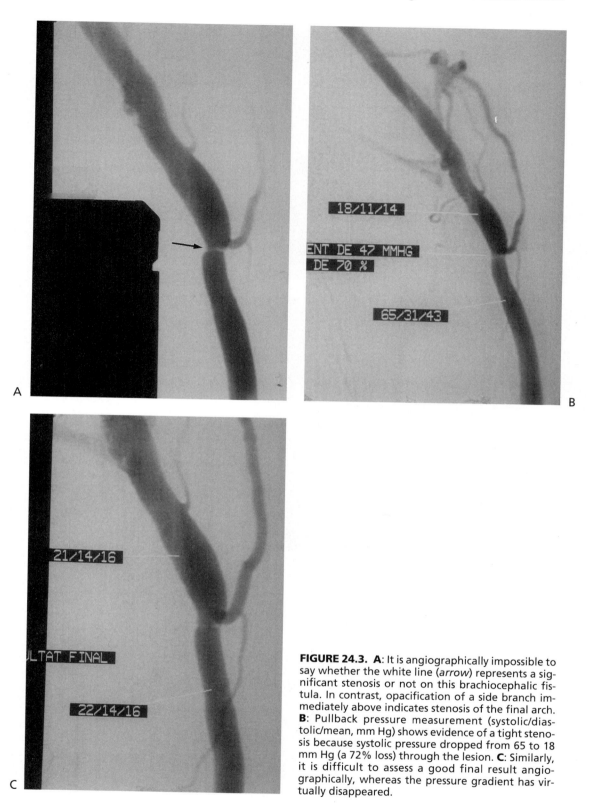

FIGURE 24.3. A: It is angiographically impossible to say whether the white line (*arrow*) represents a significant stenosis or not on this brachiocephalic fistula. In contrast, opacification of a side branch immediately above indicates stenosis of the final arch. **B**: Pullback pressure measurement (systolic/diastolic/mean, mm Hg) shows evidence of a tight stenosis because systolic pressure dropped from 65 to 18 mm Hg (a 72% loss) through the lesion. **C**: Similarly, it is difficult to assess a good final result angiographically, whereas the pressure gradient has virtually disappeared.

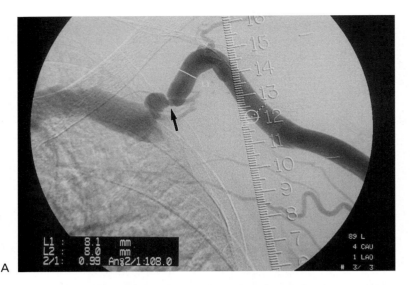

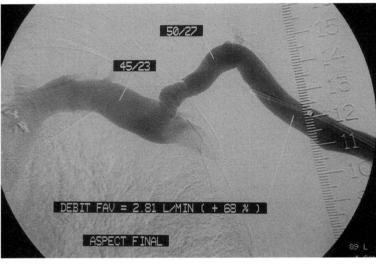

FIGURE 24.4. A: This 2-year-old brachiocephalic fistula had the classic clinical aneurysmal appearance of an excessively high-flow fistula with concomitant stenosis of the final arch (*arrow*). Dilatation was scheduled before surgical flow reduction. Predilatation flow rate was around 1.7 L per minute. **B**: Angiographic appearance looked good after dilatation to 8 mm, confirmed by minor residual pressure gradient (5 mm Hg = 10%) and by an increase in the fistula flow rate to 2.8 L per minute (+ 65%).

The dilatation balloon is inflated with a manometer filled with diluted contrast medium. Pressure is slowly increased to abolish the waist of the stenosis on the balloon, the edges of which must be *completely* parallel (Fig 24.1C and 24.5C). No residual notch should be accepted. The inflated balloon is left in place for 1 to 3 minutes. Dilatation is often painful locally. Local anesthesia can be administered when stenoses are just under the skin.

Venous stenoses are often very hard, and high-pressure balloons with bursting pressures over 25 atm must be used (Blue-Max, Medi-Tech, Natick, MA, U.S.A.; Centurion, Bard, Covington, GA, U.S.A.; Extreme, Cordis, Miami, FL, U.S.A.) (Figs. 24.1C and 24.5C). Immediate postdilatation angiography, with the guidewire left in place through the dilated area, may show several possibilities:

1. No residual stenosis and no parietal damage: The procedure is complete.
2. Minor parietal damage: 3 to 5 minutes' low-pressure ballooning is performed to try to smooth the vessel wall (Fig 24.1D and 24.5E).

3. Rupture with clear extravasation of contrast medium and creation of a hematoma: The dilatation balloon must be rapidly reinflated to 2 atm for repeated periods of 10 minutes (Figs. 24.2C, 24.6B, and 24.7A).
4. Residual stenosis: If there is no parietal damage, a new dilatation is performed with a balloon that is 1 mm greater in diameter. Less than 30% residual stenosis is acceptable at this stage only if it results from the first dilatation ever performed for this stenosis. If there is greater than 30% residual stenosis, new dilatation should be performed with a larger balloon, but more than 2 mm overdilatation is not recommended at the time of the first intervention.

Stenosis recoil is possible, especially in large veins. Recoil means that the vessel wall collapses and the stenosis reforms as soon as the balloon is removed, despite the absence of waisting on the inflated dilatation balloon. Recoil is treated by stent placement.

In cases of early recurrence in a previously dilated stenosis (<4 months), it is necessary to be more demanding

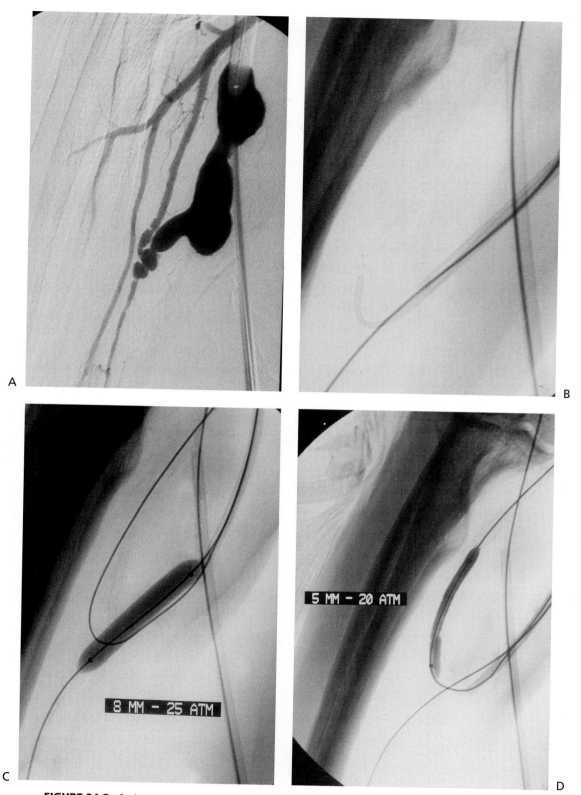

FIGURE 24.5. A: Aneurysmal sites under tension and low-flow rates were the reason for angiography of this 45-month-old radiocephalic fistula placed fairly high in the forearm of this diabetic patient. The arterial inflow was studied by reflux while the balloon was inflated on a tight elbow stenosis, showing evidence of significant stenoses both on the artery and on the postanastomotic vein. **B**: Local anatomy showed that it was possible to dilate the venous stenoses without placing the balloon across the anastomosis; however, retrograde selective catheterization of the feeding artery was performed first for placement of a safety guidewire. **C**: The stenoses of the anastomotic venous segment were dilated to 8 mm and very high pressure was required to overcome their resistance. **D**: The radial artery then was dilated to 5 mm, which was painful and limited to 20 atm.

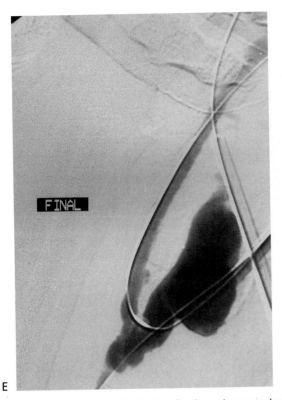

E

FIGURE 24.5. *(Continued.)* **E**: The final angiogram showed good result on the venous segment, with a small residual parietal damage on the artery.

with regard to the result. Absolutely no residual stenosis should be accepted: *Greater overdilatation* and eventual stent placement must be considered to achieve the perfect result.

Once the dilatation has been performed, the catheters and introducers are removed. The puncture site must be compressed as gently as possible to stop bleeding without stopping flow through the fistula. The outpatient then can

get up, and the vascular access is immediately usable for hemodialysis.

SPECIFIC CASES

Delayed maturation is always explained by an underlying stenosis, which is diagnosed in 100% of cases if the fistula is appropriately evaluated by puncture of the brachial artery. Our experience indicates that the best treatment is surgical or radiologic correction of the stenosis, not ligation or embolization of collaterals (Fig. 24.2) (11).

Tandem lesions are not rare. The most central stenosis must be treated first (Fig. 24.1 and 24.5). If the most peripheral stenosis were treated first and if the dilatation induced a transient rupture, secondary dilatation of the more central stenosis would create hyperpressure peripherally that would reopen the rupture on the site of the previously dilated stenosis.

Stenoses resistant to 25-bar pressures are infrequent. In our experience, they occur in 1% of forearm fistulae and 5% of upper-arm fistulae (final arch of the cephalic vein) (12). Atherectomy catheters and cutting balloons have been reported to be of some value in such cases, but they are expensive (14).

Stenoses of the feeding artery and of the arteriovenous anastomosis may be impossible to traverse using a regular retrograde fistula approach. Antegrade puncture of the brachial artery and catheterization of the feeding artery are feasible but carry a greater risk of local complications at the puncture site (Fig. 24.2). This is why, unlike Maninnen, we recommend avoiding this brachial artery route whenever possible (15,16).

Dilatation of anastomotic venous stenosis in the forearm can necessitate placing the dilatation balloon across the anastomosis. The balloon diameter must therefore be limited to 1 mm greater than the diameter of the artery, which means

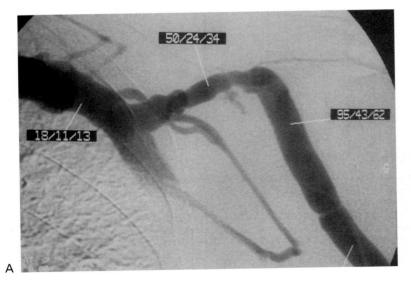

A

FIGURE 24.6. A: Tight stenosis on the final arch of this 16-month brachiocephalic fistula was confirmed by severe systolic pressure drop from 95 to 18 mm Hg (an 81% loss). **B**: Dilatation to 8 mm caused rupture, but the guidewire was left in place. **C**: The rupture was sealed by balloon tamponade, but there was a 75% residual drop in systolic pressure. **D**: Stent placement improved the result (47% final pressure drop), and the fistula remained patent for 13 months. The stent was placed correctly because it did not protrude into the subclavian vein.

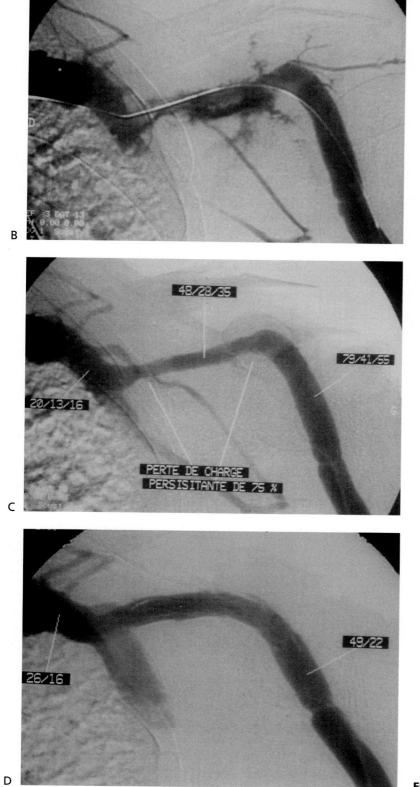

FIGURE 24.6. *(continued)*

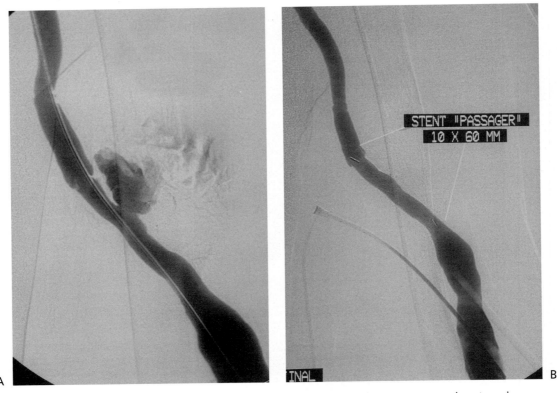

FIGURE 24.7. A: Dilatation of this transposed brachiobasilic fistula to 9 mm caused rupture despite deliberate slight underdilatation in this slightly aneurysmal fistula. The rupture was not controlled by 30 minutes' balloon tamponade. **B:** Placement of a covered stent sealed the rupture immediately. Covered stent was preferred because of presumed high flow in this fistula, but a bare stent might have worked.

that residual stenosis will be left on the vein. Because of the difference in compliance between arterial and venous walls, a vein must be larger than an artery to allow the same flow rate (for example, compare the diameter of the ascending aorta with the diameter of the two venae cavae on computed tomography scan). The diameter of the vein of a fistula should always be larger, therefore, than its proximal feeding artery and even more if the distal artery has retrograde filling and also contributes to feeding the fistula. This goal cannot be achieved when the dilatation balloon is placed across the anastomosis (Fig. 24.1). This is one of the arguments for surgical revision of such stenoses. The problem is rare with upper-arm fistulae because the most proximal feeding arteries have a greater diameter.

Upper-arm fistulae frequently tend to develop excessively high flow (Fig. 24.4), which should be suspected when the vein is aneurysmal (Fig. 24.7). Full dilatation of the stenosis to the diameter of the upstream abnormally large vein could induce rupture and secondary high flow. Deliberate residual stenosis must be accepted in such cases (e.g., after dilatation to 8 mm), although this means that redilatation will be necessary within a shorter interval. Flow measurement soon after dilatation will help to decide whether the same or a larger balloon will have to be used the next time.

Distal Ischemia

Dilatation has no place if the arteries are normal and if distal ischemia is due simply to the arterial steal of the fistula. In contrast, dilatation of an arterial stenosis before or after the arteriovenous anastomosis can significantly improve distal flow and cure the patient (17). (See also Chapter 31 for surgical management.)

COMPLICATIONS OF DILATATION

Rupture

Rupture can occur at very low pressure and is not systematically linked to the balloon bursting. The patient often reports a sudden acute pain at the dilated site as soon as the balloon is deflated (Figs. 24.2, 24.6, and 24.7). If rupture is confirmed, the balloon must be reinflated quickly to 2 atm and left in place for 10 minutes. If previously injected, heparin must be neutralized by injection of protamine (except in patients using insulin), and the hematoma can be compressed manually if clinically accessible. If extravasation continues despite three periods of 10-minute balloon tamponade, a stent must be placed (18,19). In our experience, rupture during dilatation occurred in 8% of Brescia–Cimino fistulae (Fig. 24.2) and 15% of upper-arm fistulae (Figs. 24.6 and 24.7) (12). Most were controlled by prolonged balloon inflation, however, and very few required a stent. The final arch of the cephalic vein (Fig. 24.6), the end of the transposition of brachiobasilic fistulae (Fig. 24.7), and the postanastomotic area of forearm fistulae (Fig. 24.2) are the most prone to rupture.

Pseudoaneurysms

Pseudoaneurysms can be the consequence of a dilatation-induced rupture that was initially controlled but reopened and was limited in its expansion. Such aneurysms can be treated by placement of a stent through the base except in cannulation areas where ultrasound-guided compression or surgery would be preferable.

Thrombosis

Thrombosis can occur during dilatation if the introducer is occlusive or if the balloon is left inflated too long in a patient not receiving anticoagulants. Dilatation of a juxta-anastomotic stenosis in forearm fistulae can cause transient occlusion of the feeding artery by a mechanism of extrinsic compression. When dilating such stenoses close to the anastomosis, a guidewire must be left through the anastomosis to allow rapid reopening of the artery if necessary (Fig. 24.5).

Bleeding

As after a dialysis session, the cannulation site can reopen subsequently, and control of such bleeding by manual compression is a part of the basic education of hemodialyzed patients. When a large introducer sheath has been used, U-shaped suturing can effectively prevent such secondary bleeding and pseudoaneurysms (20).

Infection

Infection is a potentially fatal complication that has been reported in all series because hemodialyzed patients have immunologic disorders. Systematic treatment with antistaphylococcal antibiotics is required when a difficult dilatation procedure has been prolonged, when several cannulations have been necessary, clots are present, the fistula was recently created, and above all in cases of breach in sterile technique.

CONTRAINDICATIONS FOR DILATATION
Absolute Contraindications

Local infection, which is much rarer than in grafts, contraindicates any endovascular procedure.

Concomitant steal syndrome is an absolute contraindication for the treatment of any stenosis located on the fistula itself because it would increase flow in the fistula and subsequent steal.

Relative Contraindications

Anastomotic stenoses in fistulae of less than 6 weeks must not be dilated because of the very high risk of rupture.

Isolated stenosis within 10 cm of the wrist in a Brescia–Cimino fistula can be dilated, but surgical creation of a new anastomosis above the stenosis is simple, minimally invasive, and usually more durable. Dilatation, however, remains the best treatment when the radial artery is occluded above the anastomosis; the fistula is being fed by the ulnar artery via the palmar arch and retrograde flow from the distal radial artery.

Long (>5 cm) stenoses and chronic occlusions can be successfully dilated in the forearm (Fig. 24.2), but stents are frequently needed in cases of recanalization at the elbow and in the final arch of the cephalic vein, allowing discussion for surgical revision.

High flow is mainly a complication of upper arm fistulae and is a relative contraindication for dilatation because treatment of the stenosis would increase the already high flow (Fig. 24.4). High flow is an underestimated problem on a world scale. In patients with normal cardiac status, there is no consensus among physicians about the upper limit of normal flow in a vascular access (somewhere between 1 and 2 L per minute).

STENTS

Indications for stent placement are *extremely unusual in forearm fistulae*, where rupture is the only valuable indication. Indications are much more frequent in the upper arm and in central veins.

Choice of the Stent

The anatomic and mechanical constraints of hemodialysis fistulae mean that flexible self-expandable stents (Wallstent type) are preferable to balloon expandable and rigid stents. Stent diameter must be 1 to 2 mm greater than the diameter of the vessel in order to cling to the intima.

When a stent has to be placed in a cannulation area, which is a rare indication, a wide mesh puncturable stent such as the Symphony* (Medi-tech) or the ZA (Cook), must be used. The disappointing results to date for covered stents lead to recommending them only for rupture control or elimination of aneurysms.

Think of the Future

Stents must not obviate further surgery and must protect the ease of making new anastomoses. For example, stent placement is contraindicated at the elbow if the stent would overlap the basilic vein and obviate future creation of a transposed brachiobasilic fistula. Also, a stent placed in the final arch of the cephalic vein must not protrude into the subclavian vein, where it could lead to stenosis (Fig. 24.6D), which would preclude future use of the basilic and axillary veins for a direct fistula or for drainage of an upper arm graft (21).

Indications

Rupture

Acute rupture is an emergency for which a stent can save the fistula. A *rupture* is a clear extravasation pushed by flow into a rapidly growing hematoma. Stent placement is necessary if the leakage persists despite three periods of 10-minute balloon tamponade. Covered stents are effective in 100% of cases (Fig. 24.7), but bare Wallstents frequently work (18, 19). Stent placement also could prevent the development of a secondary pseudoaneurysm.

Aneurysms

Aneurysms can be eliminated by placement of a (preferably covered) stent through the neck or base. The indication is valuable for aneurysms located in noncannulation areas, where surgery may be difficult. Surgery is preferable in cannulation areas.

Soft Post-Percutaneous Angiography Recoil

Recoil needs a stent when the residual stenosis is greater than 30%. It is important to have dilated enough before placing the stent, that is, for at least 5 minutes, with a slightly oversized balloon. Significant recoil is extremely unusual in forearm veins.

There are stenoses whose waisting on the dilatation balloon is not abolished despite the highest pressure applicable with the strongest balloons (25 atm). Stents are not logical in these cases, which are indications for more mechanically aggressive tools, that is, an atherectomy device, cutting balloon, or surgery.

Early Recurring Stenoses (Less than 4 Months)

There is no consensus regarding the indications for and value of stents to delay restenosis. Some multidisciplinary teams accept redilating stenoses every 4 months or sooner if necessary. We do not if there is a simple surgical alternative, but we try a stent first. In our experience (12), stents doubled the intervals between reinterventions after appropriate

placement in early recurring stenoses. Stents are valuable, however, only if no residual stenosis has been accepted after placement. This means that the stenosis has previously been sufficiently dilated and that absolutely no residual waist has been accepted on the inflated balloon.

Follow-Up

There is no need for anticoagulants or antiplatelet drugs before, during, or after stenting of a fistula. There is a high risk of restenosis, although delayed, either in stent or at its extremities.

RESULTS

There are only two studies in the international literature about dilatation of native fistulae with a sufficiently high number of patients to reach some statistical significance (12,15). *Primary patency rates after dilatation* of forearm native fistulae are very close in both studies, with 44% and 51% at 1 year. We have emphasized in our study that forearm fistulae fare significantly better than grafts because, in our experience, they have provided a 51% rate versus 29% for grafts at 1 year and 37% versus 13% at 2 years. On the other hand, upper-arm fistulae have provided intermediate results, with 35% at 1 year and 24% at 2 years (12). Compared with the forearm, these poorer results in upper-arm fistulae are due to difficulties in the management of stenoses of the final arch of the cephalic vein (rupture or resistance to dilatation, early recurrence). In all groups, significant morbidity was low (2%–4%), and the mortality of 2% was not attributable to the radiological procedures.

Primary patency rates after stent placement in our experience were 36% and 20% at 1 year in the forearm and in the upper-arm, respectively, which is low. The beneficial effect of stents is clearer when intervals between maintenance reinterventions are compared before and after stent placement. In our study, the mean interval approximately doubled from 4.1 to 9.7 months in forearm fistulae and from 2.26 to 4.22 months in the upper arm ($p < 0.05$ in both groups) (12). Manninen and colleagues reported similar findings, with a mean interval increasing from 3.4 to 6.3 months after stent placement in the forearm (15).

Secondary patency rates after dilatation and stent placement were exactly the same for forearm fisulae, that is, 85% for forearm fistulae at 1 year in the study by Manninen and colleagues and in our study. It was necessary in our experience to reintervene only every 18 months after the initial dilatation to achieve 85% at 1 year and 77% at 4 years. During the same period, the rates for grafts were 92% at 1 year and 60% at 4 years, with reinterventions every 10 months.

Rates for upper-arm fistulae were 82% at 1 year and 51% at 4 years, with reinterventions every 11 months. Upper-arm fistulae require significantly more frequent reinterventions than forearm fistulae and do not fare better than grafts after dilatation.

Finally, we recently confirmed the influence of the age of the fistula at the time of the first dilatation on its outcome after dilatation. The interval between maintenance reinterventions is significantly shorter in forearm fistulae of less than 1 year compared with those of more than 1 year (16 versus 30 months in our experience). Younger accesses recur faster than older accesses.

CONCLUSION

Treatment of native fistula dysfunction by interventional techniques achieves excellent long-term secondary patency rates, which does not mean that all stenoses are good indications for dilatation, although reports of surgical results starting from fistula revision are extremely rare in the literature. Multidisciplinary cooperation with nephrologists and surgeons is essential to determine the best therapeutic option according to stenosis location, patient history, and life expectancy. It could be said in 2001 that there is an unacceptable loss of opportunity for patients who are dialyzed in centers not working in close cooperation with an interventionist.

REFERENCES

1. Mehta S. Statistical summary of clinical results of vascular access procedures for hemodialysis. In: Sommer HM, ed. *Vascular access for hemodialysis*, part II. Precept Press, Chicago: Precept Press, 1991:145–155.
2. Schwab S, Besarab A, Beathard G, et al. NKG-DOQI clinical practice guidelines for vascular access. *Am J Kidney Dis* 1997;30 (Suppl 4).
3. Rodriguez J, Armadans L, Ferrer E, et al. The function of permanent vascular access. *Nephrol Dial Transplant* 2000;15:402–408.
4. Konner K. Primary vascular access in diabetic patients: an audit. *Nephrol Dial Transplant* 2000;15:1317–1325.
5. Sands J, Jabyac P, Miranda C, et al. Intervention based on monthly monitoring decreases hemodialysis access thrombosis. *ASAIO J* 1999;45:147–150.
6. Schwab S, Oliver M, Suhocki P, et al. Hemodialysis arteriovenous access: detection of stenosis and response to treatment by vascular access blood flow. *Kidney Int* 2001;5:358–362.
7. Strauch B, O'Connell R, Geoly K, et al. Forecasting thrombosis of vascular access with Doppler color flow imaging. *Am J Kidney Dis* 1992;19:554–557.
8. Sands J, Young S, Miranda C. The effect of Doppler flow screening studies and elective revisions in dialysis access failures. *ASAIO J* 1992;38:M524–M527.
9. Spinosa D, Angle F, Hagspiel K, et al. CO_2 and gadopentetate dimeglumine as alternative contrast agents for malfunctioning dialysis grafts and fistulas. *Kidney Int* 1998;54:945–950.
10. Ehrman K, Taber T, Gaylord G, et al. Comparison of diagnostic accuracy with carbon dioxide versus iodinated contrast material in the imaging of hemodialysis access fistulas. *J Vasc Interv Radiol* 1994;5:771–775.
11. Turmel-Rodrigues, Mouton A, Birmelé B, et al. Salvage of immature forearm fistulas for hemodialysis by interventional radiology. *Nephrol Dial Transplant* 2001;16:2365–2371.
12. Turmel-Rodrigues L, Pengloan J, Baudin S, et al. Treatment of stenosis and thrombosis in haemodialysis fistulas and grafts by interventional radiology. *Nephrol Dial Transplant* 2000;15:2029–2036.
13. Turmel-Rodrigues L, Pengloan J, Blanchier D, et al. Insufficient dialysis shunts: improved long-term patency rates with close hemodynamic monitoring, repeated percutaneous balloon angioplasty, and stent placement. *Radiology* 1993;187:273–278.
14. Vorwerk D, Adam G, Mueller-Leisse C, et al. Hemodialysis fistulas and grafts: use of cutting balloons to dilate venous stenoses. *Radiology* 1996;201:864–867.
15. Manninen HI, Kaukanen ET, Ikaheimo R, et al. Endovascular treatment of failing Brescia-Cimino hemodialysis fistulae by brachial artery access: initial success and long-term results. *Radiology* 2001;218:711–718.
16. Trerotola S, Turmel-Rodrigues L. Off the beaten path: transbrachial approach for native fistula interventions. *Radiology* 2001;218:617–619.
17. Valji K, Hye R, Roberts A, Oglevie S, Ziegler T, Bookstein J. Hand ischemia in patients with hemodialysis access grafts: angiographic diagnosis and treatment. *Radiology* 1995;196:697–701.
18. Sapoval M, Turmel-Rodrigues L, Raynaud A, et al. Cragg covered stents in hemodialysis access: initial and mid-term results. *J Vasc Interv Radiol* 1996;7:335–342.
19. Raynaud A, Angel C, Sapoval M, et al. Treatment of hemodialysis access rupture during PTA with Wallstent implantation. *J Vasc Interv Radiol* 1998;9:437–442.
20. Vorwerk D, Konner K, Schuermann K, et al. A simple trick to facilitate bleeding control after percutaneous hemodialysis fistula and graft interventions. *Cardiovasc Intervent Radiol* 1997;20:159–160.
21. Turmel-Rodrigues L, Bourquelot P, Raynaud A, et al. Primary stent placement in hemodialysis-related central venous stenoses: the dangers of a potential "radiologic dictatorship." *Radiology* 2000;217:600–602.

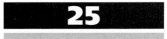

CENTRAL VEIN LESIONS: PREVENTION AND MANAGEMENT

RICHARD J. GRAY

Until the mid-1980s, there was little recognition in the medical literature that central venous lines have detrimental effects on the central veins. Over the past 15 years, however, there has been increasing recognition that central lines, especially those placed through the subclavian vein, predispose dialysis patients to central venous stenoses and occlusions. In 1997, the initial Dialysis Outcomes Quality Initiative (DOQI) (1) mandated that upper-extremity central line utilization should be minimized and that the internal jugular vein should be the vein of first choice for patients who need a tunneled central line. The guidelines further stipulated that all subclavian vein punctures should be reserved for patients with no possibility for an ipsilateral permanent upper-extremity access. Herein the incidence, etiologic factors, significance, prevention, diagnosis, treatment options, and outcomes associated with central vein lesions are presented.

INCIDENCE

The exact incidence of central venous lesions in the dialysis population is unknown but can be estimated from the existing literature. In 1992, Beathard (2) published a large angioplasty series during which 5% of the 285 patients in the referral base developed a clinically significant central venous lesion over the 5-year period that the study was conducted. In a smaller study, Schwab and colleagues (3) described a central vein lesion incidence of 11% over 3 years in a population of 110 dialysis patients. Schumacher and colleagues reported an incidence of 14% in their hemodialysis population (4). Haage and associates, in a central venous stent study, reported a 17% incidence of clinically significant central vein lesions over 10 years in the patients referred for endovascular treatment (5). Thus, these studies suggest an incidence of 5% to 17%.

Central vein lesions are actually much more common if asymptomatic lesions are included; one merely has to look for them. Venograms performed in predominantly asymptomatic dialysis patients have revealed significant stenoses

($\geq$50%) in 42% to 50% of patients with prior subclavian catheters (6–9) and in up to 10% of patients with prior internal jugular catheters (8,9). Central lesions are rare in the absence of a previous indwelling central catheter (6). Venographic studies also have suggested that multiple central vein catheterizations (8,10), longer catheter in-dwell times (7,10,), and even a longer-functioning autologous or synthetic arteriovenous (AV) access (3,11) in the ipsilateral upper extremity after a central line are all associated with a higher incidence of central venous lesions. Because virtually all dialysis patients will require catheter access at some time, it follows that every dialysis patient who lives long enough eventually will develop a central lesion. Obviously, indiscriminant central line use will hasten their occurrence.

PATHOPHYSIOLOGY

The histologic composition of central lesions has been investigated in a few studies. A human autopsy study showed that a fibrin coating (fibrin sheath) will begin to form around a subclavian line within 24 hours after insertion and typically starts at the catheter's venous puncture site (12) as well as the tip where it contacts the vein wall. Histologic examination of fibrin sheaths associated with central catheters in rats has revealed a gradual transformation from fibrin to fibrous tissue (13). Atherectomy specimens removed from stenosed and occluded subclavian veins of symptomatic dialysis patients have confirmed the presence of fibrous tissue as well as intimal hyperplasia (14). The trauma of passing a large dialysis catheter through the vein wall thus appears to be an important initiating stimulus for fibrin sheath and subsequent fibrosis in the subclavian vein, the most common site for a central vein stenosis (Fig. 25.1). Respirations, cardiac motion, and even positional changes (15,16) move the indwelling catheter within the vein, probably damaging the wall as well. Subsequent creation of an ipsilateral AV access with the associated high flows, turbulence (17), and perivascular vibrations (18) stimulate intimal hyperplasia, which can accumulate anywhere along the intra-

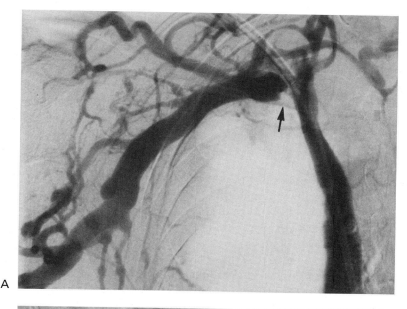

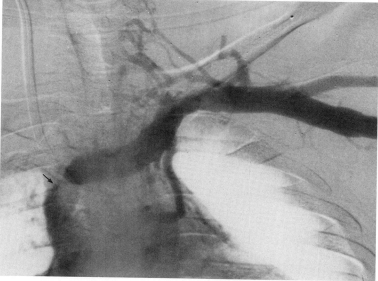

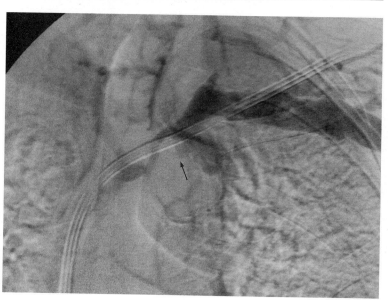

FIGURE 25.1. A: Subclavian stenosis (*arrow*) at catheter entrance site into the subclavian vein. **B**: Left innominate stenosis (*arrow*) at tip of contralateral dialysis catheter. **C**: Left innominate occlusion (*arrow*) around midpoint of dialysis catheter. (A and B are reprinted from Gray RJ. Central venous stenosis in hemodialysis patients. In: *SCVIR syllabus: venous interventions*. Fairfax, VA: Society of Cardiovascular and Interventional Radiology, 1995: 123–135, with permission; A is also reprinted from Gray RJ. The role of stent deployment for central and peripheral venous stenosis in hemodialysis access. *Seminars in Dialysis* 1998;11:365–373, with permission.)

venous course of the catheter (Fig. 25.1), even after the central line is removed. This sequence of events ultimately results in stenoses of the subclavian vein, innominate vein, or superior vena cava; it is also consistent with the observations of the aforementioned venographic studies.

CLINICAL SIGNIFICANCE

Clinical recognition of symptomatic central lesions associated with a functioning ipsilateral permanent dialysis access was first reported in the late 1970s and early 1980s (19–22). Development of an intrathoracic stenosis or occlusion in the final common pathway for venous drainage from the extremity is disastrous for patients with need for an ipsilateral upper-extremity dialysis access. High venous pressures will be transmitted to the entire extremity, including the dialysis access (3); cosmetically displeasing superficial venous dilatation of the chest wall and extremity can occur (Fig. 25.2). More importantly, painful edema often results, rendering the entire extremity useless for a permanent life-sustaining dialysis access (Fig. 25.2). Even if the swelling is minimal or not painful, any permanent access in that extremity can be predisposed to thrombosis because of elevated venous pressures (3,23) and decreased flows (24). Worse yet, depending on the lesion's severity, location and collateral development, placement of a central dialysis catheter may not even be possible.

PREVENTION

It is obvious that the key to prevention of central venous lesions lies in minimizing the necessity for central line placements, especially through the subclavian vein. This fact was emphasized in the DOQI guidelines in several ways: early creation of autologous AV fistulae or grafts for patients in whom the need for dialysis is anticipated (25); prophylactic angioplasty or surgery for failing autologous AV fistulas and grafts (26); and prompt surgical or endovascular treatment of thrombosed AV fistulas and grafts (27). If a central line is unavoidable, the internal or external jugular veins should be used first (28); the subclavian should be used only after all

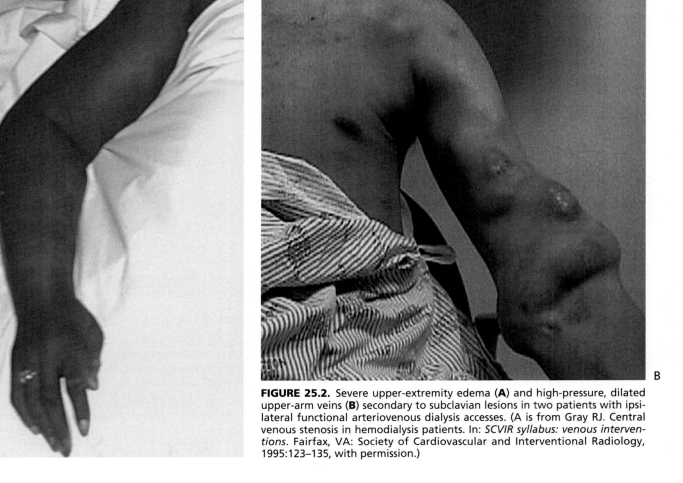

A   B

FIGURE 25.2. Severe upper-extremity edema (**A**) and high-pressure, dilated upper-arm veins (**B**) secondary to subclavian lesions in two patients with ipsilateral functional arteriovenous dialysis accesses. (A is from Gray RJ. Central venous stenosis in hemodialysis patients. In: *SCVIR syllabus: venous interventions*. Fairfax, VA: Society of Cardiovascular and Interventional Radiology, 1995:123–135, with permission.)

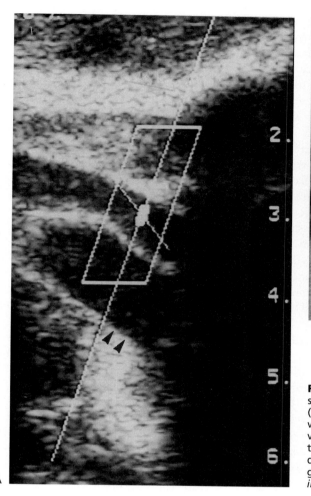

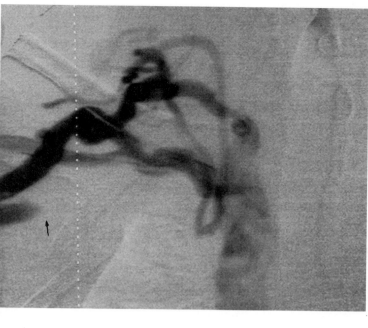

FIGURE 25.3. A: Duplex ultrasound interpreted as venous flow through a small subclavian vein (Doppler cursor) adjacent to a larger subclavian artery (*arrowheads*). **B**: Angiogram shows complete subclavian occlusion (*arrow*) with large collaterals, one of which had been mistaken for the subclavian vein in A. (B is from Gray RJ. Central venous stenosis in hemodialysis patients. In: *SCVIR syllabus: venous interventions*. Fairfax, VA: Society of Cardiovascular and Interventional Radiology, 1995:123–135, and Gray RJ. Angioplasty and stents for peripheral and central venous lesions. *Techniques in Vascular and Interventional Radiology* 1999;2:189–198, with permission.)

permanent access sites in the ipsilateral extremity are depleted (29). Although the DOQI guidelines (27) allow a single common femoral line to be inserted until patency can be restored to a clotted access, the DOQI vascular access work group believed that these too should be minimized by prompt endovascular or surgical treatment of the access.

DIAGNOSIS

Central venous stenoses and occlusions are best diagnosed by venography. Therefore, the DOQI guidelines (30) mandate venography prior to permanent access creation for all patients who have ever had a previous subclavian line. Color-flow duplex ultrasound can be insensitive to complete obstructions because well-developed collaterals can be mistaken for the obstructed vein (31,32) (Fig. 25.3). A fistulogram or venogram is therefore necessary prior to correction, and appropriate therapeutic measures can be taken at the time of the study. For these reasons, in patients with ipsilateral upper extremity edema and a functional ipsilateral permanent access, the diagnostic modality of choice is a venogram or fistulogram (31,32).

TREATMENT

A variety of treatments have been used for these lesions (Table 25.1). As one would suspect from the existence of multiple treatments, most do not work well, have an unacceptable complication rate, or are simply not desirable. Conservative measures such as elevation (33) and anticoagulation (34) may resolve the acute symptoms; however, intra-access pressures usually remain elevated (3), predisposing the access to thrombosis. Ligating (20,33) or percutaneously occluding (34) the ipsilateral access will resolve the ipsilateral extremity swelling and pain; unfortunately, the extremity then is aban-

TABLE 25.1. CENTRAL VEIN LESION TREATMENT METHODS

Conservative
Access ligation/percutaneous occlusion
Surgical veno–veno bypass
Thrombolysis
Angioplasty
Stent deployment
Covered stents
Brachytherapy

doned for dialysis access. Surgical venovenous bypasses have been reported (35–38) in small series and still are practiced by some; nevertheless, short-lived results and the often-disfiguring nature of the surgery have precluded widespread adoption of these procedures. Directional atherectomy with supplemental balloon angioplasty was reported with promising preliminary results (14); however, the spinning cable within the device occasionally traps the vein wall and results in rupture. Use of directional atherectomy is thus contraindicated in central vein locations, which cannot be easily compressed to control bleeding. This device is currently not available. Thrombolysis has been reported sporadically (39,40) and works well for acute thrombosis; however, most central vein occlusions are chronic, probably because thrombus formation is inhibited by high central venous flows and the heparin administered for every dialysis. The only treatments considered acceptable by the DOQI guidelines (41) for chronic central vein stenoses and occlusions are angioplasty with or without stent deployment, discussed later herein.

The results of the available balloon angioplasty series (2,3,38,39,42–44) that have focused on the central veins are presented in Table 25.2. The initial success rates are reasonably good, and even serious complications like rupture are rare and easily treated (45,46); however, the trend toward poor outcomes within a few months is clear. The two small studies with promising results (3,39) were followed later by a much larger report of dismal patencies (44), all from the same institution. These angioplasty studies were published before the widespread adoption of modern reporting practices. Nevertheless, the results in Table 25.2 are generally poor relative to the 38% to 63% 6-month cumulative primary patency expected after screening/angioplasty of pe-

ripheral venous stenoses (2,11,47,48). In one study that reported cumulative patencies following angioplasty of both central and peripheral vein lesions, the 6-month primary patency for subclavian and innominate lesions (28.9%) was statistically significantly lower than the 6-month primary patency for lesions at all other locations (62%) (2). In the same study, the immediate procedure success for central venous lesions (89%) was also significantly lower than for other lesions (97%). Thus, the results of angioplasty for central vein lesions are poor relative to those expected after angioplasty of peripheral venous stenoses (2,11,47,48). Furthermore, when a chronic central vein stenosis progresses to an occlusion, the lesion is even more difficult to treat; only one small study has reported an initially successful angioplasty (39) in this scenario. Despite the generally poor results of balloon angioplasty, the DOQI guidelines (41) recommend angioplasty as the preferred treatment for physiologically significant central vein *stenoses*, a term that the DOQI work group presumably intended to apply also to occlusions. Like lesions at other locations, posttreatment surveillance and repetitive angioplasty are indicated unless more than two such treatments are necessary within 3 months.

For lesions that respond poorly to balloon angioplasty, stent deployment is a logical treatment alternative, especially for lesions that fail immediately due to elastic recoil of the vein wall (Fig. 25.4). Retention of elasticity, with slow resumption of the preangioplasty configuration in the diseased central vein segment after the balloon is removed, occurs commonly after angioplasty (Fig. 25.5); 64% of the central lesions in an endoluminal ultrasound study demonstrated significant elastic recoil (49). Stents, by their ability to maintain luminal patency, can prevent immediate elastic

TABLE 25.2. CENTRAL VEIN[a] ANGIOPLASTY

Investigator	No. of Patients	Success	Patency
Glanz et al. (42)	13	76%	38% @ 6 mo[b]
Schwab et al. (3)	11	100%	82% @ 12 mo mean
Newman et al. (39)[c]	14[d]	86%	86% @ 6 mo mean
Beathard (2)	27	89%	28.9% @ 6 mo[e]
Wisselink et al. (38)	13	77%[f]	
Lund et al. (43)	18	85%	26% @ 7 mo mean[g]
Kovalik et al. (44)	30	70%	13% @ 2.9 to 7.6 mo mean

[a] Subclavian and innominate veins.
[b] Initial failures added for retabulation of published data.
[c] All occlusions; three also infused with thrombolytic infusion.
[d] Includes one axillary vein.
[e] Primary patency.
[f] Reported patency included three stents and two non–end-stage renal disease patients.
[g] Patency based on 27 procedures.
Note: Case reports and series composing fewer than ten patients not included.

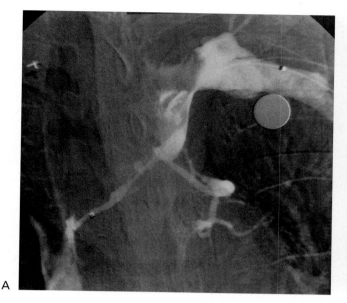

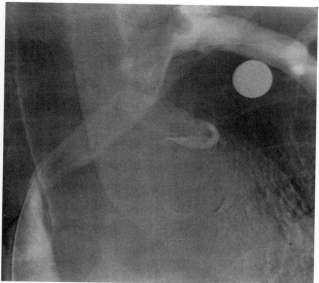

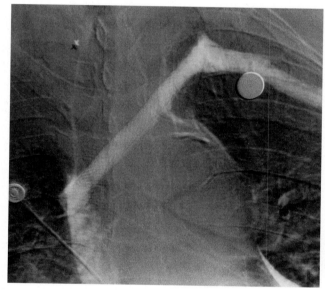

FIGURE 25.4. A: Innominate vein occlusion after recanalization and attempted angioplasty. **B**: Minimally changed after thrombolytic infusion. **C**: Widely patent after Wallstent deployment.

recoil. Table 25.3 presents the studies for stent deployment as the first-line *de novo* treatment for central vein lesions (36,37,50–53); these studies are generally small and several used a combination of stent types. Nevertheless, the initial success rates were high, and the patencies in two of the studies (50,51) suggested that stents might provide better results than angioplasty (compare with Table 25.2). These promising early results led several investigators to study stent deployment for lesions that had failed balloon angioplasty. After early disastrous experiences with Palmaz stents (J&J) in which the stent migrated (54) or was compressed between the clavicle and first rib (55), interest in a self-expandable stent, such as the Wallstent (BSCI), grew. The Wallstent is flexible enough to allow delivery to an intrathoracic posi-

tion, and the sharp flared ends with the ability to reexpand when compressed provide positional stability.

Four peer-reviewed studies of at least 20 patients have examined the outcomes of Wallstent deployment for immediate balloon angioplasty failures or early recurrences (5,40,56,57). [Although Haage and colleagues reported "primary Wallstent placement," most of their cases were actually immediate angioplasty failures because "stent placement was always performed after conventional balloon dilatation, after which most of the obstructed vessels showed considerable residual stenosis. . . ."] As shown in Table 25.4, two of the studies reported the results for central venous lesions exclusively (5,57), whereas the other two reported either a majority (40) or a significant minority (56) of central

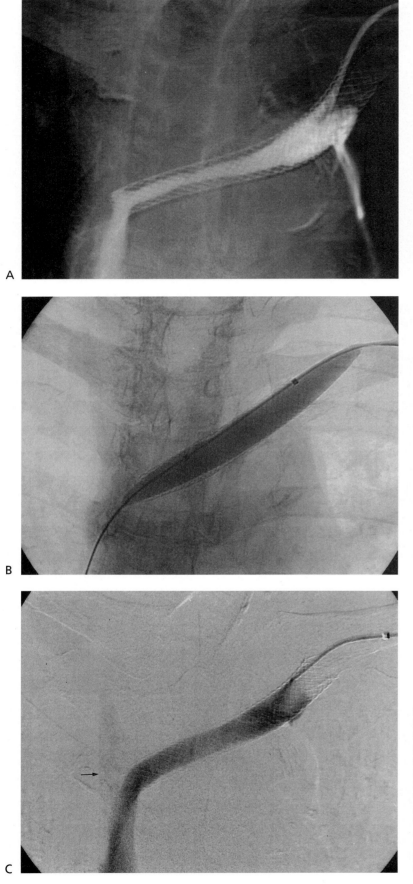

A

B

C

FIGURE 25.5. A: Innominate vein in-stent restenosis. **B**: Fully inflated angioplasty balloon within stent. Note that the balloon does not touch the entire stent. **C**: Postangioplasty contrast lumen also does not touch the entire stent because of residual in-stent intimal hyperplasia. Note that the contralateral innominate origin (*arrow*) is not compromised by the stent. (A is from Gray RJ. Central venous stenosis in hemodialysis patients. In: *SCVIR syllabus: venous interventions*. Fairfax, VA: Society of Cardiovascular and Interventional Radiology, 1995:123–135; A–C are from Gray RJ. The role of stent deployment for central and peripheral venous stenosis in hemodialysis access. *Seminars in Dialysis* 1998;11:365–373, with permission.)

TABLE 25.3. CENTRAL VEIN PRIMARY STENT TREATMENT

Investigator (Ref. No.)	No. of Patients	Stent Type	Success (%)	Primary Patency	
				3 Mo (%)	6 Mo (%)
Quinn et al. (50)	20 (10CV)	Z	90	79	65
Schoenfeld et al. (51)	19	W, P	100	90	68
Criado et al. (36)	17	W, P	76		
Quinn et al. (52)	8	Z, W	100	35	11
Bhatia et al. (37)	13	[a]	100		
Mickley et al. (53)[b]	14	W	100		

Z, Gianturco zigzag; W, Wallstent; P, Palmaz.
[a] Stents described as "rigid" (n = 6) or "flexible" (n = 7). Some patients also received a thrombolytic infusion.
[b] Reported only cumulative stent patency for 20 stents, including those placed at follow-up for recurrence.

vein lesions. Because there is no other widely used or effective treatment alternative for a central lesion that fails angioplasty, these four studies are by necessity "feasibility" in nature. Overall, 68% (129 of 191) of the lesions in these studies were centrally located, and 29% were chronic occlusions. It should be noted that Gray and colleagues (40) and Vorwerk and associates (56) could not determine any significant difference between their peripheral and central venous results. The immediate salvage rates were all high, ranging between 96% and 100%, and stent-related complications were rare. The primary patency (durability of treatment with no further intervention) at 6 months ranged broadly, from 42% to 84%, but by 12 months was less than 31% in all studies. This broad range of patencies is due to several factors: 51% of the patients in the study by Vorwerk and colleagues (56) and 70% of the patients in the study by Haage's group (5) had autologous AV fistulae in the involved extremities. This probably contributed to the better results in those studies than the others who had exclusively PTFE grafts. In addition, Haage and colleagues (5) reported "stent patency," which one would expect to be better than

the patency of the entire access circuit that was reported by the other researchers. The most common reason for recurrence was proliferation of intimal hyperplasia in or adjacent to the stent (Fig. 25.5) (5,40,56), presumably stimulated by persistent high flows, turbulence, and perivascular vibration (17). Repeat balloon angioplasty of the stents and treatment of new lesions at other locations resulted in 6-month assisted primary patencies between 62% and 76% and 6-month dialysis access patencies between 64% and 88%. When one considers that these studies were all for suboptimal lesions that otherwise would have failed endoluminal treatment, the results are remarkably good. Nevertheless, with each successive dilatation, the in-stent restenosis becomes progressively more difficult to dilate and eventually becomes untreatable (Fig. 25.5).

Recently, a series of iliac stenoses treated by Wallstent deployment after failed angioplasty reported outcomes similar to those for the upper extremities (58). Although deployment of a Wallstent will double the cost of the procedure relative to balloon angioplasty (59), the lack of another viable treatment alternative justifies the additional expense.

TABLE 25.4. WALLSTENTS FOR ANGIOPLASTY FAILURES

Investigator (Ref. No.)	# (CV)[a]	Success (%)	Primary Patency		Assisted Primary Patency		Access Patency 6 Mo (%)
			6 Mo (%)	12 Mo (%)	6 Mo (%)	12 Mo (%)	
Vorwerk et al. (56)	65 (27)[b]	100	56	31	—	—	88
Gray et al. (40)	56 (32)[c]	96	46	20	76	33	—
Vesely et al. (57)	20 (20)[c]	100	42	25	62	47	64
Haage et al. (5)	50 (50)	98	84[d]	54[d]	—	—	—

CV, Central veins (subclavian, innominate).
[a] 29% (37 of 129) CV were occluded.
[b] 33 PTFE grafts, 32 endogenous fistulae.
[c] All polytetrafluoroethylene (PTFE) grafts. Three iliac lesions.
[d] Primary "stent" patency. All other patencies in table are for the entire circuit.
Note: Case reports and series with fewer than 20 patients not included.

Wallstent deployment is an invaluable treatment for an otherwise untreatable situation; it provides reasonable additional time for successful dialysis when a central venous lesion fails balloon angioplasty. The DOQI guidelines (41) mandated central vein stent deployment as the indicated treatment after a balloon angioplasty failure because of elastic recoil or for an early recurrence (within 3 months) after an initially successful angioplasty. U.S. Food and Drug Administration approval of the Wallstent for use in the subclavian vein, innominate vein, and the superior vena cava was recently granted. New stent designs, some approved for biliary strictures, are now available but should be studied in humans only after positional stability can be demonstrated in an animal model.

TECHNICAL CONSIDERATIONS

The performance of central venous angioplasty is a natural extension of peripheral venous angioplasty and, as such, often is performed in conjunction with treatment of a more peripherally located venous outflow stenosis. Therefore, the percutaneous puncture site is most commonly directly into the dialysis graft or autologous fistula of the ipsilateral extremity. This is convenient because high-grade central venous lesions, especially occlusions, can be difficult to cross from a femoral approach (Fig. 25.6) because of the multiple collaterals that typically drain immediately central to the lesion. The choice of guidewire and catheter combination for crossing lesions is a function of operator preference; we prefer a hydrophilic guidewire, particularly for crossing occlusions. Occlusions usually can be crossed if there is a nubbin

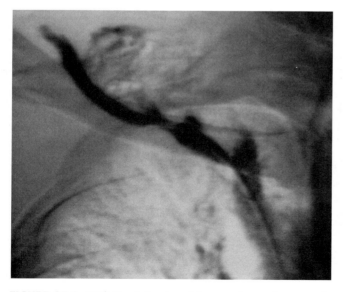

FIGURE 25.6. Catheter introduced from a femoral approach preferentially entering collateral rather than crossing the subclavian vein occlusion. (From Gray RJ. Angioplasty and stents for peripheral and central venous lesions. *Techniques in Vascular and Interventional Radiology* 1999;2:189–198, with permission.)

beyond the nearest adjacent collateral (Fig. 25.7). The exact length of an occlusion may become apparent only after the lesion is crossed because of the collaterals that maintain patency of the innominate vein (Fig. 25.8).

As for dialysis access related stenoses elsewhere, appropriate balloon diameter is typically that of the adjacent vein 1 to 2 mm larger. When in doubt, the degree of patient discomfort during balloon inflation can be used to gauge the largest size balloon that can be safely inflated. Prolonged inflations of at least 1 to 2 minutes are most commonly performed, although some operators prefer a 5-minute inflation. High-pressure balloons capable of 20 to 30 atm are also desirable and are available in balloons up to 12 mm. The subclavian and innominate veins often require a 14- or 16-mm-diameter balloon and occasionally even larger; these large balloons are rated only to 8 atm but usually can be safely inflated up to 50% higher than the rated burst pressure (i.e., an 8-atm balloon can be inflated to 12 atm). Large-diameter balloons (and stents) may require an 8 or 9 Fr sheath, which in our hands have been safe (14). Because of the sometimes-poor deflation profile of large-diameter balloons, these balloons are occasionally difficult to withdraw after dilatation. Long sheaths can minimize trauma and the resulting spasm in the intervening vein between the percutaneous puncture site and the lesion. It is also useful to be familiar with the direction in which the balloons are wrapped around the catheters during packaging; after balloon deflation, rotation of the catheter in the appropriate direction before and during withdrawal can ease the removal.

Stent deployment is performed using standard technique as elsewhere in the biliary or arterial system. We usually dilate lesions, including early recurrences, before stent deployment, to ensure that the lesion is expandable. We also dilate the stent after deployment to ensure maximal stent expansion and contact with the vein wall. The stent length should match the lesion length as closely as possible. When the Wallstent is longer than the lesion, most of the extra length of the stent should extend peripheral to the lesion for improved positional stability; this is facilitated by an ipsilateral upper-extremity approach, which allows repositioning of a partially deployed Wallstent by simple withdrawal. Leaving the excess stent in the larger vein central to the stenosis predisposes the stent to minor central slippage (10% in reported Wallstent series); this results in uncovering of the lesion (Fig. 25.9) and even could allow migration to the heart or pulmonary artery. We routinely pass a guidewire into the inferior vena cava before stent deployment to guarantee at least partial control of the stent in the unlikely event of an immediate migration. Also, we never deploy a stent from a femoral approach; withdrawal of the covering sheath or the postdeployment dilatation balloon may pull the stent centrally, with potentially disastrous consequences (Fig. 25.10). It should be noted that although future central line insertions are not precluded by a properly positioned indwelling stent (Fig. 25.11), fluoroscopic guidance might be necessary

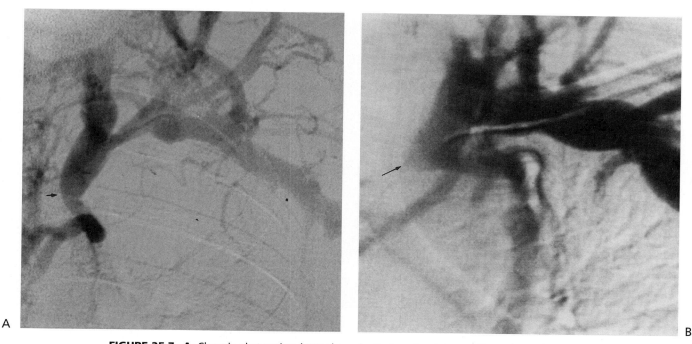

A

B

FIGURE 25.7. **A**: Chronic obstruction (*arrow*) gradually tapering into a collateral may be impassible with a guidewire. **B**: Nubbin (*arrow*) beyond the nearest adjacent collateral shows morphology that usually can be crossed with a catheter/guidewire and suggests that the lesion is likely to be treatable. Favorable morphology also is seen in Figures 25.3B and 25.8A. (A is from Gray RJ. Central venous stenosis in hemodialysis patients. In: *SCVIR syllabus: venous interventions.* Fairfax, VA: Society of Cardiovascular and Interventional Radiology, 1995:123–135.)

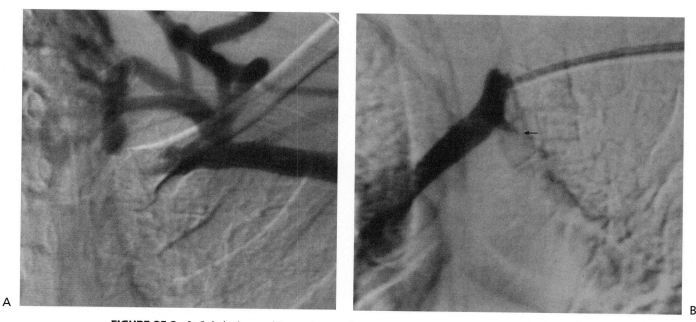

A

B

FIGURE 25.8. **A**: Subclavian and innominate veins appear completely occluded. **B**: After subclavian is crossed with a catheter, the innominate is seen to be widely patent, kept open by inflow through a mediastinal collateral (*arrow*). (A is from Gray RJ. Central venous stenosis in hemodialysis patients. In: *SCVIR syllabus: venous interventions.* Fairfax, VA: Society of Cardiovascular and Interventional Radiology, 1995:123–135, with permission; B is from Gray RJ. Angioplasty and stents for peripheral and central venous lesions. *Techniques in Vascular and Interventional Radiology* 1999;2:189–198, with permission.)

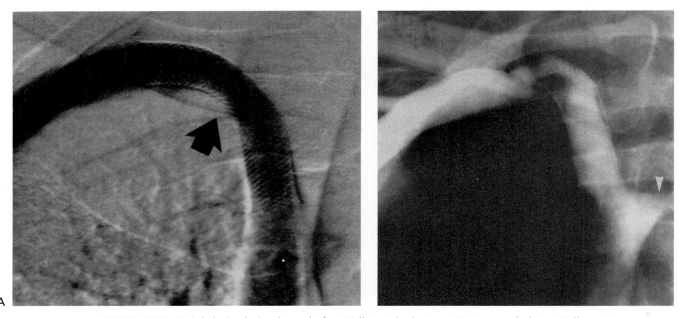

A

B

FIGURE 25.9. A: Subclavian lesion (*arrow*) after Wallstent deployment. **B**: Four weeks later, Wallstent has slipped centrally into the larger innominate vein, although the relationship of the stent to the contralateral innominate (*arrowhead*) has not changed significantly. Compare with A. (From Gray RJ. Angioplasty and stents for peripheral and central venous lesions. *Techniques in Vascular and Interventional Radiology* 1999;2:189–198; and Gray RJ, Horton KM, Dolmatch BL, et al. Use of Wallstents for hemodialysis access-related venous stenoses and occlusions untreatable with balloon angioplasty. *Radiology* 1995;195:479–484, with permission.)

to avoid stent migration or disruption (40,51). It is critical that physicians caring for the patient be aware that a central stent is present to prevent untoward events during future catheter insertions.

The endpoint of treatment mandated by the DOQI guidelines as well as the Society of Cardiovascular and Interventional Radiology (SCVIR) practice (60) and reporting (61) standards is a residual anatomic stenosis of 30% or less (preferentially as little as possible, actually) *and* resolution of

the arm swelling or high intra-access pressures that lead to the initial diagnostic angiogram. Because resolution of arm swelling will not occur for 24 to 72 hours, we rely on an intraprocedural posttreatment static venous pressure ratio less than 33% (62) (see Chapter 21) as an immediately available hemodynamic indicator of pro-

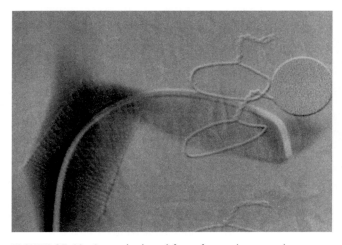

FIGURE 25.10. Stent deployed from femoral approach was unintentionally pulled centrally. This position will complicate future line insertions from both extremities. (From Gray RJ. Angioplasty and stents for peripheral and central venous lesions. *Techniques in Vascular and Interventional Radiology* 1999;2:189–198, with permission.)

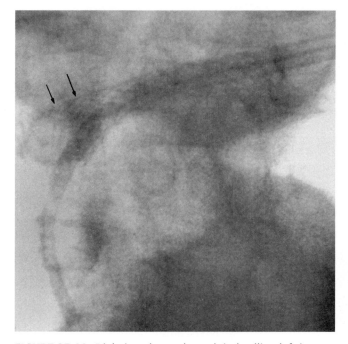

FIGURE 25.11. Dialysis catheter through indwelling left innominate vein stent (*arrows*).

cedure success. This may be an insensitive indicator, but when the posttreatment intragraft pressure is high and the anatomic result seems adequate, transcatheter pressure measurements from the superior vena cava back to the graft can localize the source of the high intragraft static pressures and indicate the need for additional treatment of the index lesion or an unsuspected second lesion. Alternatively, venous pressures can be high secondary to elevated right-sided heart pressures, and no additional therapy will be necessary. Following treatment, patients are monitored clinically for signs of recurrent arm edema or high access pressures; repeat intervention can be performed as necessary.

SUMMARY

Central venous lesions are caused primarily by central venous line insertion and are therefore partially preventable by minimizing the need for central venous lines. Central catheter utilization is decreased by appropriate planning in patients who soon will need dialysis (25), surveillance to minimize access thrombosis/replacement (see Chapter 22) and prompt surgical or thrombolytic treatment for thrombosed accesses. If a central line is needed, the internal jugular should be the vein of first choice (28), with subclavian puncture reserved exclusively for upper extremities that have no potential for a future permanent access (29). When central lesions do occur, the initial treatment of choice is balloon angioplasty, but the success rate and patency rate are low. Wallstent deployment is thus an extremely valuable addition to the treatment armamentarium and is indicated for early angioplasty recurrences, immediate angioplasty failures, and complete chronic occlusions (41). Brachytherapy (63,64) and covered stents (65–68) have been reported in preliminary animal and clinical studies. These topics are addressed elsewhere in this volume (see Chapters 43 and 44). These new treatment modalities have potential to extend the dialysis usefulness for extremities that have a lesion in the final common pathway of a central vein; the ultimate role, if any, of these new therapies and stent designs awaits further investigation.

REFERENCES

1. National Kidney Foundation Dialysis Outcome Quality Initiative (NKF-DOQI). *Clinical practice guidelines for vascular access.* New York: National Kidney Foundation, 1997.
2. Beathard GA. Percutaneous transvenous angioplasty in the treatment of vascular access stenosis. *Kidney Int* 1992;42:1390–1397.
3. Schwab SJ, Quarles LD, Middleton JP, et al. Hemodialysis-associated subclavian vein stenosis. *Kidney Int* 1988;33:1156–1159.
4. Schumacher KA, Walker B, Weidenmaier W, et al. Shuntferne venose okklusionen als storungsfaktor bei der hamodialyse. *Rofo Fortschr Geb Rontgenstr Neuen Bildgeb Verfahr* 1989;150:198–201.
5. Haage P, Vorwerk D, Piroth W, et al. Treatment of hemodialysis-related central stenosis or occlusion: results of primary Wallstent placement and follow-up in 50 patients. *Radiology* 1999;121:175–180.
6. Surratt RF, Picus D, Hicks ME, et al. The importance of preoperative evaluation of the subclavian vein in dialysis access planning. *AJR Am J Roentgenol* 1991;156:623–625.
7. Barrett N, Spencer S, McIvor J, et al. Subclavian stenosis: a major complication of subclavian dialysis catheters. *Nephrol Dial Transplant* 1988;3:423–425.
8. Cimochowski GE, Worley E, Rutherford WE, et al. Superiority of the internal jugular over the subclavian access for temporary dialysis. *Nephron* 1990;54:154–161.
9. Schillinger F, Schillinger D, Montagnac R, et al. Post catheterization vein stenosis in hemodialysis: comparative angiographic study of 50 subclavian and 50 internal jugular accesses. *Nephrol Dial Transplant* 1991;6:722–724.
10. Vanherweghem JL, Yassine T, Goldman M, et al. Subclavian vein thrombosis: a frequent complication of subclavian vein cannulation for hemodialysis. *Clin Nephrol* 1986;26:235–238.
11. Kanterman RY, Vesely TM, Pilgram TK, et al. Dialysis access grafts: anatomic location of venous stenosis and results of angioplasty. *Radiology* 1995;195:135–139.
12. Hoshal VL Jr, Ause RG, Hoskins PA. Fibrin sleeve formation on indwelling subclavian central venous catheters. *Arch Surg* 1971;102:353–358.
13. O'Farrell L, Griffith JW, Lang CM. Histologic development of the sheath that forms around long-term implanted central venous catheters. *JPEN J Parenter Enteral Nutr* 1996;20:156–158.
14. Gray RJ, Dolmatch BL, Buick MK. Directional atherectomy treatment for hemodialysis access: early results. *J Vasc Interv Radiol* 1992;3:497–503.
15. Kowalski CM, Kaufman JA, Rivitz SM, et al. Migration of central venous catheters: implications for initial catheter tip positioning. *J Vasc Interv Radiol* 1997;8:443–447.
16. Nazarian GK, Bjarnason H, Dietz CA Jr, et al. Changes in tunneled catheter tip position when a patient is upright. *J Vasc Interv Radiol* 1997;8:437–441.
17. Fillinger MF, Reinitz ER, Schwartz RA, et al. Graft geometry and venous intimal-medial hyperplasia in arteriovenous loop grafts. *J Vasc Surg* 1990;11:556–566.
18. Middleton WD, Erickson S, Melson GL. Perivascular color artifact: pathologic significance and appearance on color Doppler US images. *Radiology* 1989;171:647–652.
19. Topf G, Jenkins P, Guttmann FD, et al. Unilateral breast enlargement: a complication of an arterio-venous fistula and coincidental subclavian vein occlusion. *JAMA* 1977;237:571–572.
20. Stone WJ, Wall MN, Powers TA. Massive upper extremity edema with arteriovenous fistula for hemodialysis. *Nephron* 1982;31:184–186.
21. El-Nachef MW, Rashad F, Ricanati ES. Occlusion of the subclavian vein: a complication of indwelling subclavian venous catheters for hemodialysis. *Clin Nephrol* 1985;24:42–46.
22. Davis D, Petersen J, Feldman R, et al. Subclavian venous stenosis: a complication of subclavian dialysis. *JAMA* 1984;252:3404–3406.
23. Sullivan KL, Besarab A, Bonn J, et al. Hemodynamics failing dialysis grafts. *Radiology* 1993;186:867–872.
24. Neyra NR, Ikizler TA, May RE, et al. Change in access blood flow over time predicts vascular access thrombosis. *Kidney Int* 1998;54:1714–1719.
25. National Kidney Foundation Dialysis Outcome Quality Initiative (NKF-DOQI). *Clinical practice guidelines for vascular access.* New York: National Kidney Foundation, 1997:31.
26. National Kidney Foundation Dialysis Outcome Quality Initiative (NKF-DOQI). *Clinical practice guidelines for vascular access.* New York: National Kidney Foundation, 1997:55–56.
27. National Kidney Foundation Dialysis Outcome Quality Initiative (NKF-DOQI). *Clinical practice guidelines for vascular access.* New York: National Kidney Foundation, 1997:58–59.
28. National Kidney Foundation Dialysis Outcome Quality Initia-

tive (NKF-DOQI). *Clinical practice guidelines for vascular access.* New York: National Kidney Foundation, 1997:26–27.

29. National Kidney Foundation Dialysis Outcome Quality Initiative (NKF-DOQI). *Clinical practice guidelines for vascular access.* New York: National Kidney Foundation, 1997:28–29.

30. National Kidney Foundation Dialysis Outcome Quality Initiative (NKF-DOQI). *Clinical practice guidelines for vascular access.* New York: National Kidney Foundation, 1997:20–21.

31. Middleton WD, Picus DD, Marx M, et al.. Color Doppler sonography of hemodialysis vascular access: comparison with angiography. *AJR Am J Roentgenol* 1989;152:633–639.

32. Dousset V, Grenier N, Douws C, et al. Hemodialysis grafts: color Doppler flow imaging correlated with digital subtraction angiography and functional status. *Radiology* 1991;181:89–94.

33. Topf G, Jenkins P, Gutmann FD, et al. Unilateral breast enlargement: a complication of an arteriovenous fistula and coincidental subclavian vein occlusion. *JAMA* 1977;237:571–572.

34. Kahn D, Pontin AR, Jacobson JE, et al. Arteriovenous fistula in the presence of subclavian vein thrombosis: a serious complication. *Br J Surg* 1990;77:682.

35. Currier CB, Widder S, Ali A, et al. Surgical management of subclavian and axillary vein thrombosis in patients with a functioning arteriovenous fistula. *Surgery* 1986;100:25–28.

36. Criado E, Marston WA, Jaques PF, et al. Proximal venous outflow obstruction in patients with upper extremity arteriovenous dialysis access. *Ann Vasc Surg* 1994;8:530–535.

37. Bhatia DS, Money SR, Ochsner JL, et al. Comparison of surgical bypass and percutaneous balloon dilatation with primary stent placement in the treatment of central venous obstruction in the dialysis patient: one-year follow-up. *Ann Vasc Surg* 1996;10:452–455.

38. Wisselink W, Money SR, Becker MO, et al. Comparison of operative reconstruction and percutaneous balloon dilatation for central venous obstruction. *Am J Surg* 1993;166:200–205.

39. Newman GE, Saeed M, Himmelstein S, et al. Total central vein obstruction: resolution with angioplasty and fibrinolysis. *Kidney Int* 1991;39:761–764.

40. Gray RJ, Horton KM, Dolmatch BL, et al. Use of Wallstents for hemodialysis access-related venous stenoses and occlusions untreatable with balloon angioplasty. *Radiology* 1995;195:479–484.

41. National Kidney Foundation Dialysis Outcome Quality Initiative (NKF-DOQI). *Clinical practice guidelines for vascular access.* New York: National Kidney Foundation, 1997:57.

42. Glanz S, Gordon DH, Lipkowitz GS, et al. Axillary subclavian vein stenosis: percutaneous angioplasty. *Radiology* 1988;168:371–373.

43. Lund GB, Trerotola SO, Mitchell SE, et al. Central venous angioplasty: an exercise in futility in hemodialysis patients? *Radiology* 1993;189(P):198.

44. Kovalik EC, Newman GE, Suhocki P, et al. Correction of central venous stenoses: use of angioplasty and vascular Wallstents. *Kidney Int* 1994;45:1177–1181.

45. Rundback JH, Leonardo RF, Poplausky MR, et al. Venous rupture complicating hemodialysis access angioplasty; percutaneous treatment and outcomes in seven patients. *AJR Am J Roentgenol* 1998;171:1081–1084.

46. Funaki B, Szymski GX, Leef JA, et al. Treatment of venous outflow stenoses in thigh grafts with Wallstents. *AJR Am J Roentgenol* 1999;172:1591–1596.

47. Safa AA, Valji K, Roberts AC, et al. Detection and treatment of dysfunctional hemodialysis access grafts: effect of a surveillance program on graft patency and the incidence of thrombosis. *Radiology* 1996;199:653–657.

48. Turmel-Rodrigues L, Pengloan J, Blanchier D, et al. Insufficient dialysis shunts: improved long-term patency rates with close hemodynamic monitoring, repeated percutaneous balloon angioplasty, and stent placement. *Radiology* 1993;187:273–278.

49. Davidson CJ, Newman GE, Sheikh KH, et al. Mechanisms of angioplasty in hemodialysis fistula stenoses evaluated by intravascular ultrasound. *Kidney Int* 1991;40:91–95.

50. Quinn SF, Schuman ES, Hall L, et al. Venous stenoses in patients who undergo hemodialysis: treatment with self-expandable endovascular stents. *Radiology* 1992;183:499–504.

51. Shoenfeld R, Hermans H, Novick A, et al. Stenting of proximal venous obstructions to maintain hemodialysis access. *J Vasc Surg* 1994;19:532–539.

52. Quinn SF, Schuman ES, Demlow TA, et al. Percutaneous transluminal angioplasty versus endovascular stent placement in the treatment of venous stenoses in patients undergoing hemodialysis: intermediate results. *J Vasc Interv Radiol* 1995;6:851–855.

53. Mickley V, Gorich J, Rilinger N, et al. Stenting of central venous stenoses in hemodialysis patients: long-term results. *Kidney Int* 1997;51:277–280.

54. Gray RJ, Dolmatch BL, Horton KM, et al. Migration of Palmaz stents following deployment for venous stenoses related to hemodialysis access. *J Vasc Interv Radiol* 1994;5:117–120.

55. Bjarnason H, Hunter DW, Crain MR, et al. Collapse of a Palmaz stent in the subclavian vein. *AJR Am J Roentgenol* 1993;160:1123–1124.

56. Vorwerk D, Guenther RW, Mann H, et al. Venous stenosis and occlusion in hemodialysis shunts: follow-up results of stent placement in 65 patients. *Radiology* 1995;195:140–146.

57. Vesely TM, Hovsepian DM, Pilgram TK, et al. Upper extremity central venous obstruction in hemodialysis patients: treatment with Wallstents. *Radiology* 1997;204:343–348.

58. Funaki B, Szymski GX, Leef JA, et al. Wallstent deployment to salvage dialysis graft thrombolysis complicated by venous rupture: early and intermediate results. *AJR Am J Roentgenol* 1997;169:1435–1437.

59. Hoffer EK, Sultan S, Herskowitz MM, et al. Prospective randomized trial of a metallic intravascular stent in hemodialysis graft maintenance. *J Vasc Interv Radiol* 1997;8:965–973.

60. Aruny JE, Lewis CA, Cardella JF, et al. Quality improvement guidelines for percutaneous management of the thrombosed or dysfunctional dialysis access. *J Vasc Interv Radiol* 1999;10:491–498.

61. Gray RJ, Sacks D, Trerotola S, et al. Reporting standards for percutaneous interventions in dialysis access. *J Vasc Interv Radiol* 1999;10:1405–1415.

62. Sullivan KL, Besarab AL. Hemodynamic screening and early percutaneous intervention reduce hemodialysis access thrombosis and increase graft longevity. *J Vasc Interv Radiol* 1997;8:163–170.

63. Trerotola SO, Carmody TJ, Timmerman RD, et al. Brachytherapy for the prevention of stenosis in a canine hemodialysis graft model: preliminary observations. *Radiology* 1999;212:748–754.

64. Waksman R, Crocker IA, Kikeri D, et al. Endovascular low dose irradiation for prevention of restenosis following angioplasty for treatment of narrowed arteriovenous dialysis grafts. *J Am Coll Cardiol* 1996;27:214A(abst).

65. Crain MR, Mewisson MW, Seibold C, et al. Novel arteriovenous access graft with stented endovenous extension: initial study in a canine model. *J Vasc Interv Radiol* 1998;9(Suppl):197(abst).

66. Murphy TP, Webb MS. Percutaneous venous bypass for refractory dialysis-related subclavian vein occlusion. *J Vasc Interv Radiol* 1998;9:935–939.

67. Sapoval MR, Turmel-Rodrigues LA, Raynaud AC, et al. Cragg covered stents in hemodialysis access: initial and midterm results. *J Vasc Interv Radiol* 1996;7:335–342.

68. Farber A, Barbey M-M, Grunert J-H, et al. Access-related venous stenoses and occlusions: treatment with percutaneous transluminal angioplasty and Dacron-covered stents. *Cardiovasc Intervent Radiol* 1999;22:214–218.

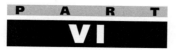

TREATMENT OF THE THROMBOSED ACCESS

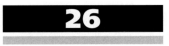

PHARMACOLOGIC THROMBOLYSIS FOR
DIALYSIS GRAFTS

PAMELA A. FLICK
CHRISTOPHER E. PIERPONT
JACOB CYNAMON

In the United States, about 155,000 patients require chronic hemodialysis (1). The number of patients undergoing hemodialysis continues to grow as technology and patient survival improve in this patient population. We know that hemodialysis grafts are plagued with multiple problems, the most common being graft failure or thrombosis. It has been reported that vascular access complications are the single largest cause of morbidity, accounting for 15% to 16% of all hospitalizations in the hemodialysis population (2). These complications cost the Medicare program between 700 and 900 million dollars annually. (3).

Native arteriovenous (AV) fistulas are the preferred forms of permanent vascular access; however, more than 80% of the permanent vascular accesses placed in the United States are expanded polytetrafluoroethylene (ePTFE) grafts (4). As we know, the 1-year patency rate for ePTFE hemodialysis grafts has been reported to be about 65% (5,6). The most common cause of graft failure is thrombosis, which is most commonly secondary to progressive venous outflow stenosis followed by occlusion (7–13). For years, traditional therapy for graft failure was surgical thrombectomy with or without graft revision or complete graft replacement or both. Surgical thrombectomy alone is usually not curative because the cause of the graft thrombosis usually has not been addressed. In the operating room, the surgeon must perform an intraoperative angiogram or a blind exploration after declotting the graft to evaluate and treat the underlying cause of thrombosis properly. By choosing to declot the graft percutaneously under direct fluoroscopic guidance, however, one can evaluate the graft thoroughly from the arterial anastomosis through to the central veins in search of an anatomic cause for the graft failure.

The challenge of determining the most effective treatment for thrombosed grafts is paramount in the minds of the nephrologists, access surgeons, and interventional radiologists. Therefore, a team approach is warranted that incorporates graft screening, percutaneous declotting, angioplasty, and surgical thrombectomy/graft revision. The goals

of this chapter are to discuss the management of the failed hemodialysis grafts.

GRAFT FAILURE

Unfortunately, despite the best intentions of the nephrologist, access surgeon, and interventional radiologist, hemodialysis grafts thrombose. Once graft failure is recognized, a decision must be made as to how to treat the patient most effectively.

Traditionally, hemodialysis graft thromboses have been treated by surgical thrombectomy with or without revision. Surgical graft salvage usually entails accessing the graft via a short incision over the venous limb of the graft or by opening the previous incision used to place the shunt. Next, thrombectomy is performed using Fogarty thrombectomy catheters. Depending on the operating room facilities, either an angiogram is performed or dilators are advanced into the veins to evaluate the graft outflow for any evidence of stenosis. If a lesion is identified, the graft is revised either by using a jump graft to a more proximal vein using PTFE or by a patch angioplasty across the stenotic lesion.

Several studies have compared the efficacy of percutaneous and surgical treatment (14,15). These studies have shown comparable patency rates with angioplasty and surgery, with no statistically significant difference between the two treatments. Primary patency rates at 1 month for angioplasty and surgery ranged from 72% to 77% and 64% to 86%, respectively (see Chapter 29 for comparison of surgery and percutaneous techniques).

Another study examined the results of graft salvage by surgical thrombectomy with or without revision. The retrospective study of 116 surgical thrombectomies or revisions found discouraging results with patency rates of 59% and 29% for revised grafts at 30 and 120 days versus 30% and 10% at the same time intervals for grafts treated only with surgical thrombectomy (16). The investigators concluded that thrombosed grafts should be abandoned in favor of a new access site. Each graft revision, extension, or new graft placement is at the expense of valuable vein, however. Percutaneous declotting using fluoroscopic evaluation and treatment of all graft lesions may spare vein and prolong the use of an extremity for hemodialysis. Treatment algorithms for the treatment and management of thrombosed grafts should include the experience of the skilled vascular surgeon and vascular interventional radiologist, of course, because their techniques should be complementary.

PHARMACOLOGIC THROMBOLYSIS

Pharmacologic thrombolysis of thrombosed hemodialysis grafts was first attempted in the mid-1980s. Initially, streptokinase was used. Streptokinase was infused into the afferent limb of the thrombosed graft. Early reports demonstrated the effectiveness of streptokinase at dissolving clot and restoring blood flow in the graft (17). Unfortunately, most patients suffered local bleeding complications from previous dialysis puncture sites, and others suffered allergic reactions. Furthermore, with repeated treatments, the patients developed drug resistance to streptokinase. These difficulties led to the abandonment of streptokinase as a thrombolytic agent for clotted grafts.

Although the initial results for thrombolysis of occluded AV grafts was not encouraging, over time, with improved techniques and a different thrombolytic agent (i.e., urokinase), thrombolytic success in the treatment of thrombosed hemodialysis grafts was achieved. At first, urokinase was used as a drip infusion through a single end-hole catheter. The initial success (patency at 24–48 hours with successful dialysis) ranged between 49% and 79%, whereas the length of infusion times varied from 2 to 20 hours (18–21). Urokinase drip infusions due to the higher systemic doses were plagued with the same local hemorrhagic complications seen with initial streptokinase studies, with up to 50% of patients experiencing bleeding complications.

PHARMACOMECHANICAL THROMBOLYSIS

In an attempt to shorten infusion times, reduce urokinase dosages, and decrease hemorrhagic complications, research began in adding a mechanical component to the already developed pharmacologic thrombolytic techniques. One group developed a novel technique termed *lacing/maceration* (22). Two 5-French dilators were placed into the midportion of the graft in a crisscross fashion. After initial graft evaluation and the exchange of dilators for two hook-shaped catheters, highly concentrated urokinase (25,000 IU/mL) was injected through the catheters, which were rotated and withdrawn through the thrombosed graft. After the catheters were repositioned at the midportion and the arterial end of the graft,

an infusion of urokinase (4,000 IU/mL) then was started at 2,000 IU per minute per catheter until the graft was clot free. Any identified stenoses then were subjected to angioplasty. The major advantages of this declotting technique were a decreased infusion time with an average infusion time of 86 minutes and a 90% initial success rate with no reported hemorrhagic complications.

The same group of investigators modified the lacing/maceration technique and eliminated the need for the supplemental urokinase infusion after the lacing. This so-called pulse-spray technique used two crossed tapered catheters with multiple side holes and forceful injections of highly concentrated urokinase into the clot (23). When the graft appeared to be relatively clot free, an angiogram was performed with subsequent angioplasty to address any stenotic lesions. This technique improved the mean infusion time from 86 minutes in the previous technique (22) to 49 minutes with the pulse-spray method. In this series, initial success was achieved in 97.9% of cases. These investigators reported a discouraging 1-year primary patency rate of 26% (24). After repeated procedures, the secondary patency rate increased to 51%, again without significant bleeding complications.

The pulse-spray technique was modified later by including early fragmentation of residual clot with a balloon catheter, intrathrombotic injection of heparin, mechanical treatment of a lysis-resistant plug at the arterial anastomosis, and the routine administration of aspirin. In 1995, the original and current techniques were compared retrospectively (25). The mean thrombolytic agent infusion time was reduced from 44 minutes to 23 minutes. The initial success rate increased from 86% to 96%, with 92% remaining patent for at least 24 hours. The complication rates between the original and current techniques did not differ significantly. Even though the modifications did not significantly improve initial success, the mean infusion time decreased dramatically. Follow-up studies using the pulse-spray technique reported the 30- and 90-day primary patencies in ranges of 70% and 50%, respectively (26–29). One study demonstrated a 30-day secondary patency rate of 92% (26).

"LYSE AND WAIT" TECHNIQUE

Other thrombolytic techniques have been reported with success. The "lyse and wait" technique first descibed by Cynamon and colleagues (Fig. 26.1) is a simplified thrombolytic method that also can be used to treat thrombosed hemodialysis grafts (30). This technique most often eliminates the need for any additional mechanical devices or pulse-spray catheters. There is significantly less time spent in the angiographic suite declotting the graft because most of the lysis occurs while the patient "waits" for the procedure. Because little or no time is spent on declotting the graft, the patient's time on the angiographic table is lessened significantly; therefore, more attention can be focused on

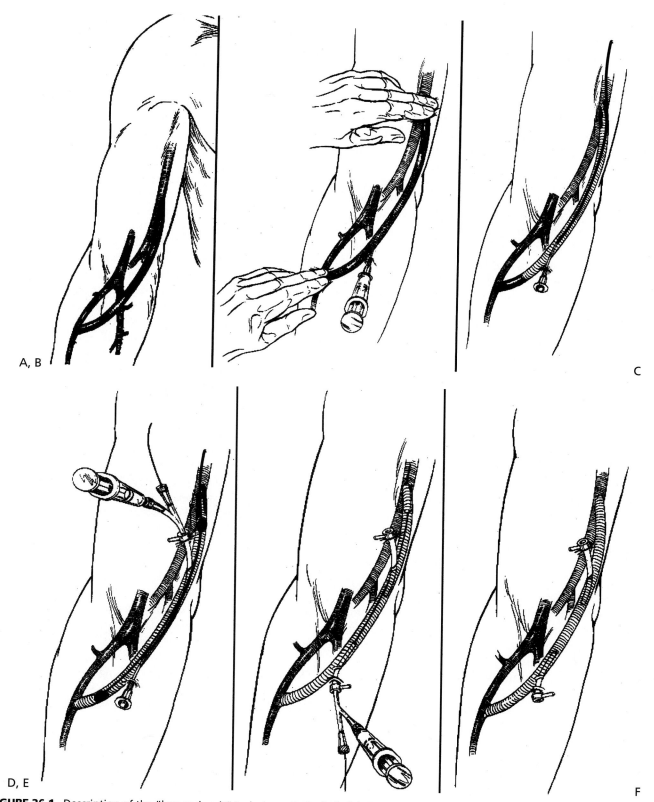

FIGURE 26.1. Description of the "lyse and wait" technique. **A**: Occluded dialysis graft. **B**: After placing a 22-gauge angiocatheter in the graft close to the arterial anastomosis pointing toward the venous anastomosis, the inflow and outflow of the graft are compressed. The lytic agent is injected into the graft. **C**: After waiting half an hour or so, an angiogram is performed. Minimal clot, an arterial plug, and a venous outflow stenosis are often encountered. **D**: After crossing the venous anastomosis and administering heparin into a central vein, a sheath is introduced toward the arterial anastomosis. A 4 French Thru-lumen Fogarty is used to mobilize the arterial plug. **E**: The venous angioplasty then is performed. Any intragraft lesion is dilated, and any residual clot is crushed or mobilized. **F**: The entire graft and outflow are evaluated. Pressures are measured to ensure low pressure in the graft.

evaluating the underlying cause for graft failure and achieving an optimal outcome to angioplasty. This is likely the most important predictor of hemodialysis graft patency.

Technique

Before the patient is brought into the angiography suite, under sterile technique, an angiocatheter is introduced into the thrombosed graft adjacent to the arterial anastomosis, pointing in the direction of the venous anastomosis. Confirmation of intragraft placement of the angiocatheter is obtained by visualizing or "milking" blood from the angiocatheter or by attempting to introduce a 0.018-inch guidewire into the graft without difficulty. The graft then is compressed at the arterial and venous anastomoses while a thrombolytic agent of the operator's choice and heparin are infused slowly over a 1- to 2-minute period into the thrombosed graft. After "waiting" for approximately 30 minutes, the patient then is brought into the angiography suite and the arm or leg is prepared and draped in the usual fashion. As with all graft evaluations, a diagnostic angiogram then is obtained, which typically shows minimal thrombus remaining within the graft and a resistant arterial plug. One must be careful to not overinject the graft, thereby avoiding reflux of any residual thrombus into the inflow artery.

As stated, an arterial plug is usually present at or close to the arterial anastomosis. Our attention then is focused to mobilizing the arterial plug. This is accomplished by introducing a short 5 or 6 French sheath into the graft via a puncture close to the venous anastomosis pointing toward the arterial anastomosis. A Fogarty balloon (Baxter) dislodges the arterial plug, and antegrade flow usually is established easily. Next, the venous lesion is dilated using a 6, 7, or 8-mm high-pressure balloon. Access from the arterial anastomosis to the right atrium then is evaluated angiographically. After the graft is free of thrombus and all lesions have been adequately dilated, a thrill is present, and intragraft pressures measure less than 40% of the systemic systolic pressure, the graft has been optimally treated and is ready for dialysis. Whether the arterial plug is mobilized first or the venous angioplasty is performed first is operator dependent. Modifications of the "lyse and wait" technique have been developed over the past few years. The lytic agent initially used for thrombolysis was urokinase (Abbokinase; Abbott Laboratories, North Chicago, IL, U.S.A.), and the original dose was 250,000 IU of urokinase along with 5,000 U of heparin into the graft.

With the withdraw of Abbokinase from the market in January 1999 by the U.S. FDA, other thrombolytic agents now being used have included reteplase (Retavase; Centacor, Malvern, PA, U.S.A.) and alteplase (rt-PA, Activase; Genentech, Inc., South San Francisco, CA, U.S.A.). *Reteplase* is a recombinant fibrinogen activator with a half-life of 14 to 18 minutes. The drug has current approval by the FDA for use in patients with acute myocardial infarction.

The dose of reteplase used for declotting grafts by pulse-spray-mechanical technique ranges from 3 to 5 U and for "lyse and wait techniques," 2 to 3 U. Dilution volumes are operator dependent. Heparin also is administered and again appears to be operator dependent, ranging from 2,000 to 5,000 U into the graft or intravenously. Note that heparin and reteplase should be administered separately because heparin appears to cause precipitation when mixed with reteplase. Numerous abstracts have been presented that have demonstrated technical and clinical success with the use of this agent. Falk and colleagues at the Society of Cardiovascular and Interventional Radiology (SCVIR) in San Antonio reported 88% success with the use of 1 U of reteplase and 4,000 U of heparin (31). Four associated complications were reported and included bleeding from old puncture sites (n = 1), embolization into the brachial artery (n = 1), and rupture of the outflow brachial vein (n = 2). At the SCVIR in San Diego, Gibbons and colleagues, using "crossing catheter pulse-spray technique" treated 64 grafts (32). Their success rate using 3 to 5 U of reteplase and varying doses of heparin (0–5,000 U) was 98% with a 1-month patency of 86%. They had no reported complications. Again, using 3 U of reteplase along with 3,000 U of heparin and the "lyse and wait" technique, Flick and associates reported at the same meeting a 94% technical success in reestablishing flow in clotted synthetic hemodialysis grafts (33). It appears in all studies that complications as well as outcomes are similar to those previously seen with urokinase.

Recombinant tissue-type plasminogen activator (rt-PA), a plasminogen activator, has now become the most widely used agent in the treatment of thrombosed grafts. Again, as with reteplase, protocol doses vary; the current doses being used for dialysis graft declots either using pulse-and-spray technique or "lyse and wait" range from 1 to 5 mg of rt-PA. Again, heparin doses vary with the individual operator (1,000–5,000 U have been reported). Heparin is incompatible with Activase; therefore, the two should not be mixed together before they are administered. Falk and colleagues reported their results using 2 mg of rt-PA, 5,000 U of heparin, and the "lyse and wait" technique (34). Their technical success rate was 96%, with two complications of minor bleeding. In a randomized study, Vogel compared 40 patients using 4 mg of alteplase "lyse and wait" to mechanical thrombectomy using the Arrow-Trerotola device (PTD) (35). All patients received 5,000 U of heparin. Results demonstrated 100% reestablishment of flow in both groups. Seven of 20 patients had prolonged bleeding or minor complications associated with bleeding. It appears both reteplase and alteplase have been efficacious and relatively safe in the treatment of thrombosed AV grafts; however, more data need to be collected and larger trials evaluated.

Another unanswered question in this patient population is: What is the role of glycoprotein (GP) IIb/IIIa platelet inhibitors, if any? As discussed in Chapter 9 on management of bleeding and clotting disorders in dialysis patients by Dr.

Alving, we know that patients who are uremic already have significant platelet dysfunction, often causing prolonging bleeding times. In this group of patients, adding an agent that blocks platelet adhesion and alters platelet function most likely would add to their potential bleeding complications. Administering additional agents adds significantly to the cost of these procedures. If, at some time, abciximab, tirofibam, and eptifibatide demonstrate properties that are beneficial to this patient population, their role most certainly will increase. (See Chapter 9 for background information on the current GP IIb/IIIa inhibitors) At this time, however, this remains to be evaluated.

At the conclusion of these procedures, after adequate treatment of "offending" lesion has been completed and the graft has been restored to complete function, if it is not now necessary to leave in the sheaths for dialysis hemostasis can be achieved simply by placing a pursestring suture.

Alternative treatment algorithms to thrombolysis include percutaneous mechanical thrombectomy, which is preferred by some, and is reviewed in Chapter 27. A randomized, prospective study comparing the Arrow-Trerotola percutaneous thrombolytic device (PTD) and pulse-spray pharmacomechanical thrombolysis found similar technical and long-term success rates between the two methods of thrombolyis, with the PTD having shorter procedure times (31).

Patient Selection

Both native AV fistulae and synthetic AV grafts can be effectively treated using the aforementioned techniques. The contraindications for treating dialysis patients with thrombolytics remain the same as for patients with acute peripheral arterial or deep vein thromboses. Other contraindications for treatment include an infected AV graft, recent surgical revision within 1 week because of the risk of bleeding, repeated graft failure after adequate declot and angioplasty, history of allergic reactions to contrast or fibrinolytics, recent history of bleeding, and patients with known severe pulmonary hypertension. One should carefully review the patient's clinical history as well as the history of previous dialysis graft intervention to prevent unnecessary complications.

CONCLUSION

In conclusion, although the results of percutaneous and surgical declotting of occluded dialysis grafts are similar, percutaneous declotting has the advantages. Percutaneous therapy has the benefit of being less invasive; it also spares the use of additional vein. Percutaneous intervention also can be easily repeated to maintain the life of the graft as long as necessary. Most importantly, it allows for the complete evaluation of the entire AV graft from the arterial anastomosis through to the right atrium, allowing treatment of all lesions found at the time of declotting.

Percutaneous declotting can be performed with mechanical devices or with thrombolysis. Both techniques readily have gained acceptance in the management of thrombosed hemodialysis grafts. Thrombolysis, both agents and techniques, has evolved over the past decade and most likely will continue to evolve with newer agents as well as improved techniques. As we have seen, the popular techniques used today for pharmacologic thrombolysis of dialysis grafts continue to be "mechanical pulse-spray" or the "lyse and wait" technique.

REFERENCES

1. United States Renal Data System (USRDS). Treatment modalities for ESRD patients. *Am J Kidney Dis* 1997;30(Suppl):54–56.
2. Feldman HI, Held PJ, Huthcinson JT, et al. Hemodialysis vascular access morbidity in the United States. *Kidney Int* 1993;43:1091–1096.
3. United States Renal Data System (USRDS). The economic cost of ESRD, vascular access procedures, and Medicare spending for alternative modalities of treatment. *Am J Kidney Dis* 1997;30(Suppl):160–177.
4. Windus DW. Permanent vascular access: a nephrologist's view. *Am J Kidney Dis* 1993;21:457–471.
5. Munda R, First MR, Alexander JW, et al. Polytetrafluoroethylene graft survival in hemodialysis. *JAMA* 1983;249:219–222.
6. Tellis VA, Kohlberg WI, Bhat DJ, et al. Expanded polytetrafluoroethylene graft fistula for chronic hemodialysis. *Ann Surg* 1979;189:101–103.
7. Kanterman RY, Vesely TM, Pilgram TK, et al. Dialysis access grafts: anatomic location of venous stenosis and results of angioplasty. *Radiology* 1995;195:135–139.
8. Beathard GA. Percutaneous transvenous angioplasty in the treatment of vascular access stenosis. *Kidney Int* 1992;42:1390–1397.
9. Turmel-Rodrigues L, Pengloan J, Blanchier D, et al. Insufficient dialysis shunts: improved long-term patency rates with close hemodynamic monitoring, repeated percutaneous balloon angioplasty, and stent placement. *Radiology* 1993;187:273–278.
10. Glanz S, Gordon DH, Butt KM, et al. The role of percutaneous angioplasty in the management of chronic hemodialysis fistulas. *Ann Surg* 1987;206:777–781.
11. Schwab SJ, Raymond JR, Saeed M, et al. Prevention of hemodialysis fistula thrombosis: early detection of venous stenoses. *Kidney Int* 1989;36:707–711.
12. Marston WA, Criado E, Jaques PF, et al. Prospective randomized comparison of surgical verus endovascular management of thrombosed dialysis grafts. *J Vasc Surg* 1997;26:373–381.
13. Brooks JL, Sigley RD, May KJ, et al. Transluminal angioplasty versus surgical repair for stenoses of hemodialysis grafts. *Am J Surg* 1987;153:530–531.
14. Bitar G, Yang S, Badosa F. Balloon versus patch angioplasty as an adjuvant treatment to surgical thrombectomy of hemodialysis grafts. *Am J Surg* 1997;174:140–142.
15. Dapunt O, Feurstein M, Rendl KH, et al. Transluminal angioplasty versus conventional operation in the treatment of hemodialysis fistula stenosis: results from a 5-year study. *Br J Surg* 1987;74:1004–1005.
16. Brotman DN, Fandos L, Faust GR, et al. Hemodialysis graft salvage. *J Am Coll Surg* 1994;178:431–434.
17. Gray RJ. Percutaneous intervention for permanent hemodialysis access: a review. *J Vasc Interv Radiol* 1997;8:313–327.

18. Mangiarotti G, Canavese C, Thea A, et al. Urokinase treatment for arteriovenous fistulae declotting in dialyzed patients. *Nephron* 1984;36:60–64.

19. Schilling JJ, Eiser AR, Slifkin RF, et al. The role of thrombolysis in hemodialysis access occlusion. *Am J Kidney Dis* 1987;10:92–97.

20. Brunner MC, Matalon TAS, Patel SK, et al. Ultrarapid urokinase in hemodialysis access occlusion. *J Vasc Interv Radiol* 1991;2:503–506.

21. Summers S, Drazan K, Gomes A, et al. Urokinase therapy for thrombosed hemodialysis access grafts. *Surg Gynecol Obstet* 1993;176:534–538.

22. Davis GB, Dowd CF, Bookstein JJ, et al. Thrombosed dialysis grafts: efficacy of intrathrombic deposition of concentrated urokinase, clot maceration, and angioplasty. *Am J Roentgenol* 1989;149:177–181.

23. Bookstein JJ, Fellmeth B, Roberts A, et al. Pulsed-spray pharmacomechanical thrombolysis: preliminary clinical results. *AJR Am J Roentgenol* 1989;152:1097–1100.

24. Valji K, Bookstein JJ, Roberts AC, et al: Pharmacomechanical thrombolysis and angioplasty in the management of clotted hemodialysis grafts: early and late clinical results. *Radiology* 1991;178:243–247.

25. Valji K, Bookstein JJ, Roberts AC, et al. Pulse-spray pharmacomechanical thrombolysis of thrombosed hemodialysis access grafts: long-term experience and comparison of original and current techniques. *AJR Am J Roentgenol* 1995;164:1495–1500.

26. Cohen MA, Kumpe DA, Durham JD, et al. Improved treatment of thrombosed hemodialysis access sites with thrombolysis and angioplasty. *Kidney Int* 1994;46:1375–1380.

27. Middlebrook MR, Amygdalos MA, Soulen MC, et al. Thrombosed hemodialysis grafts: percutaneous mechanical balloon declotting versus thrombolysis. *Radiology* 1995;196:73–77.

28. Berger MF, Aruny JE, Skibo LK. Recurrent thrombosis of polytetrafluoroethylene dialysis fistulas after recent surgical thrombectomy: salvage by means of thrombolysis and angioplasty. *J Vasc Interv Radiol* 1994;5:725–730.

29. Beathard GA. Mechanical versus pharmacomechanical thrombolysis for the treatment of thrombosed dialysis access grafts. *Kidney Int* 1994;45:1401–1406.

30. Cynamon J, Lakritz PS, Wahl SI, et al. Hemodialysis graft declotting: description of the "lyse and wait" technique. *J Vasc Interv Radiol* 1997;8:825–829.

31. Falk A, Lookstein R, Mitty H, et al. Thrombolysis of clotted hemodialysis grafts with reteplase. 26th Annual SCVIR, San Antonio. *J Vasc Interv Radiol* 2001;12(Suppl):S115.

32. Gibbens DT, Depalma J, Albanese J, et al. Percutaneous thrombolysis of hemodialysis using reteplase: 25th Annual SCVIR, San Diego. *J Vasc Interv Radiol* 2000;11(Suppl)2:250.

33. Flick PA, Das M, Horton KM, et al. Initial experience with reteplase using "lyse and Wait" technique in thrombosed dialysis grafts: 25th Annual SCVIR, San Diego. *J Vasc Interv Radiol* 2000;11(Suppl)252.

34. Falk A, Mitty H, Guller J, et al. Thrombolysis of clotted hemodialysis grafts with tissue-type plasminogen activator. *J Vasc Interv Radiol* 2001;12:3 305–311.

35. Vogel PM. "Lyse and wait" compared to mechanical thrombolysis of hemodialysis grafts: 26th Annual SCVIR, San Antonio. *J Vasc Interv Radiol* 2001;12(Suppl):S3..

36. Trerotola SO, Vesely TM, Lund GB, et al. Treatment of thrombosed hemodialysis access grafts: Arrow–Trerotola percutaneous device versus pulse-spray thrombolysis. *Radiology* 1998;206:403–414.

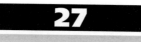

MECHANICAL THROMBECTOMY TECHNIQUES AND DEVICES

THOMAS M. VESELY
MELHEM J. SHARAFUDDIN

Throughout the past decade, there has been a plethora of published reports describing numerous percutaneous techniques for the treatment of thrombosed hemodialysis grafts and fistulae (1–12). These techniques can be divided into two broad categories; one group uses thrombolytic agents, and the other uses mechanical thrombectomy techniques. The category of mechanical thrombectomy techniques includes balloon thrombectomy, thromboaspiration, and the use of mechanical thrombectomy devices. This chapter reviews the techniques and tools used for performing mechanical thrombectomy of a thrombosed vascular access.

Treatment of a thrombosed vascular access can be a challenging experience. Experience, good judgment, and the ability to improvise are just a few of the attributes that will increase your success and make this a routine procedure to perform.

PREPROCEDURAL PATIENT ASSESSMENT

Physical Examination of the Vascular Access

The patient's vascular access should be examined before draping the extremity. The graft or fistula should be inspected carefully for signs of infection such as erythema, localized swelling, or tenderness. An infected vascular access is an absolute contraindication to an endovascular procedure.

The vascular access also should be examined to determine its location, configuration, and condition. When evaluating a loop configuration graft, the orientation of the arterial and venous limbs and the extent of a "jump" or interposition graft should be ascertained. Finally, the location and size of access-related pseudoaneurysms should be determined. The presence of a pseudoaneurysm may alter the entry site into the vascular access. A large pseudoaneurysm can present a challenge during thrombus removal.

Cardiopulmonary Disease

Before the thrombectomy procedure, it is important to determine whether the patient has a history of significant cardiac or pulmonary disease. Studies have revealed that fragments of thrombus can escape from the graft and travel to the lung as pulmonary emboli during endovascular thrombectomy procedures (13–16). Although most patients are able to tolerate these small pulmonary emboli, patients with significant pulmonary or cardiac disease are at greater risk for acute decompensation. Patients who have a history of right-sided heart failure, pulmonary hypertension, cardiac dysrhythmias, or right-to-left cardiac shunts are not good candidates for an endovascular thrombectomy procedure. It may be prudent to refer these patients for a surgical thrombectomy. The surgeon can occlude (clamp) the venous outflow to prevent embolization of thrombus during the thrombectomy procedure.

Hematologic Parameters

Ideally, the patient's hematocrit level should be ascertained before the thrombectomy procedure. Hemodialysis patients are chronically anemic, and intraprocedural blood loss may compromise the patient, thereby increasing the risk of an acute cardiac event.

Mechanical thrombectomy procedures can cause blood loss by several different mechanisms. These include bleeding from access entry sites, aspiration of blood, and, less commonly, mechanical destruction of red cells. Several thrombectomy devices, such as the Hydrolyser (Cordis, Warren, NJ, U.S.A.), the Oasis (Boston Scientific, Natick, MA, U.S.A.), and the EndoVac (Neovascular Technologies, Brooklyn, NY, U.S.A.), have powerful aspiration capabilities. Prolonged or inattentive activation of these devices can lead to substantial intraprocedural blood loss. The device activation time should be minimized and the volume of effluent fluid in the drainage bag should be monitored during the thrombectomy procedure.

Prolonged activation of mechanical thrombectomy devices can cause fragmentation and destruction of red cells. This process is more detrimental to patients with residual renal function and nonhemodialysis patients. The liberation of large amounts of plasma-free hemoglobin, secondary to the destruction of red cells, can overwhelm the binding capacity of serum haptoglobin and potentially lead to acute renal failure. The critical level of plasma-free hemoglobin that incites renal tubular damage is not known, but mechanical fragmentation of even a small amount of thrombus (< 5 cc) can cause a fourfold increase in plasma-free hemoglobin levels (12). For this reason, some mechanical thrombectomy devices should be used cautiously in patients with residual renal function, particularly when using a device to remove large volumes of thrombus.

Most chronic hemodialysis patients receive routine injections of exogenous erythropoietin (EPO). Without EPO injections, these patients typically have hematocrit levels of 23% to 27%. With regular administration of EPO, their baseline hematocrit levels can be maintained in the 30% to 35% range. Each physician should establish guidelines for acceptable hematocrit values for patients undergoing percutaneous thrombectomy procedures. For example, if the patient's hematocrit level is greater than 30%, the thrombectomy procedure can be performed in the usual manner. If the hematocrit is greater than 25% but less than 30%, the interventionalist should take particular care to limit intraprocedural blood loss; the physician may want to avoid using a high-flow aspirating thrombectomy device. If the patient's hematocrit is less than 25%, the thrombectomy procedure should be performed cautiously, and the intraprocedural blood loss must be closely monitored. If necessary, the patient should be admitted to the hospital for overnight observation following the procedure. If the patient's hematocrit is less than 23%, it is prudent to postpone the thrombectomy procedure until the patient receives a blood transfusion.

PERCUTANEOUS THROMBECTOMY PROCEDURE

There are four basic steps to perform during a percutaneous thrombectomy procedure: (a) an initial venogram to evaluate the central and peripheral veins; (b) removal of the thrombus from the vascular access; (c) treatment of all significant stenoses using angioplasty, atherectomy, or vascular stents; and (d) dislodgement of the arterial plug.

There are a variety of different types and configurations of vascular access for hemodialysis. The following description of a percutaneous thrombectomy procedure pertains to a loop-configuration, polytetrafluoroethylene (PTFE) graft located in the forearm.

Venography

The initial needle puncture is made in an antegrade (with respect to blood flow) direction into the arterial limb of the graft, approximately 2 to 3 cm from the arterial anastomosis. A multipurpose angiographic catheter is inserted into the graft over a guidewire and advanced through the venous anastomosis. A diagnostic venogram is performed to evaluate the entire native venous outflow, including the central veins. If a long-segment stenosis, multiple sequential stenoses, or occlusions are identified in the native veins, one should consider terminating the procedure (Fig. 27.1). It can be difficult to treat such venous lesions, and, even when they are successfully treated, the results may not be durable. A patient with extensive venous pathology may be best treated with a surgical revision to extend the graft above the stenotic or occluded venous segment, or the patient may need a new graft in a different location. Most commonly, the diagnostic venogram reveals a single focal stenosis at the

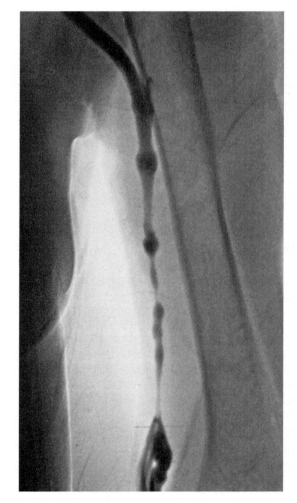

FIGURE 27.1. A long-segment, multifocal stenosis in the basilic vein located distal to the venous anastomosis of a hemodialysis graft.

venous anastomosis that can be easily treated using standard endovascular techniques.

Although several different thrombectomy techniques are available, most interventional radiologists prefer to leave the venous anastomotic stenosis intact during thrombus removal. This stenosis serves to hold the thrombus within the graft, allowing it to be more readily removed, and prevents embolization of thrombus into the native venous circulation.

Alternatively, some interventionalists prefer to dilate the venous anastomotic stenosis before removing the thrombus. Activation of a mechanical thrombectomy device may cause substantial turbulence and increase intragraft pressure, thereby increasing the risk of arterial embolization. Dilating the venous anastomotic stenosis before insertion of the thrombectomy device can provide a pathway for decompression of these forces on activation of the device.

Thrombus Removal: Venous Limb

After completion of the diagnostic venogram, the angiographic catheter is removed and replaced with a vascular sheath. A 6 or 7 French sheath will provide access for most mechanical thrombectomy devices and angioplasty balloon catheters. Heparin (2,000–5,000 U) is commonly administered at this point in the thrombectomy procedure. It can be given through a peripheral intravenous line or slowly infused into the vascular access via the sidearm of the sheath.

Removing thrombus from the venous limb of a graft can be accomplished using a single thrombectomy method or a combination of several mechanical thrombectomy techniques. These mechanical thrombectomy methods include balloon-assisted thrombectomy (BAT), thromboaspiration, or the use of mechanical thrombectomy devices. The details of these different techniques are discussed in the following section.

The mechanical thrombectomy procedure, removing thrombus from the graft, is performed under fluoroscopic observation. The speed at which the thrombectomy is performed is both operator and technique dependent. Most of the devices are pushed or pulled slowly, but others can be manipulated quickly. There is a short learning curve to understand how each technique can be most effectively performed.

It is often helpful to inject a small amount of dilute radiographic contrast material through the side arm of the sheath to visualize the thrombus within the vascular access. The thrombectomy catheter or device then can be directed to remove any residual thrombus fragments.

After removing the thrombus from the venous limb of the graft, the venous angioplasty procedures are performed. It is advantageous to complete all the venous interventions before inserting the second vascular sheath. This second sheath, inserted retrograde into the vascular access, will be used to reach the proximal arterial limb of the graft. The presence of this second sheath within the graft can interfere with movement of angioplasty balloon catheters or other endovascular devices during treatment of the venous stenoses. All venous interventions should be completed before inserting this second sheath.

Treatment of Venous Stenoses

As previously mentioned, the most common location for a stenosis is at, or just beyond, the venous anastomosis (Fig. 27.2). These neointimal hyperplastic lesions can be difficult to open, often requiring the use of high-pressure (20 atm) angioplasty balloons for effective dilatation. The diameter of the balloon should be 10% to 20% greater than the vessel diameter. Typically, a 7-mm- or 8-mm-diameter angioplasty balloon is used to dilate a venous anastomotic stenosis.

Alternatively, if the diagnostic venogram reveals a severe venous stenosis, the venous angioplasty procedure can be performed before thrombus removal. Occasionally, it may

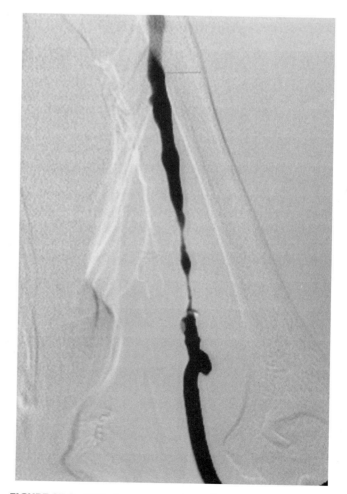

FIGURE 27.2. Typical venous anastomotic stenosis.

be advantageous to assess the results of angioplasty before performing the thrombectomy. If the angioplasty is unsuccessful, the procedure can be terminated without reestablishing blood flow within the vascular access.

Thrombus Removal: Arterial Limb

Following the venous angioplasty procedure, the interventionalist then will need to remove the thrombus from the proximal arterial limb, which is behind (downstream to) the first vascular sheath. To reach the proximal arterial limb, a second puncture is made, in a retrograde direction, into the venous segment of the graft, and a second vascular sheath is inserted. The thrombectomy catheter or device is inserted through this second sheath and advanced into the proximal arterial segment to remove the remaining thrombus. The first vascular sheath, which is within the arterial segment, can be temporarily removed over a guidewire to facilitate thrombus removal. When removing thrombus from the proximal arterial limb, one must avoid unintentional dislodgement of the arterial plug into the adjacent native artery.

Dislodgement of the Arterial Plug

The final step of the procedure is to dislodge the arterial plug. It consists of densely packed red blood cells and fibrin formed into a hard, bullet-shaped plug that is adherent to the graft wall adjacent to the arterial anastomosis. Studies have shown that the volume of the arterial plug is small (<0.5 mL) and represents minimal risk if allowed to embolize to the lung (17,18). Compliant balloons, such as a Fogarty embolectomy balloon or a balloon occlusion catheter, are commonly used to dislodge the arterial plug. A compliant balloon can variably expand, thereby exerting traction on the plug, as it is pulled through the arterial anastomosis into the vascular access. Noncompliant balloons, such as an angioplasty balloon, also can be used to dislodge the arterial plug.

To dislodge the arterial plug, the embolectomy balloon is advanced into the native artery just beyond the arterial anastomosis. Under fluoroscopic observation, the balloon is partially inflated in the artery and gently pulled back through the arterial anastomosis. As the balloon is pulled into the graft, it is further inflated to grasp and dislodge the arterial plug. The arterial plug is often firmly adherent to the graft wall. Three or four passes of the embolectomy balloon usually are required to remove the plug completely. Once dislodged, the arterial plug usually passes quickly through the graft and into the pulmonary circulation.

Lazzaro and colleagues have reported their results using the percutaneous thrombolytic device (PTD) to remove the arterial plug (19). The 9-mm nitinol basket is advanced across the arterial anastomosis in the constrained position. The basket is deployed carefully within the artery and then pulled back across the arterial anastomosis to dislodge the plug. The PTD is not activated during this maneuver. These investigators reported a 6% incidence of arterial embolization using this technique. Once the arterial plug has brought into the graft, it can be fragmented by activation of the PTD.

As previously mentioned, most interventionalists prefer to dilate the venous anastomotic stenosis before dislodging the arterial plug. Opening the venous anastomosis allows the arterial plug to exit the vascular access quickly. This prevents the plug from becoming caught within the graft or at the venous anastomosis. Some interventionalists favor dislodging the arterial plug before performing the venous angioplasty. With this technique, the venous stenosis traps the arterial plug within the graft, allowing it to be fragmented using a mechanical thrombectomy device. Again, there are different styles and techniques, each with its own benefits and risks.

After dislodgement of the arterial plug, there should be restoration of brisk blood flow through the vascular access. A final fistulogram, including examination of the arterial anastomosis, is performed to verify that all the thrombus has been removed, and the venous stenoses have been effectively dilated.

Obtaining Hemostasis

High-flow vascular sheaths can be used if the patient is scheduled for a hemodialysis treatment immediately following the thrombectomy procedure. This type of sheath has high blood flow capabilities (400–500 mL per minute), and the large-caliber side arm allows a direct connection to the blood tubing of the hemodialysis machine. Using this type of high-flow hemodialysis sheath can be advantageous for several reasons. First, the interventionist does not have to obtain hemostasis before dialysis. This saves time for both the physician and the patient. Second, the patient does not have to undergo recannulation with needles for the hemodialysis treatment. The nurse can connect the sheaths directly to the blood tubing of the hemodialysis machine. One final benefit is these high-flow hemodialysis sheaths are short, typically 4 to 6 cm long. This minimizes the amount of obstructive plastic material within the vascular access during the thrombectomy procedure.

If the patient is not going to the hemodialysis center following the thrombectomy procedure, then a pursestring suture can be used to close the vascular access sites. Several different closure methods using a pursestring suture have been reported (20,21). Although different suture materials can be used, in our hands 2-0 Vicryl (Ethicon, Somerville, NJ, U.S.A.) works well for this application. Making two or three small in-and-out bites in the skin around the sheath creates the pursestring suture. The stitch is kept superficial in the skin; it does not pass through the PTFE graft material. Once the suture has been sewn around the sheath, an assistant places a finger over the skin puncture site and removes the sheath while the pursestring suture is tightened and tied. The suture is pulled taut to cinch the tissue around the puncture site, but not too tightly, which might hurt the patient. If the site continues to bleed, lateral tugging on the pursestring suture will effectively control the puncture site until hemostasis is achieved. Typically, the stitch is removed 1 to 3 days after the thrombectomy procedure, usually at the time of the next hemodialysis treatment. This pursestring suture technique substantially reduces the time to achieve hemostasis, particularly when large-diameter vascular access sheaths have been used. Of note, a pursestring suture should not be used in PTFE grafts that are less than 2 months old. The graft must be fully incorporated ("mature") into the surrounding tissue for effective hemostasis using this technique.

MECHANICAL THROMBECTOMY TECHNIQUES

No single percutaneous thrombectomy technique has been proven to be more efficacious than the other methods. A review of the published results from multiple clinical trials reveals that all these techniques are capable of achieving a 3-month primary patency up to 35% to 45% (5–12). These similar results suggest that the long-term patency of a vascular access is independent of the method by which the thrombus is removed. The long-term patency appears to be primarily dependent on the identification and successful treatment of all significant stenoses, both venous and arterial, and the complete removal of the arterial plug.

The choice of thrombectomy technique is often dependent on the physician's expertise and cost conscientiousness. As will be discussed, patient-related variables, such as graft configuration, graft age, or the presence of thrombus in the native veins, can be important determinants in selecting the most appropriate thrombectomy technique.

Balloon Thrombectomy

The concept of "balloon-sweep" thrombectomy was the first "purely mechanical" percutaneous alternative to the then-popular pulse-spray pharmacomechanical thrombolysis technique. This approach was accomplished using a variety of devices to macerate, dislodge, or sweep thrombus from the occluded graft into the central venous circulation. The most commonly used devices were angioplasty balloons, Fogarty- and Bowman-type compliant balloons, and baskets. These purely mechanical techniques, whereby the thrombus within the graft is swept into the central venous circulation, gained popularity in the mid-1990s (22–26). Results were comparable to standard pharmacomechanical thrombolysis in terms of technical success (86%–94%), clinical success at 1 week (59%–76%), and primary patency rates. Complication profiles were also similar (1%–2%), most commonly consisting of arterial emboliza-

tion. One study comparing balloon-sweep thrombectomy to thrombolytic therapy showed shorter procedure time and equivalent efficacy and safety (27). A modified "pull-back" balloon-sweep thrombectomy technique has been proposed as a means to clear rapidly thrombosed hemodialysis grafts from an ipsilateral internal jugular vein approach (24). Objections to this technique have been raised, however, because of the added risk of thrombosis of the internal jugular vein, a significant complication in a hemodialysis patient.

Despite the controversy regarding the appropriateness of deliberate pulmonary embolization, these balloon thrombectomy techniques are generally well tolerated, primarily because the amount of thrombus contained within a thrombosed graft is small, usually less than 4 cm^3 (17,18). The occurrence of symptomatic pulmonary embolism has been very low in most reported series (1–12). One study reported two fatalities, however, that were caused by pulmonary embolism in a series of 43 patients treated with balloon-sweep mechanical thrombectomy (15). Both fatalities occurred in patients with poor cardiac or pulmonary reserve. Therefore, deliberate embolization of the entire contents of a thrombosed graft into the central venous circulation is contraindicated in patients with cardiopulmonary compromise. Other absolute contraindications include a known right-to-left intracardiac shunt, especially with pulmonary hypertension. To reduce the risk of symptomatic pulmonary embolism during balloon thrombectomy procedures, the thrombus should be macerated thoroughly by using balloons before allowing it to enter the central venous circulation.

Balloon-sweep thrombectomy techniques may never become widely accepted as a routine primary thrombectomy method for treatment of thrombosed hemodialysis grafts. The selective use of this technique as an adjunctive method to reduce the thrombus burden or to manage otherwise-resistant occlusive material can be appropriate. Indeed, interventional radiologists for the management of resistant thrombus, most notably the arterial plug, now commonly use this approach.

Thromboaspiration

Thromboaspiration is another useful technique in the armamentarium of the interventional radiologist. It is most useful with fresh thrombus, which is often soft and amenable to suction removal. A variety of thromboaspiration techniques have been described, including the use of a guide catheter or large-bore sheath (22–26) (see also Chapter 30). BAT is another valuable technique with several variations. Standard BAT used a 4 French embolectomy catheter inserted through a 7 or 8 French vascular sheath. The embolectomy balloon is advanced beyond the thrombus within the vascular access. The balloon is inflated and pulled back while aspiration is applied to the sheath, allowing removal of thrombus. An assistant can manually compress and occlude the graft behind the sheath to minimize the risk of retrograde embolization. Another variation uses dual aspiration sheaths and two balloons positioned in opposite directions. One balloon and sheath set is used to pull and aspirate thrombus, and the second balloon is inflated behind the aspiration sheath to ensure a closed system and decrease the risk of embolization.

External massage of the graft alone, or during activation of a mechanical thrombectomy device, can be a valuable adjunctive technique. For example, external massage can be used to move thrombus that is caught between two crossing sheaths. Another useful application of this technique is during treatment of a thrombosed aneurysmal segment of a native fistula. External compression can be used to massage thrombus out of an aneurysmal area so that it can be removed more easily using mechanical methods.

The adherent-clot catheter (ACC) (Edwards Lifesciences, Irvine, CA, U.S.A.) is another useful tool that assists in the removal of firmly adherent material from a vascular access (28). It is most useful for removing fibrotic, organized thrombus creating intragraft stenoses. Because of the relative rigidity the ACC, however, which may result in vascular injury, and the additional expense of this device, balloon angioplasty should be attempted first. The ACC should be reserved for situations where balloon angioplasty has failed.

Mechanical Thrombectomy Devices

Mechanical thrombectomy devices were designed to remove thrombus quickly, effectively, and safely from hemodialysis grafts. Although physicians are using these devices for other applications, including treatment of thrombus in native veins and arteries, it is important to remember that most of these devices have not received approval from the United States Food and Drug Administration (FDA) for these other applications.

Eight different mechanical thrombectomy devices have received approval for use in PTFE hemodialysis grafts (Table 27.1). These include (a) Helix (Microvena, White Bear Lake, MN, U.S.A.), (b) Xpeedior (Possis Medical, Minneapolis, MN, U.S.A.), (c) Trerotola-percutaneous thrombectomy device (PTD) (Arrow International, Reading, PA, U.S.A.), (d) Cragg thrombolytic brush and Castaneda thrombolytic brush (Micro Therapeutics, San Clemente, CA, U.S.A.), (e) Endovac, (f) Oasis catheter, (g) Hydrolyzer catheter, and (h) Thrombex PMT (Edwards Lifesciences, Irvine, CA, U.S.A.). A detailed review of the mechanical design of each device can be found in a review by Sharafuddin and Hicks (29–31).

These different mechanical thrombectomy devices can be divided into two categories based upon their mechanisms of action (29–31). Recirculation-type devices, which include the Helix, Xpeedior, Oasis catheter, Hydrolyzer catheter, and Thrombex PMT, create a hydrodynamic vortex, similar to a kitchen blender, which homogenizes the thrombus, converting it into slurry. The hydrodynamic vortex is created by either a powerful jet spray of fluid (saline) or by a rotating, high-speed micropropeller. Depending on the specific device, the residual thrombus slurry may be aspirated and removed or allowed to embolize to the pulmonary circulation. The non–recirculation-type devices, which include the Trerotola-PTD and the thrombolytic brush catheters (Cragg/Castaneda), use a rapidly spinning wire basket or plastic brush to mechanically fragment the thrombus. The particulate thrombus that remains within the graft can be aspirated through a vascular sheath, dissolved using a thrombolytic agent, or embolized to the pulmonary circulation.

There are no universally accepted techniques for using these mechanical thrombectomy devices when treating a thrombosed vascular access. On the contrary, a wide variety of styles and methods is currently used by interventionists. We may discover that each device has its own niche and is best used for certain specific situations. A busy interven-

TABLE 27.1. CHARACTERISTICS OF CURRENTLY AVAILABLE MECHANICAL THROMBECTOMY DEVICES

Device	Sheath Size (French)	Over-the-Wire	Saline Jets[a]	Aspiration	Price (U.S. $)
Helix	7	No	No	No	$550
Xpeedior	5	Yes	Yes	Yes	$600
PTD	5.5	No[a]	No	No	$600
Brushes	6	Yes	No	No	$600
Oasis	6	Yes	Yes	Yes	$600
Endo Vac	6	No	No	Yes	$350
Hydrolyzer	7	Yes	Yes	Yes	$600
Thrombex	6	Yes	No	Yes	$600

PTD, percutaneous transluminal dilatation.
[a] Catheter uses saline jets to fragment or remove thrombus.

TABLE 27.2. RESULTS USING MECHANICAL THROMBECTOMY DEVICES

Device (Ref. No.)	Tech Success	1 Mo	3 Mo	6 Mo
ATD (4)	89	47		
AngioJet (12)	73	32	15	
PTD (5)	95		39	20
Hydrolyzer (6)	84	57	48	37
Cragg brush (11)	93		37	
Oasis (10)	95	69	40	

ATD, amplatz thrombectomy device; PTD, percutaneous thrombectomy device.

tionist should be familiar with several of these devices to most effectively treat the variety of clinical problems that may be encountered.

Several patient-related variables are important determinants for selecting the optimal technique and thrombectomy device. These include (a) age of thrombus, (b) graft age, (c) graft configuration, (d) presence of thrombus in the native veins, and (e) presence of pseudoaneurysms or intragraft stenoses.

All the mechanical thrombectomy devices are effective for treating fresh thrombus, which is thrombus that is less than 3 days old. Because most thrombectomy procedures are performed within 2 or 3 days after thrombosis of a vascular access, any of these devices should prove useful in most clinical situations. The reported results for the mechanical devices are found in Table 27.2.

Over time, thrombus gradually becomes fibrotic and more resistant to mechanical fragmentation and aspiration. The EndoVac device and the Trerotola-PTD are both useful for treating hardened thrombus. EndoVac is particularly advantageous because of its ability to aspirate and remove chronic thrombus. If these thrombectomy devices fail, then pretreatment with a thrombolytic agent may be beneficial to soften the fibrotic thrombus and allow it to be removed more easily.

Old hemodialysis grafts, particularly those that have previously thrombosed, commonly have a "rind" of hard, fibrotic tissue lining the endoluminal surface (28). This fibrotic material is often densely layered at sites of needle cannulation. A focal accumulation of this tough, fibrous material can create an intragraft stenosis that may interfere with the movement of thrombectomy catheters or devices. In addition, it can be difficult to extract thrombus that is sequestered behind an intragraft stenosis. Although the Trerotola-PTD can be effective in this situation, thick accumulations of this fibrous material are often difficult to remove using conventional endovascular techniques. As previously mentioned, the ACC is a wire basket-like device that can be used to remove this adherent material. Eventually, these fibrotic segments of the graft will need to be surgically replaced.

Graft configuration is another important consideration when selecting a mechanical thrombectomy device. Loop-configuration grafts that have an acute angle at the apex can be difficult to traverse with a mechanical device. Devices that contain a mechanical drive shaft can become problematic when activated across acute angles. The rotational speed of the Trerotola-PTD and the Cragg/Castaneda brushes may be reduced when used around sharp corners. The drive shaft of the 8 French Clot Buster (Microvena, White Bear Lake, MN, U.S.A.) has a tendency to break when activated around acute angles; this problem has been remedied with the new 7 French "Helix" version of the Amplatz thrombectomy device (ATD). Thrombectomy devices that are guidewire compatible and do not contain a rotating drive shaft, such as the Xpeedior, the Oasis, and Hydrolyzer catheters, are advantageous for negotiating sharp corners and through intragraft stenoses.

When confronted with an acute angulation, such as a sharply curved graft apex, one solution is to use the "apex-stick" access approach (32). Using this technique, the graft is entered directly at the apex (Fig. 27.3). Entry into the

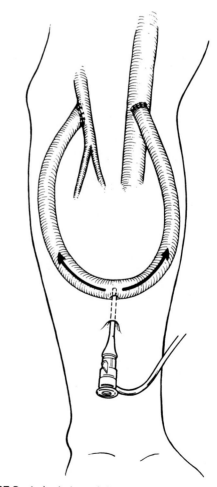

FIGURE 27.3. A depiction of the apex stick technique for access into a hemodialysis graft.

middle (equator) of the graft apex allows easier manipulation when changing directions from venous limb to arterial limb. On puncturing the graft, the needle is rotated in the horizontal plane until the tip is directed into the venous limb. The guidewire is advanced into the venous limb and a vascular sheath is inserted. After successful thrombectomy and angioplasty of the venous limb, the vascular sheath then is redirected into the arterial limb; reinserting the introducer into the vascular sheath and backing the sheath out of the graft over the introducer accomplishes this. Under close fluoroscopic observation, the introducer is carefully withdrawn until the tip can be rotated horizontally toward the arterial limb of the graft. The guidewire then is advanced out of the introducer toward the arterial anastomosis. The sheath is reinserted into the arterial limb over the introducer.

In addition to thrombus within the vascular access, thrombus can extend into the native veins. The volume of thrombus within the native veins can be substantial. When using conventional pulse-spray thrombolysis techniques, this situation presents a difficult and time-consuming chore to remove such extensive amounts of thrombus. With mechanical thrombectomy devices, the thrombus in the native veins can be quickly and easily removed, a clear advantage for using any of these devices (Fig. 27.4).

Thrombectomy devices that aspirate and have over-the-wire capabilities are advantageous when removing native vein thrombus. A guidewire can be helpful to lead the device through the thrombosed native vein and prevent the tip from catching on side branches and valve cusps.

There continues to be concern regarding the use of wall-contact thrombectomy devices, such as the Trerotola-PTD and the Cragg/Castaneda brushes, in native vessels. Although any mechanical thrombectomy device may damage the endoluminal surface of a native vessel, devices that directly contact the vessel wall have the potential to be more injurious. Hydrodynamic devices, which use saline jet sprays to fragment and remove thrombus, are probably less traumatic to the endoluminal surface of a native vein.

Pseudoaneurysms arising from a graft or fistula can present another perplexing problem. It can be difficult to maneuver a thrombectomy device into the pseudoaneurysm cavity to remove the thrombus. All the thrombectomy devices are designed to work "in-axis" with the graft and, despite considerable manipulations, it may be impossible to guide the device into a pseudoaneurysm. In addition, the thrombus within a pseudoaneurysm is often older, fibrotic, and resistant to removal. Wall-contact devices can be useful in this situation. The rapidly spinning, 9-mm-diameter

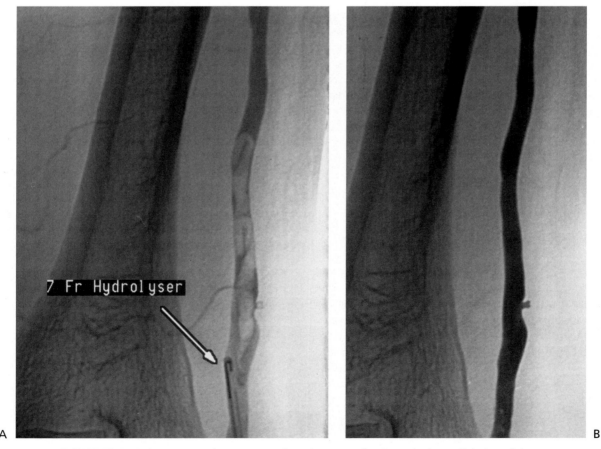

FIGURE 27.4.   **A**: A venogram demonstrates thrombus extending from the hemodialysis graft into the basilic vein. **B**: The thrombus has been removed using the Hydrolyser thrombectomy device.

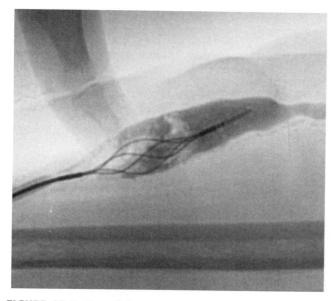

FIGURE 27.5. Use of the percutaneous thrombolytic device (PTD) to remove thrombus from a pseudoaneurysm. The thrombus within the pseudoaneurysm can be manually compressed against the basket.

nitinol basket of the Trerotola-PTD can be used to remove chronic thrombus from a pseudoaneurysm. It is helpful to compress the pseudoaneurysm manually against the spinning basket of the PTD to accelerate fragmentation of the thrombus (Fig. 27.5). The Endovac also can remove thrombus from pseudoaneurysms; suction is activated next to the "neck" of the pseudoaneurysm for a prolonged interval with or without manual compression of the pseudoaneurysm.

CONCLUSION

Mechanical thrombectomy methods can increase the speed of thrombus removal dramatically, thereby decreasing the overall procedure time, a benefit for both the interventionist and the patient. These techniques also eliminate the use of thrombolytic agents and the complications associated with these drugs. For these reasons, mechanical thrombectomy techniques will continue to play an important role in the treatment of thrombosed hemodialysis grafts and fistulae. Removing thrombus is only one part of the overall thrombectomy procedure, however. The long-term patency of the vascular access appears to be dependent on the identification and successful treatment of all hemodynamically significant stenoses and the complete removal of the arterial plug. The cause of thrombosis must be identified and repaired to provide a durable result.

The use of mechanical thrombectomy devices will continue to expand as they are approved for native arterial and venous applications. The clinical performance of these devices also continues to improve; more powerful catheters are already under development. Additional features, such as directional capabilities and variable speed control, will further increase their clinical utility.

REFERENCES

1. Valji K, Bookstein JJ, Roberts AC, et al. Pulse-spray pharmacomechanical thrombolysis of thrombosed hemodialysis access grafts: comparison of original and current techniques. *AJR Am J Roentgenol* 1995;164:1495–1500.
2. Cynamon J, Lakritz PS, Wahl SI, et al. Hemodialysis graft declotting: description of the "lyse and wait" technique. *J Vasc Interv Radiol* 1997;8:825–829.
3. Beathard GA, Welch BR, Maidment HJ. Mecahnical thrombolysis for the treatment of thrombosed hemodialysis grafts. *Radiology* 1996;200:711–716.
4. Uflacker R, Rajagopalan PR, Vujic I, et al. Treatment of thrombosed dialysis access grafts: randomized trial of surgical thrombectomy versus mechanical thrombectomy with the Amplatz device. *J Vasc Interv Radiol* 1996;7:185–192.
5. Trerotola SO, Vesely TM, Lung GB, et al. Treatment of thrombosed hemodialysis access grafts: Arrow-Trerotola percutaneous thrombolytic device versus pulse-spray thrombolysis. *Radiology* 1998;206:403–414.
6. Vorwerk D, Schürmann K, Müller-Leisse C, et al. Hemodynamic thrombectomy of haemodialysis grafts and fistulae: results of 51 procedures. *Nephrol Dial Transplant* 1996;11:1058–1064.
7. Overbosch EH, Pattynama PMT, Aarts HJCNM, et al. Occluded hemodialysis shunts: Dutch multicenter experience with the hydrolyser catheter. *Radiology* 1996;201:485–488.
8. Sofocleous CT, Cooper SG, Schur I, et al. Retrospective comparison of the Amplatz thrombectomy device with modified pulse-spray pharmacomechanical thrombolysis in the treatment of thrombosed hemodialysis access grafts. *Radiology* 1999;213:561–567.
9. Uflacker R, Rajagopalan PR, Vujic I, et al. Treatment of thrombosed dialysis access grafts: randomized trial of surgical thrombectomy versus mechanical thrombectomy with the Amplatz device. *J Vasc Interv Radiol* 1996;7:185–192.
10. Barth KH, Gosnell MR, Palestrant AM, et al. Hydrodynamic thrombectomy system versus pulse-spray thrombolysis for thrombosed hemodialysis grafts: a multicenter prospective randomized comparison. *Radiology* 2000;217:678–684.
11. Dolmatch BL, Castaneda F, McNamara TO, et al. Synthetic dialysis shunts: thrombolysis with the Cragg thrombolytic brush catheter. *Radiology* 1999;213:180–184.
12. Vesely TM, Williams D, Weiss M, et al. Comparison of the AngioJet rheolytic catheter to surgical thrombectomy for the treatment of thrombosed hemodialysis grafts. *J Vasc Interv Radiol* 1999;10:1195–1205.
13. Kinney TB, Valji K, Rose SC, et al. Pulmonary embolism from pulse-spray pharmacomechanical thrombolysis of clotted hemodialysis grafts: urokinase versus heparinized saline. *J Vasc Interv Radiol* 2000;11:1143–1152.
14. Petronis JD, Regan F, Briefel G, et al. Ventilation-perfusion scintigraphic evaluation of pulmonary clot burden after percutaneous thrombolysis of clotted hemodialysis access grafts. *Am J Kidney Dis* 1999;34:207–211.
15. Swan TL, Smyth SH, Ruffenbach SJ, et al. Pulmonary embolism following hemodialysis access thrombolysis/thrombectomy. *J Vasc Interv Radiol* 1995;6:683–686.
16. Trerotola SO, Johnson MS, Schauwecker DS, et al. Pulmonary

emboli from pulse-spray and mechanical thrombolysis: evaluation with an animal dialysis-graft model. *Radiology* 1996:200; 169–176.

17. Sharafuddin MJ, Titus JL, Gu X, et al. Dialysis grafts arterial plug: retrieval using a tulip sheath device in vitro. *Cardiovasc Intervent Radiol* 1997;20:154–158.
18. Winkler TA, Trerotola SO, Davidson DD, et al. Study of thrombus from thrombosed hemodialysis access grafts. *Radiology* 1995; 197:461–465.
19. Lazzaro CR, Trerotola SO, Shah H, et al. Modified use of the Arrow-Trerotola percutaneous thrombolytic device for the treatment of thrombosed hemodialysis access grafts. *J Vasc Interv Radiol* 1999;10:1025–1031.
20. Vesely TM. Use of a purse string suture to close a percutaneous access site after hemodialysis graft interventions. *J Vasc Interv Radiol* 1998;9:447–450.
21. Zaleski GX, Funaki B, Gentile L, et al. Purse-string sutures and miniature tourniquet to achieve immediate hemostasis of percutaneous grafts and fistulas: a simple trick with a twist. *AJR Am J Roentgenol* 2000;175:1643–1645.
22. Trerotola SO, Lund GB, Scheel PJ, et al. Thrombosed dialysis access grafts: percutaneous declotting without urokinase. *Radiology* 1994;191:721–726.
23. Sharafuddin MJA, Kadir S, Joshi SJ, et al. Percutaneous balloon-assisted aspiration thrombectomy of clotted hemodialysis access grafts. *J Vasc Interv Radiol* 1996;7:177–183.
24. Soulen MC, Zaetta JM, Amygdalos MA, et al. Mechanical declotting of thrombosed dialysis grafts: experience in 86 cases. *J Vasc Interv Radiol* 1997;8:563–567.
25. Brossman J, Bookstein JJ. Percutaneous balloon-assisted thrombectomy: preliminary in vivo results with an expandable vascular sheath system. *Radiology* 1998;206:439–445.
26. Turmel-Rodrigues L, Sapoval M, Pengloan J, et al. Manual thromboaspiration and dilatation of thrombosed dialysis access: mid-term results of a simple concept. *J Vasc Interv Radiol* 1997; 8:813–824.
27. Middlebrook MR, Amygdalos MA, Soulen MC, et al. Thrombosed hemodialysis grafts: percutaneous mechanical balloon declotting versus thrombolysis. *Radiology* 1995;196:73–77.
28. Puckett JW, Lindsay SF. Midgraft curettage as a routine adjunct to salvage operations for thrombosed polytetrafluoroethylene hemodialysis access grafts. *Am J Surg* 1988;156:139–143.
29. Sharafuddin MJ, Hicks ME. Current status of percutaneous mechanical thrombectomy devices. Part I: general principle. *J Vasc Interv Radiol* 1997;8:911–921.
30. Sharafuddin MJ, Hicks ME. Current status of percutaneous mechanical thrombectomy devices. Part II: devices and mechanisms of action. *J Vas Interv Radiol* 1998;9:15–31.
31. Sharafuddin MJ, Hicks ME. Current status of percutaneous mechanical thrombectomy devices. Part III: present and future applications. *J Vasc Interv Radiol* 1998;9:209–224.
32. Hathaway P, Vesely TM. The apex puncture technique for mechanical thrombolysis of occluded hemodialysis grafts. *J Vasc Interv Radiol* 1999;10:553–558.

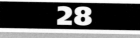

SURGICAL THROMBECTOMY AND REVISION: POLYTETRAFLUOROETHYLENE GRAFTS

AMER RAJAB
MITCHELL L. HENRY

More than 250,000 patients are treated for chronic renal failure yearly. Whereas about 5% will undergo renal transplantation, dialysis remains the only option for the remaining patients. Based on a continuously increasing number of patients on hemodialysis, vascular access surgery has become part of the daily work of many surgeons. Fifteen percent of hospitalizations of patients with end-stage renal disease (ESRD) are caused by vascular access complications. This makes it a major cost as well as a health issue. A significant number of dialysis patients run out of sites for access. Measures to improve the longevity of vascular accesses are needed.

The main complication of all types of vascular access is thrombosis. Palder and associates reported that 91% of all complications of polytetrafluoroethylene (PTFE) grafts were caused by thrombosis (1). The high rate of thrombotic graft loss was supported in a retrospective study by Glanz and colleagues (2) in which there was an 87% incidence of graft failure caused by thrombosis. Many centers report 1- and 3-year patency rates of arteriovenous (AV) grafts of 60% and 20%, respectively. Infection is the next most common cause of graft loss. Albers (3) found that 20% of graft placements were associated with infection resulting in their removal.

Before addressing strategies for the restoration of thrombosed access, it is important to emphasize some points regarding planning and monitoring of the access. Native AV fistulae have been demonstrated to be superior to the PTFE grafts, especially regarding long-term patency and durability. Strategies to increase the percentage of AV fistulae and conversely decrease the use of PTFE grafts need to be implemented to achieve these long-term advantages. Planning strategies aimed at a first attempt to place the wrist AV fistula (Brescia–Cimino), subsequently the cephalic system at the elbow, and finally consideration of using the transposed basilic vein AV fistula in the upper arm should be entertained. If these options are exhausted, then an AV PTFE graft is placed. Avoidance of peripheral vein depletion by indiscriminate placement of intravenous lines, as well as a policy not to use the subclavian vein for temporary dialysis, should be adapted widely.

NATURAL HISTORY

Several studies have outlined the natural history of prosthetic vascular access grafts. Miller and colleagues (4) evaluated prospectively the outcomes of 256 grafts placed at a single institution during a 2-year period. A salvage procedure to maintain graft patency (thrombectomy, angioplasty, or surgical revision) was required in 29% of the grafts at 3 months, 52% at 6 months, 77% at 12 months, and 96% at 24 months. Thus, primary graft survival (time from graft placement to the first intervention) was only 23% at 1 year and 4% at 2 years. A mean of 1.22 interventions per graft-year (pg-y) were required to maintain access patency, including 0.51 pg-y thrombectomies, 0.54 pg-y angioplasties, and 0.17 pg-y surgical revisions. In a longitudinal study, Leapman and colleagues (5) followed up on 387 grafts, which required a total of 261 revisions. Of these, 36% never required a repair, whereas 64% did require surgical intervention. The mean time to revision was 10.5 months after placement, and the 1-year secondary patency rate was 93%. Sicard and colleagues (6) described a 1-year secondary patency rate for PTFE grafts of 87% (n = 613). These patients underwent 894 revisions, or a revision rate of 1.46 per patient. Of these, 33% required one or two interventions, and 31% required three or more procedures to maintain patency. Sabanayagam (7) observed in 1,229 patients receiving 526 PTFE grafts that only one third of PTFE grafts are primarily patent (no revisions) after 5 years, but the secondary patency rate in the same population was 67%. The best patencies were reported by Davidson and colleagues (8) in 446 patients with PTFE grafts. The primary patency rate was

85%, 81%, and 79% at 1, 3, and 5 years, respectively (8). The secondary patency rate was 92%, 88%, and 84% at 1, 3, and 5 years, respectively (8).

SURGERY OR RADIOLOGY?

In recent years, percutaneous transluminal angioplasty (PTA) has grown considerably in popularity for treatment of vascular stenosis. PTA has been shown to be safe, easily performed, and effective (9). Beathard performed 862 cases of PTA on PTFE dialysis access grafts over 6.5 years; with initial success defined as less than 20% residual stenosis, success was obtained in 92% of cases (10). The lesion most effectively treated with percutaneous balloon angioplasty is the short (<2 cm) stenotic outflow lesion. This is the exact lesion that is simply treated surgically with a simple patch angioplasty using either native or prosthetic materials. Long strictures are treated less successfully by balloon angioplasty, and those lesions are best addressed surgically with a short, succinct jump graft. Interventional radiologists frequently refer to surgical intervention of the venous outflow as depleting "venous real estate." It is pointed out that jump grafts use long lengths of vein, which then are not available for any future access revision. Indiscriminate use of the jump graft may indeed do this; however, well-planned surgical rescue of the failing access graft need not deplete significant venous territory. In fact, placement of intravascular stents following balloon angioplasty in venous outflow do indeed render the area unavailable for further surgical therapy, thereby depleting venous real estate, and are currently not recommended.

For thrombosed grafts, nonsurgical treatments also are attempted by pharmacologic, pharmacomechanical, and mechanical thrombolysis. Pharmacologic thrombolysis uses a fibrinolytic enzyme to dissolve the thrombus. The results, however, have been disappointing, with a low success rate, long treatment time, incomplete clot dissolution, and large number of complications (10). In addition, thrombolytic enzymes carry a significant cost. Pharmacomechanical thrombolysis is composed of two phases. The first is pharmacologic, consisting of enzymatic lysis. This is immediately followed by the second phase, mechanical maceration and removal of the remaining clots. Dolmatch and colleagues (11) evaluated the effectiveness of pharmacomechanical thrombolysis with a pulsed spray (n = 34) or a thrombolytic brush catheter (n = 43). The total amount of urokinase used, including secondary interventions, was 243,657 IU with the catheter versus 476,563 IU with the pulsed. At 15 minutes, clot lysis was successful in 66% of the patients with the catheter versus in 19% with the pulsed spray. At 30 minutes, clot lysis was successful in 98% with the catheter versus 47% with the pulsed spray. Complication rates and patency at 3 months were similar for the catheter and the pulsed-spray groups; however, complica-

tions associated with the use thrombolytic enzymes remain. Mechanical thrombolysis avoids the use of thrombolytic enzymes, and early results showed success rates comparable to surgical treatment (12). Undoubtedly, however, small thrombi are being released into the circulation; therefore, the possibility of creating a dangerous pulmonary embolus has been a concern. There is undoubtedly a combined strategy of radiologic intervention plus surgical intervention that can maximally benefit the patients. These decisions need to be made based on the strength of the two disciplines at the local level. (See Chapter 29 for a presentation of the roles of surgery and angioplasty.)

SURGICAL PROCEDURES

Surgical salvage of a failed or failing graft requires an understanding of the mechanisms and anatomic sites of abnormalities. These include (a) arterial inflow, (b) conduit, (c) venous outflow, and (d) remote outflow (more proximal veins or central venous systems).

Arterial Inflow

The arterial inflow is an uncommon site for anatomic abnormalities, which cause or contribute to failing or failed access. Some studies, however, have emphasized that this problem is greater than previously recognized. Angiographic or Duplex ultrasonographic demonstration of the underlying anatomic abnormality before surgical intervention is quite helpful. A short inflow narrowing usually can be repaired easily with a short patch of native or prosthetic material, or the entire anastomosis can be revised. As the age, comorbid conditions, and incidence of diabetic patients with ESRD increase, sites of atherosclerotic arterial narrowing proximal to the access need to be considered. If identified, patch angioplasty or short bypass grafts can effectively alleviate this problem.

Conduit

Long-term studies of the function of prosthetic grafts have led to the realization that graft material can suffer from pseudoaneurysms as a result of repetitive needle sticks, from multiple intragraft stenoses, or as a result of neointimal hyperplasia. Surgical intervention can salvage grafts with either single large symptomatic pseudoaneurysms or multiple aneurysms along the entire graft. The single large symptomatic aneurysm can be easily addressed by dissecting the graft free of the aneurysm at the proximal and distal ends and by passing a short piece of PTFE material around the dilatation (or through the opened aneurysm). End-to-end anastomosis of the PTFE then restores continuity of the graft and excludes the aneurysm. The graft can be used immediately in the areas of the old graft that have not been dis-

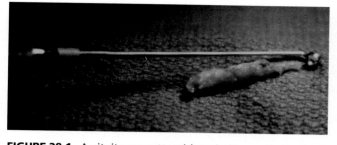

FIGURE 28.1. A pituitary curette with typical hyperplastic debris removed from a thrombosed polytetrafluoroethylene (PTFE) graft.

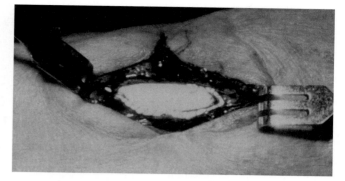

FIGURE 28.3. Goretex (W.L. Gore & Associates) patch used to correct a short stenosis of the outflow tract.

turbed. Multiple aneurysms can be cared for in a similar manner where the arterial and venous ends of the graft are preserved, and a long piece of PTFE is passed outside the existing graft. The venous and arterial ends of the old graft are dissected free and anastomosed to the new graft passed outside the old graft. The old graft can be left in place without consequences.

Surgical curettage has been demonstrated to improve the outcome of grafts undergoing surgical intervention; intragraft stenoses were identified as the cause of failure in 23% of cases in one series (13). Rigid curettes (pituitary or endocervical) passed along the axis of the grafts can clear sites of proliferative material, restoring blood flow to previous levels (Fig. 28.1). Puckett and Lindsay (13) demonstrated superior patency rates in grafts undergoing routine curettage compared with those without it.

Long tunnel infections surrounding a PTFE graft or multiple areas of the graft usually require excision of the entire graft. Local infections can be handled in two ways. The first requires a segmental resection of the infected graft and a short bypass graft placed around the previous site in an uninfected tunnel. The ends then are anastomosed and flow resumed, and the infected piece is excised. For limited surface infections or eschars over the graft, excision of the affected soft tissue and graft coverage with a V-Y skin flap are acceptable.

Venous Outflow Lesions

The most common site of lesions causing graft failure is found in the venous outflow. Pathologic stricture or occlusion of the venous outflow can be addressed surgically by patch angioplasty, intraoperative balloon angioplasty, or prosthetic jump grafting. A short stenosis of the outflow tract (Fig. 28.2) is addressed by opening the venous end of the access graft longitudinally and extending the incision through the stenotic area. Distal outflow can be assessed directly with coronary artery dilators, umbilical catheters (or similar devices), intraoperative angiography, or with angioscopy. If the distal outflow is deemed adequate, a native vein or prosthetic patch is fashioned in an ellipse and sewn to a opening created previously (Fig. 28.3). If the stricture is greater than 2 to 2.5 cm (Fig. 28.4), a short jump graft fashioned from a piece of 6 mm PTFE is used as an extension of the venous end of the graft (Fig. 28.5). Prudent restraint is necessary to preserve as much proximal vein as possible because future interventions may be warranted. Some surgeons have described the use of intraoperative balloon dilatation, which allows a surgical approach as well as the ability to optimally use other interventional techniques.

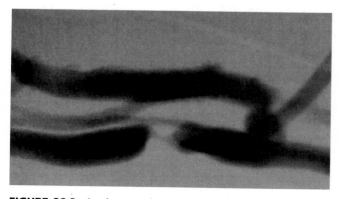

FIGURE 28.2. Angiogram demonstrating short stenosis of the outflow tract in a forearm polytetrafluoroethylene (PTFE) graft.

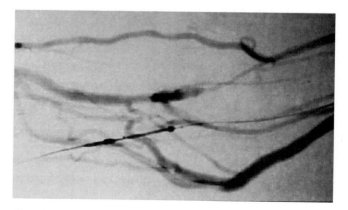

FIGURE 28.4. Angiogram demonstrating a long stenosis of the outflow tract in a forearm polytetrafluoroethylene (PTFE) graft.

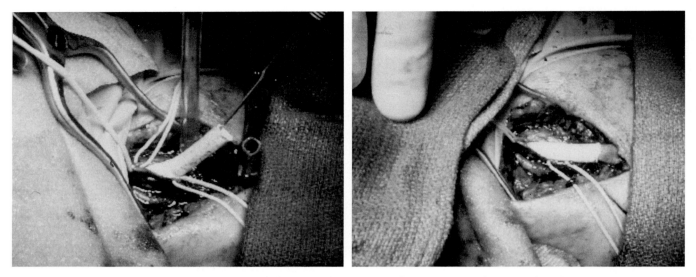

FIGURE 28.5. A short jump graft fashioned from a piece of 6-mm polytetrafluoroethylene (PTFE) is used as an extension to bypass a stenosis of the venous end of the graft.

Central Venous Stenosis

Remote outflow stenosis or occlusion have been identified with increasing frequency as the cause of graft dysfunction or failure. It is hoped that, with the realization that temporary dialysis catheters in the subclavian position cause the vast majority of these lesions, most centers have routinely discontinued the use of subclavian vein, and this will become less of a problem. It should be recognized that central vein stenosis can occur with the catheter placed via the internal jugular vein. PTA of the subclavian vein is the preferred approach, but bypass of the subclavian vein can be accomplished if the former approach fails. Prosthetic graft from the cephalic or basilic system to the ipsilateral jugular vein has been successfully demonstrated (14), often with dramatic relief of symptoms. Direct repair of the subclavian vein has been described (15) but is of a magnitude that should allow its use only after all other possibilities have failed. (See Chapter 25 for an in-depth discussion of central vein lesions.)

Thrombectomy

If the access has thrombosed before intervention, surgical thrombectomy is entertained. The venous end of the graft is isolated with proximal and distal control and opened either transversely or longitudinally. A thrombectomy balloon is passed carefully into the outflow tract and into the central circulation. The balloon is inflated and gently pulled back through the venous tract. Attention is paid to sites of tension with withdrawal of the catheter. This portion is completed when no further clot is extracted and there is good venous back bleeding. The catheter then is advanced to and through the arterial anastomosis and again withdrawn. This portion is completed when brisk arterial bleeding is accompanied by recovery of the classic platelet plug (Fig. 28.6).

We use a further step of graft curettage as well as gentle curettage of the venous outflow. It is the rule rather than the exception to recover more clots and neointimal debris with curettage. Some surgeons routinely use completion angioscopy (16) or angiography and believe that this adds significantly to their outcomes by identifying other lesions that need to be corrected. (See Chapter 29 for more on surgical thrombectomy, intraoperative angiography, and outcomes after surgical salvage.)

OUTCOMES OF SURGICAL INTERVENTION

The National Kidney Foundation has released a document addressing the Dialysis Outcome Quality Initiative (DOQI) for vascular access. These guidelines address expected outcomes for various interventions on the vascular access. The

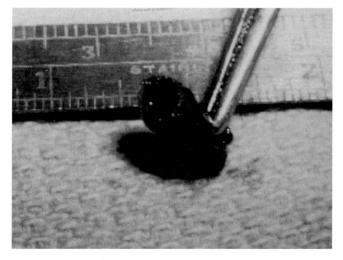

FIGURE 28.6. A platelet plug.

TABLE 28.1. SECONDARY PATENCY RATES (%) OF GRAFTS SALVAGED WITH SURGERY

	No. Patients	1-yr Secondary Patency
Miller et al. (4)	256	77
Marston et al. (17)	56	25
Anderson et al. (18)	100	87
Haimov et al. (19)	95	84
Sabanayagam et al. (20)	225	90
Rapaport et al. (21)	103	89
Raju (22)	312	93
Sterioff (23)	203	87
Mehta (24)	106–1	75
Leapman et al. (5)	397	93
Puckett and Lindsay (25)	127	95
Davidson et al. (8)	174	93
Sabanayagam (7)	1526	98

DOQI guidelines indicate that surgical thrombectomy and revision for thrombosed vascular access are considered successful if there is at least a 40% unassisted post-thrombectomy patency rate at the end of 1 year. They also recommend at least a 70% cumulative patency rate at 1 year after graft creation, regardless of the number of primary interventions or thrombectomies. Toward that end, Table 28.1 presents the 1-year secondary patency rate from several studies. These studies, in relatively large patient populations, demonstrate that surgical intervention can significantly prolong the outcomes of AV grafts used for hemodialysis and meet the 1-year goal of 70%. In fact, single-center results have demonstrated equal outcomes at 1 year when comparing grafts never requiring intervention and those rescued with surgical intervention. Several studies noted that the outcome of AV grafts treated with either patch angioplasty or bypass grafting have equivalent survival, even though they may not have treated the same pathologic lesions in both groups.

SUMMARY

Salvage of the failing or failed access graft begins at the time the access is being planned and placed. Attempts to place increased numbers of native AV fistulae, as well as an overall plan for maximizing access sites, are important. A surveillance policy in the dialysis unit is important as identification of a dysfunctional fistula or graft can allow intervention and superior outcomes to those that have thrombosed. The most common site of abnormalities in prosthetic grafts is the venous outflow.

REFERENCES

1. Palder SB, Kirkman RL, Whittemore AD, et al. Vascular access for hemodialysis: patency rates and results of revision. *Ann Surg* 1985;202:235–239.
2. Glanz S, Bashist B, Gordon DH, et al. Angiography of upper extremity access fistulas for dialysis. *Radiology* 1982;143:45–52.
3. Albers FJ. Causes of hemodialysis access failure. *Adv Renal Replace Ther* 1994;1:107–118.
4. Miller PE, Carlton D, Deierhoi MH, et al. Natural history of arteriovenous grafts in hemodialysis patients. *Am J Kidney Dis* 2000;36:68–74.
5. Leapman SB, Pescovitz MD, Thomalla JV, et al. Salvage surgery for arteriovenous conduits: does it make sense? In: Henry ML, Ferguson RM, eds. *Vascular access for hemodialysis—III.* Chicago: W.L. Gore & Associates, Inc., and Precept Press, 1993:169–185.
6. Sicard GA, Allen BT, Anderson CB. Polytetrafluroethylene grafts for vascular access. In: Sommer BG, Henry ML, eds. *Vascular access for hemodialysis.* Chicago: W.L. Gore & Associates and Precept Press, 1989:51–64.
7. Sabanayagam P. 15-year experience with tapered (4–7 mm) and straight (6 mm) PTFE angio-access in ESRD patients. In: Henry ML, Ferguson RM, eds. *Vascular access for hemodialysis—IV.* Chicago: W.L. Gore & Associates and Precept Press, 1995: 159–168.
8. Davidson IJA, Ar'Rajab A, Balfe P, et al. Long-term outcome of PTFE arteriovenous grafts. In: Henry ML, ed. *Vascular access for hemodialysis—VI.* Chicago: W.L. Gore & Associates and Precept Press, 1999:155–162.
9. Schwab SJ, Saeed M, Sussman SK, et al. Transluminal angioplasty of venous stenoses in polytetrafluoroethylene vascular access grafts. *Kidney Int* 1987;32:395–398.
10. Beathard GA. The treatment of vascular access graft dysfunction: a nephrologist's view and experience. *Adv Ren Replac Ther* 1994;1:131–147.
11. Dolmatch BL, Castaneda F, McNamara TO, et al. Synthetic dialysis shunts: thrombolysis with the Cragg thrombolytic brush catheter. *Radiology* 1999;213:180–184.
12. Uflacker R, Rajagopalan PR, Vujic I, et al. Treatment of thrombosed dialysis access grafts: Randomized trail of surgical thrombectomy versus mechanical thrombectomy with Amplatz device. *J Vasc Interv Radiol* 1996;7:185–192.
13. Puckett J, Lindsay S. Midgraft curettage as a routine adjunct to salvage operation for PTFE hemodialysis access grafts. *Am J Surg* 1988;156:139–143.
14. Polo JR, Echenagusia AMC, Polo J, et al. Bypass to a proximal vein to treat peripheral venous stenosis in PTFE grafts for hemodialysis. In: Henry ML, Ferguson RM, eds. *Vascular access for hemodialysis—V.* Chicago: W.L. Gore & Associates and Precept Press, 1997:127–134.
15. Williams LR, Flinn WR, Yao JST. Spiral vein graft bypass of subclavian obstruction complicating arm dialysis access. In: Sommer BG, Henry ML, eds. *Vascular access for hemodialysis—II.* Chicago: W.L. Gore & Associates and Precept Press, 1991:237–245.
16. Holzenbein TJ, Miller A, Gottlieb MN, et al. The role of routine angioscopy in vascular access surgery. *J Endovasc Surg* 1995;2: 10–25.
17. Marston WA, Criado E, Jaque PE, et al. Prospective randomized comparison of surgical versus endovascular management of thrombosed dialysis access grafts. *J Vasc Surg* 1997;26:373–381.
18. Anderson CB, Sicard GA, Etheredge EE. Bovine carotid artery and expanded polytetrafluoroethylene grafts for hemodialysis vascular access. *J Surg Res* 1980;29:184–188.
19. Haimov M, Burrows L, Schanzer H, et al. Experience with arterial substitutes in the construction of vascular access for hemodialysis. *J Cardiovas Surg* 1980;21:149–154.
20. Sabanayagam P, Schwartz AB, Soricelli RR, et al. A comparative study of 402 bovine heterografts and 225 reinforced expanded PTFE grafts as AVF in the ESRD patient. *Trans Am Soc Artific Intern Organs* 1980;26:88–91.
21. Rapaport A, Noon GP, McCollum CH. Polytetrafluoroethylene (PTFE) grafts for hemodialysis in chronic renal failure: assess-

ment of durability and function at three years. *Aust N Z J Surg* 1980;51:562–567.

22. Raju S. PTFE grafts for hemodialysis access. *Ann Surg* 1987;206: 666–673.

23. Sterioff S. Salvage of the failing vascular access. In: Sommer BG, Henry ML, eds. *Vascular access for hemodialysis*. Chicago: W.L. Gore & Associates and Precept Press, 1989:153–162.

24. Mehta S. Statistical summary of clinical results of vascular access procedures for hemodialysis. In: Sommer BG, Henry ML, eds. *Vascular access for hemodialysis-II*. Chicago: W.L. Gore & Associates and Precept Press, 1991:145–157.

25. Puckett JW, Lindsay SF. Graft curettage. In: Henry ML, Ferguson RM, eds. *Vascular access for hemodialysis—III*. Chicago: W.L. Gore & Associates and Precept Press, 1993:186–195.

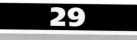

29

SALVAGE OF THE THROMBOSED DIALYSIS ACCESS GRAFT: SURGICAL VERSUS RADIOLOGIC METHODS
DOES IT MATTER?

GARY GELBFISH
WILLIAM A. MARSTON

The maintenance of functional vascular access for patients on hemodialysis is one of the most difficult problems for practitioners involved in the care of these patients. Despite concerted efforts to increase the frequency of primary arteriovenous (AV) fistula construction for hemodialysis patients, fewer than 50% of patients are being dialyzed via an AV fistula in the vast majority of hemodialysis units. Instead, a prosthetic bridge fistula is used. Unfortunately, the average primary patency of prosthetic hemodialysis grafts averages 12 to 18 months in most reports (1–4). The average hemodialysis patient can expect an episode of graft thrombosis every 12 to 15 months, and access problems are the most common reason of admission for dialysis patients, accounting for more than 500 million dollars per year in health care costs (5,6).

Currently, both open surgical and percutaneous techniques have been developed for salvage of thrombosed hemodialysis grafts. The dialysis outcome quality initiatives (DOQI) guidelines carefully outlined expected results for thrombosed hemodialysis grafts (7). Graft salvage should be performed rapidly, with the patient under local anesthesia, and in an outpatient setting unless other medical issues require hospital admission. Central venous catheters should be avoided. The expected patency after percutaneous salvage should be 40% at 3 months and for surgical salvage 50% at 6 months. A higher patency rate was set for surgical patency because open surgical techniques are more invasive and may use veins extending up the arm that would not be affected by percutaneous techniques.

An optimal protocol of management of clotted hemodialysis grafts has not been clearly defined. In this chapter, we review the primary surgical and percutaneous techniques for management of the thrombosed hemodialysis graft and describe the strengths and weaknesses of each. In most practice situations, a combination of these techniques will provide optimal results, but each dialysis center should assess available resources and professional talents to determine how best to manage the thrombosed dialysis graft. Finally, the ideal method should be as cost-effective as possible. It is imperative that centers develop protocols of management to allow effective use of manpower and resources and to preserve access sites for optimal patient care.

CAUSES OF GRAFT FAILURE

Most AV grafts thrombose because of myointimal hyperplasia of the venous outflow tract. Valji and colleagues reported that graft angiography after graft thrombectomy identified stenosis limited to the venous anastomosis in 77% of cases (Fig. 29.1). Longer-segment outflow stenosis was found in 9%. Other causes identified were arterial anastomotic stenosis in 18% and intragraft stenosis in 7% (8). In the study by Marston and colleagues comprising 115 patients, venous outflow disease was identified as the cause of graft failure in 85% (9). In this report, 55% were limited to the anastomotic area and 30% were more extensive long-segment stenoses or venous occlusions (Fig. 29.2). Again, a relatively small number of grafts failed because of other causes (Table 29.1).

SURGICAL SALVAGE TECHNIQUES

The technique of surgical salvage is critical to obtain optimal results. All graft thromboses cannot be treated with a single solution, and the theoretic advantage of open procedures is the ability to provide a specific solution to the cause of thrombosis that may have a better chance of long-term patency than balloon angioplasty of the diseased graft or venous segment. The cause of thrombosis must be determined to allow a specific solution. The technique advocated is not

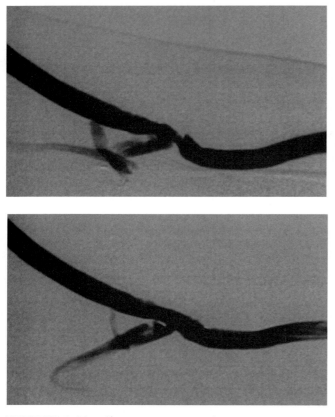

FIGURE 29.1. Top: Short-segment stenosis at venous anastomosis of polytetrafluoroethylene dialysis access graft. **Bottom**: Anastomotic region of venous anastomosis after percutaneous balloon angioplasty revealing resolution of stenotic lesion.

a blind surgical technique relying on "feel" to determine the cause of failure but instead uses elements of radiologic intervention as well.

Proper equipment is important, as always. A table, which allows unobstructed fluoroscopy of the involved extremity and venous outflow to the right atrium, is essential, as is fluoroscopic equipment, mobile or fixed, that will allow a high-quality angiogram to be performed and evaluated. Balloon thrombectomy catheters, including over-the-wire thrombectomy catheters, are essential, as are appropriate guidewires to facilitate crossing difficult lesions.

Graft salvage may be performed with the patient under local anesthesia, which is usually adequate for forearm graft revision procedures. If an upper-arm graft requires revision with a jump graft in the axilla, a regional block is often desirable for patient comfort. The graft is accessed at a superficial location with a small incision.

Graft thrombectomy is performed in standard fashion with thrombectomy balloon catheters until the inflow and outflow are reestablished. Angiography of the graft must be performed to identify the cause of thrombosis and allow a specific corrective solution. In our experience and in other reports, thrombectomy alone was rarely successful in establishing long-term graft function. In 12 patients treated with thrombectomy alone, the 3-month patency was 21% (9).

An angiogram may be performed intraoperatively using mobile fluoroscopy units. Both anastomoses and the venous outflow tract, including the central venous drainage to the right atrium, should be evaluated. Graft angiography allows the surgeon to identify the specific cause(s) of graft failure in most cases as outlined already. Of interest is the frequency of causes other than venous anastomotic stenosis and grafts with multiple areas of pathology. The performance of blind revisions based on presumed venous anastomotic stenoses often leave the true cause of shunt failure uncorrected and a predictably poor outcome. It is our strong belief that comprehensive anatomic data are necessary for accurate surgical intervention. This approach most likely will yield the maximum graft patency after a given surgical intervention.

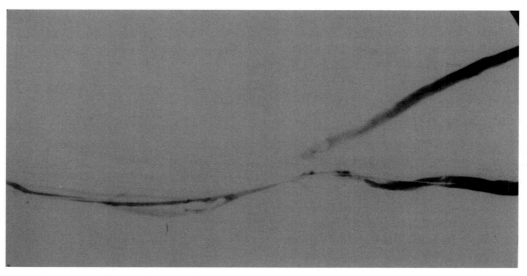

FIGURE 29.2. Polytetrafluoroethylene dialysis access graft after percutaneous thrombectomy revealing long-segment stenosis of venous outflow tract.

TABLE 29.1. CAUSE OF SHUNT THROMBOSIS BY TREATMENT GROUPS

Cause of Shunt Thrombosis	All Patients	Surgical Group	EV Group (%)
Venous anastomotic stenosis	63 (55%)	50	59
Long segment outflow stenosis	23 (20%)	16	24
Venous outflow occlusion	11 (10%)	13	7
Arterial anastomotic stenosis	7 (6%)	9	3
Central venous stenosis	17 (15%)	15	14
Intragraft stenosis	6 (5%)	5	5
Other	4 (3%)	5	2
None identified	4 (3%)	7	0

EV, endovascular.
No significant difference in any category between surg and EV groups.

In cases of venous anastomotic stenosis, we prefer to perform a short-segment jump graft, but patch angioplasty of the anastomosis also can be performed if the lesion is limited. To perform a jump graft, a new segment of vein proximal to the diseased area is exposed and prepared for anastomosis. The thrombosed graft is isolated over a 1-cm length 2 to 3 cm from the venous anastomosis and divided transversely. The old graft is oversewn on the venous side, and a short segment of new polytetrafluoroethylene (PTFE) is obtained and tunneled from this site to the newly exposed vein site. We prefer to use a ringed segment of PTFE to limit kinking across the elbow joint. The new PTFE segment is sewn end-to-end to the old shunt and end-to-side to the new segment of vein.

Grafts that thrombose because of venous outflow occlusion or long-segment outflow stenosis (extending up the arm away from the anastomosis) have a very low chance of long-term patency after salvage procedures unless a new venous outflow tract can be used. In our experience, attempted percutaneous salvage or salvage with thrombectomy alone maintained graft function in only 9% at 3 months (9). Essentially, the only patients in this group to have long-term graft function were those who had their venous outflow revised to a new patent vein. As would be expected, an angiogram or duplex scan is helpful to assess the suitability of any accessory veins for this revision. One must note, however, that in this situation, it is important to determine whether revision to another vein would prohibit the creation of a cephalic or basilic vein transposition fistula because these may be preferable to revision of the existing graft (see Chapters 14 and 31 for transposition fistulae).

In some cases, an arterial anastomotic problem or an intragraft stenosis is identified. The arterial anastomosis can be revised, or a new segment of PTFE can be inserted into the graft as needed. Occasionally, purulent material mixed with thrombus is encountered on opening the graft. A dilemma then arises concerning whether this requires graft removal or not, particularly in the patient with no systemic or external evidence of infection. We previously had not considered salvage of a graft in this situation, but there are several reports of successful salvage using a segment of cry-

opreserved vein (Cryolife, Inc.) inserted into the graft through the area of possible infection (10). This option should be considered, particularly in patients with limited remaining access sites. (See Chapter 16). After surgical salvage, there should rarely be a need for hospital admission unless a more complex revision is required or a complication occurs.

Results of Surgical Arteriovenous Graft Salvage

Detailed studies of the length of AV graft function after surgical salvage are few, and the reported results are contradictory. Earlier studies reported particularly good results, with prolonged graft function after salvage. Palder and colleagues reported on 189 episodes of graft thrombosis; flow was reestablished by thrombectomy alone in 87%. Recurrent thrombosis was common, however, and, after a second episode, a significantly longer cumulative patency was obtained by performing a bypass around an outflow stenosis than with repeat thrombectomy. Almost 60% of grafts required more than one revision, but the cumulative access patency from the time of construction was reported as greater than 60% at 3 years, similar to grafts that were not revised (2). Rizzuti and colleagues also reported that the use of graft revision extended secondary graft patency to that of unrevised grafts, approximately 50% at 3 years (11). Again, shunt angiography was deemed critical at the time of salvage to guide revision. Etheridge and colleagues reported a 54% secondary patency at 1 year after graft revision, often requiring multiple procedures for continued patency (12).

Conversely, Brotman and colleagues reported a 25% patency at 120 days for revised AV grafts after thrombosis (13), and Beathard reported a 15% patency at 6 months for thrombectomy alone and 33% patency at 6 months after thrombectomy and surgical revision (14). It is difficult to reconcile these large variations in reported results, but it is likely that population differences and selection of patients for salvage are important factors. Most investigators agree that graft revision guided by intraoperative angiography, particularly with jump extension around outflow stenoses, is preferable to thrombectomy alone. The degree of any such enhancement of surgical results by anatomic data obtained through intraoperative angiography has never been studied. It is self-evident, however, that a positive impact would be expected.

PERCUTANEOUS SALVAGE TECHNIQUES

The procedure of percutaneous declotting for AV grafts has evolved to a significant degree since lytic therapy was first used for restoring graft patency almost 20 years ago. Most innovations concern the method of treatment of the clot contained within the graft. Options include (a) traditional lysis by slow infusion, (b) pulse spray lysis, (c) lyse and wait, (d) purely mechanical means of displacing the clot; and (e) treatment of the clot via mechanical thrombectomy devices of various designs and mechanical principles. The plethora of available techniques and personal preferences yield an almost innumerable number of ways to declot an AV graft. (See Chapters 26, 27, and 30 for detailed presentations of percutaneous salvage techniques.)

Although the precise technique and sequence may vary, all methods of percutaneous declotting consist of the following steps: (a) the clot is cleared from the graft using any of the aforementioned methods; (b) balloon dilatation is performed on any noted stenosis; (c) flow is restored by dislodging the arterial plug; and (d) a complete evaluation of the arterial inflow and venous outflow is performed.

Results of Percutaneous Arteriovenous Graft Salvage

All declotting techniques have reported remarkably similar postintervention patency rates with immediate graft patency of 80% to 95% and a 3-month patency of approximately 40% (15). This is not unexpected because all clotting methods share the same endpoint: to restore graft flow without residual clot and to treat pathology via percutaneous means. It is widely accepted that graft patency after a declotting procedure is probably independent of the method used to treat the clot. Instead, patency after a procedure is a function of (a) patient selection, (b) the underlying pathology and its response to percutaneous therapy, and (c) the individual skill of the practitioner.

Outstanding Issues Regarding Percutaneous Therapy

Through significant innovation, percutaneous therapy of clotted grafts has become a viable and, according to some, a preferable alternative to open surgery. Several areas of insufficient data and controversy remain, however. These include (a) the precise role and timing of surgical intervention as an adjunct to percutaneous therapy, (b) the role of stents in poorly responsive venous stenosis, and (c) the clinical importance of recurrent subclinical pulmonary emboli. We will address each area briefly.

The first and the most important issue concerns patients with recurrent thrombosis. When does a patient cease to be a candidate for percutaneous therapy and instead is best treated by surgical revision? Associated questions include the following: What is a reasonable minimum patency for a percutaneous procedure? Also, considering that percutaneous therapy is minimally invasive and in most cases "vein-preserving," what is an appropriate differential in acceptable results when comparing percutaneous with surgical therapy for a given anatomic lesion? Because every patient presents with a unique anatomic pathology, which lesions are specifically amenable to surgical or percutaneous therapy? Furthermore, when patients with relatively benign anatomic pathology develop rethrombosis, how do we determine when to proceed with a surgical revision or, instead, to perform repeated percutaneous declotting and ascribe closure to nonanatomic causes, such as hypotension, poor cannulation technique, hypercoagulable state, and so on?

Unfortunately, there are few data to answer any of these questions or to support a firm recommendation. Each case should be decided individually using clinical experience and judgment coupled with knowledge of the precise anatomy, the patient's previous response to therapy, and input from the patient's nephrologist, surgeon, and interventionalist.

The second issue is the role of stents for venous lesions that recoil. Although several studies have explored this issue, the precise role of stents has not been defined (16,17). We are relatively restrictive in our use. We advocate the use of stents in the immediate venous outflow of grafts when not surgically accessible, in central venous stenosis only when flow is insufficient to maintain graft patency, and when significant swelling of the extremity persists despite balloon angioplasty. Venous rupture/salvage and poor surgical risk are other indications. When a stent is placed, the shortest possible length should be used.

The last area of controversy regards the potential long-term effects of recurrent pulmonary emboli. These emboli are known to occur during percutaneous declotting procedures because clot displacement is to some degree an integral component of all described percutaneous techniques. The extent to which this occurs, however, depends on the efforts of the physician to remove clot from the graft and, at times, the venous outflow of the graft. These efforts range from meticulous aspiration of clot using clot-extraction devices, to the wholesale central displacement of clot using saline or Fogarty catheters.

An editorial by Dolmatch and colleagues raised the issue of pulmonary emboli from percutaneous procedures (18). A clinical report by Swan and colleagues further highlighted the potential for pulmonary embolism by showing pulmonary perfusion abnormalities in 59% of patients undergoing percutaneous thrombectomy with urokinase lysis and also reported two deaths attributed to pulmonary embolism (19).

Some investigators have minimized the theoretic potential for harm, citing the finding of an average of 3.2 cc of clot per graft in a study of 22 thrombosed dialysis grafts (20). We take issue with such logic because the long-term effects of even a few cubic centimeters of clot is not known, particularly when macerated into multiple small fragments and then widely distributed throughout the lung vasculature, where they can plug small vessels and cause further thrombosis. There are additional reasons why this apparently small clot volume is not reassuring to us: As with any average, some patients may have a significantly greater clot burden than 3.2 cc, especially with long grafts. Second, clot may exist in the venous outflow of grafts. This native venous clot often fills the entire venous lumen and may be several centimeters long, especially in the large upper-arm veins or in more distal veins when a proximal stenosis is present. Venous clot is typically laminated and firm, unlike the poorly formed clot that exists in synthetic grafts. If not removed or adequately lysed, this clot can embolize in one piece once flow is restored. We are aware of several unpublished reports of acute pulmonary embolization and death under these circumstances. Third, many patients are chronically ill and may have a limited preexisting pulmonary reserve. This is typically not evaluated prior to referral for AV access procedures. Fourth, multiple procedures are the norm, making small, yet cumulative pulmonary damage a distinct possibility.

A study by Kinney and colleagues may provide some credibility to the prospect of long-term pulmonary sequelae. A report by these researchers compared saline and urokinase pulse spray declotting procedures and the incidence of pulmonary perfusion defects prior to and after the procedure in a cohort of 27 patients (21). This group had histories of multiple previous percutaneous thrombectomies (3.1 ± 4.3 episodes per patient.) Although the average age of the group was only 48.4 ± 18.2 years, an astounding 70.4% had abnormal perfusion defects (≥20% segmental perfusion defect) before the index procedure. The average number of affected segments was 2.3 ± 3.1. Of note is that no patients had any pulmonary symptoms during the procedure. Whereas a conclusion regarding the contribution of previous thrombectomies is not possible based on this study, we believe this report should provide the impetus for further study of this issue.

To study this issue, we first would need to control for other potential contributing factors. Patients would need to be randomized and followed up over the course of multiple thrombectomies using various declotting techniques, with baseline pulmonary studies performed before the first declotting episode or at the time of the first graft implantation. Admittedly, such a study ultimately might prove the benign nature of clot embolization. Until this occurs, however, our preferred technique is to remove clot with thrombectomy devices that extract clot rather than use maceration thrombectomy devices or lytic therapy. We pay close attention to clot in the venous outflow tract and will not restore flow to the graft until this clot is adequately removed. This approach satisfies our own aversion to intentional embolization in the absence of proof of its benign nature and especially after the data presented by Kinney and colleagues (21).

COMPARATIVE STUDIES

Several important questions concerning the comparative benefits of surgical and percutaneous graft salvage techniques require investigation with prospective randomized trials. The primary patency after a single intervention is an important question, but more relevant is the secondary, long-term graft patency after multiple interventions using a given technique. The relative cost of each technique is also critical information. The first question of primary patency after a single intervention was addressed by several prospective studies.

Marston and colleagues randomized 115 patients with thrombosed AV grafts to surgical (n = 56) or percutaneous (n = 59) salvage (9). All grafts were followed up until failure, and data were reported on an intent-to-treat basis. The results with both techniques were relatively poor, with surgical salvage rates significantly better than percutaneous, as illustrated in Figure 29.3. The incidence of long-segment

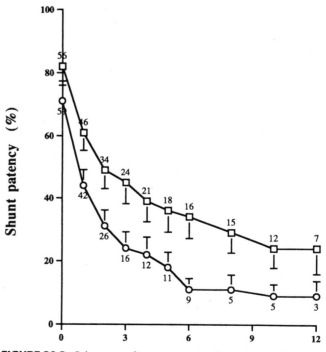

FIGURE 29.3. Primary graft patency rate after salvage of thrombosed dialysis access grafts treated with surgical (*squares*) compared with endovascular techniques (*circles*). Patency rates are significantly different by log-rank test (*p* < 0.05).

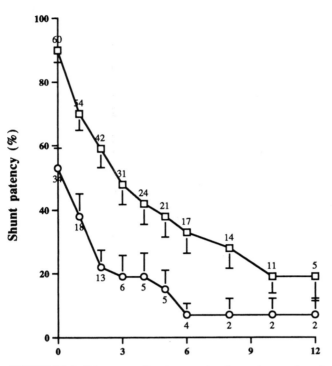

FIGURE 29.4. Primary graft patency rate after salvage of grafts that thrombosed as a result of venous anastomotic stenosis (*squares*) compared with grafts with long-segment venous outflow stenosis or occlusion (*circles*). Patency rates are significantly different by log-rank test ($p < 0.01$).

outflow stenosis or occlusion was high, and these lesions were in part responsible for the poor results of percutaneous salvage using balloon angioplasty. Figure 29.4 compares the results for these grafts with grafts that failed due to stenosis limited to the venous anastomosis.

Daugherty and colleagues randomized 80 patients prospectively to a surgical salvage procedure (using intraoperative angiography to guide the procedure) or percutaneous salvage using mechanical thrombectomy (22). Similar results to those of the previous study were obtained. At 12 months after graft salvage, 30% of the surgically revised grafts continued to function for dialysis, which was significantly higher than 14% for the percutaneous group. Of interest, in this study, the assisted primary patency after graft salvage is reported, reflecting the use of further procedures to maintain graft patency. Figure 29.5 illustrates these results.

Vesely and colleagues reported a multicenter prospective trial of the use of the AngioJet rheolytic catheter and angioplasty compared with surgical salvage procedures in 153 patients (23). There were protocol problems in each group. In the AngioJet group, a well-defined protocol for use was lacking, and there was insufficient power to remove clot in all grafts. In the surgical group, 73% were treated by thrombectomy alone with no attempted corrective procedure. Patency results were poor in each group, with only 15% of the AngioJet group and 26% of the surgical group patent at 3

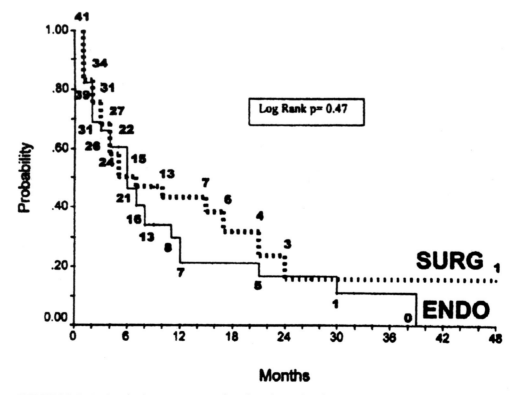

FIGURE 29.5. Assisted primary patency of grafts salvaged with surgical versus endovascular techniques reflecting function rate after repeated salvage procedures.

months. There was no statistical difference between the two groups.

These studies suggest that if primary patency after salvage is the most important goal, surgical salvage may be the preferred method. Given the results of surgical salvage in these studies, most patients will require multiple procedures for long-term graft function, and the more important question concerns the long-term secondary graft patency or the time until the graft is abandoned and a new access is required.

Beathard addressed the question of long-term graft salvage with multiple procedures in a nonrandomized, historical controlled study (14). In this large study of 466 patients with AV graft thrombosis, surgical salvage was used primarily during one 12-month period, followed by percutaneous salvage in a subsequent 12-month period. Beathard found that the use of thrombolysis as the primary method of graft salvage did not result in an increase in the number of episodes of thrombosis per graft, but it significantly reduced the need for surgical graft revision by two thirds. To date, no large prospective, randomized trials of secondary graft patency after multiple interventions have been conducted.

Only two studies comparing the cost of the two techniques have been reported. Vesely and colleagues reported a median cost for percutaneous salvage using thrombolysis plus angioplasty of $6,062, compared with $5,580 for surgical graft salvage (24). There was no significant difference in these costs. Marston and colleagues found that the median cost of percutaneous treatment was significantly lower at $2,958 using primarily mechanical thrombectomy, compared with $4,155 for surgical treatment (25). Of course, because these techniques are in continual evolution, the costs may be affected profoundly by the cost of new equipment used for each procedure. (See also introduction of Chapter 26 and Chapter 28 for additional viewpoints on surgery versus percutaneous treatments.)

COMBINED SALVAGE PROTOCOLS

As outlined by Gelbfish, a protocol using only surgical or percutaneous techniques is likely to result in suboptimal outcomes (26). Given the variety of causes of AV graft thrombosis, it would be surprising if a single technique of salvage were optimal for all patients. Minimally invasive procedures that do not require surgical incisions are clearly preferred by patients whenever possible. We believe that an approach that defines the causative problem and allows a specific solution will provide the best chance of long-term graft salvage.

Ideally, thrombosed grafts should be salvaged in a dedicated suite that is capable of both high-quality vascular imaging and open surgical procedures. The patients should be treated expeditiously to minimize the need for temporary dialysis catheters. Given the excellent initial results of percutaneous thrombectomy for clearing thrombus, the proce-

dure should be performed in this fashion to clear the graft and allow an angiogram to be performed. This should image the entire graft, the arterial and venous anastomoses, and the venous outflow tract, including the central veins.

If a lesion amenable to percutaneous angioplasty is found, it should be done. Clearly, central venous lesions and intragraft stenoses should be treated in this fashion. Venous anastomotic stenoses can be treated easily with angioplasty, and, if a good result is obtained initially, the patient should be monitored closely for recurrent graft dysfunction. If this occurs soon after angioplasty, the patient may benefit more from surgical revision than frequent repeated angioplasty. The time of benefit from angioplasty is varies with the individual patient, but we consider a patient who has recurrent graft dysfunction within 2 months a good candidate for surgical revision. If an occlusion or long-segment venous stenosis is identified, the patient is unlikely to benefit from angioplasty, and the patient should be converted to a surgical revision at that time, generally with a jump graft to a more proximal patent vein. It must be noted that the diagnosis of a long-segment stenosis must be made carefully only after flow has been restored and the appropriate angioplasty has been performed. We have found that a preliminary outflow venogram in a clotted graft often poorly predicts the quality of the venous outflow, secondary to venous spasm or the normal venous caliber reduction that often occurs in the absence of flow

Dedicated dialysis salvage units with the capabilities described herein may be relatively rare but will likely impact on the ability to provide improved graft salvage with a reduced need for temporary dialysis catheters. These protocols should be combined with surveillance programs to identify and correct graft problems before thrombosis whenever possible. Cooperative management of these difficult cases using the skills of multiple specialists will result in improved outcomes (27,28).

Unfortunately, most dialysis centers do not have the facilities described here available to them; either multispecialty expertise is not available, or timely access to radiology suites or operating rooms is difficult. In each case, individualization is necessary, and the primary requirement in each center offering dialysis access is physician interest and expertise. Unfortunately, many centers do not have the luxury of surgical and interventional experts involved in dialysis graft salvage. In these situations, nephrologists will likely seek out the practitioners with the best results to treat their patients and help maintain access patency.

SUMMARY

Minimally invasive percutaneous thrombectomy is an established method of restoring access patency. Surgical revision of unresponsive lesions can salvage percutaneous failures, especially after the precise anatomic pathology has been defined. To optimize patient care, the treating physician must be familiar with the patient's previous response to therapy and the benefits and limitations of the various declotting techniques. Further study is necessary to define precisely treatment protocols and surgical intervention guidelines. The role of stents and the long-term impact of clot embolization also require additional study.

REFERENCES

1. Munda R, First R, Alexander JW, et al. Polytetrafluoroethylene graft survival in hemodialysis. *JAMA* 1983;249:219–222.
2. Palder SB, Kirkman RL, Whittemore AD, et al. Vascular access for hemodialysis: patency rates and results of revision. *Ann Surg* 1985;202:235–239.
3. Coburn MC, Carney WI. Comparison of basilic vein and polytetrafluoroethylene for brachial arteriovenous fistula. *J Vasc Surg* 1994;20:896–904.
4. Tordoir JH, Hofstra L, Leunissen KM, et al. Early experience with stretch polytetrafluoroethylene grafts for hemodialysis access surgery: results of a prospective randomized study. *Eur J Vasc Endovasc Surg* 1995;9:305–309.
5. Lazarus JM, Huang WH, Lew NL, et al. Contribution of vascular access-related disease to morbidity of hemodialysis patients. In: Henry ML, Ferguson R, eds. *Vascular access for hemodialysis—III*. Hong Kong: Precept Press, 1993:3–13.
6. Port FK. The end-stage renal disease program: trends over the past 18 years. *Am J Kidney Dis* 1992;20(Suppl 1):3–7.
7. National Kidney Foundation Dialysis Outcome Quality Improvement (NKF-DOQI). *Clinical practice guidelines for vascular access.* New York: National Kidney Foundation, 1997:55–56.
8. Valji K, Bookstein JJ, Roberts AC, et al. Pharmacomechanical thrombolysis and angioplasty in the management of clotted hemodialysis grafts: early and late clinical results. *Radiology* 1991;178:243–247.
9. Marston WA, Criado E, Jaques PF, et al. Prospective randomized comparison of surgical versus endovascular management of thrombosed dialysis access grafts. *J Vasc Surg* 1997;26:373–381.
10. Matsuura JH, Johansen KH, Rosenthal D, et al. Cryopreserved femoral vein grafts for difficult hemodialysis access. *Ann Vasc Surg* 2000;14:50–55.
11. Rizzuti RP, Hale JC, Burkhart TE. Extended patency of expanded polytetrafluoroethylene grafts for vascular access using optimal configuration and revisions. *Surg Gynecol Obstet* 1988;166:23–27.
12. Etheridge, EE, Haid SD, Maeser MN, et al. Salvage operations for malfunctioning polytetrafluoroethylene hemodialysis access grafts. *Surgery* 1983;94:464–469.
13. Brotman DN, Fandos L, Faust GR, et al. Hemodialysis graft salvage. *J Am Coll Surg* 1994;178:431–434.
14. Beathard GA. Thrombolysis versus surgery for the treatment of thrombosed dialysis access grafts. *J Am Soc Nephrol* 1995;6:1619–1624.
15. Gray RJ. Percutaneous intervention for permanent hemodialysis access: a review. *Vasc Interv Radiol* 1997;8:313–327.
16. Gray RJ, Horton KM, Dolmatch, et al. Use of wall stents for hemodialysis access-related venous stenoses and occlusions untreatable with balloon angioplasty. *Radiology* 1995;195:479–484.
17. Vorwerk D, Gunther RW, Bohndorf K, et al. Follow-up results after stent placement in failing arteriovenous shunts: a three-year experience. *Cardiovasc Intervent Radiol* 1991;14:285–289.
18. Dolmatch BL, Gray RJ, Horton KM. Will iatrogenic pulmonary embolization be our pulmonary embarrassment? *Radiology* 1994;191:615–617.
19. Swan TL, Smyth SH, Ruffenach SJ, et al. Pulmonary embolism following hemodialysis access thrombolysis/thrombectomy. *J Vasc Interv Radiol* 1995;6:683–686.
20. Winkler TA, Trerotola SO, Davidson DD, et al. Study of thrombus from thrombosed hemodialysis access grafts. *Radiology* 1995;197:461–465.
21. Kinney TB, Valji K, Rose SC, et al. Pulmonary embolism from pulse-spray pharmacomechanical thrombolysis of clotted hemodialysis grafts: urokinase versus heparinized saline. *J Vasc Interv Radiol* 2000;11:1143–1152.
22. Dougherty MJ, Calligaro KD, Schindler N, et al. Endovascular versus surgical treatment for thrombosed hemodialysis grafts: a prospective randomized study. *J Vasc Surg* 1999;30:1016–1023.
23. Vesely TM, Williams D, Weiss M, et al. Comparison of the AngioJet rheolytic catheter to surgical thrombectomy for the treatment of thrombosed hemodialysis grafts. *J Vasc Interv Radiol* 1999;10:1195–1205.
24. Vesely TM, Idso MC, Audrain J, et al. Thrombolysis versus surgical thrombectomy for the treatment of dialysis graft thrombosis: pilot study comparing costs. *J Vasc Interv Radiol* 1996;7:507–512.
25. Marston WA. Cost effectiveness of salvage procedures for thrombosed hemodialysis shunts: a prospective study of surgical and percutaneous techniques. In: Henry ML, ed. *Vascular access for hemodialysis—VI.* Precept Press, 1999:301–306.
26. Gelbfish GA. Surgery versus percutaneous treatment of thrombosed dialysis access grafts: is there a best method? *J Vasc Interv Radiol* 1998;9:875–877.
27. Allon M, Bailey R, Ballard R, et al. A multidisciplinary approach to hemodialysis access: prospective evaluation. *Kidney Int* 1988;53:473–479.
28. Duda C, Spergel LM, Holland J, et al. How a multidisciplinary vascular access care program enables implementation of the DOQI guidelines. *Nephrology News & Issues* 2000;14:13–17.

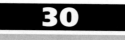

30

ENDOVASCULAR TREATMENT OF THROMBOSED AUTOLOGOUS FISTULAE

LUC TURMEL-RODRIGUES

Recent radiologic publications indicate that the endovascular approach might be clearly more effective than conventional surgery and soon should become the gold standard for the treatment of thrombosed native fistulae for hemodialysis (1,2). An underlying stenosis is unmasked in almost all cases, thus warranting stenosis-detection programs and preventive treatments (guidelines 11 and 18 of the Dialysis Outcome Quality Initiative, or DOQI) (3). A mature native fistula is, however, much less at risk of thrombosis than a prosthetic graft for two main reasons:

1. Much tighter stenoses and therefore much lower flow rates are necessary to cause thrombosis because the venous endothelial cells secrete local anticoagulant factors; veins are therefore physiologically scheduled for remaining patent in relatively low-flow conditions.
2. The presence of collaterals helps to maintain flow from the artery to the superior vena cava (SVC) even when the flow in the main vein is compromised.

These fundamental anatomic and physiologic factors also explain why early rethrombosis after native fistula declotting is less frequent than with grafts. In contrast, early (<3 months) thrombosis after creation is the weakness of native fistula construction, especially in the forearm. A tight underlying stenosis is unmasked in all cases of immature fistula thrombosis when radiologic salvage can be attempted (4). These stenoses are either the consequence of surgical misfit or are due to intrinsically poor condition of the artery or vein whose quality may have been overestimated by preoperative examinations.

The technique for declotting a polytetrafluoroethylene (PTFE) graft can be standardized easily: a thick prosthetic wall that is easy to palpate and to cannulate, a constant graft diameter, a small (mean 3.2 mL) clot volume (5), and underlying stenosis located at the venous anastomosis in the vast majority of cases. Nonetheless, clotted native fistulae can result in a wide range of difficulties: (a) the thin venous wall is difficult to palpate and is pierced through without resistance; (b) the anatomy is irregular, and it can be impossible to localize the anastomosis clinically; (c) the underlying stenosis can occur anywhere from the feeding artery to the central veins; (d) this underlying stenosis is frequently very tight and difficult to traverse; (e) the collaterals are deceptive; (f) a large volume of clots can be encountered; (g) aneurysms are more frequent than in grafts, possibly with thick layers of old wall-adherent thrombi; and (h) concomitant artery thrombosis is not rare, with a sharp arteriovenous angulation that may be impossible to traverse from the fistula.

CONTRAINDICATIONS

Local infection is the main contraindication to percutaneous declotting. Local inflammation and pain immediately upstream from the stenosis occur frequently in recently thrombosed native fistulae (this is a phlebitis), and the diagnosis of infection is not easy to make.

Immature fistulae never previously used for hemodialysis are a technical contraindication if the forearm vein is not clinically palpable because catheterization of the fistula is usually impossible.

Large aneurysms in cannulation areas are a technical contraindication (see "Specific Cases" to follow). A diameter greater than 5 cm can be suggested as the limit above which an aneurysm is too large and contraindicates endovascular declotting.

Huge clot burden (100 cc) is also probably a contraindication. This is a rare clinical situation with which we were recently confronted. A 17-year-old aneurysmal left radiocephalic fistula was associated with brachiocephalic stenosis. The patient developed considerable arm edema in a few days, and the initial angiogram showed a patent forearm cephalic vein but with a huge thrombosis in the aneurysmal basilic, axillary, and subclavian veins (estimated clot volume: >100 cc). Thrombectomy failed because of the impossibility of passing a catheter through the tortuous axillary segment, leading to vessel rupture. Safe removal of thrombi from 40 cm of vein with an average diameter of 2 cm (=126 cc) probably would have been impossible. Which thrombectomy method, radiologic or surgical, could be sure not to leave potentially fatal residual thrombi in such veins before dilating the innominate vein and reopening the route to iatrogenic pulmonary embolism? Should we use temporary SVC filters?

BASIC TECHNIQUE

A fistula can be easily declotted up to 3 weeks after thrombosis (we have achieved this in patients with a renal transplant), but this usually is done as soon as possible to avoid the need for temporary central dialysis lines.

As for the treatment of grafts, there are two mandatory stages in the treatment of a thrombosed fistula: (a) removal of clots and (b) treatment of the cause of the thrombosis, which in 99% of cases is a tight underlying stenosis. Percutaneous declotting of a dialysis fistula is an outpatient procedure. Anticoagulation (at least 3,000 U of heparin) is mandatory before initiation of any declotting maneuver (6); antistaphylococcal antibiotics are injected.

For grafts, most fistulae are treated after blind puncture of the thrombosed fistula with the patient under local anesthesia. Two introducer sheaths are placed in opposite directions to gain access to both the venous outflow and the arterial inflow. Clinical examination is essential to choose the best site for initial catheterization. When the stenosis is clinically located a few centimeters from the wrist anastomosis, with no evidence of concomitant outflow stenosis, a single retrograde approach from the vein at the elbow *after placement of a tourniquet* is sufficient to treat the whole fistula. In typical cases (Fig. 30.1), however, an initial ("venous") introducer sheath is placed a few centimeters from the anastomosis using an antegrade approach to treat the venous outflow. A small subcutaneous tunnel between the entry point of the skin and that of the vessel is recommended to facilitate final compression and prevent formation of pseudoaneurysms. A 5 French catheter is pushed over a wire up to the SVC and then slowly pulled back while contrast medium is injected under fluoroscopy to localize the downstream (central) extension of the thrombosis. The fistula is abandoned at this stage if the venous outflow cannot be traversed or recanalized *and* if no other obstruction explains fistula thrombosis.

A second ("arterial") introducer is placed with a retrograde approach some centimeters downstream from the "venous" introducer in the direction of the arterial inflow. When the artery cannot be reached because of tight stenosis or because of deceptive collaterals, opacification and sometimes catheterization of the arterial inflow are performed by puncture of the brachial artery at the elbow (see "Specific Cases" to follow). The fistula is referred for surgery if it is

impossible to traverse the arteriovenous anastomosis with a guidewire.

Once access to both the arterial inflow and venous outflow is guaranteed with a guidewire, the final success of the procedure is predictable, and the stage of thrombus removal is initiated. To avoid hyperpressure due to reestablishment of arterial flow, thrombi on the venous side are removed first, before the thrombi on the arterial side.

In France, we use the method of manual catheter-directed thromboaspiration, which is based on a simple concept (7): A slightly angulated 7 to 9 French catheter (Guider, Medi-Tech, Natick, MA, U.S.A.; Vista Brite Tip, Cordis, Miami FL, U.S.A.) with a firm wall, wide inner lumen, and soft atraumatic tip is pushed through the introducer sheath over a guidewire to make contact with the thrombus. Strong manual aspiration is created through a regular Luer-Lok 50-mL syringe while pulling back the catheter. The syringe and the aspiration catheter are flushed through gauze into a cup, and the maneuver is repeated as long as clots remain. It is essential to use angled catheters to be able to aspirate clots in large, aneurysmal, or curved vessels. The tip of the angled catheter can strip the venous wall and, by (sometimes forceful) back and forth movement, it detaches wall-adherent thrombi such as the *arterial plug*, the hard clot that frequently remains in contact with the blood flow at the anastomosis.

Once the thrombi have been removed, the unmasked underlying stenosis or stenoses must be dilated. High-pressure balloons, which can be inflated up to 25 atm, are used to abolish the stenosis when necessary, with the aim of accepting absolutely no residual stenosis. Dilatation before thromboaspiration is sometimes necessary to allow passage of the aspiration catheter to remove clots immediately upstream or downstream from the stenosis (Fig. 30.1).

The use of stents is limited to the treatment of acute ruptures not controlled by balloon tamponade, acute pseudoaneurysms, and major stenosis recoil (>50%) after dilatation.

Finally, the whole fistula must be checked from the feeding artery to the SVC to rule out residual thrombi and stenoses. Minor residual thrombi or residual stenoses of less than 50% are accepted if an excellent flow is restored. In contrast, they must be treated more aggressively when flow remains insufficient. Incidental arterial embolism must be searched for and treated (by thromboaspiration or "back-bleeding") (8,9), even when asymptomatic.

Final compression of the entry points of the introducers can be clearly shortened by purse-string suturing (10), and the fistula is immediately usable for dialysis. We recommend systematic low-molecular-weight heparin for some days or weeks both to avoid rethrombosis and to treat possible pulmonary embolism. In our experience, the mean procedure time from initial puncture to completion of the final compression was about 2 hours.

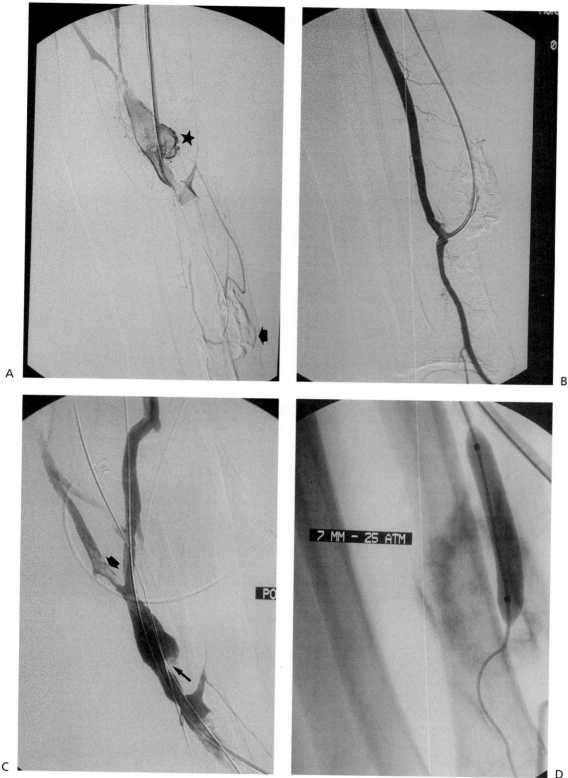

FIGURE 30.1. A: Postanastomotic stenosis explaining thrombosis of this 6-year-old radiocephalic fistula was clinically easily palpated. The fistula was accessed first in the retrograde fashion because it was obvious that traversing this stenosis and the anastomosis was the main challenge. It was very challenging because the initial "wrong way" catheterization attempt created transient extravasation (*arrow*). Clots are visible in the outflow and especially in the aneurysm (*star*) of the venous dialysis needle site. **B**: Local low-pressure injection confirmed adequate access to the artery. **C**: After antegrade cannulation of the fistula, manual aspiration was performed first in the outflow veins with an 8 French catheter. This is an intermediate stage before additional aspiration of residual clots in the aneurysm (*thin arrow*) and in the basilic vein (*wide arrow*). **D**: Dilatation of the postanastomotic stenosis was performed before thrombus removal in the anastomotic area to allow passage of the aspiration catheter.

(continued)

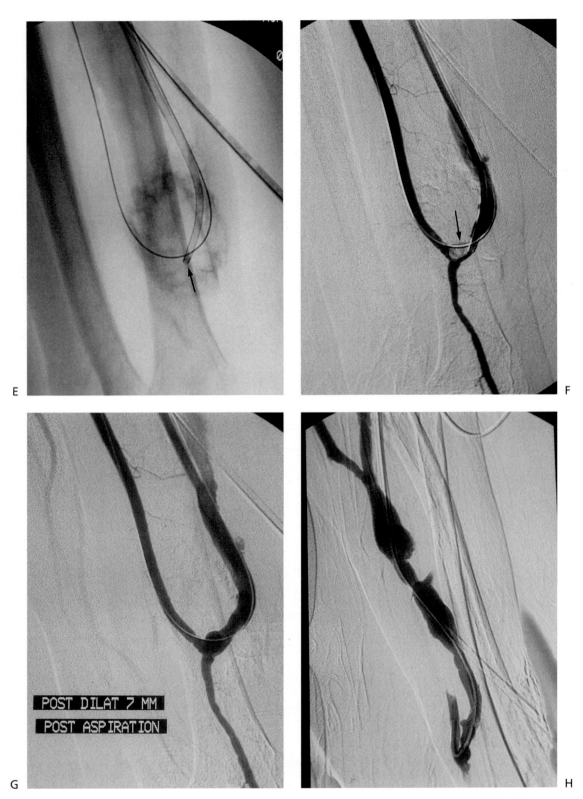

E

F

G

H

FIGURE 30.1. *(continued)* **E**: A safety guidewire was placed through the anastomosis before initiation of aspiration (*arrow* indicates the tip of the aspiration catheter). **F**: This intermediate stage showed evidence of an "arterial plug" (*arrow*), which was finally broken and aspirated. **G,H**: The final angiogram showed slight residual parietal damage in the location of the initial stenosis.

Within image G: POST DILAT 7 MM / POST ASPIRATION

SPECIFIC CASES AND TECHNICAL SUBTLETIES

Use of a Safety Guidewire

When the fistula is tortuous, with alternation of stenoses, sharp angulations, and aneurysms, or when blind predilatation is necessary to allow the passage of the thrombectomy catheter (Fig. 30.1), repeat passes with catheters or dilatation balloons are likely to be difficult. Similarly, thrombectomy or dilatation in the anastomotic area can damage the feeding artery. In such cases, a guidewire is pushed from the introducer sheath into the feeding artery or into the SVC according to the location of the area of concern. After placement of this "safety" guidewire, which must never be a hydrophilic guidewire prone to spontaneous unintentional removal, a second guidewire is pushed through the same sheath. The sheath then is removed and repositioned only over the second guidewire, leaving the safety guide wire exiting directly through the skin beside the introducer sheath. Declotting and dilatation maneuvers are performed through the sheath, but the safety guidewire is a fluoroscopic landmark of the anatomy of the fistula and guarantees rapid reopening of the fistula by pushing a dilatation balloon or a stent over it when complications develop.

Recent Forearm Fistulae

Recent forearm fistulae are relatively immature but nevertheless are used for dialysis. They are difficult to cannulate, however, especially when numerous stenoses with few clots are present. The solution is to place a tourniquet on the upper arm to make the elbow veins swell. The turgescent cephalic or basilic vein at the elbow then is easily punctured and catheterized with a retrograde approach, and it is possible to find the way back into the fistula down to the anastomosis. In such cases, this unique retrograde approach is usually sufficient to clear the fistula of thrombi and to dilate underlying stenoses. For nonpalpable, recently created upper-arm fistulae, the brachial artery approach must be used, and the fistula will be entered through its anastomosis.

Rupture of Vein

Another frequent problem with immature fistulae is the risk of rupture of the vein despite the small (5 mm) diameter of the balloons used. In several cases, controlling a large rupture by a wide strut puncturable covered stent (Passager, Medi-Tech* Europe, La Garenne-Colombes, France) (to date, not available in the United States) has proved to be durably effective, despite routine cannulation of the stent for dialysis.

When the Anastomosis Cannot Be Reached by Retrograde Approach from the Fistula

When the anastomosis cannot be reached by retrograde approach from the fistula, either because there is stenosis or because the catheter and guidewire are lost in collaterals, it is helpful to puncture the brachial artery with a 20-gauge needle to opacify the feeding artery (Figs. 30.2 through Fig. 30.4). This shows where the anastomosis is and aids catheterization by mapping. If, however, there is a postanastomotic tight stenosis that cannot be traversed in a retrograde fashion, antegrade cannulation of the brachial artery at the elbow and selective catheterization of the feeding artery (usually radial) are feasible (Figs. 30.2 and 30.3). The combination of an angled 4 French catheter ("internal mammary" type) and a (0.035-inch) hydrophilic guidewire frequently makes it possible to pass the stenosis. This approach can fail when, for example, there is a high origin of the radial artery above the elbow.

Using the hydrophilic guidewire, the next step is to enter the introducer sheath, which was previously placed in the fistula in a retrograde fashion over the guidewire that initially failed to pass the stenosis (Fig. 2C–E). The hydrophilic guidewire then is pushed selectively into the introducer on contact with the hemostatic valve while the introducer is slowly removed. This guidewire inserted via the brachial artery emerges therefore from the fistula, through the skin above the stenosis. The introducer sheath is reintroduced over the hydrophilic guidewire and makes it possible to dilate the stenosis with a balloon pushed from the fistula instead of the brachial artery (Fig. 30.2 F), thus limiting the size of the hole in the artery.

Concomitant Thrombosis of The Feeding Artery

In cases of concomitant thrombosis of the feeding artery, retrograde catheterization of the thrombosed artery from the fistula is usually possible, and thromboaspiration can be performed with a more flexible 6 French catheter if 7 or 8 French catheters do not pass. If not, aspiration also can be performed after antegrade cannulation of the feeding artery and placement of a 6 French introducer sheath in the brachial artery (Fig. 30.3). Some teams do not hesitate to try simply to detach the clots with an over-the-wire Fogarty balloon and to pull them into the fistula, with the reestablished inflow then pushing the thrombi into the lungs.

Thrombi in Aneurysms

Thrombi in aneurysms are not a problem when they are fresh. When it is difficult to direct the aspiration catheter

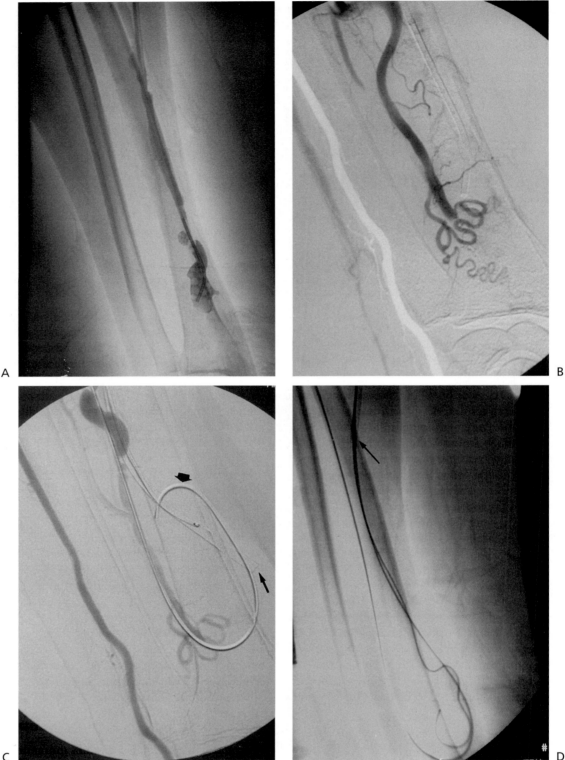

FIGURE 30.2. A: Inflow had been a long-standing problem when thrombosis occurred in this 10-year-old radiocephalic fistula in a patient with a failing renal transplant. Retrograde catheterization (after placement of a tourniquet) of this flat fistula showed no evidence of thrombus, but access to the feeding artery was impossible. **B**: Angiography of forearm arteries was performed by sticking the brachial artery and showed occlusion of the radial artery just above the anastomosis. This occlusion was the late complication of chronic stenosis as evidenced by the well-developed collateral arteries. **C**: Antegrade catheterization of the radial artery was performed after antegrade cannulation of the brachial artery at the elbow. Passage through the occluded artery and anastomosis was easy, and an angled 4 French catheter (*wide arrow*) was pushed into the vein (*thin arrow* indicates the tip of the faintly visible introducer initially placed in retrograde fashion in the fistula). **D**: The combination of this angled catheter and a hydrophilic guidewire made it possible to perform elective catheterization of the introducer initially placed in retrograde fashion in the fistula (*arrow* indicates the tip of the introducer traversed by the two guidewires, one coming from the brachial artery, the other pushed through the sheath hemostatic valve).

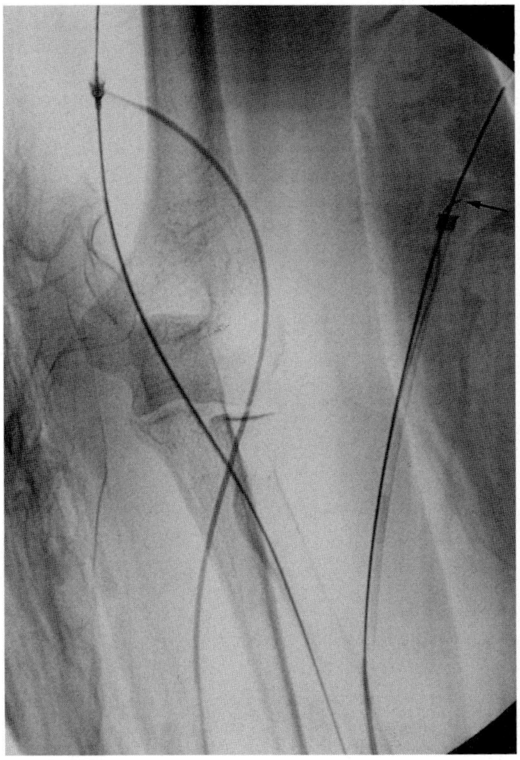

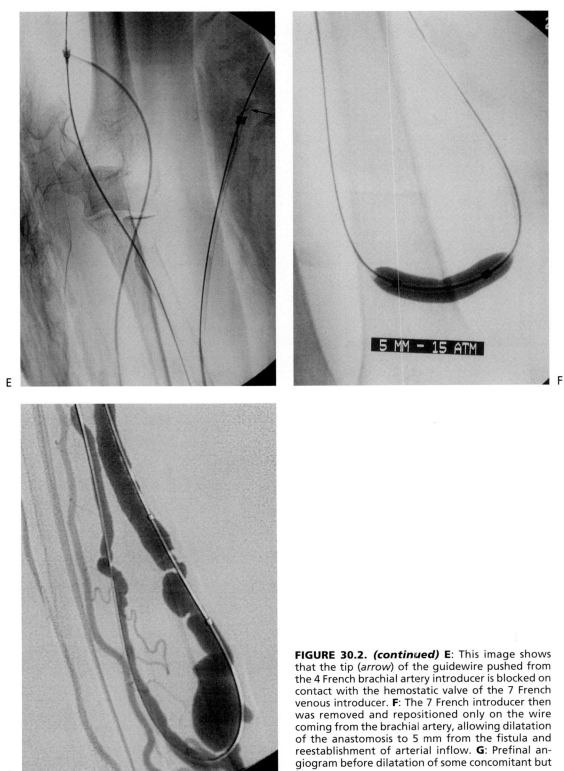

E

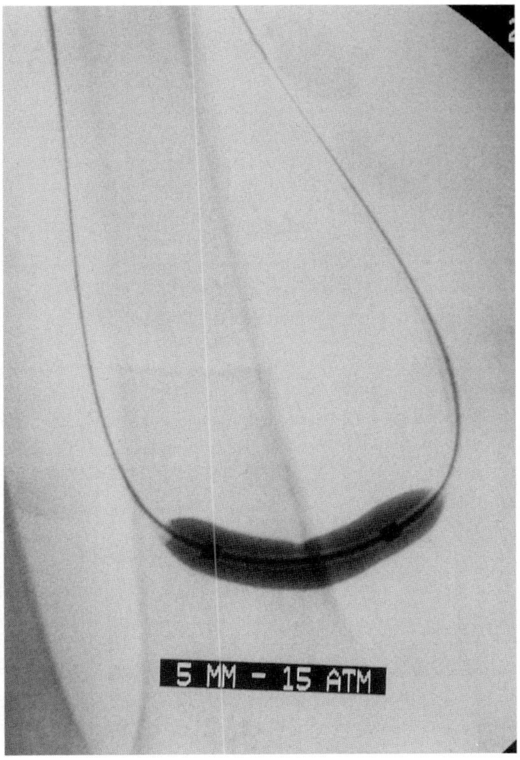

F

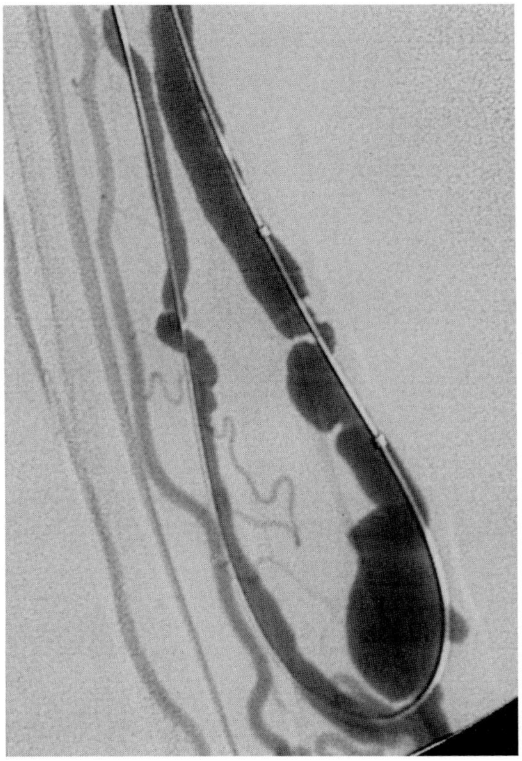

G

FIGURE 30.2. ***(continued)*** **E**: This image shows that the tip (*arrow*) of the guidewire pushed from the 4 French brachial artery introducer is blocked on contact with the hemostatic valve of the 7 French venous introducer. **F**: The 7 French introducer then was removed and repositioned only on the wire coming from the brachial artery, allowing dilatation of the anastomosis to 5 mm from the fistula and reestablishment of arterial inflow. **G**: Prefinal angiogram before dilatation of some concomitant but less severe venous stenoses.

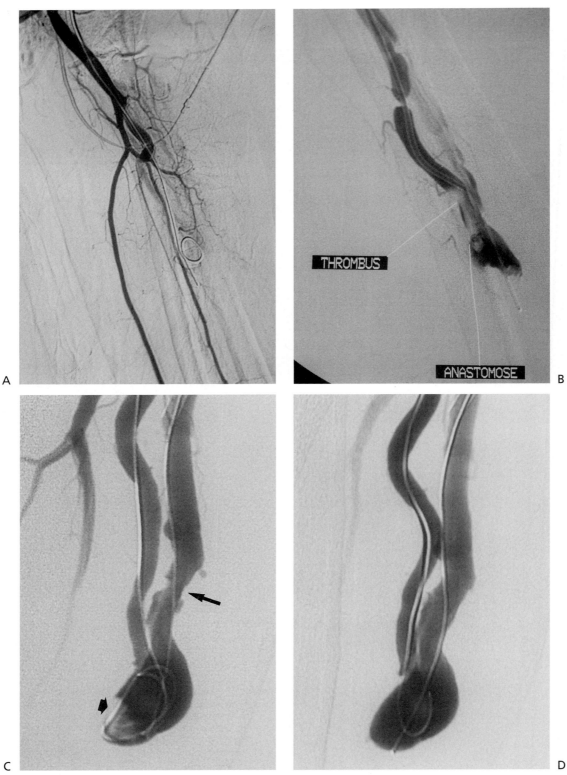

FIGURE 30.3. A: This 4-year-old fistula had not been used for dialysis for 3 years in this 50-year-old patient with a second renal transplant. Nephrologists asked for fistula declotting in view of the history of difficult fistula construction. Access to the feeding artery was impossible after retrograde catheterization of the fistula itself and opacification from the brachial artery showed evidence of concomitant thrombosis of the radial artery (the guidewire is in the vein). **B**: Antegrade cannulation of the brachial artery and selective catheterization of the radial artery showed fresh thrombi in the feeding artery immediately above the anastomosis because it was an end-to-end fistula. These thrombi then were removed through a 6 French manual aspiration catheter after placement of a 6 French introducer in the brachial artery. There was also tight postanastomotic stenosis on the vein that explained fistula thrombosis. **C**: This was the prefinal result after aspiration of arterial and venous thrombi. Some residual clots remained visible in the anastomotic culde-sac (*wide arrow*). The venous stenosis had been dilated to 7 mm (*thin arrow*). **D**: Final angiogram after complementary aspiration of the clots and venous dilatation to 8 mm.

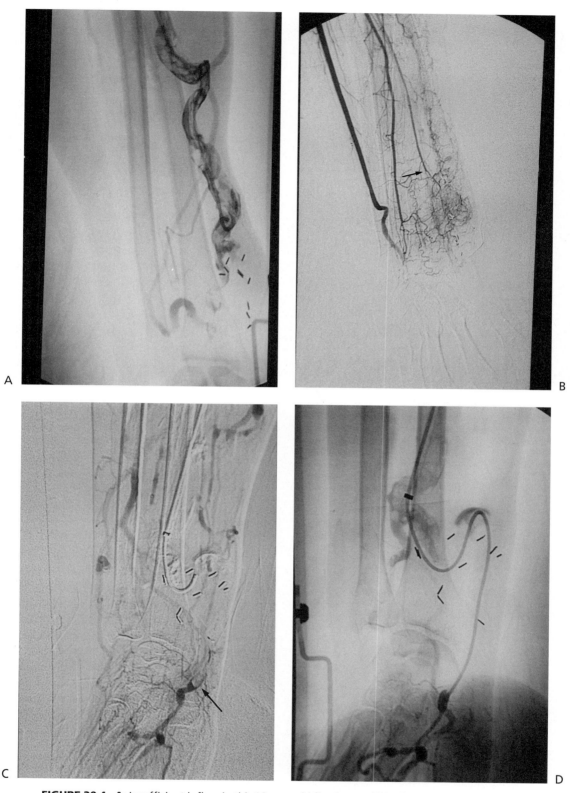

FIGURE 30.4. A: Insufficient inflow in this 16-year-old fistula was clinically masked by chronic venous outflow obstruction because of indirect drainage at the elbow responsible for development of collaterals. Dialysis was nevertheless routinely possible when the fistula thrombosed. After retrograde cannulation of the main vein, it was, however, impossible to find the way to the arterial feeding. **B**: Opacification from the brachial artery showed that the proximal radial artery was very thin and occluded before the anastomosis (*arrow*). **C**: It also showed that the feeding of the fistula relied only on the distal radial artery receiving reversed-direction flow from the ulnar artery. Clots were visible at the anastomosis (*arrow*). **D**: Selective catheterization down to the distal radial artery.

(continued)

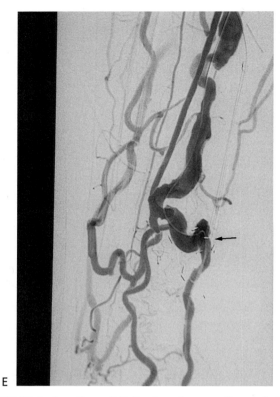

E

FIGURE 30.4. *(continued)* **E**: Final angiogram after aspiration of clots and dilatation to 7 mm of the stenosis, which was located in the first venous curve (*arrow* indicates entry point of the introducer placed to aspirate the arterial clots).

in the enlarged area, external compression of the aneurysm facilitates contact between clots and the catheter. In contradistinction, old wall-adherent thrombi are usually resistant to lysis or aspiration. Such old thrombi frequently detach during declotting maneuvers and can block the flow intermittently. Because we do not consider it acceptable to push such clots into the lungs, the only solution to ensure the safety and success of the procedure is to trap them with a stent placed across the aneurysm if the aneurysm is not too big (see preceding discussion of "Contraindications").

Concomitant Acute Thrombosis of Central Veins

Concomitant acute thrombosis of central veins is a problem common to native fistulae and grafts, but with native fistulae, they share the technical problem of removing huge clots without inducing significant pulmonary embolism. From the experience gained with native fistulae, catheter-directed thromboaspiration can be effective in thrombosed subclavian and brachiocephalic veins if the clot burden is not too high (See discussion of "Contraindications").

SPECIFIC COMPLICATIONS OF PERCUTANEOUS THROMBECTOMY TECHNIQUES

Non–Procedure-Related Deaths

Such deaths are not uncommon during the first month's follow-up in these patients, who often have underlying cardiovascular diseases that frequently facilitate development of access thrombosis.

Pulmonary Embolism

The risk of pulmonary embolism is greater with native fistulae than with grafts because a large volume of thrombus can be encountered in native veins. The technique of thrombus removal or lysis must therefore be adapted to large vessels and larger volumes of clots.

Arterial Embolism

Injection of a thrombolytic agent or contrast medium in a thrombosed fistula or graft creates high pressure, which can push clots into the outflow or into the inflow. Passing the arteriovenous anastomosis with a catheter also means a risk of pushing back clots into the arterial system. Although usually asymptomatic, these arterial emboli must be treated whenever possible by thromboaspiration, Fogarty balloon, back-bleeding technique, or thrombolytic infusion because, at the occasion of future thromboses, additional emboli would lead to chronic ischemia of the hand.

Infection

Thrombi in a clotted fistula are just under the skin in a vessel punctured twice 1 or 2 days before. The risk of septic colonization is high. Furthermore, percutaneous declotting usually requires more than 1 hour. Long guidewires have to be handled in two directions, which means a high risk of breaches in sterile technique because their ends can easily touch the patient's face or the floor. For all these reasons, systemic antistaphylococcal antibiotics must be injected before any declotting procedure, and the patient's local and general status must be checked carefully during the following days. The use of vancomycin is extremely controversial.

Secondary Bleeding and Pseudoaneurysms

Secondary bleeding and pseudoaneurysms from the introducer sheath entry points are probably underreported, although the risk is smaller in native veins than in prostheses. When the sheaths are initially placed for declotting, a good prevention technique is the creation of a small subcutaneous tunnel between the skin entry point and the graft entry point: It facilitates final compression. Another excellent "trick" is to close the sheath holes by a pursestring suture (10).

Local and General Hemorrhagic Complications

Local and general hemorrhagic complications can occur when patients are treated with fibrinolytics and when patients receive high-dose heparin. Accidents are reputed to be rare with thrombolytics at the low doses currently used if contraindications are respected (e.g., recent surgery, recent cerebrovascular accident, severe hypertension).

Early Rethrombosis

Early rethrombosis is a frequent complication in grafts but is rare in forearm fistulae, and residual clots in a native fistula are less a problem than in grafts if excellent flow has been restored. As an illustration, our success rate in the declotting of forearm fistulae is 93%, with an excellent 89% primary patency rate at 1 month. In grafts, the 100% success rate drops to 78% at 1 month (1).

OTHER TECHNIQUES IN THE LITERATURE

In 1994, Trerotola and colleagues published a controversial article that was a milestone in the history of hemodialysis access declotting because it explained everything that occurred before and after the procedure (11). This article was titled "Percutaneous Declotting without Urokinase," which was euphemistic, because the title should have been "Declotting by Deliberate Embolization of the Clots into the Lungs." After placing the two introducers, these researchers first pulled the clots from the arterial side of the graft to the venous side with the help of a Fogarty balloon and then pushed the clots from the venous side into the lungs. They justified this technique by the fact that the average volume of thrombus in a clotted graft is only 3.2 mL (5), which explains why this modest iatrogenic pulmonary embolism is asymptomatic in the vast majority of cases.

This key article explains why so many declotting methods have been reported for the declotting of prosthetic grafts: Everybody can claim to remove clots with more or less efficient devices or drugs because residual clots can be pushed into the lungs with a low risk of complications. The question remains, however, of who actually experiences the risk of complication: the physician or the patient?

From this experience gained with grafts, some teams use this technique of deliberate pulmonary embolization of clots when the volume of thrombus in the native fistula is presumed to be equivalent to the mean 3 cc encountered in

grafts. An 82% to 100% success rate and no complications were reported in the series of Haage and associates and that of Zaleski and colleagues, but they included only 17 and 20 patients, respectively (2,12).

In an editorial published concomitantly with the article by Trerotola and colleagues, Dolmatch and associates emphasized that even a small pulmonary embolism can induce bronchospasm, which can be particularly deleterious in debilitated patients (13). Trerotola and colleagues stopped using this "rough" technique soon after, when they experienced a casualty (14). Other casualties have since been reported in the literature, from pulmonary or septic embolism and from hemiplegia due to paradoxic embolism in patients with a patent foramen ovale and a right-to-left shunt (15–18). Because it is likely that not all the fatal complications are reported in the literature, these courageous reports make techniques recommending intentional embolization of clots or residual thrombi questionable.

The first teams to report the feasibility of percutaneous declotting of native fistulae used urokinase infusion for some hours before crushing or aspiration of residual clots, with success rates ranging from 36% to 65% (19–21). This was our first approach as well, but it was rapidly abandoned because thrombolytic infusion proved unnecessary and had drawbacks such as incorrect placement of needles with oozing of urokinase into adjacent tissues, local pain, bleeding from reopening recent dialysis puncture sites, and inconsistent effectiveness, especially when urokinase escaped through collaterals. An American team using local infusions of thrombolytics published good results in a small series of patients (22), and we are aware of an unpublished Japanese experience of more than 100 patients that also had an apparently good success rate. In both series, however, our opinion again is that the treatment of residual clots by crushing with a dilatation balloon or detachment with a Fogarty balloon is questionable.

Small series have been reported using the Hydrolyser (Cordis), the Amplatz-Thrombectomy-Device (ATD) (Microvena-Bard, Covington, GA, U.S.A.), and the Arrow-Trerotola Percutaneous Thrombectomy Device (PTD) (Arrow, Reading, PA, U.S.A.) (2,23–25).

Haage and colleagues reported an 89% success rate using the Hydrolyser and the ATD (2). In seven cases, the devices were not able to break up the thrombus material, a cause of failure that is extremely unusual in our experience with manual catheter-directed thromboaspiration, which confirms our personal skepticism concerning the cost-effectiveness of these devices. Vorwerk and colleagues reported that it was necessary to trap residual clots left by the Hydrolyser with stents, which is of course an expensive solution (26). Using also the Hydrolyser, the groups of Overbosch and Rousseau achieved good success rates but reported frequent residual clots (23,24). Overbosch and colleagues simply crushed the clots with a balloon, which meant a major risk of detachment and pulmonary embolization, whereas Rousseau and associates used manual aspiration, as we did. Rocek and colleagues reported a 90% clinical success rate with the PTD in a short series of ten fistulae, with, however, significant residual thrombus in three cases and some selection bias (25). In all ten fistulae (seven in the forearm, three in the upper arm), the thrombosed segment was more than 10 cm long and the diameter was greater than 6 mm. Finally, Schmitz-Rode and colleagues reported a 100% success rate and no complications in 15 fistulae (27) by using a purely mechanical method of fragmentation of the thrombus with a cheap "rotating mini-pigtail catheter" (Cook, Bjaeverskov, Denmark).

Results

Most series reported in the literature are small and do not provide statistically reliable patency rates. In addition, many series mix grafts and native fistulae or forearm fistulae with upper-arm fistulae, whose outcome are different in our personal experience. Only two recent series in the literature have included more than 50 patients and have some statistical significance. We have reported success rates of 93% in the forearm and 76% in the upper arm, comparable to the 89% rate reported by Haage and colleagues in a series that mixed some upper-arm fistulae with a majority of forearm fistulae. They reported a 27% primary patency rate at 1 year, whereas we had a 49% patency rate in the forearm and only 9% in the upper arm. Our 1-year secondary patency rates were 81% and 50% in the forearm and in the upper arm, respectively, whereas Haage's group reported a rate of 51%.

Our personal comparative experience indicates that declotting forearm fistulae is more difficult than declotting grafts because the immediate success rate is slightly inferior (93% versus 100%), with failures due to stenoses that were impossible to traverse or to immaturity of the veins. Rethrombosis and the need for prophylactic redilatations are, however, clearly less frequent than for grafts, as underlined by the clearly higher primary patency rates (49 versus 14% at 1 year).

Although secondary patency rates after declotting are similar for forearm fistulae and grafts in our series (81% and 83% at 1 year, respectively), the clearly greater interval between maintenance reinterventions in forearm veins (19.6 months versus 6.4 months for grafts) confirms that, whereas declotting a forearm fistula is more difficult, the results are more durable and the need for reintervention is three times less that of grafts. These radiologic findings confirm that forearm fistulae are the vascular access of choice.

On the other hand, we reported results in upper-arm fistulae, which were clearly poorer than in the forearm and similar to those reported with prostheses, with a poor primary patency rate of 9% at 1 year and the need for reintervention every 5.7 months. This poorer outcome is due mainly to problems encountered in the management of stenoses of the final arch of the cephalic vein (ruptures, resistance to dilatation, early recurrence). It is even more regrettable that interventional techniques work less well in the upper arm because it is also in this location that surgical alternatives are the most limited and vein consuming.

SURGERY OR RADIOLOGY?

Few surgical reports have described the outcome of thrombosed native fistulae after surgical treatment, and the results reported are poor: A relatively low success rate of 65% was reported by Oakes and colleagues and a primary patency of 50% at 4 months by Hodges and associates (28,29).

CONCLUSION

The recent literature indicates much better results for interventional techniques compared with surgery in the treatment of thrombosed fistulae, with the overall advantage of less invasiveness and better preservation of the patient's venous capital. There is, however, a learning curve, and not all declotting techniques used for grafts can be used for native fistulae. In view of the advantages of the percutaneous approach, our opinion is that, except for isolated stenoses at the wrist, percutaneous radiologic treatment should be attempted first and should be initiated in all dialysis centers so long as the local radiologists are trained and enthusiastic.

ACKNOWLEDGMENTS

Thanks to Doreen Raine for editing the English.

REFERENCES

1. Turmel-Rodrigues L, Pengloan J, Rodrigue H, et al. Treatment of failed native arterio-venous fistulae for hemodialysis by interventional radiology. *Kidney Int* 2000;57:1124–1140.
2. Haage P, Vorwerk D, Wildberger J, et al. Percutaneous treatment of thrombosed primary arteriovenous hemodialysis access fistulae. *Kidney Int* 2000;57:1169–1175.
3. Schwab S, Besarab A, Beathard G, et al. NKG-DOQI clinical practice guidelines for vascular access. *Am J Kidney Dis* 1997;30 (Suppl 4).
4. Turmel-Rodrigues, Mouton A, Birmelé B, et al. Salvage of immature forearm fistulas for hemodialysis by interventional radiology. *Nephrol Dial Transplant* 2001;16:2365–2371.
5. Winkler T, Trerotola S, Davidson D, et al. Study of thrombus from thrombosed hemodialysis access grafts. *Radiology* 1995;197: 461–465.
6. Trerotola S, Lund G, Scheel P, et al. Thrombosed hemodialysis access grafts: percutaneous mechanical declotting without urokinase. *Radiology* 1994;191:721–726.

7. Turmel-Rodrigues L, Sapoval M, Pengloan J, et al. Manual thromboaspiration and dilation of thrombosed dialysis access: mid-term results of a simple concept. *J Vasc Interv Radiol* 1997; 8:813–824.

8. Trerotola S, Johnson M, Shah H, et al. Backbleeding technique for treatment of arterial emboli resulting from dialysis graft thrombolysis. *J Vasc Interv Radiol* 1998;9:141–143.

9. Turmel-Rodrigues L, Beyssen B, Raynaud A, et al. Thromboaspiration to treat inadvertent arterial emboli during dialysis graft declotting. *J Vasc Interv Radiol* 1998;9:849–850.

10. Vorwerk D, Konner K, Schuermann K, et al. A simple trick to facilitate bleeding control after percutaneous hemodialysis fistula and graft interventions. *Cardiovasc Intervent Radiol* 1997;20: 159–160.

11. Trerotola S, Lund G, Scheel P, et al. Thrombosed hemodialysis access grafts: percutaneous mechanical declotting without urokinase. *Radiology* 1994;191:721–726.

12. Zaleski G, Funaki B, Kenney S, et al. Angioplasty and bolus urokinase infusion for the restoration of function in thrombosed Brescia-Cimino dialysis fistulas. *J Vasc Interv Radiol* 1999;10: 129–136.

13. Dolmatch B, Gray R, Horton K. Will iatrogenic pulmonary embolization be our pulmonary embarrassment? *Radiology* 1994; 191:615–617.

14. Trerotola S, Vesely T, Lund G, et al. Treatment of thrombosed hemodialysis access grafts: Arrow-Trerotola percutaneous thrombolytic device versus pulse-spray thrombolysis. *Radiology* 1998; 206:403–414.

15. Soulen Zaetta J, Amygdalos M, Baum R, et al. Mechanical declotting of thrombosed dialysis grafts: experience in 86 cases. *J Vasc Interv Radiol* 1997;8:563–567.

16. Swan T, Smyth S, Ruffenach S, et al. Pulmonary embolism following hemodialysis access thrombolysis/thrombectomy. *J Vasc Interv Radiol* 1995;6:683–686.

17. Owens C, Yaghmai B, Aletich V, et al. Fatal paradoxic embolism during percutaneous thrombolysis of a hemodialysis graft. *AJR Am J Roentgenol* 1998;170:742–744.

18. Briefel G, Regan F, Petronis J. Cerebral embolism after mechanical thrombolysis of a clotted hemodialysis access. *Am J Kidney Dis* 1999;34:341–343.

19. Hunter D, Castaneda-Zuniga W, Coleman C, et al. Failing arteriovenous dialysis fistulas: evaluation and treatment. *Radiology* 1984;152:631–635.

20. Mangiarotti G, Canavese C, Thea A, et al. Urokinase treatment for arteriovenous fistulae declotting in dialyzed patients. *Nephron* 1984;36:60–64.

21. Poulain F, Raynaud A, Bourquelot P, et al. Local thrombolysis and thromboaspiration in the treatment of acutely thrombosed arteriovenous hemodialysis fistulas. *Cardiovasc Intervent Radiol* 1991;14:98–101.

22. Schon D, Mishler R. Salvage of occluded arteriovenous fistulae. *Am J Kidney Dis* 2000;36:804–810.

23. Overbosch E, Pattynama P, Aarts H, et al. Occluded hemodialysis shunts: Dutch multicenter experience with the Hydrolyser catheter. *Radiology* 1996;201:485–488.

24. Rousseau H, Sapoval M, Ballini P, et al. Percutaneous recanalization of acutely thrombosed vessels by hydrodynamic thrombectomy (Hydrolyser). *Eur Radiol* 1997;7:935–941.

25. Rocek M, Peregrin J, Lasovickova J, et al. Mechanical thrombolysis of thrombosed hemodialysis native fistulas with use of the Arrow-Trerotola percutaneous thrombolytic device. *J Vasc Interv Radiol* 2000;11:1153–1158.

26. Vorwerk D, Guenther R, Schuermann K. Stent placement on fresh venous thrombosis. *Cardiovasc Intervent Radiol* 1997;20: 359–363.

27. Schmitz-Rode T, Wildberger J, Hübner D, et al. Recanalization of thrombosed dialysis access with use of a rotating mini-pigtail catheter: follow-up study. *J Vasc Interv Radiol* 2000;11:721–727.

28. Hodges T, Fillinger M, Zwolak R, et al. Longitudinal comparison of dialysis access methods: risk factors for failure. *J Vasc Surg* 1997;26:1009–1019.

29. Oakes D, Sherck J, Cobb L. Surgical salvage of failed radiocephalic arteriovenous fistulae: techniques and results in 29 patients. *Kidney Int* 1998;53:480–487.

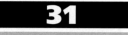

SURGICAL MANAGEMENT OF AUTOLOGOUS FISTULAE

EARLY AND LATE THROMBOSIS, MATURATION FAILURE, AND OTHER COMPLICATIONS

JAN H. M. TORDOIR

The native radiocephalic arteriovenous fistula (AVF) continues to be regarded as the primary choice for hemodialysis vascular access when this method can be used (1–3). The reasons for this preference include factors such as superior long-term patency rates and a low incidence of infection and other complications (e.g., thrombosis and aneurysm formation). After a period of maturation, the arterialized vein has a dilated, thickened wall that is suitable for repeated puncturing and resists thrombosis. Once established, native AVFs can function for many years. A considerable number of native AVFs will thrombose directly after operation, however, or will fail to mature, which results in inadequate hemodialysis treatment. Also, difficult cannulation and low blood flow jeopardize the functioning of the native AVF.

Alternative autologous access sites in patients who lack adequate vessels for radiocephalic fistula creation or have developed an unsalvageable thrombosis of such a fistula have proved very valuable, with long-term patency rates comparable to radiocephalic fistulae. For this purpose, the brachiocephalic and brachiobasilic fistula with transposition of the basilic vein to a superficial position have been advocated more and more in recent years. This chapter discusses the surgical management and strategies for treatment of dysfunctional and thrombosed autologous fistulae.

EARLY FAILURE OF AUTOLOGOUS FISTULAE

Early thrombosis (within 4 weeks after placement) of radiocephalic fistulae is reported with an incidence from 4% to 24% (Table 31.1). Clotting may be already noted in the operating room after completion of the anastomosis. It is recognized by the absence of a palpable thrill, and a technical problem must be considered if there is only a palpable pulse without thrill. Most frequently, thrombosis is due to selection of an inadequate artery or vein for anastomosis. A radial

artery and cephalic vein at least 2 mm in diameter at the site of the wrist and continuity of the cephalic vein for more than 10 cm in the forearm are recommended for a successful creation of the radiocephalic fistula (14–17). For brachiobasilic AVFs, brachial artery and basilic vein diameters greater than 3 mm are recommended (18).

The reasons for failure in order of frequency are (a) technical problems at the anastomosis and positioning of the artery and vein relative to another including rotation and angulation; (b) a sclerotic vein segment in the proximal forearm; (c) calcification of the arterial wall causing difficulty at the anastomosis, such as elevation of an intimal flap, lack of distensibility, or poor flow because of proximal occlusive disease; (d) hypotension usually associated with low blood volume from recent dialysis resulting in a poor flow through the anastomosis.

Surgical Management

Technical factors are often responsible for thrombosis of the newly placed fistula. One must be careful not to narrow the lumen of the artery or vein during suturing and to avoid dissection of the radial artery. Twisting or kinking of the cephalic vein in an end-of-vein to side-of-artery anastomosis must be avoided by sufficient vein dissection and marking the vein to prevent it from rotating. Turbulent flow is a feature of AVFs, but rapid flow across the fistula is usually adequate to prevent early thrombosis. A competent venous valve in the caudal venous limb of a side-to-side AVF produces a cul-de-sac in which there is turbulence but no flow. Thrombosis with propagation across the fistula is almost inevitable. To prevent this problem, a probe should be passed along the caudal limb, and when obstruction is encountered, the distal limb should be ligated (19). A side-to-side anastomosis may predispose to thrombosis in the proximal venous limb, resulting in a dilated plexus on the back of the

TABLE 31.1. EARLY FAILURE OF RADIOCEPHALIC AVFS: RESULTS OF SURGICAL TREATMENT

Author (Ref. No.)	No. AVFs	Early Failure (%)	Successful Revision (%)
Reilly et al. (4)	145	11	33
Erasmi et al. (5)	299	14	24
Tordoir et al. (6)	129	14	55
Louridas et al. (7)	137	13	—
Wedgwood et al. (8)	71	10	14
Palder et al. (9)	99	24	66
Kherlakian et al. (10)	100	12	58
Braun and Polith (11)	277	20	57
Burger et al. (12)	208	6	27
Konner (13)	202	4	90

AVFs, arteriovenous fistulae.

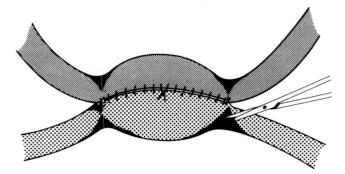

FIGURE 31.2. Release of the vein strictures in a side-to-side radiocephalic arteriovenous fistula.

hand. If a side-to-side anastomosis is preferred, the distal venous limb can be ligated, with leads to augmented flow up the cephalic vein (2).

Declotting by Fogarty thrombectomy is performed by introducing the catheter through a transverse venotomy near the anastomosis or through the distal limb of a side-to-side fistula. Vasospasm in patients undergoing construction of AVFs is relatively common and often impairs the arterial blood supply to the cephalic vein. Prophylaxis with intravenous nicardipine may be effective in preventing vasospasm (20). Otherwise, gentle dilatation of the radial artery or cephalic vein proximal to the site of the anastomosis with a Fogarty catheter or coronary probes overcomes spasm and assures a wide anastomosis. Vein strictures and fibrous bands may cause narrowing and should be released (Figs. 31.1 and 31.2). If there is any doubt about patency, the anastomosis must be taken down to look for errors; if an adequate reanastomosis is not possible, a more proximal new anastomosis can be performed. The success of surgical intervention of thrombosed radiocephalic AVFs by means of thrombectomy and revision of anastomoses varies from 14% to 90% (Table 31.1).

Microsurgical techniques either with magnification glasses or the operation microscope are very useful in the res-

cue of failed AVFs. Microsurgery permits a precise assessment of the lesion, atraumatic handling of the vessels, and an accurate removal of the adventitia, leading to a lower rate of complications and improved outcome of the revision operation. With the use of microsurgery, AVF salvage can be obtained in 80% of cases (21,22).

Superficial repositioning of the brachial or radial artery is an alternative method for vascular access creation in patients with frequent early thrombosis of AVFs. The brachial/radial artery at the elbow is exposed over a length of 10 cm; after ligation of small side branches, the aponeurosis is sutured under the artery. In this way, the superficialized artery can be cannulated within 2 weeks of operation. The returning blood from the artificial kidney reaches the patient through any of the veins in the ipsilateral or contralateral arm (23). Good results with this method were reported in 28 of 35 patients (80%); mean access survival was 65 months (range 3–84 months).

The incidence of early thrombosis of brachiocephalic and basilic AVFs is lower (i.e., 2%–13%) compared with that of radiocephalic AVFs (Table 31.2). Surgical treatment is more difficult, however, and has a lower success rate compared with radiocephalic AVFs. Low blood pressure and kinking or torsion of the basilic vein in its subcutaneous tunnel are usually the causes for thrombosis. Also, hematoma, compressing the vein, may be responsible for AVF clotting. For a successful declotting, it is usually necessary to remove the vein from the tunnel. After derotation, thrombectomy, and tunneling, it is reanastomosed with the brachial artery.

FAILURE OF ARTERIOVENOUS FISTULA MATURATION

Successful access through an autologous AVF depends on a sufficient blood flow and size of the vein that will allow uncomplicated repeated cannulations. To minimize the chance of recirculation, the needles should be placed with at least a 5 cm interspace. This means that an accessible vein with a length of more than 5 cm must be present.

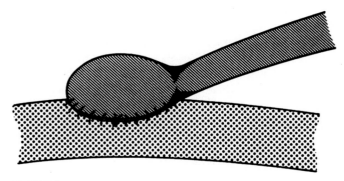

FIGURE 31.1. Vein strictures in an end-to-side radiocephalic arteriovenous fistula.

TABLE 31.2. EARLY FAILURE AND LATE THROMBOSIS OF BRACHIOCEPHALIC AND BASILIC AVFS

Author	Type AVF	No. AVFs	Early Failure (%)	Late Thrombosis (%)
Cantelmo et al. (24)	BB	68	7	20
	BC	31	6	10
Dunlop et al. (25)	BC	81	—	30
Zibari et al. (26)	BC	48	—	10
Nazzal et al. (27)	BC	42	—	9
Rivers et al. (28)	BB	65	2	40
Coburn and Carney (29)	BB	59	—	7
Hakaim et al. (30)	BB	26	—	—
Humphries et al. (31)	BB	67	—	16
Ascher et al. (18)	BC	22	9	—
	BB	30	13	—
Murphy et al. (32)	BB	74	3	19

AVFs, arteriovenous fistulae; BB, brachiobasilic AVF; BC, brachiocephalic AVF.

Usually, the high shear stress induced by the augmented blood flow through the AV anastomosis will cause venous dilatation and vessel-wall thickening, which make repeated cannulations possible. Not only venous dilatation but also arterial remodeling and dilatation are of utmost importance for a sufficient inflow (in radiocephalic fistulae >500 mL per minute). The time required for fistula maturation varies among patients; at least 6 to 8 weeks is ideal. After this period, the chance of maturation is nil. An early cannulation may result in a higher incidence of hematoma with associated compression and risk of fistula loss. An AVF may remain patent in face of a relatively low blood flow. For effective dialysis treatment, the AVF has to deliver only a blood flow that is greater than the pump flow. The dialysis may not be technically possible, however, when the AVF does not mature to a size adequate for cannulation.

Preoperative vessel assessment with duplex ultrasonography results in an increase of the number of newly created autologous AVFs and a decrease in the number of immature AVFs (15,18). Inadequate preoperative evaluation leads to high percentages of failed radiocephalic AVFs, however, ranging from 31% to 70 % (30,33,34).

Surgical Management

Insufficient radial artery blood flow, AV anastomotic stenosis, or diversion of blood away from the cephalic vein predisposes to immature AVFs. Flow into the distal limb of side-to-side radiocephalic fistulae may deprive the proximal cephalic vein. By simple ligation with the patient under local anesthesia, the flow in the proximal cephalic vein is augmented. When AV anastomotic stenosis is the cause for AVF failure to mature, either percutaneous transluminal angioplasty (PTA) or surgical revision is amenable. Creation of a new proximal anastomosis is usually the only option in radial artery stenotic lesions. Failure of AVF development has been attributed to a combination of venous stenosis or the presence of venous side branches (19). The optimum venous anatomy for AVF development may be a single cephalic vein running from the wrist to the antecubital space. Usually the cephalic vein has several side branches that may divert blood from the cephalic vein, resulting in reduced blood flow and less dilation and arterialization. Ligation of these side branches alone or in combination with angioplasty could redirect the flow in the cephalic vein and may have a beneficial effect on AVF maturation. Using this specific strategy, salvage was achieved in 82.5% of 63 patients with nonfunctional fistulae (35).

Patients with immature AVFs resulting from an insufficient arterial inflow because of remodeling failure of the radial artery (inability to dilate in anatomically small or atherosclerotic vessels) are not cured by AVF revision but need a new AVF, constructed using larger vessels (36). (See also Chapter 14.)

CANNULATION COMPLICATIONS

Difficult Cannulation

Among the unsuccessful fistula systems are some that fail because the arterialized vein, despite adequate size and flow, lies too deep, or is too tortuous, or because the overlying skin is too tough. For two-needle dialysis, an accessible vein segment at least 10 cm long is preferable. Short vein segments make cannulation of these fistulae difficult or even impossible. Brittle veins and large venous branches, adding confusion about where to puncture, may cause hematoma and discomfort to the patient. AVF thrombosis following large local hematomas after cannulation may occur (37).

Bleeding Complications

Usually, AVFs require minimal aftercare once the needles are withdrawn. Bleeding usually subsides within 15 min-

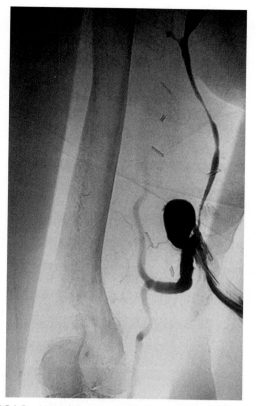

FIGURE 31.3. Cannulation complication in a brachiobasilic arteriovenous fistula. The needles have been stuck into a small vein segment, resulting in perforation of the back wall and the formation of a pseudoaneurysm.

utes, and AVF puncture sites clot faster than graft puncture sites. Prolonged bleeding from the puncture site may be the first sign of increased venous pressures caused by an outflow stenosis. The risk of bleeding complications, hematoma, and aneurysm formation is greater in brachiobasilic AVFs and eventually may lead to loss of the access site (29). Cannulation difficulty resulting in perforation of the back wall of the basilic vein is usually the cause for this complication (Fig 31.3).

Surgical Management

Improvement of accessibility can be accomplished by transposition of the arterialized cephalic vein to a more superficial and convenient position for puncture. The cephalic vein is dissected from the wrist up to the antecubital area through a continuous or interrupted longitudinal incision. The side branches are ligated, and the vein is transected 2 cm beyond the anastomosis with the radial artery. The proximal site of the vein remains attached, and after irrigating with heparin, it is repositioned in a new subcutaneous tunnel and anastomosed to the previously transected vein at the wrist.

Reported outcome of vein repositioning showed marked improvement in accessibility in 20 of 22 patients (38). Further, long-term durability without complications was ob-

tained in 80% of patients. Another beneficial effect of vein repositioning may be the elimination of large side branches that divert runoff from the main vein. AVFs with too-short vein segments may be repaired by vein transposition, either from a vein adjacent to the AVF or the forearm basilic vein (39).

LOW FLOW IN ARTERIOVENOUS FISTULAE

Intra-access flow inadequate to meet the blood flow needed for the amount of dialysis prescribed leads to recirculation, decreased dialysis efficiency, and finally AVF thrombosis. In autologous AFVs, inadequate flow can be detected by sequential monitoring of Kt/V, inline flow methods, or looking for signs of underdialysis. A blood flow of less than 400 to 500 mL per minute or a decline in flow of 20% between two measurements is likely to increase the risk of AVF thrombosis and to jeopardize dialysis efficiency (40).

The most common cause for low flow is a stenotic lesion or vessel segment induced by intimal hyperplasia. In radiocephalic AVFs, 75% of these stenoses are located at the AV anastomosis and 25% in the venous outflow track (41). Stenoses distal to the placement of the venous needle usually produce, in the absence of collateral vessels, a high venous pressure. In brachiocephalic and basilic AVFs, the typical location for stenosis is at the junction of the cephalic with the subclavian vein or the basilic with the axillary vein, respectively.

Surgical Management

The surgical treatment of low-flow AVFs depends on the location of the stenosis or occlusion.

Anastomotic Stenosis

Intimal hyperplasia at the AV anastomosis is best managed by one of three methods: widening of the lumen with a patch angioplasty, interposition of a short segment of prosthetic graft, or transferring the vein to the more proximal radial artery. In most cases, the stenotic lesion is located in the proximal cephalic vein just adjacent to the anastomosis. Surgical treatment is carried out by dissection of the proximal and distal radial artery and cephalic vein. After clamping of these vessels, a longitudinal incision is made, starting from a normal vein segment with prolongation toward the anastomosis. After opening the stenosed vessel segment, a vein or prosthetic patch is sutured in place (Fig. 31.4). In case of a more proximally located stenotic segment, the same technique can be used.

If the proximal radial artery is stenosed, it is easier to perform a new proximal AV anastomosis or to transfer the radial artery to the cephalic vein. Radial artery transposition is an attractive alternative method in patients with low flow

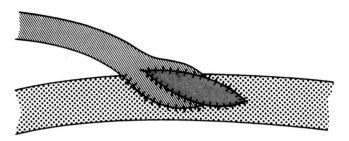

FIGURE 31.4. Patch plasty for an anastomotic stenotic lesion in an arteriovenous fistula.

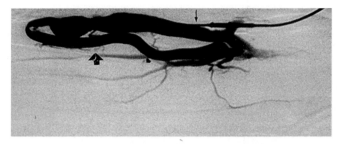

FIGURE 31.6. Radial artery transposition. The distal radial artery (*large arrow*) has been transected and turned in a smooth loop to the cephalic vein (*small arrow*) and subsequently anastomosed.

and an occluded distal artery (Figs. 31.5 and 31.6). The radial artery is dissected over a distance of 5 cm from the anastomosis upwards. After transection, it is turned in a smooth loop and anastomosed in an end-to-end fashion to the cephalic vein (42).

In severely diseased vessels or when the intimal hyperplasia extends over a length greater than 3 cm, a graft interposition is the best option. The disadvantage of this method is the inability to cannulate the access site immediately.

Venous Outflow Stenosis/Occlusion

The primary choice for treatment of short-segment outflow stenoses (<2 cm) is PTA. The best treatment for long-segment stenoses or occlusions is by using graft interposition or basilic vein transposition.

This latter method has several advantages: Only one anastomosis has to be performed, and the risk of intimal hyperplasia occurring at the graft–venous anastomosis is avoided. The surgical technique consists of dissection of the basilic vein in the forearm and, after removal, rerouting it in a smooth subcutaneous tunnel from the medial aspect of the elbow to the cephalic vein with an end-to-end anastomosis. When the basilic vein is not suitable, because of a small diameter, an externally ringed polytetrafluoroethylene (PTFE) interposition graft is sutured between the cephalic vein in the forearm and the basilic or deep vein in the upper arm (Figs. 31.7 and 31.8).

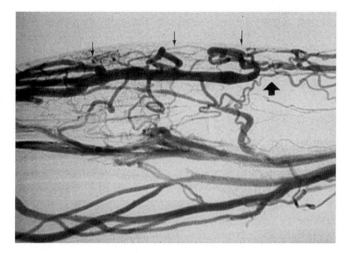

FIGURE 31.7. Distal cephalic vein occlusion (*large arrow*) at the elbow in a patient with a radiocephalic arteriovenous fistula. Notice the numerous side branches (*small arrows*), which divert blood flow from the cephalic vein.

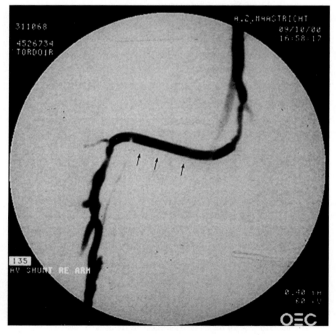

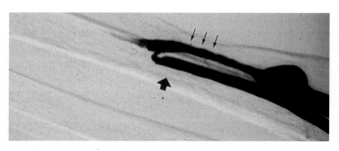

FIGURE 31.5. Proximal radial artery stenosis (*large arrow*) and distal radial artery occlusion in an end-to-side radiocephalic arteriovenous fistula (*small arrows*, cephalic vein).

FIGURE 31.8. Proximal cephalic vein obstruction. A 6-mm prosthetic (polytetrafluoroethylene) graft (*small arrows*) has been interposed between the cephalic vein (left side) and the basilic vein (right side). Same patient as Figure 31.7.

TABLE 31.3. LATE FAILURE OF RADIOCEPHALIC AVFS: RESULTS OF SURGICAL TREATMENT

Author (Ref. No.)	No. AVFs	Follow-up (yr)	Late Thrombosis (%)	Successful Revision (%)
Paruk et al. (45)	113	3	11	—
Rohr et al. (46)	126	3	24	58
Reilly et al. (4)	145	5	9	23
Erasmi et al. (5)	299	9	28	26
Tordoir et al. (6)	129	3	21	11
Wetzig et al. (47)	100	4	11	—
Kherlakian et al. (10)	100	4	17	—
Zibari et al. (26)	112	5	11	—
Ktenidis et al. (48)	165	5	22	32
Tautenhahn et al. (49)	210	6	13	20
Enzler et al. (50)	412	14	21	—
Konner (13)	202	5	13	—

AVFs, arteriovenous fistulae.

Junctional Stenosis (Brachiocephalic/Basilic Arteriovenous Fistula)

In brachiocephalic and basilic AVFs, junctional stenoses occur very frequently. PTA is the first option for treatment of basilic vein junctional stenosis. A surgical patch plasty may be needed after failed PTA. The primary surgical management of stenoses at the site of the cephalic vein entering into the subclavian vein is advisable because of the risk of rupture after PTA. Because a patch plasty can be a difficult operation, an alternative procedure, such as transposition of the proximal cephalic vein to the axillary vein, is recommended.

Central Vein Stenosis/Occlusion

Only rarely will central vein stenosis or occlusion cause low flow in an autologous AVF. Usually, the first signs of central vein obstruction are swelling and pain resulting from venous hypertension. The treatment options of this entity are discussed in Chapter 25.

LATE THROMBOTIC OCCLUSION

Clotting of the autologous fistula after the first postoperative month usually is caused by anastomotic or outflow vein stenosis, jeopardizing blood flow through the fistula. Repetitive puncture of the fistula in the same area with extravasation of blood and hematoma also may lead to fibrosis and stenoses. Anastomotic intimal hyperplasia has been attributed to mechanical endothelial cell damage by the high shear stress and pulse pressure of arterial blood flowing into the venous system. Hypotension during hemodialysis treatment or major surgery can induce fistula thrombosis. Severe fluid restriction and a hypercoagulable state may contribute to this complication (43,44).

The incidence of late thrombotic occlusion of radiocephalic AVF varies between 9% and 28% over a mean follow-up of 5.4 years (range 3–14 years) (Table 31.3). Although an underlying stenosis gradually develops, a significant number of thrombotic failures may be preventable by careful monitoring. Regular clinical examination, measurement of venous pressures, inline flow methods, and determination of dialysis efficacy by calculating Kt/V may identify access dysfunction. Duplex scanning or fistulography can detect stenotic lesions, which may be amenable to treatment with angioplasty or elective surgical revision [see Part IV (chapters 17–21)].

Surgical Management

The type of access and the site of thrombosis are important determinants of treatment outcome. Thrombosis may affect the postanastomotic vein segment as result of anastomotic stenosis, or it may begin at the needle site. When the clot is localized to the anastomosis in radiocephalic and brachiocephalic fistulae, the outflow vein may be patent because of the natural sidebranches that continue to deliver venous flow.

The surgical treatment options for thrombosed radiocephalic and brachiocephalic fistulae are (a) thrombectomy, (b) thrombectomy with patch plasty, (c) new proximal anastomosis, or (d) graft interposition. Surgical exploration of the AV anastomosis is performed under local or regional anesthesia. The proximal and distal artery and the cephalic vein are dissected, and vessel loops are admitted. After clamping the artery, the cephalic vein is opened longitudinally, and clots are removed from the inflow and outflow vessels by using a Fogarty catheter. Simple thrombectomy may be sufficient to restore blood flow, but when a stenosis is detected (which is usually the case), patch plasty with vein or prosthetic material must be performed. In case of stenosis over a long segment, a graft interposition between the

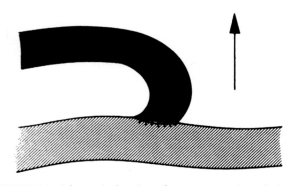

FIGURE 31.9. Schematic drawing of an anastomotic occlusion of an arteriovenous fistula.

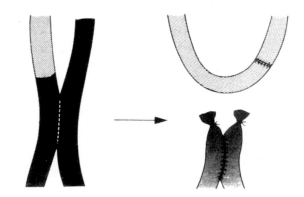

FIGURE 31.11. Thrombosed artery and vein of an arteriovenous fistula. Conversion of a side-to-side in an end-to-end anastomosis.

artery and outflow vein may be necessary. For the common postanastomotic stenosis in radiocephalic fistulae, revision of the anastomosis by mobilizing the cephalic vein and performing a new more proximal anastomosis with the radial artery are good options (Figs. 31.9 and 31.10). This is a simple operation, with its main advantage being that the already dilated proximal vein can be directly accessed for cannulation. In published series reporting on the use of this technique for a new proximal anastomosis in the ipsilateral forearm, success percentages of 50% to 72% are reported (51–53). When both the artery and vein are thrombosed, conversion of a side-to-side to an end-to-end anastomosis can be carried out with the possibility of using this new AVF immediately for cannulation (Fig. 31.11). This technique of arterialized cephalic vein anastomosis to the radial artery in previously thrombosed AVFs yielded a success rate of 57% in 72 patients with deterioration of kidney transplant function. Preoperative examination of the nonfunctioning AVF in these patients usually reveals a thrombosis of the AVF only to the first side branch with no evidence of proximal vein occlusion (54).

Successful surgical thrombectomy with or without AVF revision is reported with an incidence between 11% and 58%. From these publications, however, it is not always clear which kind of revision was carried out (Table 31.3).

Late occlusion in brachiocephalic and basilic AVFs occurs in 7% to 40% of fistulae (Table 31.2). Thrombosis in fistulae with transposed basilic veins usually leads to clot

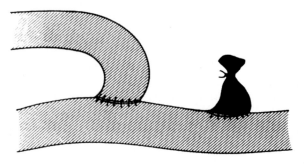

FIGURE 31.10. New proximal anastomosis between radial artery and cephalic vein.

propagation into the entire vein. This is the result of the fact that all side branches have been ligation during fistula creation, with the result that collateral venous inflow is impossible. An attempt at successful thrombectomy of a brachiobasilic fistula must be performed within several hours after clotting. Obstructing stenoses are the cause for thrombosis, and usually these are located at the AV anastomosis or at the junction of the basilic with the deep vein. Basilic vein compression by hematoma caused by cannulation difficulty also can result in thrombosis.

After declotting with a Fogarty catheter, additional repair of stenoses must be performed by patch plasty or PTA in the operating room. The results of surgical thrombectomy of brachiobasilic AVFs are worse, and often salvage of the AVF is not attempted, but a new AVF is created.

It may be obvious that completion angiography in the operation room after revision surgery of thrombosed autologous fistulae is mandatory to detect residual clots and stenoses.

SUMMARY

Autologous AVFs remain the first option for the creation of primary vascular access in dialysis patients. Early failure and nonmaturation in this type of AVF may occur in a high percentage of patients and can be beneficially influenced by careful vessel selection by means of preoperative duplex scanning. When an autologous fistula has an initial good function and uncomplicated cannulations, however, it may run for years with only a slight risk of dysfunction or thrombosis. The options for surgical intervention in thrombosed fistulae are thrombectomy with or without patch plasty or graft interposition. A new proximal anastomosis offers a good alternative in these cases.

Improvement of autologous AVF outcome may be accomplished by initiating of a routine surveillance program to detect failing AVFs (AVF with low flow), which may successfully respond to elective interventional or surgical treatment.

REFERENCES

1. Kinnaert P, Vereerstraeten P, Toussaint C, et al. Nine years' experience with internal arteriovenous fistulas for haemodialysis: a study of some factors influencing the results. *Br J Surg* 1977;64: 242–246.
2. Uldall R. Prevention of thrombosis in arteriovenous fistulas. *Blood Purif* 1985;3:89–93.
3. Windus DW. Permanent vascular access: a nephrologist's view. *Am J Kidney Dis* 1993;21:457–471.
4. Reilly DT, Wood RF, Bell PR. Prospective study of dialysis fistulae: problem patients and their treatment. *Br J Surg* 1982;69: 549–553.
5. Erasmi H, Horsch S, Schmidt R, et al. Complications of arteriovenous fistulas and surgical intervention. In: Kootstra, Jorning, eds. *Access Surgery*, Lancaster, UK: MTP Press, 1984:163–167.
6. Tordoir JH, Kwan TS, Herman JM, et al. Primary and secondary access surgery for haemodialysis with the Brescia-Cimino fistula and the polytetrafluoroethylene (PTFE) graft. *Neth J Surg* 1983; 35:8–12.
7. Louridas G, Botha JR, Levien L, et al. Vascular access for haemodialysis—experience at Johannesburg Hospital. *S Afr Med J* 1984;66:637–640.
8. Wedgwood KR, Wiggins PA, Guillou PJ. A prospective study of end-to-side vs. side-to-side arteriovenous fistulas for haemodialysis. *Br J Surg* 1984;71:640–642.
9. Palder SB, Kirkman RL, Whittemore AD, et al. Vascular access for hemodialysis: patency rates and results of revision. *Ann Surg* 1985;202:235–239.
10. Kherlakian GM, Roedersheimer LR, Arbaugh JJ, et al. Comparison of autogenous fistula versus expanded polytetrafluoroethylene graft fistula for angioaccess in hemodialysis. *Am J Surg* 1986;152:238–243.
11. Braun L, Polith J. Der Ciminishunt. *Chir Praxis* 1989;40:293–302.
12. Burger H, Kluchert BA, Kootstra G, et al. Survival of arteriovenous fistulas and shunts for haemodialysis. *Eur J Surg* 1995;161: 327–334.
13. Konner K. Primary vascular access in diabetic patients: an audit. *Nephrol Dial Transplant* 2000;15:1317–1325.
14. Wong V, Ward R, Taylor J, et al. Factors associated with early failure of arteriovenous fistulae for haemodialysis access. *Eur J Vasc Endovasc Surg* 1996;12:207–213.
15. Silva MB Jr, Hobson RW 2nd, Pappas PJ, et al. A strategy for increasing use of autogenous hemodialysis access procedures: impact of preoperative noninvasive evaluation. *J Vasc Surg* 1998;27: 302–307.
16. Lemson MS, Leunissen KM, Tordoir JH. Does pre-operative duplex examination improve patency rates of Brescia-Cimino fistulas? *Nephrol Dial Transplant* 1998;13:1360–1361.
17. Sands JJ. Increasing AV fistulas: revisiting a time-tested solution. *Semin Dial* 2000;13:351–353.
18. Ascher E, Gade P, Hingorani A, et al. Changes in the practice of angioaccess surgery: impact of dialysis outcome and quality initiative recommendations. *J Vasc Surg* 2000;31:84–92.
19. Klauber GT, Belitsky P, Morehouse DD, et al. Preventable problems with arteriovenous fistulas for hemodialysis. *Surg Gynecol Obstet* 1971;132:457–459.
20. Owada A, Saito H, Mochizuki T, et al. Radial arterial spasm in uremic patients undergoing construction of arteriovenous hemodialysis fistulas: diagnosis and prophylaxis with intravenous nicardipine. *Nephron* 1993;64:501–504.
21. Bourquelot P, Cussenot O, Corbi P, et al. Microsurgical creation and follow-up of arteriovenous fistulae for chronic haemodialysis in children. *Pediatr Nephrol* 1990;4:156–159.
22. Cavallaro G, Taranto F, Cavallaro E, et al. Vascular complications of native arteriovenous fistulas for hemodialysis: role of microsurgery. *Microsurgery* 2000;20:252–254.
23. Yasunaga C, Nakamoto M, Fukuda K, et al. Superficial repositioning of the artery for chronic hemodialysis: indications and prognosis. *Am J Kidney Dis* 1995;26:602–606.
24. Cantelmo NL, LoGerfo FW, Menzoian JO. Brachiobasilic and brachiocephalic fistulas as secondary angioaccess routes. *Surg Gynecol Obstet* 1982;155:545–548.
25. Dunlop MG, Mackinlay JY, Jenkins AM. Vascular access: experience with the brachiocephalic fistula. *Ann R Coll Surg Engl* 1986;68:203–206.
26. Zibari GB, Rohr MS, Landreneau MD, et al. Complications from permanent hemodialysis vascular access. *Surgery* 1988;104: 681–686.
27. Nazzal MM, Neglen P, Naseem J, et al. The brachiocephalic fistula: a successful secondary vascular access procedure. *Vasa* 1990;19:326–329.
28. Rivers SP, Scher LA, Sheehan E, et al. Basilic vein transposition: an underused autologous alternative to prosthetic dialysis angioaccess. *J Vasc Surg* 1993;18:391–397.
29. Coburn MC, Carney WI Jr. Comparison of basilic vein and polytetrafluoroethylene for brachial arteriovenous fistula. *J Vasc Surg* 1994;20:896–902.
30. Hakaim AG, Nalbandian M, Scott T. Superior maturation and patency of primary brachiocephalic and transposed basilic vein arteriovenous fistulae in patients with diabetes. *J Vasc Surg* 1998;27:154–157.
31. Humphries AL Jr, Colborn GL, Wynn JJ. Elevated basilic vein arteriovenous fistula. *Am J Surg* 1999;177:489–491.
32. Murphy GJ, White SA, Knight AJ, et al. Long-term results of arteriovenous fistulas using transposed autologous basilic vein. *Br J Surg* 2000;87:819–823.
33. Hodges TC, Fillinger MF, Zwolak RM, et al. Longitudinal comparison of dialysis access methods: risk factors for failure. *J Vasc Surg* 1997;26:1009–1019.
34. Miller PE, Tolwani A, Luscy CP, et al. Predictors of adequacy of arteriovenous fistulas in hemodialysis patients. *Kidney Int* 1999; 56:275–280.
35. Beathard GA, Settle SM, Shields MW. Salvage of the nonfunctioning arteriovenous fistula. *Am J Kidney Dis* 1999;33:910–916.
36. Albers F. Causes of hemodialysis access failure. *Adv Ren Replace Ther* 1994;1:107–118.
37. Lindfors O, Eklund B, von Numers H, et al. Experience with different types of fistulas and shunts for hemodialysis. *Scand J Urol Nephrol* 1975;6–7(29 Suppl):81–82.
38. Foran RF, Levin PM, Cohen JL, et al. Delayed vein repositioning: a procedure for improving inadequate radial-cephalic arteriovenous fistulas. *Arch Surg* 1976;111:675–677.
39. Silva MB Jr, Hobson RW 2nd, Pappas PJ, et al. Vein transposition in the forearm for autogenous hemodialysis access. *J Vasc Surg* 1997;26:981–986.
40. Schwab SJ, Oliver MJ, Suhocki P, et al. Hemodialysis arteriovenous access: detection of stenosis and response to treatment by vascular access blood flow. *Kidney Int* 2001;59:358–362.
41. Langeveld APM, Leunissen KML, Eikelboom BC, et al. Duplex ultrasound detection of stenoses in newly created hemodialysis AV fistulas. In: Tordoir, Kitslaar, Kootstra, et al., eds. *Progress in access surgery*. Maastricht: Datawyse, 1990:145–154.
42. Karmody AM, Lempert N. "Smooth loop" arteriovenous fistulas for hemodialysis. *Surgery* 1974;75:238–242.
43. Brenowitz JB, Williams CD, Edwards WS. Major surgery in patients with chronic renal failure. *Am J Surg* 1977;134:765–769.
44. Berger A, Rosenberg N. Hypotension and closure of hemodialysis access shunts. *Am Surg* 1983;49:551–553.
45. Paruk S, Koenig M, Levitt S, et al. Arteriovenous fistulas for

hemodialysis in 100 consecutive patients. *Am J Surg* 1976;131: 552–555.

46. Rohr MS, Browder W, Frentz GD, et al. Arteriovenous fistulas for long-term dialysis. Factors that influence fistula survival. *Arch Surg* 1978;113:153–155.

47. Wetzig GA, Gough IR, Furnival CM. One hundred cases of arteriovenous fistula for haemodialysis access: the effect of cigarette smoking on patency. *Aust N Z J Surg* 1985;55:551–554.

48. Ktenidis K, de Vleeschauwer P, Horsch S. Komplikationen der subkutanen arteriovenosen dialysefisteln. *Phlebologie* 1991;20: 35–38.

49. Tautenhahn J, Heinrich P, Meyer F. Arteriovenous fistulas for hemodialysis—patency rates and complications—a retrospective study. *Zentralbl Chir* 1994;119:506–510.

50. Enzler MA, Rajmon T, Lachat M, et al. Long-term function of vascular access for hemodialysis. *Clin Transplant* 1996;10(6 Pt 1):511–515.

51. Romero A, Polo JR, Morato EG, et al. Salvage of angioaccess after late thrombosis of radiocephalic fistulas for hemodialysis. *Int Surg* 1986;71:122–124

52. Nakagawa Y, Ota K, Sato Y, et al. Complications in blood access for hemodialysis. *Artif Organs* 1994;18:283–288.

53. Oakes DD, Sherck JP, Cobb LF. Surgical salvage of failed radiocephalic arteriovenous fistulae: techniques and results in 29 patients. *Kidney Int* 1998;53:480–487.

54. Grochowiecki T, Szmidt J, Galazka Z, et al. Usefulness of arterialized cephalic vein of forearm of previously thrombosed arteriovenous fistula for creating a new vascular access for hemodialysis in patients with renal allograft insufficiency. *Transplant Proc* 2000;32:1375–1376.

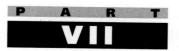

CENTRAL DIALYSIS CATHETERS

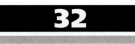

THE USE OF CATHETERS FOR HEMODIALYSIS: OVERVIEW

JOHN H. RUNDBACK
PATRICK C. MALLOY

HISTORY AND BACKGROUND

The use of catheters for chronic hemodialysis parallels the history of dialysis itself (1). The first report of arterial and venous cannulation for prolonged hemodialysis was by Quinton and colleagues in 1960 (2). Shortly afterward, in 1961, Shaldon and associates described the use of femoral artery catheterization for hemodialysis (3). Subsequent developments in the early 1970s included the use of a single-lumen catheter with a reciprocating pump to alternate inflow and outflow (4) and the practice of inserting separate transfemoral catheters into both renal veins (5). In 1979, Uldall and colleagues reported the first use of guidewire exchange techniques and a subclavian vein puncture for the insertion of temporary dialysis catheters (6). In the late 1980s, Schwab and colleagues introduced the concept of a cuffed catheter for long-term access (7). Refinements of this early device resulted in the tunneled cuffed catheters available today.

Chronic hemodialysis requires stable high-flow circulatory access, conditions that are fulfilled, when necessary, by the use of central venous catheters. As a result, venous catheters have become a critical component in the management of patients requiring long-term renal replacement therapy. This chapter outlines some of the general principles—indications, functional requirements, considerations for catheter selection and insertion, and complications—governing the use of central venous catheters in the hemodialysis population.

COSTS, PRACTICE PATTERNS, AND INDICATIONS

In the United States, at the turn of the millennium, almost 200,000 patients are receiving chronic hemodialysis each year, and an incident 54,000 persons are starting therapy annually (8). Close to 20% of patients starting hemodialysis have a tunneled cuffed catheter as their initial form of venous access (9), with a presumably much larger number beginning dialysis via temporary catheters. The number of catheters still in use 1 month after initiating hemodialysis has increased since 1991 from fewer than 15% to almost 40% (10).

Until recently, the placement of catheters has increased steadily each year. In 1996, temporary and permanent catheter insertion accounted for 12% of all part B hemodialysis expenditures and 29% of outpatient vascular access costs (8). This represents a 2.4-fold increase for temporary catheters and a 1.4-fold increase for permanent catheters compared with 1991 values, disproportionate to the growth of the dialysis patient population over the same interval. An additional 24% of outpatient vascular access costs were due to catheter revision or removal (8). Catheter placement by nephrologists accounted for a significant percentage of these overall increases. To help reverse these trends, the National Kidney Foundation in 1997 published the Dialysis Outcomes Quality Initiative (DOQI) vascular access guidelines (guidelines 3 and 30). These guidelines discouraged the use of chronic hemodialysis catheters and suggested that fewer than 10% of patients receiving renal replacement therapy should have indwelling catheters as their permanent access (11). Although these guidelines have been widely incorporated into quality improvement programs, their ultimate impact on access patterns has not yet been determined (12).

With projections that 520,000 Americans will be dialysis dependent by the year 2010 (8), the prevalence of and costs associated with dialysis catheter insertion and maintenance will more than likely continue to grow. Although it appears that catheter survival and complication rates are similar regardless of the specialty of the inserting physician (13–15), radiologically guided insertion has been shown to decrease costs (16) as well as reduce catheter failures (17,18). Consequently, DOQI (guideline 5) recommends real-time ultrasound-guided venous puncture for catheter insertion and mandates fluoroscopy for catheter insertion and positioning (11).

Indications for the use of both temporary and permanent hemodialysis catheters have been defined by DOQI (guide-

TABLE 32.1. CLINICAL INDICATIONS FOR DIALYSIS CATHETERS

Nontunneled (temporary) catheters
  Acute renal failure
  Poisoning
  Plasmapharesis
  ICU setting (i.e., CVVHD in patient requiring bedside
    catheter insertion)
  Short-term bridge to permanent access (<3 wk)
Tunneled-cuffed (chronic) catheters
  Temporary dialysis during AV fistula maturation
  Temporary access during peritoneal catheter maturation
  Interim access during graft revision or treatment of
    graft infection
  Bridge to permanent access (>3 wk)
  Unavailability of permanent AV access site
  Repeated failure of permanent AV access
  Multiple comorbid medical conditions limiting life expectancy
  Severe left ventricular dysfunction
  Elderly patients
  Daily home dialysis requiring frequent access

ICU, intensive care unit; CVVHD, chronic veno-venous hemodialysis; AV, arteriovenous.

lines 5 and 6), and appropriate clinical applications are shown in Table 32.1 (11). Noncuffed temporary catheters are suitable for acute vascular access of less than 3 weeks' duration, should be inserted immediately prior to use, and must be removed at the earliest sign of infection (9,11). Tunneled cuffed catheters can be used as a bridge to permanent access exceeding 3 weeks [i.e., during arteriovenous (AV) fistula or peritoneal dialysis access maturation), in frail elderly patients with multiple medical problems limiting life expectancy (19,20), or in patients who have no remaining sites for a permanent AV access (fistula or autogenous graft) placement. Despite the recognized role of dialysis catheters as a temporary bridge to permanent AV access availability, this may be associated with increased mortality (21) and should be discouraged. Thus, early referral to a nephrologist for end-stage renal disease (ESRD) counseling and access planning is recommended by DOQI (guideline 8) (11).

GENERAL FUNCTIONAL PRINCIPLES

Recent reviews (9,22) identified many of the characteristics of the "ideal" hemodialysis catheter (Table 32.2). (See Chapter 42 for more on catheter design, materials, and hemodynamics.) Unfortunately, no currently available de-

vice fulfills all these criteria. Despite their deficiencies, catheters must possess several properties that are uniformly recognized as necessary for acceptable dialysis. The most critical of these is the ability to provide consistently high blood flow with low rates of recirculation. With the increasing use of ambulatory hemodialysis and the resulting need to enhance patient throughput, the capability to maintain flows sufficient for high-flux hemodialysis is the rate-limiting step for successful catheter usage. DOQI (guideline 23) has established the minimal acceptable flow rate to be 300 mL per minute (10), although recently introduced high-flow catheters probably should be expected to sustain reliably flow rates exceeding 350 or even 400 mL per minute (21, 23). Other investigators evaluated the urea reduction ratio (URR) or achieved Kt/V as a measure of the adequacy of catheter dialysis (9,24,25). Regardless of the technique used, it is important to recognize that the actual or effective blood flow (Qb_{eff}) as determined by ultrasound dilution techniques is frequently less than the recorded or prescribed dialyzer pump speed (Qb_{meas}), particularly at higher flow rates (9,22). This is due to the tendency for partial collapse of the arterial lumen of the catheter at lower (more negative) prepump pressures. In fact, the discrepancy between Qb_{eff} and Qb_{meas} may be as large as 30% with the dialyzer blood pump set at 400 mL per minute (9). In these circumstances, it may be necessary to set the catheter pump speed at 350 to 400 mL per minute to achieve the minimum Qb_{eff} of 300 mL per minute as defined by DOQI.

The two major determinants of the Qb_{eff} for chronic tunneled hemodialysis catheters are *functional lumen size* and *tip location*. For the purpose of this discussion, the functional lumen size is the actual diameter of the arterial lumen during use at prescribed dialysis flow rates and (as discussed already) may differ from the measured lumen diameter before insertion or when not receiving dialysis. In general, thin-walled polyurethane catheters manufactured with larger luminal calibers will maintain a better functional lumen size during use than will silicone catheters. Functional lumen size also may be affected by the shape (or type) of the catheter as well as by the catheter insertion site. In one study (23), the presence of discrete lumina (i.e., split lumen and twin catheters) provided better flow than catheters with an internal septum. With regard to insertion site, several reports suggested that catheters placed via the left internal jugular vein have worse flows than catheters inserted via other upper-extremity sites (26,27). Most likely, this is the result of compromise of the lumen as a result of the greater

TABLE 32.2. CHARACTERISTICS OF THE "IDEAL" CATHETER

Biologically inert	→	Does not induce venous thrombosis or fibrin sheath formation
Resistant to infection	→	Catheter surface prevents bacterial migration and seeding
High flow	→	Able to consistently maintain dialysis flows ≥350 to 400 mL/min
Atraumatic	→	Soft, easily inserted, durable, comfortable
Inexpensive	→	Lower economic burden of chronic hemodialysis

angulation and number of turns the catheter must take to reach the right atrium. Subclavian catheters are also subject to compression at the junction of the clavicle and first rib ("pinch-off" syndrome), which also may reduce the functional lumen size (28).

The position of the catheter tip is the other critical factor determining the Qb_{eff}. Catheters should be positioned with their tips in the mid right atrium (RA) or at the cavoatrial junction to maximize flow. A more peripheral catheter tip location adversely affects catheter function, causing both diminished flow rates and higher recirculation (29). This effect is even more pronounced in volume-depleted patients with predialysis central venous pressures below 5 mm Hg, probably because of collapse of the vein caused by prepump pressures (30). Technical malpositioning of the tip in the upper superior vena cava (SVC) also may result in initial catheter malfunction because of wedging of the tip against the vein wall and is more likely to occur with left-sided access. This effect can be minimized by rotating the catheter at the time of placement so that the side holes of the arterial lumen are directed toward the middle of the SVC (31). In obese patients or patients with large breasts, the catheter tip will frequently retract cephalad as the patient assumes an erect position, and the catheter should therefore be secured deeper into the SVC or RA at the time of placement (31). (See Chapters 33 and 36 for additional information on catheter position)

Recirculation refers to a pattern of circular flow in which filtered blood returned from the dialyzer is immediately reaspirated through the arterial or "draw" lumen of the catheter. As a result, less unfiltered blood is passed through the dialyzer, and the efficiency of dialysis is reduced. To prevent this, dialysis catheters with staggered tips are designed with the arterial port 2 to 3 cm proximal to the venous port, and twin catheters are inserted with the tips at least 4 cm apart. Nevertheless, recirculation occurs to some extent with all hemodialysis catheters and is in part dependent on catheter position and blood flow in the surrounding vein (9). Thus, catheters positioned with their tips in a smaller vein are prone to greater recirculation than catheters positioned in larger central veins or the RA. Recirculation is aggravated in cases when it is necessary to reverse the "draw" and "return" (venous) ports because of insufficient arterial lumen flows (24). Other causes of increased recirculation include fibrin sheath formation, partial venous thrombosis, and catheter breakdown (32). Rates of recirculation exceeding 15% considerably reduce dialysis efficiency and mandate catheter exchange or revision.

TYPES OF CATHETERS AND CATHETER MATERIALS

Hemodialysis catheters have evolved into two distinct classes of device that encompass the vast majority of clinical practice: (a) temporary, or acute catheters; and (b) tunneled cuffed, or chronic catheters (Fig. 32.1).

Acute Catheters

Temporary venous access devices for hemodialysis are designed to provide rapid, safe access that is suitable for up to 3 weeks. Current coaxial lumen catheters have become the clinical standard and have replaced the previous single lumen,

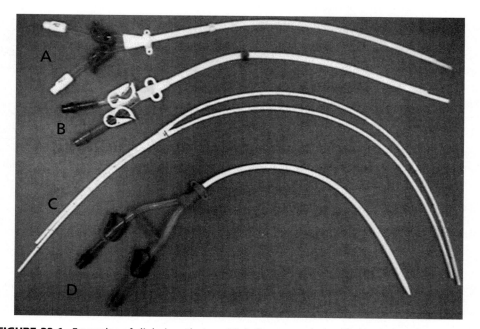

FIGURE 32.1. Examples of dialysis catheters. High-flow tunneled cuffed polyurethane catheter (*A*). Tunneled cuffed dual-lumen silicone catheter (*B*). Tunneled split catheter (*C*). Temporary non-cuffed catheter (*D*).

dual catheters, and trocar methods formerly in use. Contemporary designs utilize construction with polyurethane or polyvinyl, which provide adequate stiffness at room temperature for insertion using over-the-wire Seldinger technique but become more pliable at body temperature to avoid vascular complications.

Temporary catheters are available in a wide variety of lengths that make them suitable for placement in jugular, subclavian, and femoral locations. The catheters can be inserted at the bedside, allowing rapid access without the necessity for fluoroscopic support. Blood flow is generally limited to 200 to 250 mL per minute, providing adequate functionality only for short-term use. Whereas the nontunneled design allows for simplicity and ease of insertion, strict catheter maintenance is critical to avoid infectious complications, which may lead to catheter-related sepsis and an increased incidence of pericatheter thrombosis.

Chronic Tunneled Cuffed Catheters

Tunneled hemodialysis catheters were introduced more than 10 years ago as an alternative to temporary catheters in an effort to provide higher flow rates and prolonged vascular access without vascular or infectious complications. These devices differ significantly from temporary catheters with respect to size, catheter construction, subcutaneous cuffed design, and method of insertion. Tunneled catheters are generally larger, ranging from 13.5 French to 20 French and allow for extracorporeal flow rates that meet or exceed the 300 mL per minute established by the DOQI (11). Catheters usually are constructed using silicone or Silastic elastomer, which results in a catheter that is much softer and more pliable than the typical acute type catheter. A bonded cuff is placed along the subcutaneous portion of the device that, after fibrous incorporation, serves to anchor the catheter to the chest wall and prevent bacterial migration to the tunnel or intravascular portion of the catheter.

Insertion of tunneled catheters is more complex than placement of acute catheters and requires fluoroscopy to ensure proper positioning of the tip within the right atrium to achieve maximum blood flow. The flexible silicone or Silastic construction precludes the use of Seldinger technique and requires use of a peel-away sheath. Although placement of the peel-away sheath necessitates overdilation of the vascular cannulation site, bleeding complications are uncommon because of the relatively low pressure of the venous circulation. The peel-away sheath insertion technique, however, does increase the risk of air embolus during insertion, and care must be taken to avoid this potential complication.

Multiple-cuffed catheters are now available for clinical use (Table 32.3) and new catheter designs are regularly introduced. The catheters are distinguished by their designs, including catheter material, tip configuration, and lumen size and geometry. Single- or fused-lumen catheters have stepped or staggered tips to prevent recirculation and are inserted using the peel-away technique without significant procedural differences between catheters. The Tesio catheter (MedComp, Harleysville, PA, U.S.A.) requires two separate cannulation sites thereby increasing the complexity of insertion and the potential for complications (33,34). A hybrid device, the Ash split catheter (MedComp), has separation of the intravascular portions of the catheter but is inserted via a single insertion site with a fused subcutaneous portion. Several catheter lumen configurations are also available (Fig. 32.2), each of which is claimed by their manufacturer to maximize blood flow.

INSERTION SITES

A detailed description of the techniques and considerations for hemodialysis catheter insertion is provided in Chapter 33. Several general considerations regarding the choice of access site warrant discussion here, however.

TABLE 32.3. CURRENTLY AVAILABLE HEMODIALYSIS CATHETERS

Name/Manufacturer[a]	Design	Shape	OD	Material
Hickman/Bard Access Systems	Double D	Round	13.5 F	Silicone
Vaxel/Boston Scientific	Double D	Round	16 F Tapered to 14 F	Polyurethane
Mahurkar/Quinton	Double D	Round	13.5	Silicone
Oval/Quinton	Side by side	Oval	16 F (oval)	Silicone
Ash Split Cath/Medcomp	Split Dual catheters	Round	14 F	Silicone
Tesio/Medcomp	Separate Dual catheters	Round	10 F	Silicone
Neostar/Horizon Medical Products	Circle C	Oval	13.5 F	Polyurethane

OD, outer diameter; F, French.
[a] Bard Access Systems, Salt Lake City, UT; Boston Scientific Corporation, Watertown, MA; Quinton Instrument Company, Seattle, WA; Neostar, Horizon Medical Products, Manchester, GA; MedComp, Harleysville, PA.

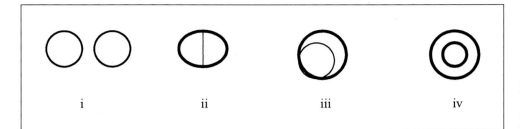

FIGURE 32.2. Configurations of catheter lumens. Twin or split lumens (*i*), double D (*ii*), circle C (*iii*), and coaxial (*iv*) lumen configurations are shown.

Upper Extremity

The right internal jugular vein is the preferred insertion site for permanent dialysis catheters. Catheters placed via this route have a direct path to the distal SVC and RA and can be tunneled with a gently sloping course toward either a lateral chest wall or parasternal exit site. Catheter insertion via the left internal jugular vein is less desirable because of the increased number of curves and the need to traverse the innominate vein, thereby potentially jeopardizing left upper-extremity venous outflow. Real-time ultrasound guidance for vein cannulation is strongly recommended by DOQI (guideline 5) (11) and clearly reduces cannulation failures and insertion related complications (11,35,36,37). Subclavian vein insertion is associated with less technical success and greater complications (38) and should be used only when jugular options are not available or the ipsilateral extremity cannot be used for a permanent AV fistula of graft. Finally, tunneled catheters should not be placed on the same side as a maturing AV access unless other sites are not available.

Femoral

In general, transfemoral catheter insertion is restricted to acute noncuffed catheters in bedridden patients, with the primary advantage being the ability for rapid, easy bedside insertion without fluoroscopic monitoring. This may be particularly advantageous in patients in whom upper-extremity central venous access is compromised by the presence of a tracheostomy cuff or multiple central venous catheters for hemodynamic monitoring and support. DOQI has determined that femoral catheters need to be at least 19 cm long to avoid unacceptably high recirculation rates (11). Much longer catheters (40–50 cm) actually may be needed for the tip to reside fully within the inferior vena cava (IVC) (9). Because of the risk of infection, these catheters should not be left in place for longer than 5 days (DOQI guideline 6) (11). At least two reports have described the use of permanent cuffed tunneled femoral catheters for ambulatory hemodialysis (39,40). These need to be even longer (60–70 cm) for the tip to be at the IVC–right atrial junction or in the RA. As might be expected, these were associated with lower flow rates, more frequent reintervention, and an increased rate of infection compared with upper-extremity placement. Nevertheless, it appears that femorally inserted catheters may be considered as another option for patients lacking other access sites.

Alternative Access Routes

The repeated placement of catheters in the upper-extremity veins not infrequently results in venous thrombosis or stricture formation. In severe instances, this leads to extensive upper-extremity venous occlusion and unavailability of a suitable patent large-vein conduit for cannulation. Although technically more demanding, catheter insertion via occluded central veins as well as through the external jugular and collateral veins has been described and does not appear to jeopardize catheter function (41,42). Other alternative access sites include direct translumbar puncture of the inferior vena cava (43) and hepatic veins (44) (see Chapter 34). These routes are associated with increased risks, including bleeding and catheter dislodgement (45).

COMPLICATIONS OF DIALYSIS CATHETERS

As with any percutaneously introduced device, the insertion of dialysis catheters is subject to potential procedural risks. Based on consensus methodology and a critical evaluation of the English language literature, the Society of Cardiovascular and Interventional Radiology (SCVIR) has established standards of practice for central venous access (46). Reported rates for successful internal jugular vein catheter placement approach 96%, and a suggested threshold of 95% has been defined by SCVIR. Procedure-related minor and major complications occur in about 7% of cases; the SCVIR recommended threshold for major procedural complications is 3%. Thresholds for specific complications such as pneumothorax or hemothorax, air embolism, and procedure-induced sepsis are set at 2% to 3%.

Although immediate insertion-related complications of hemodialysis catheters are low, these devices are plagued by early and delayed complications that limit long-term use. These events often result in device failure or loss of the venous access site. Reporting standards from the SCVIR have defined device failure as "any limitation in catheter function despite technically successful catheter placement," including inadequate blood flow or occlusion of one lumen (47). Inadequate dialysis flow rates requiring device removal occur in 50% to 90% of implanted venous dialysis catheters within 1 year of placement, resulting in an overall catheter use-life inferior to all other methods of dialysis (31,48). In contradistinction, "technique" or "modality" failure represents cumulative (*secondary*) catheter survival and is delineated by abandonment of the access site. Catheter revision using techniques such as guidewire exchange, repositioning, or stripping may result in secondary 1-year technique survival exceeding 80% (49).

The major adverse events resulting in catheter loss or revision are catheter-related infection and occlusion. In addition, thrombosis or stenosis of the access vein or veins traversed by the catheter may impede subsequent catheter placement or affect ipsilateral creation of an autogenous fistula or graft.

Infection

Catheter-related infection may manifest as asymptomatic colonization, exit-site or tunnel infections, bacteremia, or overt clinical sepsis. The management of the infected catheter depends on the severity of the infection, and a detailed review can be found in Chapter 35. DOQI guideline 26 also provides general principles for treatment of infection of the tunneled cuffed catheter (11). Timely and appropriate therapy is necessary to avoid potentially significant morbidity, including endocarditis, osteomyelitis, sepsis, and death.

Asymptomatic colonization probably occurs in most catheters left in place for more than several weeks, with one study identifying positive catheter cultures in 68% of tunneled catheters by 1 month (50). Although seeding with *Staphylococcus epidermidis* is most common (51), infections with *Staphylococcus aureus* pose a greater risk for subsequent bacteremia and occur as a result of the frequent nasal carriage of this organism in patients with ESRD (52). Careful catheter handling and dressing guidelines are suggested by DOQI (guideline 15) to help reduce colonization resulting in symptomatic infections (11). Infections occurring at the exit site usually are treated without threatening catheter loss using local care as well as topical and oral antibiotics. More serious infections involving the subcutaneous catheter tunnel generally respond to a course of parenteral antibiotics, although guidewire exchange with creation of a new tunnel and exit site may be necessary.

Catheter related bacteremia occurs at a rate of 0.15 to 0.55 per 100 catheter days (31,53,54) and is the most common reason for technique failure. More recently, salvage of the access site has been reported using a 3-week course of parenteral antibiotics, with catheter exchange over a guidewire 48 hours after initiating antibiotic therapy (55,56). Using this strategy, preservation of the access site has been described in more than 80% of cases (54,56,57). Patients with overt clinical sepsis require catheter removal (57).

Catheter Occlusion

Catheter occlusion may occur secondary to intrinsic thrombosis or the development of a fibrin sheath and is the most frequent cause for device failure. A detailed review of fibrin sheath formation and treatment can be found in Chapter 36. Thrombosis of the catheter lumen is due to inadequate heparin filling of the catheter between dialysis sessions and can be treated safely and effectively in most cases by the intracatheter instillation of a thrombolytic agent. When thrombolysis fails, the cause of the catheter occlusion is usually formation of a fibrin sheath at the catheter tip. This fibrin sheath is histologically composed of laminated proteinaceous material with eosinophilic and inflammatory infiltrates consistent with organizing thrombus (58). Fibrin sheaths that do not respond to thrombolytic therapy have been treated by either transfemoral catheter stripping using a percutaneously introduced snare catheter (59) or catheter exchange over a guidewire (60). DOQI guideline 23 supports either approach (11). A recent prospective randomized trial suggested that catheter exchange is associated with better patency (61) than stripping. More importantly, repeated catheter exchange does not appear to affect adversely cumulative catheter patency or increase the risk of infectious complications (60,62).

Venous Stenosis and Thrombosis

Insertion-site trauma or repetitive injury of the vascular intima by catheter movement may induce venous thrombosis or stenosis (63). Access-site thrombosis is lower when using percutaneous ultrasound-guided techniques compared with using surgical cutdown (64,65). The choice of access site is also critical in determining the risk and possible sequelae of venous thrombosis. Catheters inserted via the internal jugular vein produce venous thrombosis in only 3% of instances, which is rarely symptomatic (66). In contrast, subclavian vein cannulation is associated with thrombosis in 13 % and, moreover, the late development of subclavian venous stenosis in up to 50% (38,67,68). As a result, subclavian catheter placement is essentially precluded in any patient who may subsequently be offered an ipsilateral arteriovenous fistula or graft (see Chapter 25).

FUTURE DEVELOPMENTS

The use of venous catheters for temporary or permanent hemodialysis is likely to remain an important part of the care of patients with ESRD. Several approaches to reducing the risk of catheter-associated infections are being evaluated.

One strategy is modification of the catheter surface or impregnation with specific antimicrobial agents to prevent bacterial adherence or surface migration. Although one study using silver-coated catheters did not reduce the rate of catheter colonization or clinical infection (69), modifications of this method or the use of other substances may prove to be effective (70). Similar techniques may be used to prevent catheter-related thrombosis or fibrin sheath formation.

With the goal of reducing infectious complications of hemodialysis access, several manufacturers have developed totally implanted hemodialysis access devices (see Chapter 42). Dialysis ports are similar in concept to existing venous access devices now widely in use for infusion therapy. Their specific design differs significantly from infusion ports because of the requirements for repetitive large-bore access. Two different devices are currently under investigation. The Dialock Port (BioLink, Middleboro, MA, U.S.A.) is a single titanium rectangular container with two thin-walled reinforced silicone catheters normally inserted by two separate jugular insertion sites (71). The device is accessed with specifically designed Dialock needles. There have been over 250 worldwide implants. The LifeSite device (Vasca, Inc., Tewksbury, MA, U.S.A.) is a stainless steel port connected to a single 12 French silicone catheter. The device is accessed using standard fistula needles. Clinical trials of this device have demonstrated superior function compared with the Tesio device, with an overall reduction in catheter-related infection. The long-term results of these devices are yet to be assessed.

REFERENCES

1. Kapoian T, Sherman RA. A brief history of vascular access for hemodialysis: an unfinished story. *Semin Nephrol* 1997;17: 239–245.
2. Quinton, WE, Dillard D, Scribner BH. Cannulation of blood vessels for prolonged hemodialysis. *Trans Am Soc Artif Intern Organs* 1960;6:104–113.
3. Shaldon S, Chianussi L, Higgs B. Hemodialysis by percutaneous catheterization of the femoral artery and vein with regional heparinization. *Lancet* 1961;2:857–858.
4. Kopp K, Gotch C, Kolff W. Single needle dialysis. *Trans Am Soc Artif Intern Org* 1972;18:75–81.
5. Nidus B, Matalon R, Katz L, et al. Hemodialysis using femoral vessel cannulation. *Nephrology* 1974;13: 416–420.
6. Uldall R, Dyck R, Woods F. A subclavian cannula for temporary vascular access for hemodialysis or plasmapharesis. *Dialysis Transplantation* 1979;8:963–968.
7. Schwab S, Buller G, McCann R, et al. Prospective evaluation of a Dacron cuffed hemodialysis catheter for prolonged use. *Am J Kidney Dis* 1988;11:166–169.
8. United States Renal Data Systems (USRDS). Incidence and prevalence of ESRD. In: *2000 Annual Data Report/Atlas*. Available at: http://www.usrds.org. Accessed January 17, 2002.
9. Schwab SJ, Beathard G. The hemodialysis catheter conundrum: hate living with them, but can't live without them. *Kidney Int* 1999;56:1–17.
10. Swartz RD, Boyer CL, Messana JM. Central venous catheters for maintenance hemodialysis: a cautionary approach. *Adv Ren Replace Ther* 1997;4:275–284.
11. Schwab S, Besarab A, Beathard G, et al. NKF-DOQI clinical practice guidelines for vascular access. *Am J Kidney Dis* 1997;30 (Suppl 3):150–191.
12. Eknoyan G, Levin NW, Steinberg EP. The dialysis outcomes quality initiative: history, impact, and prospects. *Am J Kidney Dis* 2000;35:S69–S75.
13. Mauro MA, Jaques PF. Radiologic placement of long-term central venous catheters: a review. *J Vasc Interv Radiol* 1993;4: 127–137.
14. Lund GB, Trerotola SO, Scheel PF, et al. Outcome of tunneled hemodialysis catheters placed by radiologists. *Radiology* 1996; 198:467–472.
15. Choudhury D, Ahmed Z, Girgis HI, et al. Percutaneous cuffed catheter insertion by nephrologists. *Am J Nephrol* 1999;19: 51–54.
16. Noh HM, Kaufman JA, Rhea JT, et al. Cost comparison of radiologic versus surgical placement of long-term hemodialysis catheters. *AJR Am J Roentgenol* 1999;172:673–675.
17. Lameris JS, Post PJM, Zonderland HM, et al. Percutaneous placement of Hickman catheters: comparison of sonographically guided and blind techniques. *AJR Am J Roentgenol* 1990;155: 1097–1099.
18. Mallory DL, McGee WT, Shawker TH, et al. Ultrasound guidance improves the success rate of internal jugular vein cannulation. *Chest* 1990;98:157–160.
19. Mosquera DA, Gibson SP, Goldman MD. Vascular access surgery: a 2-year study and comparison with PermCath. *Nephrol Dial Transplant* 1992;7:1111–1115.
20. Akoh JA. Use of permanent dual lumen catheters for long-term haemodialysis. *Int Surg* 1999;84:171–175.
21. Chesser AMS, Baker LRI. Temporary vascular access for first dialysis is common, undesirable and usually avoidable. *Clin Nephrol* 1999;51:228–232.
22. Trerotola SO. Hemodialysis catheter placement and management. *Radiology* 2000;215:651–658.
23. Trerotola SO, Shah H, Johnson M, et al. Randomized comparison of high-flow versus conventional hemodialysis catheters. *J Vasc Interv Radiol* 1999;10:1032–1038.
24. Atherikul K, Schwab SJ, Conlon PJ. Adequacy of haemodialysis with cuffed central-vein catheters. *Nephrol Dial Transplant* 1998;13:745–749.
25. Tonelli M, Muirhead N. Access type as a predictor of dialysis adequacy in chronic hemodialysis patients. *ASAIO J* 2000;46: 279–282.
26. De Meester J, Vanholder R, De Roose J, et al. Factors and complications affecting catheter and technique survival with permanent single-lumen dialysis catheters. *Nephrol Dial Transplant* 1994;9:678–683.
27. Swartz R, Messana J, Boyer C, et al. Successful use of cuffed central venous hemodialysis catheters inserted percutaneously. *J Am Soc Nephrol* 1994;4:1719–1725.
28. Hinke DH, Zandt-Stastny DA, Goodman LR, et al. Pinch-off syndrome: a complication of implantable subclavian venous access devices. *Radiology* 1990;177:353–356.
29. Abidi SM, Fried LF, Chelluri L, et al. Factors influencing function of temporary dialysis catheters. *Clin Nephrol* 2000;53: 199–205.
30. Jean G, Chazot C, Vanel T, et al. Central venous catheters for haemodialysis: looking for optimal blood flows. *Nephrol Dial Transplant* 1997;12:1689–1691.
31. Trerotola SO, Johnson MS, Harris VJ, et al. Outcome of tunneled hemodialysis catheters placed via the right internal jugular vein by interventional radiologists. *Radiology* 1997;203:489–495.

32. Sarnak MJ, Halin N, King AJ. Severe access recirculation secondary to free flow between the lumens of a dual-lumen dialysis catheter. *Am J Kidney Dis* 1999;33:1168–1170.

33. Caridi JG, Grundy LS, Ross EA, et al. Interventional radiology placement of twin Tesio catheters for dialysis access: review of 75 patients. *J Vasc Intervent Radiol* 1999;10:78–83.

34. Perini S, LaBerge JM, Pearl JM, et al. Tesio catheter: radiologically guided placement, mechanical performance, and adequacy of delivered dialysis. *Radiology* 2000;215:129–137.

35. Lameris JS, Post PJM, Zonderland HM, et al. Percutaneous placement of Hickman catheters: comparison of sonographically guided and blind techniques. *AJR Am J Roentgenol* 1990;98: 157–160.

36. Denys BG, Uretsky BF, Reddy PS. Ultrasound-assisted cannulation of the internal jugular vein: a prospective comparison to the external landmark-guided technique. *Circulation* 1993;87: 1557–1562.

37. Troianas CA, Jobes DR, Ellison N. Ultrasound-guided cannulation of the internal jugular vein: a prospective randomized study. *Anesth Analg* 1991;12:823–826.

38. Cimochowski GE, Worley E, Rutherford WE, et al. Superiority of the internal jugual over the subclavian access for temporary hemodialysis. *Nephron* 1990;54:154–161.

39. Weitzel WF, Boyer CJ, El-Khatib MT, et al. Successful use of indwelling cuffed femoral vein catheters in ambulatory hemodialysis patients. *Am J Kidney Dis* 1993;22:426–429.

40. Zaleski GX, Funaki B, Lorenz JM, et al. Experience with tunneled femoral hemodialysis catheters. *AJR Am J Roentgenol* 1999;172:493–496.

41. Horton MG, Mewissen MW, Rilling WS, Crain MR, Bair D. Hemodialysis catheter placement directly into occluded central vein segments: a technical note. *J Vasc Interv Radiol* 1999;10: 1059–1062.

42. Forauer AR, Brenner B, Haddad LF, et al. Placement of hemodialysis catheters through dilated external jugular and collateral veins in patients with internal jugular vein occlusions. *AJR Am J Roentgenol* 2000;174:361–362.

43. Lund GB, Trerotola SO, Scheel PJ. Percutaneous translumbar inferior vena cava cannulation for hemodialysis. *Am J Kidney Dis* 1995;25:732–737.

44. Crummy AB, Carlson P, McDermott JC, et al. Percutaneous transhepatic placement of a Hickman catheter [Letter]. *AJR Am J Roentgenol* 1989;153:1317–1318.

45. Biswal R, Nosher JL, Siegel RL, et al. Translumbar placement of paired hemodialysis catheters (Tesio catheters) and follow-up in 10 patients. *Cardiovasc Interv Radiol* 2000;23:75–78.

46. Lewis CA, Allen TE, Burke DR. Quality improvement guidelines for central venous access: Society of Cardiovascular and Interventional Radiology Standards of Practice Committee. *J Vasc Interv Radiol* 1997;8:475–479.

47. Silberzweig JE, Sacks D, Khorsandi AS, et al. Reporting standards for central venous access. *J Vasc Interv Radiol* 2000;11:391–400.

48. Hodges TC, Fillinger MF Zwolak RM, et al. Longitudinal comparison of dialysis access methods: risk factors for failure. *J Vasc Surg* 1997;26:1009–1019.

49. McLaughlin K, Jones B, Mactier R, et al. Long-term vascular access for hemodialysis using silicon dual-lumen catheters with guidewire replacement of catheters for technique salvage. *Am J Kidney Dis* 1997;29:553–559.

50. Dittmen ID, Sharp D, McNulty AM, et al. A prospective study of central venous hemodialysis catheter colonization and peripheral bacteremia. *Clin Nephrol* 1999;51:34–39.

51. Almirall J, Gonzalez J, Rello J, et al. Infection of hemodialysis catheters: incidence and mechanism. *Am J Nephrol* 1989;9: 454–459.

52. Cheesbrough JS, Finch RG, Burden RP. A prospective study of the mechanisms of infection associated with hemodialysis catheters. *J Infect Dis* 1986;154:579–589.

53. Stevenson KB, Adcox MJ, Mallea MC, et al. Standardized surveillance of hemodialysis vascular access infections: 18-month experience at an outpatient, multifacility hemodialysis center. *Infect Control Hosp Epidemiol* 2000;21:200–203.

54. Saad TF. Bacteremia associated with tunneled, cuffed hemodialysis catheters. *Am J Kidney Dis* 1999;34:1114–1124.

55. Tanriover B, Carlton D, Saddekni S, et al. Bacteremia associated with tunneled dialysis catheters: comparison of two treatment strategies. *Kidney Int* 2000;57: 2151–2155.

56. Robinson D, Suhocki P, Schwab SJ. Treatment of infected tunneled venous access hemodialysis catheters with guidewire exchange. *Kidney Int* 1998;53:1792–1794.

57. Beathard G. Management of bacteremia associated with tunneled-cuffed hemodialysis catheters. *J Am Soc Nephrol* 1999;10: 1045–1049.

58. Suojanen JN, Brophy DP, Nasser I. Thrombus on indwelling central venous catheters: the Histopathology of "fibrin sheaths". *Cardiovasc Intervent Radiol* 2000; 23: 194–197.

59. Johnstone RD, Stewart GA, Akoh JA, et al. Percutaneous fibrin sleeve stripping of failing haemodialysis catheters. *Nephrol Dial Tranplant* 1999;14:688–691.

60. Garofalo RS, Zaleski GX, Lorenz JM, et al. Exchange of poorly functioning tunneled permanent hemodialysis catheters. *AJR Am J Roentgenol* 1999;173:155–158.

61. Merport M, Murphy TP, Egglin TK, et al. Fibrin sheath stripping versus catheter exchange for the treatment of failed tunneled hemodialysis catheters: randomized clinical trial. *J Vasc Interv Radiol* 2000;11:1115–1120.

62. Duszak R, Haskal ZJ, Thomas-Hawkins C, et al. Replacement of failing tunneled hemodialysis catheters through pre-existing subcutaneous tunnels: a comparison of catheter function and infection rates for de novo placements and over-the-wire exchanges. *J Vasc Interv Radiol* 1998;9:321–327.

63. Kohler TR, Kirkman TR. Central venous catheter failure is induced by injury and can be prevented by stabilizing the catheter tip. *J Vasc Surg* 1998;28:59–66.

64. Lund GB, Trerotola SO, Scheel PF, et al. Outcome of tunneled hemodialysis catheters placed by radiologists. *Radiology* 1996; 198:467–472.

65. Agraharkar M, Isaacson S, Mendelssohn D, et al. Percutaneously inserted Silastic jugular hemodialysis catheters seldom cause jugular vein thrombosis. *ASAIO J* 1995;41:169–172.

66. Trerotola SO, Kuhn-Fulton J, Johnson MS, et al. Tunneled infusion catheters: increased incidence of symptomatic venous thrombosis after subclavian versus internal jugular venous access. *Radiology* 2000;217:89–93.

67. Schwab SJ, Quarles LD, Middleton JP, et al. Hemodialysis-associated subclavian vein stenosis. *Kidney Int* 1988;33:1156–1159.

68. Schillinger F, Schillinger D, Montagnac R, et al. Post catheterization vein stenosis in haemodialysis: comparative angiographic study of 50 subclavian and 50 internal jugular accesses. *Nephrol Dial Transplant* 1991;6:722–724.

69. Trerotola SO, Johnson MS, Shah H, et al. Tunneled hemodialysis catheters: use of a silver-coated catheter for prevention of infection - a randomized study. *Radiology* 1998;207:491–496.

70. Bach A. Prevention of infections caused by central venous catheters - established and novel measures. *Infection* 1999;27: S11–S15.

71. Canaud B, My H, Morena M, et al. Dialock: a new vascular access device for extracorporeal renal replacement therapy. Preliminary clinical results. *Nephrol Dial Transplant* 1999;14:692–698.

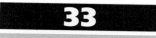

CATHETER INSERTION: TECHNIQUES, COST, AND OUTCOMES

JACK WORK

The tunneled cuffed catheter, frequently referred to as the Permcath,[1] is used for a variety of reasons, including the following:

1. As a bridge access to allow time for maturation of a permanent access, such as an autogenous fistula or prosthetic bridge graft
2. As a temporary vascular access for patients with acute renal failure
3. As a backup vascular access
4. As a permanent vascular access for patients for whom all other options have been exhausted

Twenty-three percent of all patients in the sample analyzed for the 2000 Clinical Performance Measures collected by the End Stage Renal Disease (ESRD) Networks were using tunneled cuffed catheters for dialysis. Of this group of patients, 20% "had all fistula or graft sites in their body exhausted" and were using the catheter as permanent access (1).

In evaluating the uses of the tunneled cuffed catheter as vascular access for the patient with ESRD, it is important to compare the catheter with the other vascular access options that are currently available. The characteristics of the "ideal" vascular access, along with how currently available options for vascular access match up to the "ideal vascular access," are outlined in Table 33.1. From the perspective of both the nephrologist and the patient, the tunneled cuffed catheter has several advantages. Unfortunately, the catheter also has several disadvantages (see Chapters 32, 35, and 42). This chapter examines catheter insertion techniques, costs, and outcomes of catheter placement.

OPTIMAL SITE FOR INSERTION

The choice of access location influences the function of the catheter, the long-term complications associated with catheter location, and potential future sites for permanent surgical access placement. The preferred site for insertion of the tunneled cuffed catheter is the right internal jugular vein, which is generally accepted as the preferred site for upper-body catheter placement because the rate of complications encountered during and after placement is lower than when other upper-body locations are used (2). The right internal jugular location offers a direct route to the right atrium, the preferred site for location of the catheter tip. It also is important in decreasing the development of central venous stenosis, which occurs more frequently with placement in the subclavian vein (3,4). Several studies examined the incidence of central vein stenosis associated with either the subclavian or internal jugular venous access site. Cimochowski and colleagues reported a 50% incidence of stenosis associated with the subclavian insertion site and no stenosis with the internal jugular insertion site after temporary catheter placement (3). In a similar study, Schillinger and associates reported a 42% incidence of stenosis with subclavian insertion sites and 10% with internal jugular insertion sites (4). In a retrospective study, Trerotola and colleagues compared the incidence of symptomatic venous thrombosis by site of insertion in 774 catheter placements. There was a 13% incidence of venous thrombosis with the subclavian catheters compared with a 3% incidence with the internal jugular catheters (5). The frequency of asymptomatic thrombosis is higher, however. Two studies in patients not undergoing dialysis found that asymptomatic thrombosis occurs in about 65% of subclavian central venous catheters (6,7).

The use of the right internal jugular vein location has other potential consequences. The human internal jugular veins have a valve located directly above the termination of the internal jugular vein in the inferior bulb, usually located directly posterior to the head of the clavicle (5). The valve prevents backward blood flow toward the brain. It is thought to be important in protecting the brain from acute increases in intrathoracic pressure that occur during coughing or positive-pressure ventilation (5). Wu and co-workers noted that incompetence of the internal jugular valve frequently was induced by cannulation of the internal jugular vein and that valvular incompetence persisted after catheter removal for up to 2 years of follow-up (8).

---

[1] Permcath is a registered trademark of Quinton catheters, but it has become part of the nephrologist's lexicon, analogous to *xerox*.

TABLE 33.1. CHARACTERISTICS OF THE "PERFECT" VASCULAR ACCESS

Characteristic of Perfect Access	Current Options
Instant or rapid maturation	Cuffed, tunneled catheter, implantable port
Long survival	Autogenous fistula (only if it matures)
High blood flow rates	Autogenous fistula, graft, implantable port and some cuffed, tunneled catheters
Small risk of thrombosis	Autogenous fistula
Small risk of infection	Autogenous fistula
Easy to cannulate	Cuffed, tunneled catheter, implantable port
Quick hemostasis at conclusion of dialysis	Cuffed, tunneled catheter, implantable port
Concealed from view with clothing	Cuffed, tunneled catheter, implantable port
Permits comfortable arm position during dialysis	Cuffed, tunneled catheter, implantable port
No needles	Cuffed tunneled catheter, implantable port

The second choice for cuffed tunneled catheter insertion is not so clearly established. Site selection is dependent on the patient's individual circumstances. The left or right subclavian veins appear to have fewer flow-related problems and perhaps less thrombosis than the left internal or external jugular vein (7). If a patient has exhausted all left upper-extremity vascular access sites, then the left subclavian vein is the preferred insertion site when the right external jugular vein is occluded. On the other hand, if the left upper extremity has a potential vascular access site, the right subclavian vein would be the site of choice (when the right internal jugular is not available). Kohler and Kirkman suggested that catheter injury to the vein wall is the direct cause of central vein thrombosis and subsequent stenosis (9). Therefore, selecting a site that minimizes contact with the vein wall appears prudent until new catheter designs that stabilize the catheter tip become available.

Hemodialysis catheters must be able to deliver more than 300 mL per minute of blood flow to provide adequate dialysis. To obtain a blood flow consistently greater than 300 mL per minute, the cuffed tunneled catheter tip should be placed in the right atrium, ideally in the middle of the right atrium. In a study of 141 patients with central venous access devices, Petersen and associates found that catheter tip position was the only factor that was predictive of malfunction (10). In another prospective study of 25 dialysis patients with central venous catheters, adequate blood flow was found more frequently in the group of patients with the catheter tip in the right atrium (11).

The cuffed tunneled catheter is placed with the patient in the supine position. When the patient is sitting in a dialysis chair for treatment, the tip of the catheter may retract up as much as 1 to 2 cm, depending on the patient's body habitus (12,13). Advancing the catheter into the lower right atrium may increase the frequency of dysrhythmias (12). Therefore, the middle of the right atrium appears to be the optimal position for placing the tip of the hemodialysis catheter. Table 33.2 lists the recommended placement criteria for cuffed tunneled catheters.

CATHETER INSERTION IMAGING TECHNIQUES

The use of ultrasound guidance to assist cannulation of the internal jugular vein was first reported in a series of studies in the mid-1980s (14). The 1997 Dialysis Outcomes Quality Initiatives (DOQI) recommended "real-time ultrasound guided insertion to reduce insertion related complications" based on both evidence and opinion (2). Since 1997, several studies have documented more fully the importance of using ultrasound guidance for internal jugular vein cannulation. In a prospective study, Denys and colleagues evaluated an ultrasound-guided method for cannulation of the internal jugular vein in 302 patients compared with an external landmark technique in 302 patients (15). Successful cannulation was achieved in 100% of the ultrasound-guided group and in 88.1% of the landmark technique group. An important finding was that the vein was punctured on the first attempt in 78% of the ultrasound-guided group but in only 38% of the landmark guided group. Complications were significantly fewer in the ultrasound-guided group, with carotid

TABLE 33.2. CUFFED TUNNELED CATHETER PLACEMENT

Preferred location
    Right internal jugular[a] > right external jugular > left internal jugular > left external jugular > subclavian veins[b] > femoral veins > translumbar
Length
    Upper-body placement: should extend into mid right atrium
    Femoral: should extend above iliac junction
Approach
    Supraclavicular site: low approach allows for smooth catheter curve
    Real-time ultrasound guidance for insertion mandatory
    Fluoroscopy is mandatory for optimal tip positioning

[a] Second choices after right internal jugular site may depend on previous vascular access sites.
[b] Subclavian not used unless all permanent access sites in ipsilateral extremity exhausted.

TABLE 33.3. COMPARISON OF ULTRASOUND (U) AND ANATOMIC LANDMARK (L) APPROACHES FOR CATHETER INSERTION VIA THE INTERNAL JUGULAR VEIN

Study	No. of Patients	% Success		% Success		% CCA	
		U	L	U	L	U	L
Denys et al.	1230	100	88	78	38	2	8
Trojanos	160	100	96	73	54	1	8
Armstrong	115	98	91	76	53	6	5

CCA, common carotid artery.
Modified from Caridi JG, Hawkins IF, Weichmann BN, et al. Sonographic guidance when using the right internal jugular vein for central vein access. *AJR Am J Roentgenol* 1998;171:1259–1263, with permission.

artery puncture occurring in 1.7%, brachial plexus irritation in 0.4%, and hematoma in 0.2% compared with the land-mark-guided group, with carotid artery puncture occurring in 8.3%, brachial plexus irritation in 1.7%, and hematoma in 3.3%. Finally, the average time taken to access the vein was less in the ultrasound-guided group (15). These observations were confirmed in another prospective study of 100 patients undergoing routine internal jugular vein cannulation. Access time, failure rates, and complications were significantly fewer with the ultrasound-guided technique compared with the anatomic landmark group (16). Numerous other studies have examined the ultrasound-guided approach compared with the landmark approach. These studies established ultrasound guidance as the standard of care for the insertion of cuffed, tunneled catheters (17). Table 33.3 illustrates a comparison of ultrasound to landmark approaches.

The higher failure rate in the landmark-guided group may be explained by the anatomic variations of the internal jugular vein location. Several studies documented the degree of anatomic variation in the location of the internal jugular vein (15,17). The internal jugular vein is located in the "normal" position as located by the external landmark-guided approach in 71% to 92% of studies. Thus, variant anatomy occurs frequently. These variations in anatomy are illustrated in Figure 33.1. Ultrasound examination done before placement of jugular vein cuffed tunneled catheters in long-term hemodialysis patients is particularly important. Forauer and Glockner examined 100 consecutive hemodialysis catheter placements in 79 patients who had been on dialysis for a mean of 19.6 months. Of these patients, 35%

had a significant ultrasound finding that altered access approach. These findings included total occlusion, nonocclusive thrombus, stenosis, and anatomic variation (18). Ultrasound-guided cannulation of the femoral vein for either acute or chronic hemodialysis access also has been shown to be efficacious. Cannulation of the femoral vein was successful in 100% of patients using ultrasound compared with 89.5% of patients using the landmark-guided technique. Using ultrasound, femoral artery puncture occurred in 7.1% and hematoma in 0% of patients compared with 15.8% femoral artery puncture and 2.6% hematoma in the external landmark group (19).

Based on opinion, the DOQI guidelines state that "fluoroscopy is mandatory for insertion of all cuffed dialysis catheters (2)." There is little evidence to support this recommendation. The use of fluoroscopy during catheter insertion does allow for placement of the guidewire into the inferior vena cava, thus decreasing the possibility for dysrhythmias, and ensures that the catheter tip is located in the right atrium. In a study of 188 cuffed tunneled catheter placements, the use of fluoroscopy was compared with an external landmark technique using the right fourth intercostal space as the landmark. All catheter insertions used ultrasound guidance. There were no differences in procedure success, complications, or catheter function with or without the use of fluoroscopy. Comparing postprocedure upright chest x-rays for tip position, 97% of the fluoroscopy group achieved a right atrial position compared with 92% in the landmark group (20). Fluoroscopy may not be necessary for cuffed tunneled catheter insertion in

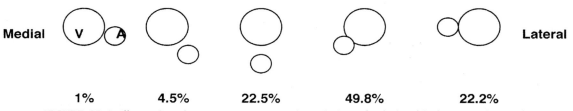

FIGURE 33.1. Illustration shows percent anatomic variation of relationship between internal jugular vein (*V*) and common carotid artery (*A*). Modified from Caridi JG, Hawkins IF, Weichmann BN, et al. Sonographic guidance when using the right internal jugular vein for central vein access. *AJR Am J Roentgenol* 1998;171:1259–1263, with permission.

selected patients without a history of prior catheters or venous abnormalities.

The necessity of postprocedure chest radiography has been questioned when the cuffed tunneled catheter is placed using fluoroscopy. Only seven procedural complications were identified in 937 consecutive central venous access procedures, of which 670 were cuffed, tunneled catheters. These included four air emboli, two pneumothoraces, and one innominate vein laceration. All of these complications were noted with fluoroscopy. Postprocedure radiography failed to reveal any unknown complications but did detect one malpositioned catheter (21). This suggests that postprocedure radiography is of little clinical benefit if fluoroscopy is used during cuffed, tunneled catheter insertion. Its continued use may be for historic or medicolegal purposes.

COMPLICATIONS OF CUFFED, TUNNELED CATHETER INSERTION

Significant immediate complications with cuffed, tunneled catheter insertion are associated almost entirely with the use of the anatomic landmark technique (or blind insertion). The success of the landmark-guided placement of the catheter depends on the target vein being in its expected position, being patent, and being of normal caliber. As discussed, the target vein fails to meet these requirements in a significant number of patients. The most common complications of cuffed, tunneled catheter placement include unintentional puncture of the carotid artery, air embolism, hemothorax, and pneumothorax (22). The extent of reported complications is impressive, however, and includes hemopericardium (23), phrenic nerve palsy (24), pseudoaneurysm of thyrocervical trunk (25), right atrial endocarditis (26), and pulmonary abscess (27). Cuffed, tunneled catheter insertion also has been implicated in the development of bilateral ophthalmoplegia and exophthalmos (28), unilateral breast enlargement (29), and bleeding of esophageal varices (30). It is important to point out that these complications are all from the era before ultrasound imaging.

TECHNIQUES OF CATHETER INSERTION

Cuffed, tunneled catheters used for hemodialysis vascular access can be placed safely in an outpatient setting using conscious sedation and strict sterile technique. This makes dialysis possible immediately after catheter placement. The right internal jugular vein is the preferred site for insertion. The rationale for choosing this site was discussed in detail already herein and in Chapter 32. Real-time ultrasound with guided puncture using a micropuncture needle and fluoroscopic guidance for insertion and positioning are the requirements for safe, effective insertion. Catheter tip position is somewhat design dependent. Typically, the red lumen is away from the vessel wall. The tip of the catheter should be placed in the middle right atrium to accommodate the inherent retraction of the catheter. After insertion but before the patient leaves the procedure room, the catheter function should be evaluated using the so-called three-T test. Using fluoroscopy, check the *tip* to ensure that it is in the right atrium, and then check the *top* to ensure that the catheter makes a smooth curve without any kinks that will restrict flow. Finally, the *tug* test is performed to check flow by placing a 10-mL syringe on each of the hubs of the catheter and rapidly withdrawing blood into the syringe without hesitation. If any problems are identified, they should be corrected before the patient leaves the procedure room.

Placement of the cuffed, tunneled catheter requires a maximum barrier protection environment for placement. This operating room type of environment is readily available in hospitals, free-standing vascular laboratories, or ambulatory surgery centers. Before surgical scrub, it is useful to examine the selected site using ultrasound to ensure that the patient has a suitable vein in the selected location. The insertion site and surrounding areas, including shoulder and chest wall, should be cleansed with surgical scrub and draped appropriately. The ultrasound probe should be covered with a sterile sheath, and the insertion site should be insonated to identify the vein. The ultrasound probe can be placed parallel to the long axis of the vessel and the cannulation needle inserted adjacent to the end or short axis of the probe. Alternatively, the probe can be placed perpendicular to the long axis of the vessel. This approach gives the vein the more typical appearance of a circle but limits visualization of the needle. The vein usually can be identified easily because it typically collapses with gentle pressure of the probe, whereas the artery does not. A Valsalva or sniffing maneuver by the patient will enlarge or decrease, respectively, the size of the vein, further enabling distinction of the vein from the artery (31). Occasionally, to identify the vein optimally, it is necessary to insonate, beginning high in the neck and continuing down to the clavicular groove. Assuming the right internal jugular vein is to be cannulated, the ultrasound probe is placed parallel and superior to the clavicle, over the groove between the sternal and clavicular heads of the sternocleidomastoid muscle (the Selldot triangle). It is important to avoid inserting the catheter through the muscle because this is uncomfortable for the patient on a long-term basis.

Once the insertion site is selected, the site for insertion is infiltrated with local anesthesia. If a peripheral intravenous catheter is available, it is advantageous to administer conscious sedation agents such as midazolam and fentanyl, which in combination provide adequate amnesia and analgesia before cannulation of the vein. Using real-time ultrasound guidance, a 21-gauge micropuncture needle with an attached syringe is inserted into the vein. The small needle limits potential complications if the carotid artery is inadvertently punctured compared with a larger 18-guage needle. In addition, ultrasound visualization makes it more likely that only the anterior wall of the vein is punctured (32). Frequently, under direct visualization, the vein will be seen to push gently in before needle penetration of the anterior wall of the vein. The ultrasound probe then is peeled away from the needle guide while carefully maintaining the position of the needle. The syringe is removed, and a 0.018-inch guidewire is inserted through the needle. The guidewire is advanced and the position of the guide wire is confirmed by fluoroscopy. The needle then is removed. If necessary, a small stab wound is made at the insertion site, where the guidewire enters the skin. A coaxial 5-French dilator then is inserted over the guidewire. The guidewire and 3-French inner translational dilator are removed, leaving the 5-French outer dilator in place. A flow switch or stopcock is attached to the dilator to prevent the possibility of an air embolism. If peripheral intravenous access has not been obtained, one can administer conscious sedation at this time through the dilator. At this point, one can insert a guidewire and then create the subcutaneous tunnel or create the tunnel before guidewire placement. The latter course of action minimizes the amount of time a guidewire is in the circulation. A 1-cm incision is made, extending laterally at the insertion site. The subcutaneous tissue is exposed by blunt dissection, creating a small subcutaneous pocket. This helps to ensure that the catheter bend will be kink free. Further dissection is performed to ensure that the soft tissue around the 5-French dilator is free and no skin tags are attached. The catheter exit site then is identified by the landmark technique (20) or by laying the catheter on the patient's chest to approximate the final position in the right atrium. The catheter length may be selected based on patient body habitus and the type of catheter used. The desired length of the subcutaneous tunnel can be determined by using the guidewire to measure the distance from the insertion site to the middle right atrium. Using this measurement as a guide, the length of tunnel can then be determined.

Once the exit site for the dual lumen-type catheter is identified, the area is infiltrated with local anesthesia and a puncture is made through the skin using a knife blade. A long needle such as the micropuncture needle then is used to infiltrate the tunnel tract extending from the exit site to the insertion site. The appropriately sized catheter is mounted on the end of the tunneling device, which may be made of either metal or plastic. The tunneling device with the catheter then is passed from the exit site subcutaneously to the insertion site. Alternatively, an appropriate size dilator with sheath can be used to create the subcutaneous tunnel, and the catheter can be passed through the sheath (33). The cuff of the catheter is pulled into the tunnel, and the tunneling device is removed from the catheter.

After tunnel preparation, attention is turned toward dilatation of the soft-tissue tract and vein for insertion of the catheter into the right internal jugular. A guidewire such as the Benson (or the guidewire provided in most catheter kits) is passed through the 5-French dilator into the inferior vena cava. Placement of the guidewire into the inferior vena cava decreases the likelihood of cardiac arrhythmias. The 5-French dilator is removed, and then in a stepwise fashion, serial dilators are passed over the guidewire to dilate the soft tissue and venous tract. The dilator should move freely over the guidewire. It is possible for the dilator to get off axis, impinge on the guidewire, and perforate the vein or the mediastinum. If there is any doubt as to location of the dilator or if there is hesitancy or difficulty in dilating the tract, the fluoroscope should be used to verify proper positioning.

After the final dilatation, the dilator with the peel-away sheath is inserted using the same caution concerning the guidewire. As one inserts the sheath, resistance is felt as the sheath goes through the soft tissue, and then a final resistance is felt as it enters the vein. The peel-away sheath then is advanced slightly and the dilator is removed. It is always safest to leave the guidewire in place. The dilator and guidewire can be removed together for right internal jugular catheter placement because the right internal jugular vein permits direct catheter placement into the right atrium. If any difficulties arise, the guidewire should be left in place to ensure that access is available. For catheter placement on the left side or other alternative sites, the guidewire is left in place so that the catheter can be inserted over the guidewire and tract directly into the right atrial position. Once the dilator is removed, the operator or an assistant should occlude the sheath between the finger and thumb. This prevents bleeding or aspiration of air while leaving enough length of the sheath to insert the catheter.

Once the dilator and guidewire have been removed, the catheter tip is inserted into the opening of the sheath in such a way to avoid twisting the catheter. The catheter is fed through the sheath, and as soon as the catheter occludes the sheath, the assistant or physician can release the sheath. The catheter is pushed further into the sheath, and the sheath is peeled downward toward the skin. As soon as the catheter is advanced maximally, the sheath is pulled out and then pealed down outside the venotomy, which avoids the sheath creating a larger venotomy. Once the sheath has been removed completely, the catheter is pulled back into the tunnel so that the cuff now is approximately 1 to 1.5 cm from the exit site. The three-T test is now performed as described previously to ensure that the catheter is functioning properly.

After confirmation of adequate flow, the venotomy site is closed using appropriate suture. The exit site is closed using a pursestring suture wrapped around the catheter to provide a harness for the catheter at the skin surface. Additional suture is used to hold the catheter at the hub. Topical antibiotic ointment and gauze dressing then can be applied to the incisions and needle puncture sites. Although frequently used, the need for prophylactic antibiotics for this procedure never has been established. Each catheter lumen is filled with the appropriate amount of heparin just to fill the catheter lumen. The manufacturer specifies the internal volume of each lumen. Heparin in a concentration of 1,000 U per cubic centimeter is used if the patient is going to undergo dialysis immediately to decrease the systemic leakage of heparin. Heparin in a concentration of 5,000 U per cubic centimeter is used if the patient will not undergo dialysis within 24 hours.

CATHETER TYPES

The Tesio catheter consists of two separate 10-French silicone catheters. Each catheter has a Dacron retention cuff fixed around a football-shaped widening of the catheter 22 cm from the distal tip. This prevents the catheter from being pulled out of the exit site. The Tesio catheter system usually requires two separate insertion sites. The catheters are usually inserted first into the right atrium, followed by construction of the tunnels. The tunneling device has a football-shaped extension that is pulled from the insertion site to the skin exit site to allow for the Dacron cuffed "football" to be pulled partially through the tunnel. By constructing the tunnel from the insertion site toward the skin exit site, the retention cuff is proximal to the catheter exit site and acts as a retention cuff. The 10-French catheter then can be pulled through the skin and does not require a skin suture at the exit site. The removable Luer-lock hubs then are attached to the catheters.

The Schon catheter is similar to the Tesio system except that it uses a connector to retain two catheters at a single venous insertion site rather than separate "football" retention cuffs. This catheter requires a single cut-down incision for removal.

The Ash split catheter is similar to a single dual-lumen catheter for cannulation of the central vein and creation of the subcutaneous tunnel but acts as two separate catheters within the central vasculature. This is accomplished by a "double-D" design that allows splitting of the catheter at the distal tips into two separate catheters. Insertion technique is similar to other single dual-lumen catheters. The catheter must be split prior to insertion. The Ash split catheter can be introduced over a single guide by taking advantage of its tip design. A guidewire is first passed into the venous tip and then brought out of the side hole of the venous catheter located on the flat side of the "D." The guidewire then is passed into the tip of the arterial catheter and brought out through the arterial hub. The Ash split catheter can then be advanced over the guidewire, taking care not to twist the catheter.

OUTCOMES AND COST

Outcome studies evaluating the efficacy and safety of cuffed, tunneled catheters are limited. Most available studies retro-

spectively report short-term placement outcomes (34,35). Although they are useful in documenting the safety and efficacy of nonsurgical percutaneous catheter placement, these reports fail to compare placement techniques directly or to provide insight into either short-term or long-term catheter effectiveness (36). Trerotola and colleagues evaluated 250 consecutive cuffed, tunneled catheter placements in 175 patients. Initial technical success was 100%, with complications including only two clinically unimportant air emboli (36). The catheter-related infection rate was 0.08 per 100 catheter days, the rate of malfunction requiring removal was 0.22 per 100 catheter days, and catheter thrombosis requiring removal was 0.16 per 100 catheter days (36). Although several different catheter types were used in this study, no differentiation of long-term outcome was made. Unfortunately, late failure resulting from inadequate blood flow was not defined rigorously.

Blood flow has been studied in the Canaud TwinCath in 33 chronic hemodialysis patients using the ultrasound dilution technique. The Tesio catheter system, more commonly used in the United States, is a modification of the Canaud twin catheter system. The Canaud TwinCath 10-French lumen catheters delivered a "true" blood flow as measured by ultrasound dilution of 5% to 10% lower than the indicated blood flow on the dialysis blood pump (37). The initial performance of 66 Tesio catheters was examined in 49 patients. Only 43% of catheters provided adequate blood flow, defined as greater than 250 mL per minute in the first five hemodialysis sessions after placement. Right-sided catheters performed better than left-sided catheters (38). In another study of the Tesio catheter system, 79 catheters were placed in 71 patients. Technical success in placement was 99%; however, the complication rate was 9% with one fatal air embolism. Primary catheter patency was only 66% at 6 months (39). In one of the few studies to compare functional characteristics of various types of catheters, the flow rate and hydraulic resistance were measured in Mahurkar, Tesio, and Ash split catheters. Hydraulic resistance was defined as the venous pressure divided by the blood flow rate: PV/Qb. Average blood flow rates were 295 ± 42 for Ash split, 279 ± 38 for Mahurkar, and 300 ± 39 for the Tesio. Hydraulic resistance for the Ash split catheter was less than the other two catheter types (40).

A paucity of published data is available on the costs of cuffed, tunneled catheters. Only one study is available that analyzes the cost of cuffed, tunneled catheter placement. Variable direct costs that represent supplies and short-term labor costs, fixed direct costs that reflect overhead costs, and fixed indirect costs reflecting allocated hospital overhead costs were analyzed for 47 radiologically placed cuffed, tunneled catheters and for 25 surgically placed catheters. Professional fees were not included in the analysis. The average total hospital cost was $926 and $1,849 for the radiologically placed and the surgically placed catheters, respectively (41). The $923 per catheter cost saving resulted from lower

TABLE 33.4. COST ANALYSIS OF PLACEMENT AND MAINTENANCE OF VARIOUS CUFFED, TUNNELED CATHETERS[a]

Catheter Type	Number	Initial Cost ($)	% Failed	Median Cost per HD Treatment	Median Days Used
Hemoflow	11	290	18	18	243
Quinton Permcath	10	198	20	21	182
Quinton Mahurkar	55	198	40	34	134
Ash Split Cath	36	550	8	50	103
Vaxcel	45	473	4	68	71

HD, hemodialysis.
[a] See text for definition of failure.

costs in each cost category. This study points out the potential cost savings most hospitals will obtain by not using an operating room, with its high ancillary costs for cuffed, tunneled catheter placements.

The cost of placement and maintenance of various cuffed, tunneled catheters was analyzed for 165 catheters placed during a single year by the Nephrology Vascular Service at our institution. The initial catheter cost, the cost of placement, and the cost of maintenance such as use of a thrombolytic and change of catheter for nonfunction were normalized by the number of dialysis treatments. Thus, the catheter with the least likelihood of failure, defined as blood flow less than 300 mL per minute for three consecutive hemodialysis treatments, was associated with the lowest cost per treatment (Table 33.4). Diabetes, gender, age, site of insertion, and prior catheter history were not associated with increased cost of maintaining a functional cuffed, tunneled catheter (42). The cost of placement and maintenance of a cuffed tunneled catheter for hemodialysis appears to vary with each type of catheter and increased the overall portion of costs attributed to vascular access.

SUBCUTANEOUS VASCULAR PORT AS AN ALTERNATIVE TO THE CUFFED TUNNELED CATHETER

As previously discussed, large numbers of patients are becoming dependent on catheters for hemodialysis because they have lost other sites that would support either an autogenous fistulae or synthetic graft. Although the cuffed tunneled catheter has several advantages, its primary disadvantage is infection and thrombosis. The development of a subcutaneous port that is durable, offers high flow, and is fully implanted subcutaneously may become an alternative hemodialysis device for chronic use. (See Chapter 42 for a detailed review of ports.) The Vasca LifeSite system obtained approval by the U. S. Food and Drug Administration. This subcutaneous port provides immediate central venous access for hemodialysis. The system consists of an access valve and silicone cannula, which is implanted like a

typical central venous catheter, preferably within the right internal jugular vein. The access valve is designed so that a standard 14-gauge fistula needle activates an internal pinch valve, allowing blood to flow. On removal of the needle, the pinch valve closes and flow stops. The valve is accessed repeatedly through a single cannulation site in the patient's skin, which eventually forms a pain-free tissue tract referred to as a *buttonhole*. The valve is about 2.5 cm in diameter and 0.68 cm high and is constructed of a titanium alloy. The valve entry site is in the center of the dome. The circular ring surrounding the injection port at the top of the valve serves as a guide to the needle that is being inserted into the valve. The valve stem accepts a 12-French silicone cannula. The bottom plate of the valve has suture holes to allow anchoring of the device at the time of implantation. The mechanical pinch clamp opens and closes when the dialysis needle is inserted or removed. This prevents any leakage of blood when the dialysis needle is not seated in the valve and allows for maintaining the heparin lock within the cannula. The channel for blood passage through the device is without constrictions or dead space. Therefore, there is no opportunity for the creation of turbulence in the blood flow or for sequestration of blood product that might increase the risk of infection. Prophylactic infection control, which involves disinfecting the valve pocket and buttonhole tract, is performed with isopropyl alcohol before and after entering the device with a dialysis needle. This is accomplished by using a 25-gauge needle and syringe with isopropyl alcohol. A 25-gauge needle can enter the valve chamber easily, without activating the pinched valve mechanism.

Implantation of the LifeSite system is similar to implanting a Port-a-cath for chemotherapy, except that the ports require a larger pocket. As with any central venous catheter used for hemodialysis vascular access, maximum barrier protection at the time of implantation is used. The LifeSite system requires that two separate valves be implanted for hemodialysis, one device for blood withdrawal and one for blood return. The device is designed to provide the flexibility of using two separate implantation sites, if needed, and to permit the replacement of only half of the assembly if a problem occurs.

The initial results using a LifeSite hemodialysis access system appear to be promising. The mean duration of device survival in 23 patients was 6.8 ± 0.97 months. The device achieved the hemodialysis prescription with blood flow rates averaging 384.7 ± 78.9 mL per minute (43). In a study comparing the efficacy and safety of the device with the Tesio catheter, device-related infections were 1.3 versus 3.3 per 1,000 patient-days compared with the Tesio catheter (44). The subcutaneous port may offer another alternative for hemodialysis vascular access with fewer infectious complications compared with the external catheter.

REFERENCES

1. Health Care Financing Administration (HCFA). 2000 Annual Report, ESRD Clinical Performance Measures Project. Department of Health and Human Services, HCFA, Office of Clinical Standards and Quality, Baltimore, MD; December 2000.
2. Schwab S, Besarab A, Beathard G, et al. NKF-DOQI clinical practice guidelines for vascular access. *Am J Kidney Dis* 1997;30: S150–S190.
3. Cimochowski GE, Worley E, Rutherford WE, et al. Superiority of the internal jugular over the subclavian access for temporary dialysis. *Nephron* 1990;54:154–161.
4. Schillinger F, Schillinger D, Montagnac R, et al. Post catheterization vein stenosis in haemodialysis: comparative angiographic study of 50 subclavian and 50 internal jugular accesses. *Nephrol Dial Transplant* 1991;6:722–724.
5. Trerotola SO, Kuhn-Fulton J, Johnson MS, et al. Tunneled infusion catheters: increased incidence of symptomatic venous thrombosis after subclavian versus internal jugular venous access. *Radiology* 2000;217:89–93.
6. Haire WD, Liegerman RP, Lund GB, et al. Thrombotic complications of silicone rubber catheters during autologous marrow and peripheral stem cell transplantation: prospective comparison of Hickman and Groshong catheters. *Bone Marrow Transplant* 1991;7:57–59.
7. DeCicco M, Matovic M, Balestreri L, et al. Central venous thrombosis: an early and frequent complication in cancer patients bearing long-term Silastic catheter-a prospective study. *Thromb Res* 1997;86:101–113.
8. Wu X, Studer W, Erb T, et al. Competence of the internal jugular vein valve is damaged by cannulation and catheterization of the internal jugular vein. *Anesthesiology* 2000;93:319–324.
9. Kohler TR, Kirkman TR. Central venous catheter failure is induced by injury and can be prevented by stabilizing the catheter tip. *J Vasc Surg* 1998;28:59–66.
10. Petersen J, Delaney JH, Brakstad MT, et al. Silicone venous access devices positioned with their tips high in the superior vena cava are more likely to malfunction. *Am J Surg* 1999;178:38–41.
11. Jean G, Chazot C, Vanel T, et al. Central venous catheters for haemodialysis: looking for optimal blood flow. *Nephrol Dial Transplant*1997;12:1689–1691.
12. Nazarian GK, Bjarnason H, Dietz CA, et al. Changes in tunneled catheter tip position when a patient is upright. *J Vasc Interv Radiol* 1997;8:437–441.
13. Kowalski CM, Kaufman JA, Rivita SM, et al. Migration of central venous catheters: implications for initial catheter tip positioning. *J Vasc Interv Radiol* 1997;8:443–447.
14. Denys, BG, Uretsky, BF. Anatomical variations of internal jugular vein location: impact on central venous access. *Crit Care Med* 1991;19:1516–1519.

15. Denys BG, Uretsky BF, Reddy PS. Ultrasound-assisted cannulation of the internal jugular vein. *Circulation* 1993;87:1557–1562.
16. Teichgraber UKM, Benter T, Gebel M, et al. A sonographically guided technique for central venous access. *AJR Am J Roentgenol* 1997;169:731–733.
17. Caridi JG, Hawkins IF, Weichmann BN, et al. Sonographic guidance when using the right internal jugular vein for central vein access. *AJR Am J Roentgenol* 1998;171:1259–1263.
18. Forauer AR, Glockner JF. Importance of US findings in access planning during jugular vein hemodialysis catheter placements. *J Vasc Interv Radiol* 2000;11:233–238.
19. Kwon TH, Kim YL, Cho DK. Ultrasound-guided cannulation of the femoral vein for acute haemodialysis access. *Nephrol Dial Transplant* 1997;12:1009–1012.
20. Saad T. Tunneled-cuffed venous hemodialysis catheter insertion with or without use of fluoroscopy. *J Am Soc Nephrol* 2000;11: 196A.
21. Caridi JG, West JH, Stavropoulos SW, et al. Internal jugular and upper extremity central venous access in interventional radiology: is a postprocedure chest radiography necessary. *AJR Am J Roentgenol* 2000;174:363–366.
22. Skolnick ML. The role of sonography in the placement and management of jugular and subclavian central venous catheters. *AJR Am J Roentgenol* 1994;163:291–295.
23. Jean G. Haemopericardium associated with disruption of a clot using a flexible J-guide-wire in a haemodialysis catheter. *Nephrol Dial Transplant* 1998;13:1898.
24. Islek G, Akpolat T, Danaci M. Phrenic nerve palsy caused by subclavian vein catheterization. *Nephrol Dial Transplant* 1998;13: 1023–1025.
25. Peces R, Navascues RA, Baltar J, et al. Pseudoaneurysm of the thyrocervical trunk complicating percutaneous internal jugular-vein catheterization for haemodialysis. *Nephrol Dial Transplant* 1998;13:1009–1011.
26. Tarng D, Huang T. Internal jugular vein haemodialysis catheter-induced right atrium endocarditis—case report and review of the literature. *Scand J Urol Nephrol* 1998;411–414.
27. Dittmer I, Tomson C. Pulmonary abscess complicating central venous hemodialysis catheter infection. *Clin Nephrol* 1998;49: 66.
28. Varelas P, Bertolrini T, Halford H. Bilateral ophthalmoplegia and exophthalmos complicating central hemodialysis catheter placement. *Am J Kidney Dis* 1999;33:966–969.
29. Phillips G, Scheel P, Zeiger M. Unilateral breast enlargement: four case reports of an "unusual" presentation of central vein stenosis in patients undergoing hemodialysis. *Surgery* 1998;123: 699–701.
30. Pop A, Cutler A. Bleeding downhill esophageal varices: a complication of upper extremity hemodialysis access. *Gastrointest Endosc* 1998;47:299–303.
31. Longley DG, Finlay DE, Letourneau JG. Sonography of the upper extremity and jugular veins. *AJR Am J Roentgenol* 1993;160: 957–962.
32. Hull JE, Hunter CS, Luiken GA. The Groshong catheter: initial experience and early results of imaging-guided placement. *Radiology* 1992;185:803–807.
33. Caridi JG, Grundy LS, Ross EA, et al. Interventional radiology placement of twin Tesio catheters for dialysis access: review of 75 patients. *J Vasc Interv Radiol* 1999;10:78–83.
34. Lund GB, Trerotola SO, Scheel PF, et al. Outcome of tunneled hemodialysis catheters placed by radiologists. *Radiology* 1996; 198:468–472.
35. Caridi JG, Grundy LS, Ross EA, et al. Interventional radiology placement of twin Tesio catheters for dialysis access: review of 75 patients. *Society of Cardiovascular and Interventional Radiology* 1999;10:78–83.

36. Trerotola SO, Johnson MS, Harris VJ, et al. Outcome of tunneled hemodialysis catheters placed via the right internal jugular vein by interventional radiologists. *Radiology* 1997;203:489–495.

37. LeBlanc M, Bosc JY, Vaussenat F, et al. Effective blood flow and recirculation rates in jugular vein twin catheters: measurement by ultrasound velocity dilution. *Am J Kidney Dis* 1998;31:87–92.

38. Hassell DD, Vesely TM, Pilgram TK, et al. Initial performance of Tesio hemodialysis catheters. *Society of Cardiovascular and Interventional Radiology* 1999;10:553–558.

39. Perini S, LaBerge JM, Santiestiban HL, et al. Tesio catheter: radiologically guided placement, mechanical performance, and adequacy of delivered dialysis. *Radiology* 2000;215:129–137.

40. Mankus RA, Ash SR, Semon JM. Comparison of blood flow rates and hydraulic resistance between the Mahurkar catheter, the Tesio twin catheter, and the Ash split cath. *ASAIO J* 1998;44:M532–M534.

41. Noh HM, Kaufman JA, Rhea JT, et al. Comparison of radiologic versus surgical placement of long-term hemodialysis catheters. *AJR Am J Roentgenol* 1999;172:673–675.

42. Zaman F, Antonious G, Murphy S, et al. Cost analysis of placement and maintenance of various tunneled catheters. *J Invest Med* 2001;49:135S.

43. Beathard GA, Posen GA. Initial clinical results with the LifeSite hemodialysis access system. *Kidney Int* 2000;58:2221–2227.

44. Moran JE. Subcutaneous vascular access devices. *Semin Dial* 2001;14:452–457.

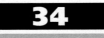

EXOTIC CATHETER ACCESS

HYUN S. KIM
GUNNAR B. LUND

Patients on chronic venous hemodialysis (HD) will require multiple venous catheters with large diameters, required to sustain the high flows needed for effective HD. These patients are therefore at high risk for central venous occlusion. Patients with prior radiation therapy, surgery, infection, congenital abnormalities, or in hypercoagulable state also carry a high risk for neck or chest venous occlusion. The venous occlusion precludes catheter placement via traditional routes and presents a challenge to interventional radiologists and nephrologists. Maintaining adequate venous access for these patients is crucial, and various alternative techniques have been developed. The purpose of this chapter is to review and describe the alternative techniques for venous access in patients with occlusion of traditional venous access. In the past, only surgical procedures provided venous access for patients who lacked traditional venous access. With advancement of interventional radiology, many additional alternative techniques have been developed (1). The following techniques have been described:

1. Surgical techniques
   a. Direct catheter placement into the right atrium (RA)
   b. Direct catheter placement into the azygos vein and hemiazygos vein
   c. Direct catheter placement into the superior vena cava (SVC)
   d. Direct catheter placement into the internal mammary vein
   e. Surgical catheter placement into the inferior vena cava (IVC) via infraumbilical veins
2. Percutaneous techniques
   a. Recanalization of occluded vein
   b. Bypassing occlusion via collateral veins
   c. Infraumbilical IVC placement
   d. Translumbar IVC placement
   e. Transhepatic IVC placement
   f. RA placement via transhepatic venous access

SURGICAL TECHNIQUES

Right Atrium, Superior Vena Cava, Azygos Vein, Internal Mammary Vein Direct Cannulation

Reported surgical techniques to obtain central venous access in the setting of occlusion of jugular and subclavian veins include direct catheter placement into the RA (2), azygos vein (3–5), or SVC (5). These techniques require thoracotomy, and catheter removal can be difficult. Recent developments now afford placement using minimally invasive surgery by thoracoscopy (6). These are the procedures of last resort. Direct cannulation of intercostal veins also can achieve access into the azygos vein, hemiazygos vein, and SVC (4,7–9). Cannulation of intercostal vein can be performed by open surgical exposure of the intercostal vein (8,10) or by percutaneous access to the intercostal vein (7). Direct cannulation of the internal mammary vein for central venous access also has been reported (11).

With the development of successful percutaneous IVC cannulation techniques, the need for surgical placement of catheters directly into the RA, SVC, or azygos vein has declined. In case of IVC thrombosis or abnormality, percutaneous access of azygous and hemiazygous veins have been described (12,13). The intercostal, internal mammary, azygous and hemiazygous veins, however, are unlikely to be useful for HD access because of the large size of the catheters relative to the size of these veins.

Inferior Vena Cava through Infraumbilical Veins

The IVC is the alternative to the SVC because it is a large-caliber vein with high venous flow. IVC access can be achieved from infrarenal, intrahepatic, or suprahepatic approaches. Surgical approaches include infrarenal IVC access via the inferior epigastric vein (14–17), femoral vein

(18–41), external iliac vein (42,43), the deep circumflex iliac vein (44), gonadal vein (18,45–47), saphenous vein (22–25,48–60), and lumbar vein (61). The infrarenal methods are not well tolerated by some patients because of tunneling in the groin. Iliofemoral thrombosis leading to pulmonary embolism and catheter infection is also a concern with this approach. Intrahepatic and suprahepatic IVC access are discussed in the following section on percutaneous techniques.

PERCUTANEOUS TECHNIQUES

Recanalization of Venous Occlusions

Recanalization of chronic venous occlusion for tunneled central catheter placement is an acceptable and safe technique (9,62,63). The chronic occlusion can be crossed safely by using a hydrophilic steerable guidewire and 4-French or 5-French directional catheter with hydrophilic coating (Fig. 34.1). With the availability of ultrasound, the jugular vein,

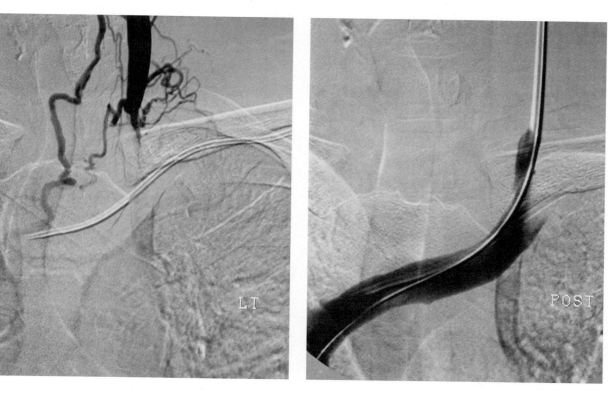

A

B

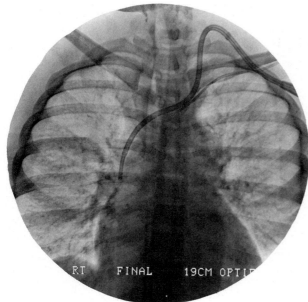

C

FIGURE 34.1. Patient with occluded bilateral internal jugular veins. Initial venogram from the left internal jugular vein (**A**) demonstrated occlusion at the left internal jugular and left subclavian vein junction with venous collateralization. The occlusion was successfully traversed and recanalized after percutaneous transluminal angioplasty, and flow was restored (**B**). Tunneled hemodialysis catheter was placed via recanalized left internal jugular vein (**C**).

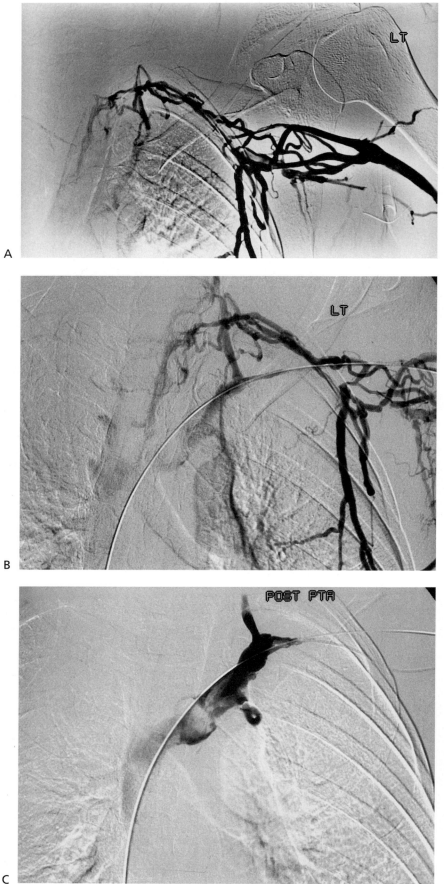

A

B

C

FIGURE 34.2. Patient with bilateral occlusion of the internal jugular and subclavian veins. Left brachial vein was accessed, and a venogram (**A**) demonstrated occluded left subclavian vein and extensive venous collateralization. Occlusion was successfully traversed with hydrophilic steerable guidewire (**B**). Residual thrombus was seen after percutaneous transluminal angioplasty (**C**). Recanalized left subclavian vein was punctured under fluoroscopic guidance targeting the traversing guidewire (**D**). Tunneled hemodialysis catheter was placed via recanalized left subclavian vein (**E**).

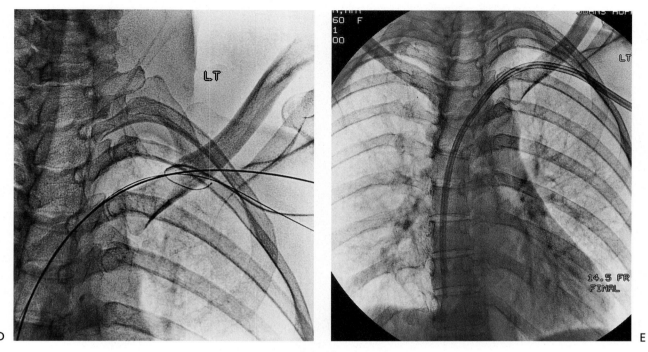

D

E

FIGURE 34.2. *(continued)*

subclavian vein, axillary vein, collateral vein, common femoral vein, or superficial femoral vein can be accessed with a 21-gauge micropuncture needle (Cook, Bloomington, IN, U.S.A.), and with contrast injection high-quality digital images can be obtained for guidance. In most instances, recanalization can be performed successfully in antegrade fashion, although sharp-needle recanalization in retrograde fashion may be needed (64). Getrajdman and colleagues reported an 89% technical success in recanalizing occluded veins for central venous catheter placement using hydrophilic steerable guidewires and catheters (63). Farrell and colleagues reported technical success for sharp-needle recanalization in five of six patients who had chronic central venous occlusion not amenable to simple recanalization with thrombolysis (64); one patient had an occlusion too long to traverse safely. In principle, if placing a guidewire across a venous occlusion is successful, a catheter can be introduced after dilating the occlusion with a balloon angioplasty catheter or dilators. In rare instances, a chronic web or elastic recoil after dilatation may preclude placing a large-caliber catheter and may require stent placement. Access to both ends of the wire (through-and-through technique) may be needed to provide a mechanical advantage and tension on the wire during catheter passage. An intravascular snare or retrieval basket can be used to grab the tip of the catheter or wire to cross the obstruction (9). Possible complications of dislodging clot-causing emboli, occluding collaterals, or causing fresh thrombus behind the obstruction have not been a significant problem in our practice (Fig. 34.2).

Catheter Placement Via Collateral Channels

Availability of high-quality digital imaging equipment and ultrasound in interventional radiology suites permits access to collateral vessels; one can follow collateral vessels around an obstruction and reenter the central vein. Familiarity with catheter and guidewire technology is required. These techniques are best suited for placement of small-caliber catheters, such as infusion catheters and ports (65).

Percutaneous Infraumbilical Inferior Vena Cava Catheters

In common clinical practice, an infraumbilical IVC HD catheter is limited to a femoral route (Fig. 34.3). Common femoral venous access is most common, although cannulation of any vein leading to IVC potentially can be used. Left gonadal vein access for a HD catheter has been described (47). In the context of acute renal failure, common femoral venous access for temporary nontunneled HD catheter is widely used. In these setting, however, patients are usually bedridden, and hospital or nursing home care can reduce the risk of infection. Tunneling of femoral catheters decreases the infection risk relative to nontunneled catheters (66); nevertheless, tunneled femoral dialysis catheters have not been widely reported. Some ambulatory patients do not tolerate a tunneled femoral catheter because of discomfort and inconvenience. Groin catheter site also compromises the sterility of catheter use, increasing the infection rate. We

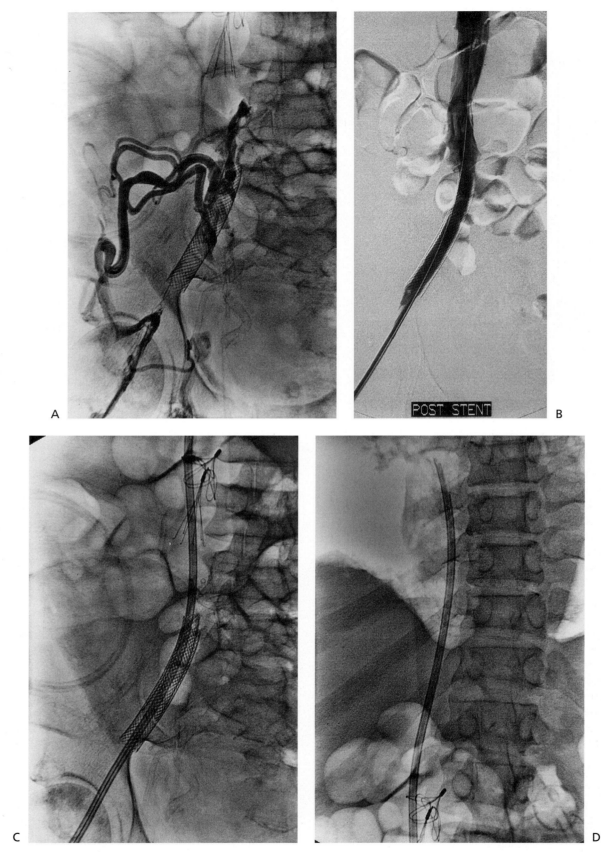

FIGURE 34.3. Patient with no central venous access and an indwelling inferior vena cava filter. Venogram (**A**) from the right common femoral venous access demonstrated occluded right common and external iliac veins with collaterals draining into the inferior vena cava. After successful recanalization with percutaneous transluminal angioplasty and an additional stent, the flow was restored (**B**). Hickman hemodialysis catheter (Bard, Murray Hill, NJ, U.S.A.) was carefully placed through the indwelling filter (**C**). The tip of the catheter was placed in the right atrium for maximal flow (**D**).

believe that the potential for ileofemoral thrombosis or stenosis also precludes its use in patients who are candidates for renal transplant or lower-extremity arteriovenous shunt access. On the other hand, Zaleski and colleagues (67) inserted 41 tunneled dialysis catheters in 21 patients and reported 30- and 180-day primary patencies (no additional treatment) of 78% and 55%; secondary patencies were 95% and 61%, respectively, at the same time intervals. There were 2.4 infections per 1,000 catheter days that required catheter removal, one partial IVC thrombosis, and no pulmonary emboli.

Translumbar Cannulation of the Inferior Vena Cava

The initial clinical experiences with translumbar IVC catheters involving small-diameter infusion catheters were reported in the late 1980s (68,69). Kenney and colleagues (68) reported the first translumbar access for total parenteral nutrition (TPN) administration in an adult. The catheter remained in place for 11 months and was removed for suspected catheter sepsis. Robards and colleagues (69) reported the first experience of placing an infusion catheter via a translumbar route in a 2-year-old child. Several early experiences indicated that placing a small-caliber infusion catheter via the translumbar route was safe (68–72). Large-diameter catheter placement for apheresis and HD via the translumbar route were possible only after documentation of safety in placement and removal of such catheters. Lund and associates (73) reported clinical, autopsy, and computed tomography findings that demonstrated a normal-appearing retroperitoneum without evidence of hemorrhage in a series of 46 apheresis catheters (15-French outer diameter) placed in 40 patients. Haire and co-workers (74–76) reported the safety and patency of translumbar IVC apheresis catheters used for peripheral stem-cell collection and infusion for the period of bone marrow recovery from autologous stem-cell transplantation. This technique also has been effective for infusion therapy in infants and children (69,71,72,77–79). The best translumbar route for avoiding complication from puncturing nearby organs has been described by a computed tomography (CT) study (80). A large series of 230 IVC catheters were reported in abstract form (81). Other uses of the translumbar technique includes parenteral nutrition, chemotherapy, placement of a LeVeen shunt (82), and access port implantation (83).

For HD, the experience with these access routes is limited. Lund and colleagues (84) reported placement of 17 translumbar IVC HD catheters in 12 patients. Technical success was 100%. The HD catheter functions best when the catheter tip is positioned in the RA. For extra length, special-order extra-long (50 and 55 cm) catheters were used (Bard Access Systems, Salt Lake City, UT, U.S.A.). Cumulative probability of patency was 0.52 at 6 months and 0.17

at 12 months. Other smaller series have been documented (85–88), reporting variable results. Markowitz and colleagues (87) reported their experience with Tesio catheters (Medcomp, Harleysville, PA, U.S.A.) via translumbar route in four patients, maintaining HD for 13 to 26 weeks.

Placement Technique

The placement of a translumbar IVC catheter is an adaptation of the translumbar aortography technique. The procedure includes four stages (Fig. 34.4):

1. Localization of the IVC
2. Direct IVC puncture
3. Subcutaneous tunneling of the catheter
4. Tract dilatation and catheter placement

Localization of the Inferior Vena Cava

The IVC localization techniques include (a) simple fluoroscopic localization and bone landmarks in a technique similar to translumbar aortography; (b) opacification with small angiographic catheter placed via the femoral vein; (c) use of radiopaque instruments, such as guidewires, catheters, wire baskets, or intravascular snares placed via the femoral vein; (d) ultrasound localization (especially in infants); (e) CT guidance. In a patient with IVC filter in placed or suspects the anomalies, occlusion, or compression, venographic evaluation of the IVC for anatomy and patency is mandatory. In our institution, most procedures are performed under fluoroscopic guidance using bony landmarks or a 0.035-inch Bentson guidewire in IVC as stationary targets. CT guidance is rarely used.

Inferior Vena Cava Puncture

In a prone position, an initial skin incision is made just above the right iliac crest 3 to 4 inches from the midline. A more medial approach than that used for translumbar aortography is recommended to avoid traversing the unusual case of medially situated colon (80). The tract is directed medially and cranially to puncture IVC at L3 level. The exact angle depends on the patient's body habitus, but care must be given to avoid sharp angulation that may cause kinking on the catheter. Delivery of a copious amount of local anesthetics along the tract using 22-gauge Chiba needle is advised to help controlling discomfort during tract dilatation and placement of peel-away sheath subsequently. To puncture the IVC, an 18-gauge trocar needle is preferred because small-caliber needles bend and make it difficult to target deep structure, especially in large patients. Complex angulation using a C-arm can be invaluable, although not necessary, as the operator gains experience. Care should be taken not to advance the needle too deep (anterior). When the trochar needle is advanced to expected position, the stylet is removed. Free flow of blood with gentle suction in-

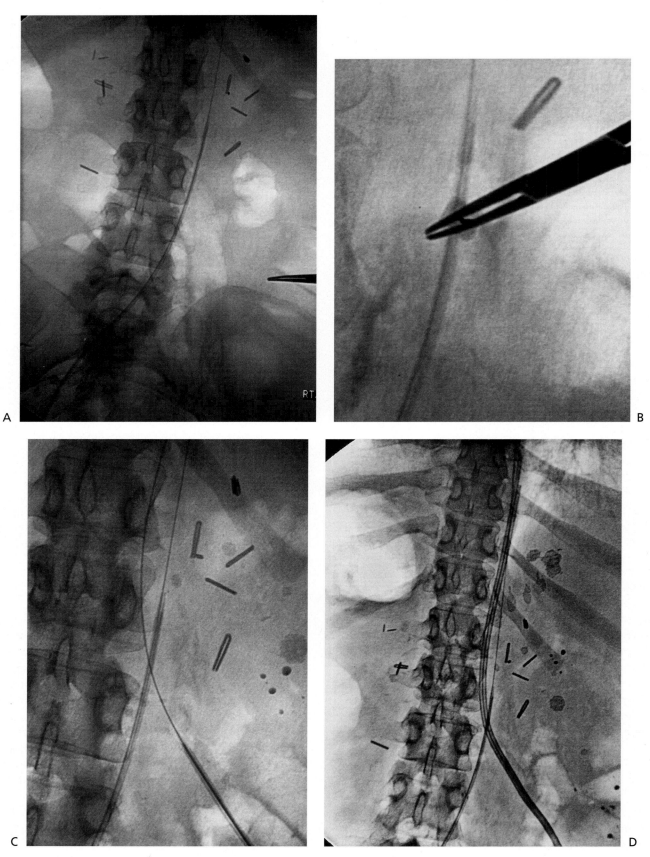

FIGURE 34.4. Translumbar inferior vena cava (IVC) hemodialysis catheter placement. Guidewire was placed via right common femoral venous access and advanced to the IVC as a localizer, and the patient was placed in prone position. The skin access site was marked under fluoroscopic guidance (**A**). Under careful fluoroscopic guidance, the IVC was punctured, targeting the guidewire and catheter in the IVC (**B**). After vena caval access was achieved, the track was dilated using serial dilators (**C**). A 55-cm-long hemodialysis catheter was placed with the tip in the right atrium (**D**).

dicates the needle position in the IVC. A soft-tipped Bentson guidewire is advanced up to the IVC, and a 5-French angiographic catheter is advanced over the guidewire after removal of the needle.

Subcutaneous Tunneling of the Catheter

A permanent exit site is established in the right flank as far anteriorly as possible. The tunnel is outlined from the permanent exit site in the flank to the posterior temporary stab incision site. Care should be taken not to create a sharp bend or not to create the track superficial to the right iliac bone because it may cause discomfort and pain to the patient and impaired catheter function by iliac bone compression on the catheter. Local anesthetic is used. Appropriate length of the catheter can be measured using a guidewire. We use 45-cm, 5-cm, and 55-cm-length custom-ordered HD catheters for various patients' body habitus. The appropriate-length catheter then is tunneled subcutaneously in the standard fashion. In a case of central venous access, a catheter, such as the Hickman catheter, can be trimmed to correct length after tunneling, similar to internal jugular or subclavian catheters. The Dacron cuff is placed in the subcutaneous tunnel about 1 to 2 inches from the skin site.

Tract Dilatation and Catheter Placement

Using stiff wire for track dilatation is advised. We prefer to use a Rosen wire or super stiff Amplatz wire for added support. The guidewire is advanced via the angiographic catheter, and sequential dilatation of the track is performed with vascular dilators. A peel-away sheath appropriate for the catheter is advanced. It is not necessary to advance the peel-away sheath too far into the IVC because to do so may cause kinking of the sheath. A sheath placed just inside the IVC is ideal. The IVC catheter is advanced via the sheath after removal of the inner dilator and the guidewire. The sheath may be kinked at the entry site of the peel-away sheath. This can be straightened by peeling back the sheath gently. Alternatively, guidewire can be exchanged with a slippery wire, such as an angle-glide Terumo wire or a stiff-angled glide Terumo wire, and the catheter can be advanced over the glide guidewire via a peel-away sheath. This technique provides extra support for the catheter and added secure access to the IVC. This technique is recommended for operators learning this procedure. Beyond the entry site of the sheath into the IVC, the catheter always passes without problems. The peel-away sheath is removed, and the catheter tip is positioned in the RA for maximum flow. The catheter tip is confirmed by contrast administration, and flow can be tested using manual suction. The puncture site is secured by a suture, and the catheter is flushed with heparinized saline.

Complications

Discomfort, soreness, and stiffness in the back are common immediately after catheter placement. Temporary right leg pain or weakness is not uncommon for several days after the procedure. There has not been a report of perioperative complication of injury to ureters, kidneys, or bowel, although late perforation of an infusion catheter tip into the right ureter has been reported (89). Inadvertent puncture of the aorta and the superior mesenteric vein without clinical consequences was reported (73).

The complications most frequently reported include thrombosis (73,78,81,84), infection (71–73,78,81,83,84), catheter defects (72,73,84), and malposition (72,73,84,89). The IVC thrombosis (Fig. 34.5) and infection occur about the same rate as for jugular and subclavian catheters. Lund and colleagues (84) reported seven episodes of access failure attributable to clot in 17 HD catheters. This represents 41% of the catheters for a rate of 0.33 episodes per 100 catheter days at risk. Urokinase infused via the catheter successfully resolved five of seven episodes. Six episodes of infection occurred (0.28 in 100 days) that required three catheter removals. Lund and colleagues (73) studied 46 single-lumen 14-French apheresis catheters and reported eight cases of thrombosis-related catheter dysfunction (18%) at a rate of 0.22 events per 100 catheters days at risk. They also reported five episodes of infection, including two subcutaneous tunnel infection and one patient with septic thrombophlebitis. Three catheters required removal. The latter series of 230 catheters from the same institution, reported by McCowan and associates (81), described 43 cases of catheter malfunction, with thrombosis of 137 catheters with available follow-up, representing 18% of total catheters and 31% of catheters with follow-up. This represents a thrombosis rate of 0.31 per 100 catheter days at risk. Of 43 catheter dysfunction from thrombosis, 37 catheters were treated successfully with thrombolysis using urokinase. They also reported 11 catheter infections that required removal. Markowitz and colleagues (87) had two complications from five paired Tesio catheters in four patients. One hemodynamically stable patient developed a retroperitoneal hematoma on day 1 that did not require treatment. The other patient developed sepsis and fluid collection around the subcutaneous cuff. The patient responded to removal of the catheter and intravenous antibiotics. Bennett and colleagues reported three complications of 29 translumbar procedures in 22 patients (83). The complications include one groin hematoma, one retroperitoneal hematoma, and one renal artery branch violation without clinical consequences. Catheter-tip dislodgment from the IVC can occur from a change in patient position, inadequate anchoring sutures, or patient growth spur. Positioning the tip of the catheter in the RA or atrium–caval junction provides maximal flow to the catheter and excess intravascular length for stability. Malpositioning of the catheter tip in hepatic veins, renal veins, and common iliac

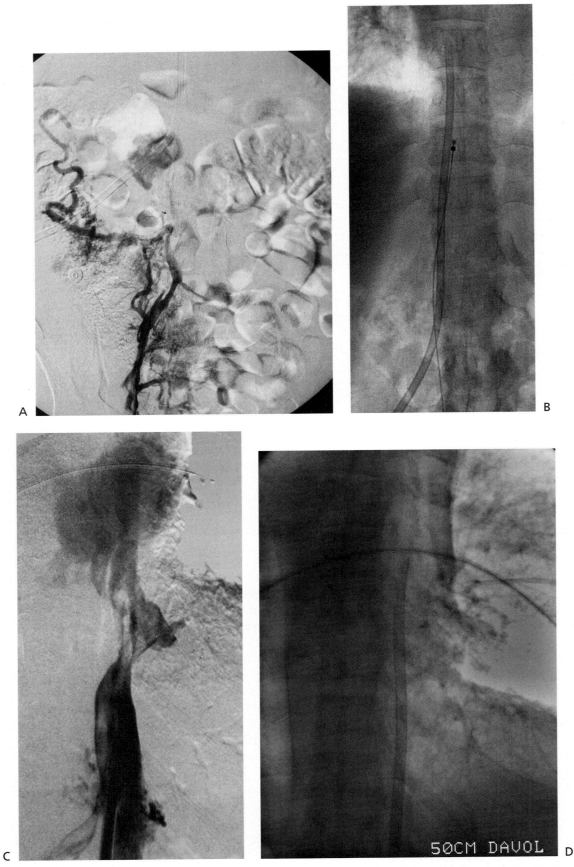

FIGURE 34.5. Patient with poor vascular access because of hypercoagulable state. Poor dialysis function was noted in the indwelling translumbar inferior vena cava (IVC) hemodialysis catheter. Initial venogram (**A**) via the right common femoral access demonstrated an occluded IVC with extensive collateralization. Mechanical thrombolysis (**B**) was performed using Amplatz thrombectomy device (Microvena, White Bear Lake, MN, U.S.A.) in an attempt to increase the flow to the catheter for improved function. The IVC flow was restored (**C**), and a 50-cm-long hemodialysis catheter was repositioned to the right atrium with the patient in a prone position (**D**) for maximal function.

veins was reported (73). Malpositioning frequently occurs with a change in the patient's position and thrombosis. Treatment for IVC catheter thrombosis is the same as that for jugular or subclavian catheters, including thrombolytic therapy, guidewire manipulations, snaring and stripping the catheter tip, and catheter exchange.

To prevent thrombosis, the catheter should be placed with its tip in a position where high blood flow can be expected. The catheter should not be placed where the blood flow can be compromised. We prefer not to place the catheter in the intrahepatic IVC. Caudate lobe hypertrophy in cirrhotic patient also can compromise intrahepatic IVC blood flow. We advise placement of the tip of the catheter in the RA or atrium—caval junction. Anticoagulation can help long-term patency of the catheter. Haire and co-workers (74) reported a significant reduction in the rate of catheter thrombosis from 20% to 3.2 % with administration of 325 mg per day of aspirin. Subcutaneous heparin administration, heparin medication, mixing heparin in an infusion, and coumadin administration all have been tried in an effort to prevent catheter thrombosis. Markowitz and colleagues (87) recommend withholding heparin from immediate postplacement dialysis session because of concern about retroperitoneal hemorrhage. Caution also should be used with patients who are at risk for gastrointestinal bleed.

The experience with translumbar IVC catheter is limited. The perioperative complication rate is minimal. The long-term complication rate, including thrombosis, infection, and catheter dysfunction, has been acceptable and does not differ significantly from that of jugular or subclavian HD catheters. The translumbar IVC catheter is a safe and valuable alternative for patients with restricted jugular and subclavian access.

In the setting of IVC thrombosis or abnormality (Fig. 34.6), case reports of percutaneous puncture of azygous and hemiazygous veins have been reported. Percutaneous puncture of the hemiazygos vein with the placement of a Broviac catheter has been reported (12). Direct translumbar percutaneous puncture of the azygos vein with placement of a Hickman catheter also has been reported (13). The experience is very limited.

Transhepatic Inferior Vena Cava and Hepatic Vein Catheters

The IVC can be punctured through the liver in an intrahepatic segment through a hepatic vein or directly, and the catheter can be placed through the access into the IVC (Fig. 34.7). The access can be achieved either by ultrasound or fluoroscopic guidance from the flank or anteriorly. The tip of the catheter can be placed in the RA for maximal flow rate. Alternatively, the tip can be placed down in the IVC. The first clinical experience involving small-diameter catheter was reported in the late 1980s (88). This technique has been used extensively in infants and children (72,78,

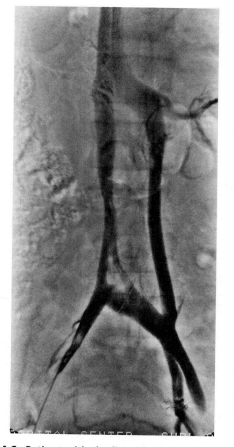

FIGURE 34.6. Patient with duplicated inferior vena cava (IVC), uncommon normal variant. Vena caval anatomic variants should be considered in infraumbilical and translumbar IVC catheter placement procedures.

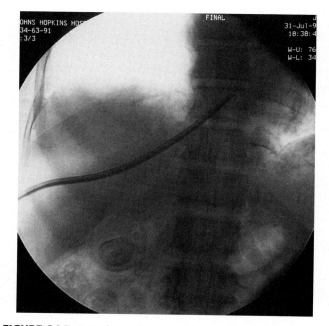

FIGURE 34.7. Transhepatic hemodialysis catheter. This 45-cm-long catheter was placed percutaneously via the right hepatic vein, and the tip was placed in the right atrium.

79,91–94). The transhepatic IVC catheter is an important alternative in a patient who has occluded infrarenal IVC or compression or an anomaly of the infrarenal IVC. The experience of this technique in HD is limited with few reported cases (47,88,95).

This technique, however, carries potential risk of significant bleeding and biliary track communication (96). Potential complication from transhepatic vein and transhepatic IVC catheters also includes infection, hepatic dysfunction from hepatic vein thrombosis, and dislodgement by extra strains on catheter from growth spurts, excessive movement and respiratory excursion. Acute Budd–Chiari syndrome caused by acute hepatic vein thrombosis from a 10-French transhepatic IVC Hickman catheter also has been reported (91). Putnam and colleagues (96) reported dislodgment of the catheter during the coughing episode; it became unstable as a result of documented intraperitoneal hemorrhage and required resuscitation. They also described a case with biliary communication from the transhepatic track, requiring coil and Gelfoam embolization on removal. Po and associates (47) reported one case of access failure and one case of infection on catheter exchange. Duncan and colleagues (95) reported a case of small intrahepatic hematoma adjacent to catheter track that required percutaneous drainage. The patient eventually died of enterococcal sepsis. Bile leak, hemorrhage, hepatic artery pseudoaneurysm formation, and discomfort by a catheter placed through intercostal space are also known risks. For these reasons, this technique is the last effort for central venous access in our institution. This technique is performed only when all other access, including translumbar IVC cannulation, cannot be achieved safely.

CONCLUSION

With advancement of medicine and dialysis, life expectancy for patients with renal failure has been increasing. As more patients receive long-term HD, and therefore resort to fewer available venous access sites, interventional radiologists should be more creative and aggressive about finding suitable venous access. Traditional venous access sites should be used. When venous occlusion occurs in traditional access sites, attempts should be made to recanalize the occluded vein or to access collaterals directly that bypass the obstruction. When these efforts fail, use of infraumbilical IVC access, translumbar IVC access, or transhepatic vein access is warranted. Among the many techniques described, the best vascular access for each patient is the least invasive one that provides adequate access without jeopardizing future access sites.

REFERENCES

1. Kaufman JA, Kazanjian SA, Rivitz SM, et al. Long-term central venous catheterization in patients with limited access. *AJR Am J Roentgenol* 1996;167:1327–1333.
2. Oram-Smith JC, Mullen JL, Harken AH, et al. Direct right atrial catheterization for total parenteral nutrition. *Surgery* 1978;83:274–276.
3. Pokorny WJ, McGill CW, Harberg FJ. Use of azygous vein for central catheter insertion. *Surgery* 1985;97:362.
4. Meranze SG, McLean GK, Stein EJ, et al. Catheter placement in the azygos system: an unusual approach to venous access. *AJR Am J Roentgenol* 1985;144:1075–1076.
5. Malt RA, Kempster M. Direct azygos vein and superior vena cava cannulation for parenteral nutrition. *JPEN J Parenter Enteral Nutr* 1983;7:580–581.
6. Birnbaum PL, Michas C, Cohen SE. Direct right atrial catheter insertion with video assisted thoracic surgery. *Ann Thorac Surg* 1996;62:1197.
7. Andrews JC. Percutaneous placement of a Hickman catheter with use of an intercostal vein for access. *J Vasc Interv Radiol* 1994;5:859–861.
8. Lammermeier D, Steiger E, Cosgrove D, et al. Use of an intercostal vein for central venous access in home parenteral nutrition: a case report. *JPEN J Parenter Enteral Nutr* 1986;10:659–661.
9. Torosian MH, Meranze S, McLean G, et al. Central venous access with occlusive superior central venous thrombosis. *Ann Surg* 1986;203:30–33.
10. Newman B, Cooney D, Karp M, et al. The intercostal vein: an alternate route for central venous alimentation. *J Pediatr Surg* 1983;18:732–733.
11. Jaime-Solis E, Anaya-Ortega M, Moctezuma-Espinosa J. The internal mammary vein: an alternate route for central venous access with an implantable port. *J Pediatr Surg* 1994;29:1328–1330.
12. Denny DF Jr. Central venous access via the hemiazygous vein. In: Trerotola SO, Savader S, Durham J, eds. *Venous interventions.* Society of Vascular and Interventional Radiology, 1995:507.
13. Patel NH. Percutaneous translumbar placement of Hickman catheter into the azygos vein. *AJR Am J Roentgenol* 2000;175:1302–1304.
14. Sutherland FR, Graham J. Long-term central venous access through the inferior epigastric vein. *Can J Surg* 1995;38:283–284.
15. Krog M, Gerdin B. An alternative placement of implantable central venous access systems. *JPEN J Parenter Enteral Nutr* 1989;13:666–667.
16. Donahoe PK, Kim SH. The inferior epigastric vein as an alternate site for central venous hyperalimentation. *J Pediatr Surg* 1980;15:737–738.
17. Maher JW. A technique for the positioning of permanent central venous catheters in patients with thrombosis of the superior vena cava. *Surg Gynecol Obstet* 1983;156:659–660.
18. Serrao PR, Jean-Louis J, Godoy J, et al. Inferior vena cava catheterization in the neonate by the percutaneous femoral vein method. *J Perinatol* 1996;16:129–132.
19. Cogliati AA, Dell'utri D, Picardi A, et al. Central venous catheterization in pediatric patients affected by hematological malignancies. *Haematologica* 1995;80:448–450.
20. Talbott GA, Winters WD, Bratton SL, et al. A prospective study of femoral catheter related thrombosis in children. *Arch Pediatr Adolesc Med* 1995;149:288–291.
21. Shefler A, Gillis J, Lam A, et al. Inferior vena cava thrombosis as a complication of femoral vein catheterisation. *Arch Dis Child* 1995;72:343–345.
22. Hogan L, Pulito AR. Broviac central venous catheters inserted via the saphenous or femoral vein in the NICU under local anesthesia. *J Pediatr Surg* 1992;27:1185–1188.
23. Stenzel JP, Green TP, Fuhrman BP, et al. Percutaneous femoral venous catheterizations: a prospective study of complications. *J Pediatr* 1989;114:411–415.

24. Williard W, Coit D, Lucas A, et al. Long term vascular access via the inferior vena cava. *J Surg Oncol* 1991;46:162–166.

25. Nour S, Puntis JW, Stringer MD. Intraabdominal extravasation complicating parenteral nutrition in infants. *Arch Dis Child Fetal Neonatal Ed* 1995;72:F207–F208.

26. Kwon TH, Kim YL, Cho DK. Ultrasound guided cannulation of the femoral vein for acute haemodialysis access. *Nephrol Dial Transplant* 1997;12:1009–1012.

27. Montagnac R, Bernard C, Guillaumie J, et al. Indwelling silicone femoral catheters: experience of three haemodialysis centres. *Nephrol Dial Transplant* 1997;12:772–775.

28. Kirkpatrick WG, Culpepper RM, Sirmon MD. Frequency of complications with prolonged femoral vein catheterization for hemodialysis access *Nephron* 1996;73:58–62.

29. Harden JL, Kemp L, Mirtallo J. Femoral catheters increase risk of infection in total parenteral nutrition patients. *Nutr Clin Pract* 1995;10:60–66.

30. Trottier SJ, Veremakis C, O'Brien J, et al. Femoral deep vein thrombosis associated with central venous catheterization: results from a prospective, randomized trial. *Crit Care Med* 1995;23:52–59.

31. Queiros J, Cabrita A, Maximino J, Lobato L, et al. Central catheters for hemodialysis: a six month experience of 103 catheters. *Nephrologie* 1994;15:113–115.

32. Swartz RD, Messana JM, Boyer CJ, et al. Successful use of cuffed central venous hemodialysis catheters inserted percutaneously. *J Am Soc Nephrol* 1994;4:1719–1725.

33. Weitzel WF, Boyer CJ Jr., El Khatib MT, et al. Successful use of indwelling cuffed femoral vein catheters in ambulatory hemodialysis patients. *Am J Kidney Dis* 1993;22:426–429.

34. Murr MM, Rosenquist MD, Lewis RW, et al. A prospective safety study of femoral vein versus nonfemoral vein catheterization in patients with burns. *J Burn Care Rehabil* 1991;12:576–578.

35. Williams JF, Seneff MG, Friedman BC, et al. Use of femoral venous catheters in critically ill adults: prospective study. *Crit Care Med* 1991;19:550–553.

36. Tavecchio L, Bedeini AV, Lanocita R, et al. Long term infusion in cancer chemotherapy with the Groshong catheter via the inferior vena cava. *Tumori* 1996;82:372–375.

37. Gouge SF, Paulson WD, Moore J Jr. Inferior vena cava thrombosis due to an indwelling hemodialysis catheter. *Am J Kidney Dis* 1988;11:515–518.

38. Lazarus HM, Creger RJ, Bloom AD, et al. Percutaneous placement of femoral central venous catheter in patients undergoing transplantation of bone marrow. *Surg Gynecol Obstet* 1990;170:403–406.

39. Kitamoto Y, Fukui H, Iwabuchi K, et al. A femoral vein catheter with immobilized urokinase (UKFC) as an antithrombotic blood access. *ASAIO Trans* 1987;33:136–139.

40. Nidus BD, Neusy AJ. Chronic hemodialysis by repeated femoral vein cannulation. *Nephron* 1981;29:195–197.

41. Kjellstrand CM, Merino GE, Mauer SM, et al. Complications of percutaneous femoral vein catheterizations for hemodialysis. *Clin Nephrol* 1975;4:37–40.

42. Mathur MN, Storey DW, White GH, et al. Percutaneous insertion of long term venous access catheters via the external iliac vein. *Aust N Z J Surg* 1993;63:858–863.

43. Ikeda S, Sera Y, Ohshiro H, et al. Transiliac catheterization of the inferior vena cava for long-term venous access in children. *Pediatr Surg Int* 1998;14:140–141.

44. White SA, Doughman T, Hayes P, et al. The deep circumflex iliac vein for secondary central venous access and haemodialysis. *Nephrol Dial Transplant* 2000;15:244–245.

45. Coit DG, Turnbull AD. Long term central vascular access through the gonadal vein. *Surg Gynecol Obstet* 1992;175:362–364.

46. Fukui S, Coggia M, Goeau-Brissonniere O, et al. [Introducing an implantable central venous catheter via the right gonadal vein]. *Presse Med* 1995;24:1608–1609.

47. Po CL, Koolpe HA, Allen S, et al. Transhepatic PermCath for hemodialysis. *Am J Kidney Dis* 1994;24:590–591.

48. Lussky RC, Trower N, Fisher D, et al. Unusual misplacement sites of percutaneous central venous lines in the very low birth weight neonate. *Am J Perinatol* 1997;14:63–67.

49. Ohki Y, Nako Y, Morikawa A, et al. Percutaneous central venous catheterization via the great saphenous vein in neonates. *Acta Paediatr Jpn* 1997;39:312–316.

50. Neubauer AP. Percutaneous central i.v. access in the neonate: experience with 535 Silastic catheters. *Acta Paediatr* 1995;84:756–760.

51. Hollyoak MA, Ong TH, Leditschke JF. Critical appraisal of surgical venous access in children. *Pediatr Surg Int* 1997;12:177–182.

52. Leibundgut K, Muller C, Muller K, et al. Tunneled, double lumen Broviac catheters are useful, efficient and safe in children undergoing peripheral blood progenitor cell harvesting and transplantation. *Bone Marrow Transplant* 1996;17:663–667.

53. Pippus KG, Giacomantonio JM, Gillis DA, et al. Thrombotic complications of saphenous central venous lines. *J Pediatr Surg* 1994;29:1218–1219.

54. Statter MB. Peripheral and central venous access. *Semin Pediatr Surg* 1992;1:181–187.

55. Kohli Kumar M, Rich AJ, Pearson AD, et al. Comparison of saphenous versus jugular veins for central venous access in children with malignancy. *J Pediatr Surg* 1992;27:609–611.

56. Eastridge BJ, Lefor AT. Complications of indwelling venous access devices in cancer patients. *J Clin Oncol* 1995;13:233–238.

57. Treiman GS, Silberman H. Chronic venous access in patients with cancer. Selective use of the saphenous vein. *Cancer* 1993;72:760–765.

58. Curtas S, Bonaventura M, Meguid MM. Cannulation of inferior vena cava for long term central venous access. *Surg Gynecol Obstet* 1989;168:121–124.

59. Appelqvist P, Pantzar P. A new site for totally implanted central venous access system in patients with malignancy: long term results of 10 cases. *J Surg Oncol* 1988;38:1–3.

60. Fusetti C, Renggli JC, Wellensiek B, et al. Chronic saphenous venous access: an interesting alternative in the case of vena cava superior syndrome. *Chirurgie* 1999;70:1036–1040.

61. Boddie AW Jr. Translumbar catheterization of the inferior vena cava for long term angioaccess. *Surg Gynecol Obstet* 1989;168:54–56.

62. Ferral H, Bjarnason H, Wholey M, et al. Recanalization of occluded veins to provide access for central catheter placement. *J Vasc Interv Radiol* 1996;7:681–685.

63. Getrajdman GI, Brown KT, Brody LA, et al. Simple central venous catheter placement in patients with occluded central veins. *J Vasc Interv Radiol* 2000;11:1043–1046.

64. Farrell T, Land EV, Barnart W. Sharp recanalization of central venous occlusions. *J Vasc Interv Radiol* 1999;10:149–154.

65. Kaufman JA, Crenshaw WB, Kuter I, et al. Percutaneous placement of a central venous access device via an intercostal vein. *AJR Am J Roentgenol* 1995;164:459–460.

66. Timsit JF, Bruneel F, Cheval C, et al. Use of tunneled femoral catheters to prevent catheter-related infection: a randomized, controlled trial. *Ann Intern Med* 1999;130:729–735.

67. Zaleski GX, Funaki B, Lorenz JM, et al. Experience with tunneled femoral hemodialysis catheters. *Am J Roentgenol* 1999;172:493–496.

68. Kenney PR, Dorfman GS, Denny DF Jr. Percutaneous inferior vena cava cannulation for long term parenteral nutrition. *Surgery* 1985;97:602–605.

69. Robards JB, Jaques PF, Mauro MA, et al. Percutaneous translumbar inferior vena cava central line placement in a critically ill child. *Pediatr Radiol* 1989;19:140–141.

70. Denny DF Jr, Dorfman GS, Greenwood LH, et al. Translumbar inferior vena cava Hickman catheter placement for total parenteral nutrition. *AJR Am J Roentgenol* 1987;148:621–622.

71. Denny DF Jr, Greenwood LH, Morse SS, et al. Inferior vena cava: translumbar catheterization for central venous access. *Radiology* 1989;172:1013–1014.

72. Robertson LJ, Jaques PF, Mauro MA, et al. Percutaneous inferior vena cava placement of tunneled Silastic catheters for prolonged vascular access in infants. *J Pediatr Surg* 1990;25:596–598.

73. Lund GB, Lieberman RP, Haire WD, et al. Translumbar inferior vena cava catheters for long term venous access. *Radiology* 1990; 174:31–35.

74. Haire WD, Lieberman RP, Lund GB, et al. Translumbar inferior vena cava catheters: experience with 58 catheters in peripheral stem cell collection and transplantation. *Transfus Sci* 1990;11: 195–200.

75. Haire WD, Lieberman RP, Lund GB, et al. Translumbar inferior vena cava catheters: safety and efficacy in peripheral blood stem cell transplantation. *Transfusion* 1990;30:511–515.

76. Haire WD, Lieberman RP, Lund GB, et al. Translumbar inferior vena cava catheters. *Bone Marrow Transplant* 1991;7:389–392.

77. Malmgren N, Cwikiel W, Hochbergs P, et al. Percutaneous translumbar central venous catheter in infants and small children. *Pediatr Radiol* 1995;25:28–30.

78. Azizkhan RG, Taylor LA, Jaques PF, et al. Percutaneous translumbar and transhepatic inferior vena caval catheters for prolonged vascular access in children. *Pediatr Surg* 1992;27:165– 169.

79. Wesley JR. Permanent central venous access devices. *Semin Pediatr Surg* 1992;1:188–201.

80. Cazenave FL, Glass-Royal MC, Teitelbaum GP, et al. CT analysis of a safe approach for translumbar access to the aorta and inferior vena cava. *AJR Am J Roentgenol* 1991;156:395–396.

81. McCowan TC, Lieberman RP, Goertzen TC, et al. Radiologic placement of inferior vena cava access catheters. *J Vasc Interv Radiol* 1993;4:35(abst).

82. Cooper SG, Iannone JP. LeVeen shunt insertion with use of a percutaneous translumbar approach to the inferior vena cava. *J Vasc Interv Radiol* 1993;4:667–668.

83. Bennett JD, Papadouris D, Rankin RN, et al. Percutaneous inferior vena caval approach for long term central venous access. *J Vasc Interv Radiol* 1997;8:851–855.

84. Lund GB, Trerotola SO, Scheel PJ Jr. Percutaneous translumbar inferior vena cava cannulation for hemodialysis. *Am J Kidney Dis* 1995;25:732–737.

85. Gupta A, Karak PK, Saddekni S. Translumbar inferior vena cava catheter for long term hemodialysis. *J Am Soc Nephrol* 1995;5: 2094–2097.

86. D'Angelo F, Ramacciato G, Aurello P, et al. Inferior vena cava implant of permanent central venous access devices. *J Chemother* 1997;9:157–158.

87. Markowitz DG, Rosenblum DI, Newman J, et al. Translumbar inferior vena caval Tesio catheter for hemodialysis. *J Vasc Interv Radiol* 1998;9:145–147.

88. Raja RM, Po CL. Reply. *Am J Kidney Dis* 1995;25:973.

89. Dimasi MH, Reid SK, Pagan-Marin H, et al. Migration of translumbar inferior vena cava catheter into the right ureter. *AJR Am J Roentgenol* 1997;169:1753–1754.

90. Crummy AB, Carlson P, McDermott JC, et al. Percutaneous transhepatic placement of a Hickman catheter. *AJR Am J Roentegenol* 1991;153:1317–1318.

91. Pieters PC, Dittrich J, Prasad U, et al. Acute Budd Chiari syndrome caused by percutaneous placement of a transhepatic inferior vena cava catheter. *J Vasc Interv Radiol* 1997;8:587–590.

92. Kaufman JA, Greenfield AJ, Fitzpatrick GF. Transhepatic cannulation of the inferior vena cava. *J Vasc Interv Radiol* 1991;2: 331–334.

93. De Csepel J, Stanely P, Padua EM, et al. Maintaining long term central venous access by repetitive hepatic vein cannulation. *J Pediatr Surg* 1994;29:56–57.

94. Shim D, Lloyd TR, Cho KJ, et al. Transhepatic cardiac catheterization in children: evaluation of efficacy and safety. *Circulation* 1995;92:1526–1530.

95. Duncan KA, Karlin CA, Beezley M. Percutaneous transhepatic PermCath for hemodialysis vascular access. *Am J Kidney Dis* 1995;25:973.

96. Putnam SG III, Ball D, Cohen GS. Transhepatic dialysis catheter tract embolization to close a venous biliary peritoneal fistula. *J Vasc Interv Radiol* 1998;9:149–151.

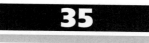

35

MANAGEMENT OF THE INFECTED CATHETER

PAUL J. SCHEEL, JR.
DORENE KUHN

In the United States, about 300,000 patients receive chronic outpatient hemodialysis (1). Because of the favorable longevity and low incidence of thrombotic and infectious complications, the preferred vascular access for these patients is an arteriovenous (AV) native fistula (2). Unfortunately, because of the underlying anatomy, late referral, or both, only 27% of patients have functioning AV native fistulas as their primary dialysis access (3).

Alternatively, a synthetic bridge graft or central venous catheter can be used. Both devices allow for adequate blood flow, but the synthetic bridge graft is preferable because of the higher incidence of thrombotic and infectious complications of central venous catheters. This chapter reviews these infectious complications and focuses on the management of central venous catheter infections.

OVERVIEW

Central venous catheters used for hemodialysis access traditionally are classified as either *temporary* or *long-term* catheters. Temporary catheters are inserted in either the internal jugular, subclavian, or femoral vein. These devices are nontunneled, are not equipped with a Dacron cuff, and are intended to be used for less than 14 days. Long-term catheters are preferentially placed in the internal jugular vein, are tunneled subcutaneously, and are equipped with a Dacron cuff. These devices can be used as a bridge to either AV native fistula or synthetic graft maturation or, if neither is technically possible, used for long-term vascular access.

Infectious complications of these devices historically have been classified based on the anatomic location of the infection. Borrowing from the peritoneal dialysis catheter literature, these infections are categorized as exit-site, tunnel, or blood-borne infections. Exit-site infections occur at the skin–catheter interface. For temporary catheters, this is at the insertion site, and for tunneled catheters, this will be the location where the catheter exits from the tunnel, including that portion of the tunnel that extends from the

Dacron cuff distal to the exit site. These exit-site infections are diagnosed clinically by some combination of swelling, erythema, fluctuance, and tenderness (Fig. 35.1).

Tunnel infections (tunneled catheters only) are located anatomically between the Dacron cuff, subcutaneously beneath the skin, and the venous insertion site. They have symptoms similar to those of exit-site infections; however, because these infections may be in a closed space and do not

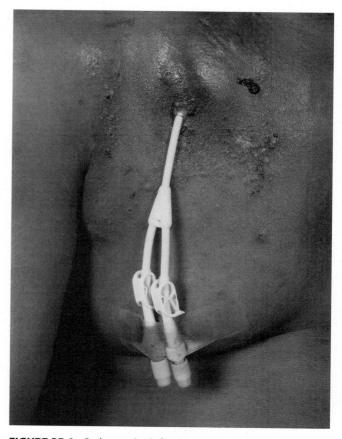

FIGURE 35.1. Catheter-site infection. Right internal jugular tunneled catheter. The subcutaneous tunnel distal to the cuff is edematous, the overlying skin is erythematous, and purulent material is draining from the exit site.

284 *Central Dialysis Catheters*

have adequate drainage through an exit site, these infections behave like an abscess.

MICROBIOLOGY

Not surprisingly, the organisms causing exit-site and tunnel infections are those typically found on the skin and include *Staphylococcus aureus, Staphylococcus epidermidis, and Enterococcus* organisms. Because these exit sites may be exposed to water, water-borne organisms also may include *Pseudomonas, Klebsiella,* and yeast.

The mechanism of these infections is one of bacteria migrating along the external part of the catheter and infecting the enclosed surrounding skin (4). Bloodstream infection secondary to indwelling catheters is the second leading cause for morbidity and mortality among patients on hemodialysis (1). Although rates for reported bloodstream infections vary from center to center, based on definition and culture technology, rates have been reported on as low as 1.5 episodes per 1,000 catheter days up to 5.5 episodes per 1,000 catheter days (5–9).

Risk factors for bloodstream infections associated with central venous catheters have long been known to be duration of placement and manipulation of ports (10,11). For patients with central venous catheters for a limited period, such as for antibiotic administration, these risk factors can be managed. For patients with central venous catheters for hemodialysis, the duration of the catheter may be for years, and these ports must be accessed by definition at least thrice weekly.

Endoluminal colonization is the mechanism by which these devices lead to bloodstream infections. Dittmer and colleagues documented that 68% of catheters were colonized with *S. epidermitis* on the intraluminal surface. The mean time to colonization was 27 days after insertion (12) (see Chapter 42). (*Editors note*: This may be promoted by a biofilm coating.)

Organisms responsible for bloodstream infections are those listed in Table 35.1. The percent of those organisms may vary by center, but the growing concern is the percentage of organisms that are becoming resistant to methicillin and vancomycin (13)

TABLE 35.1. MICROBIOLOGY OF CATHETER-ASSOCIATED INFECTIONS

Staphylococcus aureus
Staphylococcus epidermidis
Klebsiella spp
Enterobacter spp
Pseudomonas aeruginosa
Corynebacteria spp
Candida spp

TABLE 35.2. CLINICAL MANIFESTATIONS CATHETER-ASSOCIATED BACTEREMIA

Mild
  Fever
  Rigors
  Positive blood culture for typical bacteria (Table 35.1)
  Localized infection at exit site
  Elevated WBC with left shift

Severe (any or all of mild symptoms)
  Hypotension
  Lack of defervescence with appropriate antibiotic coverage
  Disseminated intravascular coagulation

WBC, white blood cell count.

The diagnosis of catheter-related bacteremia is based on clinical and laboratory parameters (Table 35.2). Patients may present to the dialysis unit febrile or develop fever and chills within the first hour on dialysis. Blood cultures should be obtained through the catheter and from a peripheral vein if feasible. If no peripheral vein is accessible, reasonable microbiologic information still can be obtained by obtaining two sets of blood cultures via the central line. Tunneson and colleagues reported on concordance between central line cultures and peripheral cultures in 143 patients (14). They found a 92% concordance rate between the central-line cultures and the peripheral vein cultures. There was a 5% false-positive rate from the central-line culture, usually *S. epidermidis,* with a 2% false-negative rate.

If the decision has been made to remove the line, the tip should be cultured according to the technique described by Maki and colleagues (15). In brief, the point at which the catheter enters the skin should be marked, and the catheter should be removed from the vein using aseptic technique. Using sterile scissors, the tunneled portion of the catheter is severed and dropped into a sterile container and forwarded to the laboratory for qualitative and quantitative cultures.

TREATMENT

Undoubtedly, the primary treatment for any infection is prevention. These preventative strategies can be implemented at the time of insertion and during repeated access. For temporary catheters, the primary decision as to where to place a catheter has been influenced by operator experience and possibly the patient's underlying coagulation profile.

Within the past several years, placement of any subclavian catheter has been discouraged secondary to concerns surrounding subclavian stenosis and thrombosis precluding ipsilateral AV access (16). Recently, Oliver and colleagues prospectively analyzed infectious complications of temporary catheters by anatomic location (17). Largely opinion based, the National Kidney Foundation's Dialysis Outcome Quality Initiative (DOQI) recommended that temporary femoral catheters remain in place no longer than 5 days, with subclavian and internal jugular catheters in place less than 21 days. The study by Oliver and colleagues supported these recommendations with data. For femoral catheters, the rate of bacteremia was 3% up to 1 week, increasing to 10.7%, 18.1%, and 29.1% at 2, 3, and 4 weeks, respectively. For internal jugular catheters, the rates for bacteremia were 1.7%, 4.6%, 5.4%, and 10.3% during the first 4 weeks of follow-up. These investigators concluded that femoral catheters should be discontinued within 1 week and internal jugular catheters by 3 weeks.

After determining the location of insertion, the insertion site should be thoroughly disinfected with chlorhexidine, povidone iodine, or tincture of iodine (18). There are conflicting reports of superiority of these different agents in skin disinfection (19,20). All catheters should be inserted with the operator observing full barrier precautions (sterile gloves, long-sleeved sterile gown, mask, cap, and large sterile drapes). These precautions reduce the incidence of bloodstream infections from 0.58 per 1,000 catheter days to 0.05 per 1,000 catheter days (21).

Once inserted, the temporary catheter exit site should be covered with povidone ointment, especially in patients known to be carriers for *S. aureus* (22). The catheter exit site should be covered with either sterile gauze or transparent dressings. Several studies found no difference between catheter-related infections based on type of covering (23,24).

Injection hub and connection port manipulation is documented to be a risk factor for catheter-related bacteremia (10,11). Unfortunately, for dialysis patients, this may occur daily in the case of acute renal failure or thrice weekly for outpatients receiving hemodialysis. To reduce bloodstream infections, catheter hubs should be disinfected before they are accessed. Alcohol, povidone iodine, chlorhexidine have all shown to be effective (25). Other measures that may prove effective include the use of nasal mupirocin ointment for those patients who are *S. aureus* carriers. Given the rapid resistance of *S. aureus* to mupirocin, this strategy may be advisable only in the acute setting to prevent temporary catheter-related infections (26). (*Editor's note*: Prophylactic catheter instillation, that is, "locking," of solutions that include antibiotics, citrate, taurolidine, and others, are being investigated. See Chapter 42.)

It has been clearly documented that several different components of a thrombus increase the adherence of *S. aureus, S. epidermidis,* and *Candida* organisms to the catheter (27–29). Very-low-dose warfarin (1 mg) reduces venographic documentation of thrombus in nondialysis, long-term catheters (30). This study led some to advocate the use of very-low-dose warfarin to prevent catheter-related bacteremia (31). No prospective randomized trial has been performed to test this hypothesis.

Temporary Catheters: Exit-Site Infection

For temporary catheters with exit-site infections, the catheter should be removed. Any purulent material should be cultured and, based on the clinical status of the patient, intravenous antibiotics should be administered, and a new catheter should be inserted in a different location. If the patient has bacteremia, all efforts should be made to have the patient's catheter free for at least 24 hours while on antibiotics before insertion of a new one (32).

Tunneled Catheters

Treatment of exit-site infections for long-term catheters is twofold. First, exit-site care must be intensified. Routine cleaning of the exit site is increased from thrice weekly to once or twice a day. Site care entails cleansing the exit site with chlorhexidine, povidone iodine, or alcohol, followed by application of a sterile dressing. Antibiotic therapy is directed at gram-positive organisms. Combined with local wound care, both parenteral and enteral antibiotics are effective in eradicating exit site infections (33–34).

Patients with catheter-related bacteremia may present with mild fever, increased white cell count, or severe symptoms, such as hypotension and other manifestations of the sepsis syndrome. For patients with severe symptoms, immediate catheter removal with appropriate antibiotic coverage is the current recommendation. For patients with milder symptoms, various strategies have been attempted to preserve the catheter and the catheter insertion site.

Antibiotic Salvage

In 1993, Capdevila and colleagues reported on 13 patients with catheter-related bacteremia (35). No patient displayed evidence of septic shock. *S. epidermidis* and *Pseudomonas aeruginosa* were the two most common organisms (73%). All patients received antibiotics (vancomycin and ciprofloxacin) without catheter removal or guidewire exchange. Follow-up blood cultures 2 weeks after the last dose of antibiotics revealed no evidence of recurrent bacteremia. A larger study by Marr and colleagues reported more discouraging results (36). In this study, 62 episodes of catheter-related bacteremia were reported. Twenty-four catheters were removed immediately, with 38 catheters being treated with antibiotics (vancomycin, gentamicin) for a minimum of 2 weeks. Ninety percent of infections were caused by gram-positive organisms, predominantly methicillin-resistant *S. aureus* (MRSA) or *S. aureus* (69%). Of the 38 attempted catheter salvage patients, 26 catheters failed treatment and required eventual removal. Of greater concern was the number of metastatic infections. Five of 38 patients had septic arthritis, osteomyelitis, or subacute bacterial endocarditis. In a subsequent report, the same researchers reported on five of these 38 patients who developed an epidural abscess (37). Therefore, based on these results, catheter salvage with antibiotics alone is not currently recommended.

Guidewire Exchange

The technique of guidewire exchange of a central venous catheter in a patient with bacteremia has not been shown to be effective in the intensive care unit (ICU) patient with a nondialysis catheter (38). For patients on hemodialysis with a long-term catheter, this is an attractive option given the unacceptable cure rates with antibiotic treatment alone and the high cost and prolonged hospitalization rates associated with catheter removal and subsequent insertion in a new site.

Carlisle and colleagues first reported their success in 1991 in 12 patients with 13 episodes of catheter-related bacteremia (39). All 13 episodes were treated successfully with intravenous antibiotics followed by guidewire catheter exchange. No patient had evidence of recurrent positive cultures or clinical evidence of infection. All patients were treated with intravenous antibiotics for 2 weeks plus catheter exchange.

Schaffer reported similar results in ten patients with 13 episodes of catheter-related bacteremia (40). All patients in this series defervesced with intravenous antibiotics for 48 hours before catheter exchange and received intravenous antibiotics for 1 to 2 weeks after the procedure. Three patients had recurrent episodes of bacteremia at 2.5, 3.0, and 13 months. Schaffer did not believe these infections represented a recurrence but rather represented *de novo* infections because in two thirds of these cases, a new organism was cultured, and in the third case a negative blood culture was documented between episodes of infection.

Robinson and colleagues described their success in 23 exchange procedures in 21 patients (41). Like the patients reported by Schaeffer, patients in this series had defervesced during the first 48 hours of receiving antibiotics. None of the patients had evidence of exit or tunnel infection. Following catheter exchange, patients received antibiotics for 3 to 4 weeks. They reported four failures within 90 days. These failures occurred at days 4, 19, 63, and 78.

Beathard reported the largest series of catheter exchanges for catheter-related bacteremia (42). In this series, treatment failure was defined as recurrence of positive blood cultures within 45 days of guidewire exchange. Forty-nine patients were entered into the study only if they clinically defervesced within 48 hours on antibiotics. No patient had recurrence of catheter-related bacteremia from the original organism. Six patients died, had a catheter removed for an unrelated reason, or became infected with a different organism. None of these six patients were thought to represent treatment failure.

Unlike reports from previous studies, Beathard also reported on patients treated with catheter-related bacteremia who also had evidence of an exit-site or tunnel infection. In this group, the guidewire exchanges were performed and a new tunnel and exit were created either medial or lateral to the old infected site. In this group, 28 patients were de-

scribed. Seventy-five percent of these patients were free of catheter-related bacteremia at 45 days. Eight percent had a recurrent infection, and 5% either died or had catheter removed for another reason. None of the deaths was thought to be related to the original infection.

Figure 35.2 outlines a treatment scheme for patients with suspected catheter-related bacteremia. It is crucial to em-

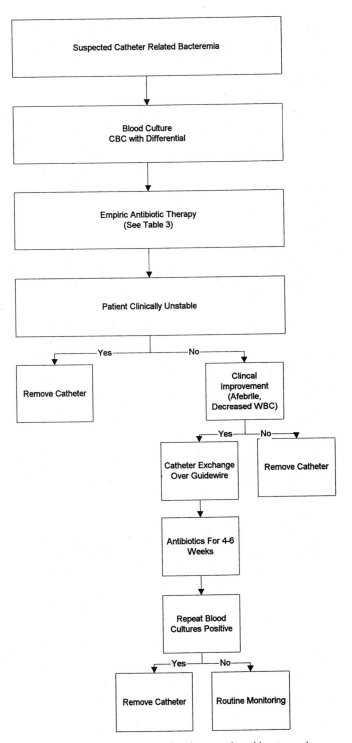

FIGURE 35.2. Management of catheter-related bacteremia.

phasize that this scheme is designed for the patient who is clinically stable and who displays only mild to moderate symptoms of bacteremia. Additionally, this treatment scheme assumes that the patient will clinically defervesce within 36 to 48 hours on antibiotics before catheter exchange over a guidewire. Equally important is appropriate follow-up after catheter exchange. Antibiotics directed against the offending microorganism should be continued for 3 to 4 weeks. One week after discontinuing antibiotics, follow-up blood cultures should be obtained to document the presence or absence of ongoing bacteremia.

ANTIBIOTICS

Kidney failure requiring hemodialysis may have a significant impact on the bioavailability, distribution, metabolism, and excretion of many of the antibiotics given for treatment of catheter-related infections. Therefore, for most of these compounds, dosing or interval adjustment will be necessary to ensure therapeutic levels while avoiding toxicity. Table 35.3 reviews two commonly used protocols for empiric antibiotic treatment for suspected catheter-related infections.

Historically, vancomycin and gentamicin were used because of their broad antimicrobial coverage and favorable pharmacokinetic profile, allowing for intravenous dosing during the outpatient dialysis procedure. Given the emergence of vancomycin-resistant enterococcus (VRE) in the dialysis population, this practice has been called into question (13). An alternative strategy using cefazolin instead of vancomycin has been shown to provide adequate drug levels in the outpatient setting while providing excellent coverage directed at gram-positive organisms (43).

As with all patients receiving vancomycin or aminoglycoside, drug levels should be followed to avoid toxicity. Dosing schedules for administering aminoglycoside to patients on hemodialysis are well established (Table 35.4). Hemodialysis removes a significant quantity of the aminoglycoside; therefore, a portion of the loading dose needs to be read-

ministered following each dialysis session. Predialysis levels should be obtained at least weekly to avoid toxicity.

Vancomycin is not removed by conventional hemodialysis (44). Patients should receive 1 g delivered intravenously as initial therapy, and levels should be checked before the fifth dialysis session. For patients receiving high-flux dialysis using polysulphone membranes, up to 40% of the drug may be removed by each session (45). Therefore, for these patients, frequent therapeutic monitoring is required with supplemental dosing given postdialysis, or the patient should be changed to a low-flux dialysis membrane during the period of vancomycin administration.

As with all infections, the antibiotic with the greatest sensitivity and the least toxicity should be used once culture results and sensitivities are established. Table 35.4 provides antibiotic dosing for commonly used antibiotics in this setting.

CONCLUSION

Catheter-related infections are a common cause of morbidity and mortality for patients undergoing hemodialysis. These infections may present as a localized infection (exit-site or tunnel) or bacteremia. The most common pathogens are those found on the skin and include *Staphylococcus* species and gram-negative organisms such as *Pseudomonas* and *Klebsiella*. For exit-site infections, therapy includes intensified wound care combined with antibiotic therapy. Tunnel infections require removal of the catheter from that tunnel with appropriate antibiotic coverage. The treatment of catheter-related bacteremia depends on the severity of the manifestations of the infection. Patients who are unstable or who do not respond to empiric antibiotic therapy should have the catheter removed. For patients who are initially stable and respond to antibiotic therapy, changing the catheter over a guidewire can salvage the catheter site.

TABLE 35.4. ANTIBIOTIC DOSING GUIDELINES FOR PATIENTS RECEIVING HEMODIALYSIS

Agent	Initial Dose	Interval
Amikacin	7.5 mg/kg i.v.	3.25 mg/kg after each dialysis
Gentamicin	1.0–2.0 mg/kg i.v.	1.0 mg/kg after each dialysis
Tobramycin	1.7 mg/kg i.v.	0.85 mg/kg after each dialysis
Cefazolin	1.0 g i.v.	1.0 g after dialysis
Cefotaxime	1.0 g i.v.	1.0 g after dialysis
Azithromycin	250–500 mg p.o.	q 24 h
Vancomycin	1.0 g i.v.	1.0 g i.v. q5–7 d
Ciprofloxacin	500 mg p.o.	q 12 h
Gatifloxacin	400 mg p.o.	200 mg p.o. q d
Levofloxacin	250 mg p.o.	q 48 h

i.v., intravenously; p.o., orally; q, every.

TABLE 35.3. EMPIRIC ANTIBIOTIC THERAPY FOR SUSPECTED CATHETER-RELATED BACTEREMIA

Agent	Initial Dose	Dosing Interval
Vancomycin	1.0 g i.v.	Every 5–7 d[a]
	+	
Gentamicin	1.5–2.0 mg/kg	1.0 mg/kg after each dialysis[b]
	Or	
Cephazolin	1.0 g i.v.	Following each dialysis
	+	
Gentamicin	1.5–2 mg/kg i.v.	1.0 mg/kg after each dialysis[b]

[a] Suggest predialysis level day 5.
[b] Suggest predialysis level day 3.

REFERENCES

1. U.S. Renal Data System (USRDS). 1999 USRDS Annual Data Report, Bethesda, MD: National Institutes of Health, National Institute of Diabetes and Suggestive Kidney Disease, April 1999: 25.

2. National Kidney Foundation Dialysis Outcome Quality Initiative (NKF-DOQI). *Clinical practice guidelines for vascular access.* New York: National Kidney Foundation, 1997:57.

3. Health Care Finance Administration (HCFA). 2000 Annual Report. End Stage Renal Disease Clinical Performance Measures Project. Baltimore, MD: Department of Health and Human Services, HCFA Office of Clinical Standards and Quality, December 2000.

4. Bach A. Prevention of infections caused by central venous catheters—established and novel measures. *Infection* 1999;27 (Suppl 1):S11–S15.

5. Swartz RD, Messana JM, Boyer CJ, et al. Successful use of cuffed central venous hemodialysis catheters inserted percutaneously. *J Am Soc Nephrol* 1994;4:1719–1725.

6. Lund GB, Trerotola SO, Scheel PJ, et al. Outcome of tunneled hemodialysis catheters placed by radiologists. *Radiology* 1996; 198:467–472.

7. Saad TF. Bacteremia associated with tunneled, cuffed hemodialysis catheters. *Am J Kidney Dis* 1999;34:1114–1124.

8. Kessler M, Hoen B, Mayeux D, et al. Bacteremia in patients on chronic hemodialysis. *Nephron* 1993:64:95–100.

9. Marr KA, Sexton DJ, Conlon PJ, et al. Catheter related bacteremia and outcome of attempted catheter salvage in patients undergoing hemodialysis. *Ann Intern Med* 1997;127:275–277.

10. Linares J, Sitges-Ser A, Garau J, et al. Pathogenesis of catheter sepsis: a prospective study with quantitative and semi-quantitative cultures of catheter hub in segments. *J Clin Microbiol* 1985; 21:357–360.

11. Salzman MB, Isenberg HD, Shapiro JF, et al. A prospective study of catheter hub as a portal of entry for microorganisms causing catheter related sepsis in neonates. *J Infect Dis* 1993;167:487–490.

12. Dittmer ID, Sharp D, McNulty CAM, et al. A prospective study of central venous hemodialysis catheter colonization in peripheral bacteremia. *Clin Nephrol* 1999;51:34–39.

13. Atta MG, Eustace JA, Xiaoyan S, et al. Outpatient vancomycin use in vancomycin resistant enterococcal colonization in maintenance hemodialysis patients. *Kidney Int* 2001;59:718–724.

14. Tonnesen A, Peuler M, Lockwood W. Cultures of blood drawn by catheters versus venipuncture. *JAMA* 1976;235:1877.

15. Maki D, Welsa C, Sarafin H. A semiquantitative method for identifying intravenous catheter-related infections. *N Engl J Med* 1977;296:1305–1309

16. National Kidney Foundation Dialysis Outcome Quality Initiative (NKF-DOQI). *Clinical Practice guidelines for vascular access.* New York: National Kidney Foundation, 1997:57.

17. Oliver MJ, Callery SM, Thorpe KE, et al. Risk of bacteremia from temporary hemodialysis catheters by site of insertion and duration of use: a prospective study. *Kidney Int* 2000;58:2543–2545.

18. Maki DG, Ringer M, Elvarado CJ. Prospective randomized trial of povidone iodine, and chlorhexidine for prevention of infections associated with central venous and arterial catheters. *Lancet* 1991;338:339–343.

19. Strand CL, Wajbort RR, Sturmann K. Effective iodophor vs. iodine tincture skin preparation on blood culture contamination rate. *JAMA* 1993;269:1004–1006.

20. Little JR, Murray PR, Traynor PS, et al. A randomized trial of povidone iodine compared with iodine tincture for venopuncture

site disinfection: effect on rates of blood culture contamination. *Am J Med* 1999;107:119–125.

21. Rad IL, Hone DC, Gilbreath J, et al. Prevention of central venous catheter related infections by using maximal sterile barrier precautions during insertion. *Infect Control Hosp Epidemiol* 1994;15: 231–238.

22. Levin A, Mason AJ, Jindal KK, et al. Prevention of hemodialysis subclavian vein catheter infections by topical providone iodine. *Kidney Int* 1991;40:934–938.

23. Maki DG, Stolz S, Wheeler S, et al. A prospective, randomized trial of gauze and two polyurethane dressings for site care of pulmonary artery catheters: implications for catheter management. *Crit Care Med* 1994;22:1729–1739.

24. Maki DG, Will L. Colonization and infection associated with transparent dressings for central venous, arterial and Hickman catheters: a comparative trial. In: *Programs and Abstracts of the 24th Interscience Conference on Antimicrobial Agents and Chemotherapy,* 8–10 October 1984; Washington, DC: American Society for Microbiology; 1984:230(abst).

25. Pearson ML. Guidelines for prevention of intravascular device-related infections. Hospital Infection Control Practices Advisory Committee. *Infect Control Hosp Epidemiol* 1996;17:438–473.

26. Zakrzewska-Bode A, Myutjens HL, Liem KD, et al. Mupirocin resistance in coagulase negative staphylococci, after prophylaxis for the reduction of colonization of central venous catheters. *J Hosp Infect* 1995;31:189–193.

27. Herrmann M, Suckard SJ, Boxer LA, et al. Thrombospondin binds to *Staphylococcal aureus* and promotes staphylococcal adherence to surfaces. *Infect Immun* 1991;59;279–288.

28. Nilson M, Frykberg L, Flock JL, et al. A fibrinogen binding protein of *Staphylococcus epidermidis. Infect Immun* 1998;66:266–273.

29. DeMuri GP, Hostetter MK. Evidence for a beta I integrin fibronectin receptor in *Candida tropicalis. J Infect Dis* 1996;174: 127–132.

30. Bern MN, Lokich JJ, Wallach SR, et al. Very low doses of warfarin can prevent thrombosis in central venous catheters: a randomized prospective trial. *Ann Intern Med* 1990;112:423–428.

31. Mermel LA. Prevention of intravascular catheter-related infections. *Ann Intern Med* 2000;132:391–402.

32. National Kidney Foundation Dialysis Outcome Quality Initiative (NKF-DOQI). *Clinical practice guidelines for vascular access.* New York: National Kidney Foundation, 1997:28

33. Schwab SJ, Buller GL, McCann RL, et al. Prospective evaluation of a Dacron cuffed hemodialysis catheters for prolonged use. *Am J Kidney Dis* 1988;11:166–169.

34. Shusterman NH, Kloss K, Mullen JL. Successful use of double lumen, silicon rubber catheters for permanent hemodialysis access. *Kidney Int* 1989;35:887–890.

35. Capdevila JA, Segarra A, Planes AM, et al. Successful treatment of hemodialysis catheter-related sepsis without catheter removal. *Nephrol Dial Transplant* 1993; 8:231–234.

36. Marr KA, Sexton DJ, Conlon PJ, et al. Catheter-related bacteremia and outcome of attempted catheter salvage in patients undergoing hemodialysis. *Ann Intern Med* 1997;127:275–280.

37. Kovalik EC, Raymond JR, Albers FJ, et al. The clustering of epidural abscesses in chronic hemodialysis patients: risks of salvaging access catheters in cases of infection. *J Am Soc Nephrol* 1996;7:2264–2267.

38. Cook D, Randolph A, Kernerman P, et al. Central venous catheter replacement strategies: a systematic review of the literature. *Crit Care Med* 1997;25:1417–1424.

39. Carlisle EJ, Blake P, McCarthy F, et al. Septicemia in long-term jugular hemodialysis catheters: eradicating infection by changing the catheter over a guide wire. *Int J Artif Organs* 1991;14:150–153.

40. Schaffer D. Catheter-related sepsis complicating long-term, tunneled central venous dialysis catheters: management by guide wire exchange. *Am J Kidney Dis* 1995;25:5935.

41. Robinson D, Suhocki P, Schwab SJ. Treatment of infected tunneled venous access hemodialysis catheters with guide wire exchange. *Kidney Int* 1998;53:1792–1794.

42. Beathard GA. Management of bacteremia associated with tunneled-cuffed hemodialysis catheters. *J Am Soc Nephrol* 1999;10:1045–1049.

43. Marx MA, Frye GR, Matzke GR, et al. Cefazolin as empiric therapy in hemodialysis-related patients: efficacy and blood concentrations. *Am J Kidney Dis* 1998;32:410–414

44. Melikian DA, Flaherty JF. Antimicrobial agents. In: Schrier RW, Gamnrtyoglio, eds. *Handbook of drug therapy in liver and kidney disease.* Boston: Little, Brown and Company, 1991.

45. Lanese DM, Alfrey PS, Molitoris BA. Markedly increased clearance of vancomycin during hemodialysis using polysulphone dialyzers. *Kidney Int* 1989;35:1409–1412.

36

MANAGEMENT OF CATHETER MALFUNCTION

RICHARD J. GRAY

Dialysis catheter malfunction is extremely common, affecting 3% to 10% of all dialysis sessions (1,2) and 87% of all catheters at some time before their removal (3). Although various maneuvers have been reported that can restore immediate catheter function, up to 28% of dialysis catheters ultimately are removed simply because they do not work (1,2,4–8). Intact catheters are removed for malfunction at a frequency similar to that for infection and far more frequently than that for symptomatic pericatheter thrombus (1,2,4–8) (Table 36.1). Chapter 35 covers the treatment of catheter infection. Herein the evaluation and current treatment approaches for the malfunctioning dialysis catheter are reviewed.

DIALYSIS CLINIC

Until its removal from the market by the U.S. Food and Drug Administration in January 1999, simple urokinase instillation at the dialysis clinic was the first-line therapy for dialysis catheters with suboptimal flow rates (<300 mL per minute) (9) unresponsive to simple positional maneuvers and port reversal. A small quantity of urokinase (Abbokinase, Abbott Laboratories, Abbott Park, IL, U.S.A.) was injected into the catheter and left to indwell for periods up to 20 minutes (1,3,10). This was tried several times, if necessary, and restored immediate function to 74% to 95% of dialysis catheters (1,3,10). Although this measure was performed blindly and the durability was unknown, it was effective enough to be the appropriate first-line therapy (9) because it was safe, inexpensive, and expediently allowed dialysis to resume during the same scheduled dialysis session after a minimal delay.

Alternative thrombolytic agents, including the recombinant tissue plasminogen activator alteplase (rt-PA, Activase, Genentech, South San Francisco, CA, U.S.A.) and the recombinant fibrinogen activator reteplase (Retavase, Centacor, Malvern, PA, U.S.A.), have been commercially available since urokinase was removed; however, they were available only in quantities far larger than the doses likely to be appropriate for catheter instillation. This necessitated

that these alternative agents be aliquoted into small doses, a procedure requiring the sterile techniques available in a hospital pharmacy. Unfortunately, the sterility requirement precluded them from being available in dialysis clinics for several years. This changed recently when rt-PA received approval for low-dose (2-mg) packaging.

Although currently little data are available for the short-term instillation of rt-PA into malfunctioning dialysis catheters, promising results (87.5%–94% immediate success) have been reported for long indwell times (2–96 hours) (11,12). However, such long indwell times are impractical as they do not allow same-session dialysis routinely. If similar efficacy data become available for short indwell times, thrombolytic instillation in the dialysis clinic, now using rt-PA, again will become the first-line treatment for dialysis catheter malfunction unresponsive to port reversal and positional maneuvers. Catheters that still malfunction will continue to be referred, following the National Kidney Foundation's Dialysis Outcomes Quality Initiative (DOQI) recommendations, for a transcatheter venogram to evaluate for mechanical problems or the presence of pericatheter fibrin sheath or thrombus (9).

MECHANICAL MALFUNCTION

Mechanical causes of poor catheter function include kinking, malposition of the catheter tip in a branch vein or against the venous wall, central vein stenosis at the catheter tip, and unintentional partial or complete catheter removal. Typically, mechanical problems are encountered in catheters that have been recently inserted, and overall these problems are much less common than pericatheter fibrin sheath or clot formation (3,4,13,14) (Table 36.2). Standard interventional catheter techniques using fluoroscopic guidance readily correct most mechanical problems (3,15).

Kinked Catheter

Kinking is more common with thin-walled, high-flow catheters such as the Ash Split-Cath (Medcomp, Harleysville,

TABLE 36.1. DIALYSIS CATHETER REMOVAL

Study	Catheters	Malfunction (%)[a]	Infection (%)	CV Thrombosis (%)
McDowell et al. (6)	172	5	5	0
Cappello et al. (7)	107	5	5	0
Moss et al. (1)	168	7	8	0
Gibson and Mosquere (2)	94	9	28	1.6
Schwartz et al. (8)	118	17	19	0
Lund et al. (5)	222	28	11	1.2
Trerotola et al. (4)	250	19	7	0
Duszak et al. (17)	77	—	13	0

CV, central vein.
[a] Variable definitions.
Adapted from Gray RJ, Levitin A, Buck D, et al. Percutaneous fibrin sheath stripping versus transcatheter urokinase infusion for malfunctioning well-positioned tunneled central venous dialysis catheters: a prospective randomized trial. *J Vasc Interv Radiol* 2000;11:1121–1129, with permission.

PA, U.S.A.), especially when the catheter tract is acutely angled because of a high internal jugular puncture. In our experience, high punctures are more common when catheters are placed without the benefit of ultrasound, which is contrary to the DOQI guidelines (16). We also see kinks more commonly after conversion of a blindly inserted nontunneled catheter to a tunneled one (Fig. 36.1). Simply rotating the catheter lumens to lie in the anteroposterior plane sometimes can correct a kink. Alternatively, over-the-wire exchange for a thicker-walled catheter such as the Hickman (Bard Access Systems, Salt Lake City, UT, U.S.A.) or Vaxcel (SCI-Meditech, Watertown, MA, U.S.A.), or creation of a new tunnel with a smaller angle at the venous lumen entry site may restore catheter function. If these maneuvers fail, a new catheter insertion site will be necessary.

Malpositioned Catheter

Malposition of the catheter tip in a vein branch or against the superior vena cava (SVC) wall usually can be solved easily by exchanging the catheter over a guidewire under fluoroscopic guidance and redirecting the catheter tip to the SVC–right atrial junction or into the right atrium (9). Catheters that unintentionally have been partially pulled back are similarly replaced. Even catheters that have been completely removed from the body can be replaced by recannulating the same tract (15) (Fig. 36.2). In such in-

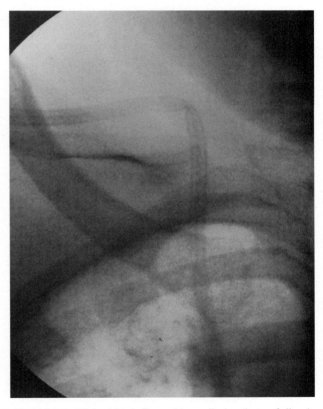

FIGURE 36.1. Kinked high-flow, thin-walled catheter following conversion of a nontunneled to a tunneled catheter.

TABLE 36.2. ETIOLOGY OF CATHETER MALFUNCTION[a]

Study	No. of Catheters	Episodes	Mechanical	Sheath/Clot
Crain et al. (13)	24	44	4	40
Suhocki et al. (3)	–	42	4	38
Rockall et al. (14)	29	31	7	24
Trerotola et al. (4)	63	63	23	40

[a] Most S/P failed urokinase instillation.
Adapted from Gray et al (29).

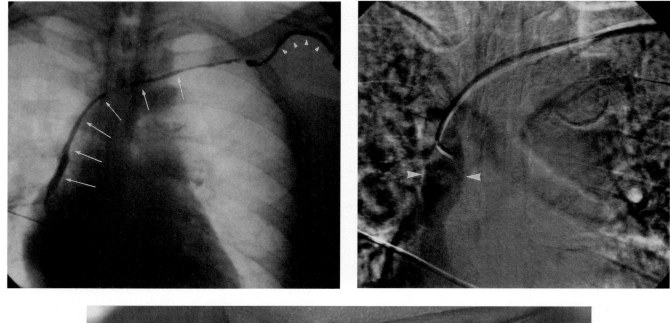

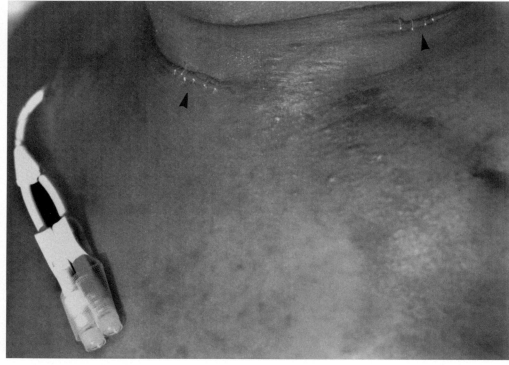

FIGURE 36.2. Catheter reinsertion via tract after unintentional removal **A**: Contrast injection outlines the subcutaneous tract (*arrowheads*) and fibrin sheath (*arrows*). **B**: Catheter in superior vena cava (SVC) (*arrowheads*) after catheter–guidewire negotiation. This is now easily exchanged for a dialysis catheter. **C**: Another patient with surgical clips (*arrowheads*) from attempts to insert a new catheter, shown here after a new catheter was reinserted by cannulating a mature catheter tract that had been without an indwelling catheter for longer than 2 weeks.

stances, it may be necessary to dilate the tract with a balloon, especially if the venous entry site is into subclavian and the catheter has been out for more than 24 hours. For patients with few remaining sites, this can be invaluable (Fig. 36.2C).

For all catheter replacements and exchanges, we prefer hydrophilic wires, as suggested by Duszak and colleagues

(17); depending on the maturity of the tract and the type of catheter, either one or two hydrophilic wires will be necessary. We use local lidocaine with epinephrine (17) for all catheter exchanges and *de novo* insertions. This practice, in combination with aspiration of the heparin from the catheter before transcatheter contrast injection or manipulation (18) has made immediate postprocedure pericatheter oozing a rare event at our institution. As a further precaution against bleeding, patients undergoing dialysis on the same day as a catheter manipulation or *de novo* catheter insertion receive a one-time heparin-free dialysis. We also administer antibiotics for all catheter manipulations and insertions unless the patient is already appropriately covered.

FIBRIN SHEATH

Catheter malfunction in well-positioned catheters (see section on Prevention to follow) typically is due to the presence of a thin pericatheter coating of fibrin (fibrin sheath) or a small amount of thrombus about the catheter tip (3,4,13,14). Pericatheter fibrin sheath formation has been shown in a human autopsy study (19) to occur as early as 24 hours following placement and is thought to occur in 80% to 100% of central venous catheters within 2 to 7 days after insertion (19–21). Fibrin sheaths propagate from the venous insertion site and from the catheter tip toward the center of the catheter and can persist for weeks, even after the catheter is removed (19). Based on observations in rats, the sheath is thought to undergo a gradual transformation from a fibrin-containing material to organized fibrous connective tissue (22). When the pericatheter sheath or associated thrombus infringes on the functional end hole(s) of the catheter, decreased dialysis flow rates result.

Diagnosis

Fibrin sheaths can be demonstrated by intravascular ultrasound (23) but usually are diagnosed by transcatheter venographic studies with (21) or without (3,13,24,25) pulling the catheter back before contrast injection (Fig. 36.3). The sensitivity of transcatheter venography for the detection of fibrin sheaths is unknown. We believe it is very important to inject contrast through the catheter slowly to avoid creating a hole in the fibrin sheath near the catheter tip. An iatrogenic fenestration in the fibrin sheath from rapid contrast (or saline) injection can hinder angiographic diagnosis of the sheath because contrast can pass preferentially through the fenestration. Furthermore, a subsequently administered transcatheter thrombolytic agent (see later discussion) also will run through the iatrogenic fenestration instead of bathing the catheter from the tip proximally to the nearest naturally occurring fenestration (Fig. 36.3); this will decrease the total surface area of the fibrin sheath exposed to the agent.

Treatment

Pericatheter fibrin sheaths or thrombus have been treated by a variety of methods, including percutaneous fibrin sheath stripping (3,13,14,24,25), thrombolytic infusion through the dialysis catheter (1,4,5,26), and catheter exchange (17,18,27), with return of catheter function for at least one dialysis session in most patients. The original DOQI (9) and the Kidney Disease Outcomes Quality Initiative (K-DOQI) recognize all these treatments. Each of these methods is discussed separately in the following sections.

Fibrin Sheath Stripping

This technique (3,13,14,24,25,28) is performed by passing a loop snare (Amplatz Goose Neck, Microvena, White Bear Lake, MN, U.S.A.) around the catheter from a remote percutaneous puncture site, usually the common femoral vein. The snare is tightened around the dialysis catheter and pulled off of the catheter to remove any obstructing pericatheter material (Fig. 36.4) The published results of pericatheter fibrin sheath stripping (13,14,24,25,27–29) are shown in Table 36.3. The initial success rates in these series are generally high, and the overall complication rate is 6.3% (18 of 284). Brady and colleagues (25) and Crain and associates (13) reported primary patencies of 63% and 45%, respectively, at 3 months; Crain also used repetitive stripping and reported that 81% of the treated catheters functioned satisfactorily for at least 1 year after the initial catheter insertion. Similarly, Suhocki and colleagues (3) emphasized that most treated catheters remained functional for their intended duration of use. Other investigators have been less optimistic. Merport and colleagues (27) reported a 31% 30-day primary patency, and all their catheters failed by 4 months. Gray and colleagues (29) found somewhat better durability, with 35% of catheters maintaining primary patency for 45 days; nevertheless, their patients greatly disliked the additional groin puncture. Haskal and associates (24) experienced dismal patencies, finding that 92% (22 of 24) of catheters returned to the pretreatment blood-liter process rate by the fifth post-stripping dialysis session. As a result of their studies, the groups of Merport, Gray, and Haskal (24,27,29) abandoned routine use of the stripping procedure.

Thrombolytic Infusion

In a thrombolytic infusion, the lytic agent is delivered through the dialysis catheter ports for several hours, which distinguishes infusion from the simple low-dose instillation performed in the dialysis clinic. The results of studies reporting thrombolytic infusion (1,4,5,26,29,30) are presented in Table 36.4. Whereas most of these studies used urokinase, alteplase and reteplase, administered in dose-equivalent infusions to urokinase, should be similar in effectiveness and safety and may be faster than urokinase. For urokinase, immediate success, defined as restoration of satisfactory function for at least one dialysis session, ranges from 55% to 97%. One investigator used a bolus of a total of 250,000 U of concentrated urokinase in both ports and reported that this "nearly always" worked for restoring

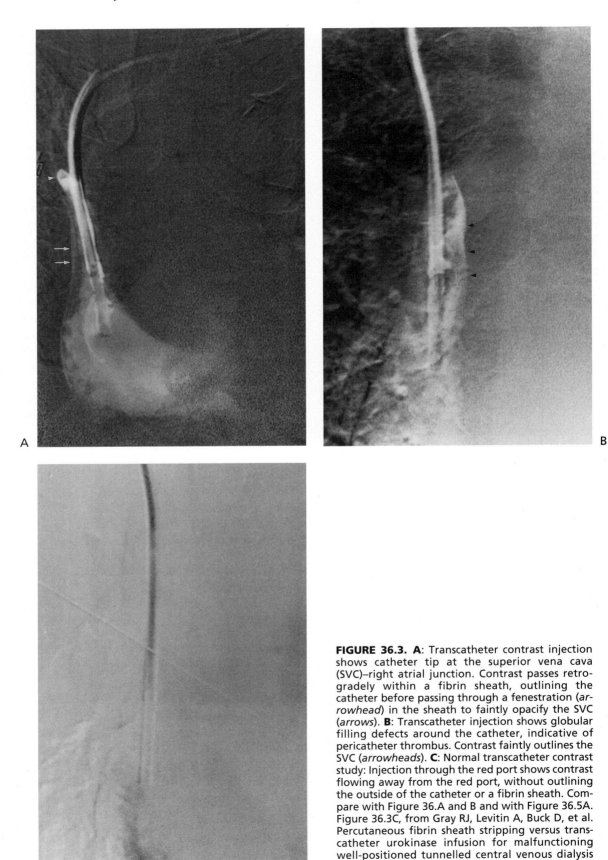

FIGURE 36.3. A: Transcatheter contrast injection shows catheter tip at the superior vena cava (SVC)–right atrial junction. Contrast passes retrogradely within a fibrin sheath, outlining the catheter before passing through a fenestration (*arrowhead*) in the sheath to faintly opacify the SVC (*arrows*). **B**: Transcatheter injection shows globular filling defects around the catheter, indicative of pericatheter thrombus. Contrast faintly outlines the SVC (*arrowheads*). **C**: Normal transcatheter contrast study: Injection through the red port shows contrast flowing away from the red port, without outlining the outside of the catheter or a fibrin sheath. Compare with Figure 36.A and B and with Figure 36.5A. Figure 36.3C, from Gray RJ, Levitin A, Buck D, et al. Percutaneous fibrin sheath stripping versus transcatheter urokinase infusion for malfunctioning well-positioned tunnelled central venous dialysis catheters: a prospective randomized trial. *JVIR* 2000; 11:1121–1129.

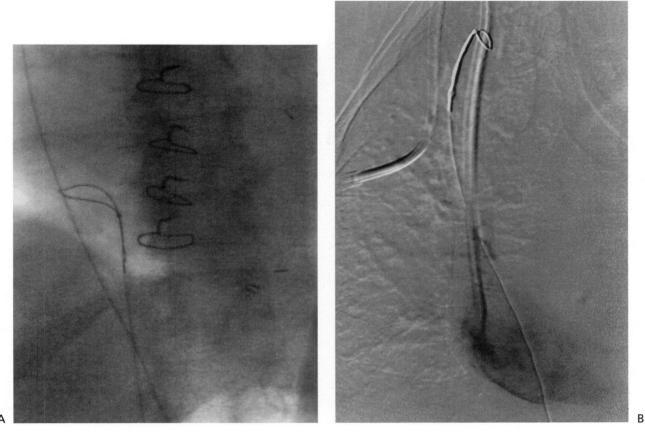

FIGURE 36.4. A: Open snare around guidewire in right atrium. **B**: Snare tightened around catheter during a stripping pass.

immediate catheter function (26). These treatments appear to be safe; no bleeding complications attributed to the thrombolytic agent occurred in any of these studies. The studies reporting cumulative primary patencies (29,30) suggest that about half of treated catheters will maintain uninterrupted function for an additional 45 to 90 days after transcatheter thrombolytic infusion. These studies are small, however. Savader and co-workers (31) recently presented less optimistic results for 124 thrombolytic infusions, with only 25% of the infused catheters still functioning at 90 days; with retreatment, 46% continued to function at 60 days. Although modest, this additional period of function will allow permanent access creation or maturation in many patients.

TABLE 36.3. FIBRIN-SHEATH STRIPPING

Study	No. of Treatments	Clinical Success (%)[a]	Additional Patency
Crain et al. (13)	40	98	45% at 3 mo (primary)
Haskal et al. (24)	24	92	8% (2/24) at 2 wk
Suhocki et al. (3)	38	95	3 mo (mean)
Rockall et al. (14)	31	61[b]	4.25 mo (median)
Brady et al. (25)	91	96	51% at 3 mo (primary)
Gray et al. (29)	28	89	35% at 45 d (primary)
Merport et al. (27)	15	94	31% at 1 mo, 7% at 3 mo (primary)
Johnstone et al. (28)	16	75	40% at 6 wk (primary)

[a] At least one successful dialysis using variable criteria for success.
[b] Includes some mechanical catheter malfunctions.
Adapted from Gray RJ, Levitin A, Buck D, et al. Percutaneous fibrin sheath stripping versus transcatheter urokinase infusion for malfunctioning well-positioned tunneled central venous dialysis catheters: a prospective randomized trial. *J Vasc Interv Radiol* 2000;11:1121–1129, with permission.

TABLE 36.4. THROMBOLYTIC INFUSION[a]

Study	No. of Treatments	Agent/Dose	Clinical Success (%)	Additional Patency
Moss et al. (1)	58	Streptokinase (12 h)	97	—
Uldall et al. (26)	103	Urokinase (250,000 U bolus)	"Nearly always"	—
Lund et al. (5)	39	Urokinase (250,000 U/6 h)	79.5	—
Trerotola et al. (4)	11	Urokinase (250,000 U/6 h)	55	31 d (mean)
Gray et al. (29)	29	Urokinase (250,000 U/4 h)	97	48% at 45 d (primary)
Savader et al. (30)	28	rtTPA (5 mg/3 h)	96	51% at 90 d (primary)

[a] No bleeding complications of 268 cases.
Adapted from Gray RJ, Levitin A, Buck D, et al. Percutaneous fibrin sheath stripping versus transcatheter urokinase infusion for malfunctioning well-positioned tunneled central venous dialysis catheters: a prospective randomized trial. *J Vasc Interv Radiol* 2000;11:1121–1129, with permission.

Catheter Exchange

After poor results for stripping (24) were demonstrated at their institution, Duszak and colleagues (17) began changing catheters through the same tract over a guidewire while making an attempt to position the catheter tip beyond or outside the confines of the fibrin sheath. This was done either by repositioning the tip more centrally or by manipulating a guidewire and the catheter tip through a fenestration in the fibrin sheath to a position outside of the sheath (Fig. 36.5). They were successful in restoring immediate function in most cases, and half of the catheters functioned without interruption for an additional 3 months (Table 36.5). They compared these catheter exchanges in a nonrandomized fashion with *de novo* catheter placement in the same patient population and found no significant differences in catheter patency or complication rates, including infections. (All patients received periprocedural antibiotics.) Merport and colleagues (27) prospectively evaluated catheter exchange and were initially successful in all cases, but their results were shorter-lived than those of Duszak and colleagues, possibly because a mechanical attempt to correct a fibrin sheath was performed in only a minority of the cases. On the other hand, Garofalo and colleagues (18) made no effort to demonstrate or disrupt a fibrin sheath, believing that any obstructive fibrin sheath would be "at least partially disrupted" during the catheter exchange procedure. In a retrospective study, they reported a 52% 90-day primary patency and used repeated exchanges to attain an 86% 90-day secondary patency. They administered periprocedural antibiotics and found no procedure-related complications. The cumulative infection rate was 1.1 per 1,000 catheter days, identical to the experience reported by Duszak's group.

Which Treatment Is Best?

Fibrin stripping, thrombolytic infusion, and catheter exchange each have their proponents, and the DOQI guidelines do not recommend any one method over another. Two studies have directly compared fibrin stripping with over-the-wire catheter exchange (27) and thrombolytic infusion (29). Merport and colleagues (27) randomized malfunctioning dialysis catheters to fibrin stripping or catheter exchange and found a large 1-month patency advantage for catheter exchange (compare Tables 36.3 and 36.5) that was statistically significant ($p < 0.01$). In addition, they also showed that the outpatient charges were statistically lower for the catheter exchange group ($p < 0.01$). Gray and associates (29) prospectively randomized well-positioned catheters to fibrin sheath stripping or a urokinase infusion and showed no statistically significant difference for either treatment in either immediate restoration of catheter function or maintenance of long-term patency (compare Tables 36.3 and 36.4). Nevertheless, they recommended a thrombolytic infusion for several reasons. First, their patients preferred the thrombolytic infusion; many refused to undergo stripping after hearing about the lysis option. Second, transcatheter infusion is noninvasive; stripping requires a venous puncture. Third, transcatheter administration of thrombolytics (1,4,5,26,29,30) at low doses has been complication free, whereas stripping has been associated with potentially disastrous complications, including septic pulmonary embolus (32), catheter infection (28), asymptomatic common femoral puncture site thrombus (13), groin hematoma requiring admission (27), and symptomatic pericatheter innominate vein thrombosis (29). As stated, the groups of Merport and Gray now rarely perform the stripping procedure.

Catheter exchange and thrombolytic infusion have never been directly compared. Catheter exchange over a guidewire spares vein (17) and usually allows a more expedient return to dialysis than a 3- to 6-hour thrombolytic infusion (4,5,29,30). As currently reimbursed by Medicare, a single catheter exchange is much less costly than an infusion (29). Nevertheless, it is an invasive procedure that can be complicated by prolonged pericatheter tract oozing (17) or cardiac arrhythmia (17). Patients probably prefer a noninvasive thrombolytic infusion; however, thrombolytic infusion probably will lose effectiveness after longer catheter indwell

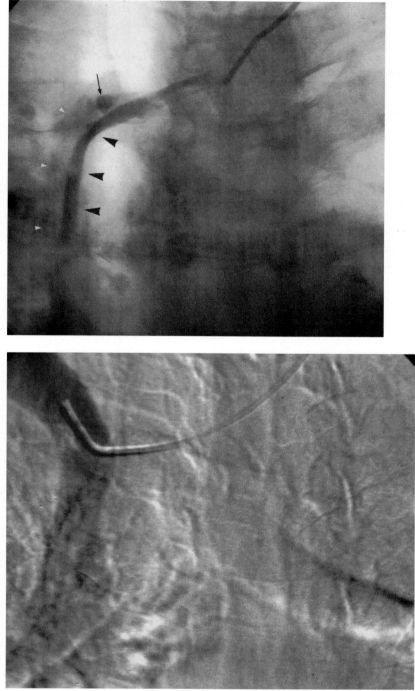

FIGURE 36.5. A: Following dialysis-catheter exchange for a diagnostic catheter, contrast injection through the diagnostic catheter in the left innominate vein shows fibrin sheath (*black arrowheads*) extending into the superior vena cava (SVC) and contrast spilling through a fenestration in the fibrin sheath (*black arrow*) to outline faintly the SVC (*white arrowheads*). **B**: After a diagnostic catheter was manipulated, with the aid of a guidewire through the fenestration in the fibrin sheath, contrast injection shows diagnostic catheter tip in the right innominate vein, outside the confines of the fibrin sheath, with free flow of contrast into the SVC. Catheter subsequently was exchanged for a new dialysis catheter (not shown).

TABLE 36.5. CATHETER EXCHANGE

Study	No. of Treatments	Clinical Success[a]	Additional Patency
Duszak et al. (17)	42	93%	51% at 3 mo (primary)
Merport et al. (27)	22	100%	27% at 3 mo (primary)
Garofalo et al. (18)	88	100%	52% at 3 mo (primary)
			86% at 3 mo (secondary)

[a] At least one successful dialysis using variable criteria for success.

times because of the gradual transformation of the peri-catheter sheath from a fibrin-containing material to an organized fibrous connective tissue (22). Currently, most of the reported infusion experience is for urokinase (Table 36.3). The feasibility study by Savader and co-workers suggests that rt-PA is as effective and safe as urokinase, and their infusion was only 3 hours long (30). If an even shorter thrombolytic infusion or bolus could provide similar results (26), more patients could be treated and return for dialysis on the same day. Comparison trials and larger studies with rt-PA and reteplase are needed to define the roles for catheter exchange and thrombolytic infusion.

Some researchers have suggested balloon dilatation (24,33) or mechanical disruption (4,24) of the fibrin sheath as adjuncts during catheter exchange. As described, other researchers (18) have considered these unnecessary. These maneuvers need to be systematically studied as well.

PREVENTION

Immediate catheter failure attributable to mechanical problems is preventable in most or all cases by using ultrasound, fluoroscopy, and standard catheter–guidewire techniques for insertion, as recommended by the DOQI document (16). Trerotola and colleagues reported 100% initial clinical success for insertion of right internal jugular catheters (4). They emphasize the importance of orienting the arterial port of stepped-tip catheters toward the lumen and away from the vessel wall. For catheter tips in the SVC, they recommend that the arterial port be oriented laterally unless the tract is parasternal, in which case medial orientation of the arterial port was suggested. For catheters positioned in the atrium, they recommend orienting the arterial port medially, that is, toward the tricuspid valve. In an abstract, Oncay and colleagues retrospectively examined the orientation of catheter ports with respect to the need for subsequent intervention (34). They found that right internal jugular catheters with the arterial port oriented laterally at any level, that is, the right atrium or SVC, were more predisposed to malfunction than catheters with the red port oriented medially or in an anteroposterior plane (34). Their preliminary numbers were too small to draw firm conclusions but are somewhat contradictory to the recommendations of Trerotola and colleagues.

Because delayed catheter malfunction is most commonly related to a fibrin sheath, the best method to preserve catheter function would be to prevent formation of a fibrin coating on the catheter. Warfarin (Coumadin) or aspirin have been reported for this purpose (26). Low-dose warfarin (1 mg per day) was shown in one study (35) to decrease the incidence of symptomatic pericatheter thrombosis and has become widely used for problematic patients in an effort to decrease catheter malfunction. Nevertheless, the effective-

ness of warfarin for fibrin sheath inhibition and maintenance of catheter function is unproved.

In rats, a fibrin sheath does not envelop the catheter tip if it is in the right atrium (22). This is not the case for humans. Nevertheless, there is a growing consensus that the catheter tip should be positioned at the SVC–right atrial junction or in the right atrium (16). The aforementioned abstract by Oncay and colleagues reported finding no difference in malfunction rates for catheters with tips placed at the SVC–right atrial junction compared with catheters with tip placement in the atrium (34). Although their numbers were small, their preliminary results agreed with the DOQI vascular access work group's opinion (16) by suggesting that catheter tips above the SVC–right atrial junction are more likely to malfunction. Although central catheter tips have been shown to withdraw proximally in the upright position compared with the supine position (36,37) associated deleterious effects on dialysis catheter function have not been demonstrated. (See also Chapters 32 and 33 for catheter position discussion.)

SUMMARY

Although the optimal position and orientation of the catheter tip to maintain function and minimize fibrin sheath formation are still unclear, ultrasound and fluoroscopic guidance during insertion will prevent most immediate mechanical problems. Malfunction that does not respond to simple positional changes, port reversal, and thrombolytic instillation in the dialysis clinic should be investigated with a transcatheter contrast study to evaluate for kinks and malposition, both of which can be corrected easily by standard interventional catheter–guidewire techniques. Although some practitioners still may favor fibrin sheath stripping, we believe that thrombolytic infusion and catheter exchange are better treatment options for well-positioned catheters with suspected or venographically proven pericatheter fibrin sheath or clot formation. Both these treatment options as well as new catheter materials, catheter designs, and prophylactic pharmacologic interventions deserve further study.

ACKNOWLEDGMENTS

I thank Mrs. Nancy Carnes for editorial assistance and Mr. Peter Brandt for preparation of the photographs.

REFERENCES

1. Moss AH, Vasilakis C, Holley JL, et al. Use of a silicone dual-lumen catheter with a Dacron cuff as a long-term vascular access for hemodialysis patients. *Am J Kidney Dis* 1990;26:211–215.

2. Gibson SP, Mosquera D. Five years experience with the Quinton Permcath for vascular access. *Nephrol Dial Transplant* 1991;6: 269–274.

3. Suhocki PV, Conlon PJ Jr, Knelson MH, et al. Silastic cuffed catheters for hemodialysis vascular access: thrombolytic and mechanical correction of malfunction. *Am J Kidney Dis* 1996;28: 379–386.

4. Trerotola SO, Johnson MS, Harris VJ, et al. Outcome of tunneled hemodialysis catheters placed via the right internal jugular vein by interventional radiologists. *Radiology* 1997;203:489–495.

5. Lund GB, Trerotola SO, Scheel PF Jr, et al. Outcome of tunneled hemodialysis catheters placed by radiologists. *Radiology* 1996;198:467–472.

6. McDowell DE, Moss AH, Vasilakis C, et al. Percutaneously placed dual-lumen silicone catheters for long-term hemodialysis. *Am Surg* 1993;59:569–573.

7. Cappello M, DePauw L, Bastin G, et al. Central venous access for haemodialysis using the Hickman catheter. *Nephrol Dial Transplant* 1989;4:988–992.

8. Schwartz RD, Messana JM, Boyer CJ, et al. Successful use of cuffed central venous hemodialysis catheters inserted percutaneously. *J Am Soc Nephrol* 1994;4:1719–1725.

9. Dialysis Outcomes Quality Initiative (DOQI) 23. *NKF-DOQI clinical practice guidelines for vascular access.* New York: National Kidney Foundation, 1997:61.

10. Schwab SJ, Buller GL, McCann RL, et al. Prospective evaluation of a Dacron cuffed hemodialysis catheter for prolonged use. *Am J Kidney Dis* 1988;11:166–169.

11. Daeihagh P, Jordan J, Chen GJ, et al. Efficacy of tissue plasminogen activator on patency of hemodialysis access catheters. *Am J Kidney Dis* 2000;36:75–79.

12. Paulsen D, Reisaether A, Aasen M, et al. Use of tissue plasminogen activator for reopening of clotted dialysis catheters. *Nephron* 1993;64:468–470.

13. Crain MR, Mewissen MW, Ostrowski GJ, et al. Fibrin sleeve stripping for salvage of failing hemodialysis catheters: technique and initial results. *Radiology* 1996;198:41–44.

14. Rockall AG, Harris A, Wetton CWN, et al. Stripping of failing haemodialysis catheters using the Amplatz gooseneck snare. *Clin Radiol* 1997;52:616–620.

15. Egglin TKP, Rosenblatt M, Dickey KW, et al. Replacement of accidentally removed tunneled venous catheters through existing subcutaneous tracts. *J Vasc Interv Radiol* 1997;8:197–202.

16. Dialysis Outcome Quality Initiative (DOQI) 5 and DOQI 23. *NKF-DOQI clinical practice guidelines for vascular access.* New York: National Kidney Foundation, 1997:26–27.

17. Duszak R Jr, Haskal ZJ, Thomas-Hawkins C, et al. Replacement of failing tunneled hemodialysis catheters through pre-existing subcutaneous tunnels: a comparison of catheter function and infection rates for de novo placements and over-the-wire exchanges. *J Vasc Interv Radiol* 1998;9:321–327.

18. Garofalo RS, Zaleski GX, Lorenz JM, et al. Exchange of poorly functioning tunneled permanent hemodialysis catheters. *AJR Am J Roentgenol* 1999;173:155–158.

19. Hoshal VL Jr, Ause RG, Hoskins PA. Fibrin sleeve formation on indwelling subclavian central venous catheters. *Arch Surg* 1971; 102:353–358.

20. Ahmed N, Payne RF. Thrombosis after central venous cannulation. *Med J Aust* 1976;1: 217–220.

21. Brismar BO, Hardstedt C, Jacobson S. Diagnosis of thrombosis by catheter phlebography after prolonged central venous catheterization. *Ann Surg* 1981;194:779–783.

22. O'Farrell L, Griffith JW, Lang CM. Histologic development of the sheath that forms around long-term implanted central venous catheters. *JPEN J Parenter Enteral Nutr* 1996;20:156–158.

23. Bolz K-D, Fjermeros G, Wideroe TE, et al. Catheter malfunction and thrombus formation on double-lumen hemodialysis catheters: an intravascular ultrasonographic study. *Am J Kidney Dis* 1995;25:597–602.

24. Haskal ZJ, Leen VH, Thomas-Hawkins C, et al. Transvenous removal of fibrin sheaths from tunneled hemodialysis catheters. *J Vasc Interv Radiol* 1996;7:513–517.

25. Brady PS, Spence LD, Levitin A, et al. Efficacy of percutaneous fibrin sheath stripping in restoring patency of tunneled hemodialysis catheters. *AJR Am J Roentgenol* 1999;173:1023–1027.

26. Uldall R, Besley ME, Thomas A, et al. Maintaining the patency of double-lumen Silastic jugular catheters for haemodialysis. *Int J Artif Organs* 1993;16:37–40.

27. Merport M, Murphy TP, Egglin TK, et al. Fibrin sheath stripping vesus catheter exchange for the treatment of failed tunneled hemodialysis catheters: randomized clinical trial. *J Vasc Interv Radiol* 2000;11:1115–1120.

28. Johnstone RD, Stewart GA, Akoh JA, et al. Percutaneous fibrin sleeve stripping of failing haemodialysis catheters. *Nephrol Dial Transplant* 1999;14:688–691.

29. Gray RJ, Levitin A, Buck D, et al. Percutaneous fibrin sheath stripping versus transcatheter urokinase infusion for malfunctioning well-positioned tunneled central venous dialysis catheters: a prospective randomized trial. *J Vasc Interv Radiol* 2000;11:1121–1129.

30. Savader SJ, Haikal LC, Ehrman KO, et al. Hemodialysis catheter-associated fibrin sheaths: treatment with a low-dose rt-PA infusion. *J Vasc Interv Radiol* 2000;11:1131–1136.

31. Savader SJ, Ehrman KO, Porter DJ, et al. Treatment of hemodialysis catheter associated fibrin sheaths by TPA infusion: critical analysis of 124 procedures. *J Vasc Interv Radiol* 2001;12: S62(abst).

32. Winn MP, McDermott VG, Schwab SJ, et al. Dialysis catheter 'fibrin-sheath stripping': a cautionary tale! *Nephrol Dial Transplant* 1997;12:1048–1050.

33. Mauro MA. Delayed complications of venous access. *Tech Vasc Interv Radiol* 1998;1:158–167.

34. Oncay ST, Levitin A, Dolmatch BL, et al. Tunneled hemodialysis catheter level and orientation predicts intervention. *Radiology* 1998;209(P):453.

35. Bern MM, Lokich JJ, Wallach SR, et al. Very low doses of warfarin can prevent thrombosis in central venous catheters: a prospective randomized trial. *Ann. Intern Med* 1990;112:423–428.

36. Kowalski CM, Kaufman JA, Rivitz SM, et al. Migration of central venous catheters: Implications for initial catheter tip positioning. *J Vasc Interv Radiol* 1997;8:443–447.

37. Nazarian GK, Bjarnason H, Dietz CA Jr, et al. Changes in tunneled catheter tip position when a patient is upright. *J Vasc Interv Radiol* 1997;8:437–441.

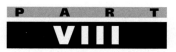

PERITONEAL DIALYSIS

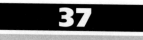

PRINCIPLES OF PERITONEAL DIALYSIS

PHYSIOLOGY, PATIENT SELECTION, AND CATHETER MAINTENANCE

JACK MOORE, JR.
PRZEMYSLAW HIRSZEL

Patients with end-stage renal disease (ESRD) have several methods of renal replacement therapy (RRT) available to them. Hemodialysis is the most widely prescribed method of RRT, and it includes both in-center and at-home options. Renal transplantation, whether from a cadaver or living donor, has now become accepted as the method of RRT associated with the most superior outcomes. Peritoneal dialysis (PD) is a less widely used, albeit well-established, method of providing dialysis for patients with ESRD. Despite being less frequently prescribed for ESRD than hemodialysis or transplantation, PD represents a viable option for many patients. It is particularly attractive to patients who wish to participate more actively in their therapy; for whom the scheduling requirements of in-center hemodialysis represent a barrier to continued employment or other daily activities; or for whom no suitable kidney for transplantation is available. PD is delivered in a number of formats, including continuous ambulatory PD (CAPD) as well as several different forms of automated PD that use an automated PD machine (a cycler) to provide dialysis to patients during their sleep. Although PD is simple conceptually, as with all forms of RRT, there are problems that make it less than an ideal form of therapy for patients with ESRD. The major challenges for PD programs include delivery of an adequate quantity of dialysis (1), preservation of the integrity of the peritoneal membrane, prevention of technique failure, and prevention or treatment of infection.

PHYSIOLOGY OF PERITONEAL DIALYSIS

Peritoneal dialysis is performed by instillation of dialysis solution (dialysate) into the peritoneal cavity to promote the movement of solutes and water from blood (and to a lesser degree from other body fluid compartments) by diffusive and convective processes. Dialysate is a sterile, balanced salt solution to which different concentrations of dextrose can be added. Dextrose is used as an osmotic agent that promotes the transport of nitrogenous waste, electrolytes, and water from the body into the fluid. Dialysate typically contains sodium, chloride, calcium, and magnesium, with lactate as a bicarbonate precursor. Although acetate can be used as a bicarbonate precursor, it is associated with some discomfort during infusion as well as long-term adverse effects on the peritoneal membrane, such as peritoneal sclerosis. A base precursor is required because bicarbonate cannot be added to dialysate without precipitating it with either the calcium or magnesium.

Drainage of the PD fluid from the abdomen results in loss of substances from the body. Obviously, urea nitrogen, creatinine, potassium, metabolic acids, and other molecules not excreted in ESRD must be removed. Conversely, dialysate can be used to provide substances for the body. Thus, PD removes bicarbonate, and the acetate in the dialysate is metabolized to bicarbonate, replacing the lost base. Proteins also can be lost in the peritoneal dialysate, and this undoubtedly is a substantial contributor to malnutrition in some patients on PD.

The peritoneal membrane consists of several heterogeneous anatomic and physiologic barriers against the movement of substances from the lumen of peritoneal capillaries into the peritoneal cavity. Several lines of evidence indicate that the major resistance to mass transport takes place in the capillary wall, followed by that of interstitial tissue and to a lesser degree by the mesothelial barrier (2). It is noteworthy that the mesothelial cells secrete surface-active phospholipid, which may have an enhancing role in ultrafiltration (UF) (3). Moreover, anionic sites have been demonstrated on the different components of the peritoneum, and they in turn may play a role in the transport of charged molecules such as albumin (4).

A three-pore model has been proposed to explain the function of the human peritoneal membrane. The capillary walls are considered the principal structures governing bidirectional blood–peritoneal exchanges. Large numbers of small pores located at the endothelial tight junctions represent pathways for small solutes; small numbers of large pores identified with endothelial gaps are involved in the transport of macromolecules. Finally, ultrapores of a very small size (subsequently identified as aquaporin I) subserve the transcellular transport of water (5).

Diffusion, convection, and peritoneal absorption are the three components of peritoneal mass transport. Diffusive transport is dependent on the concentration gradient between blood and dialysate as well as the molecular size of the solute. Convective transport occurs by means of dextrose-induced UF, whereby a large number of molecules are moving together with water through the pores of the membranes. Molecular sieving takes place during this process because aquaphorin channels transport a portion of the water. Thus, the sodium concentration in the osmotically induced PD ultrafiltrate is about 50 % of its plasma values (6).

Lymphatic absorption subtracts from gross UF volume (7). It is the primary pathway for isotonic dialysate absorption as well as a route for transport of macromolecules, particles, and formed blood elements. The normal rate of lymphatic absorption is 0.5 to 1.5 mL per minute, and it markedly increases during peritonitis.

Peritoneal Equilibration Test

Because of the great variability in peritoneal transport rates among PD patients, a peritoneal equilibration test (PET) was developed to quantify PD membrane characteristics (8). This subsequently was found to have a powerful influence on the specific method of PD that should be prescribed. Some patients require long exchanges of several hours and are served best by performing CAPD 24 hours each day. Others are served best by shorter exchanges and are able to use the automated cycling machine at night. Some patients require a mixture of ambulatory and cycling methods. Unfortunately, it is not possible to predict the membrane characteristics an individual patient will exhibit before formal PET testing. Moreover, the results of PET testing have not been validated except for patients who have been using their peritoneal membrane for a few weeks. Thus, we advise new patients that they need to be prepared to do continuous ambulatory dialysis, and we do not offer the promise of dialysis only on the cycler at night until the PET test results are available.

After a patient has been on PD for about 4 weeks, we perform the first PET test. The test, which requires 4 hours, starts with the instillation of 2 L of 2.5% dextrose dialysis solution into the abdomen. Dialysate (D) samples are obtained at 0, 2, and 4 hours, and plasma (P) samples are drawn at 2 and 4 hours. Glucose and creatinine concentra-

tions then are measured in each sample. By plotting D/P creatinine ratios and D/D0 glucose dialysate ratios versus time, patients can be characterized as high/high–average or low/low–average peritoneal transporters. Simple commercial software is available for the computation of PET results. Patients with more rapid transport rates have better dialysis with shorter cycle lengths and are switched to the cycler. Patients with slower transport rates require longer cycle lengths and continue with ambulatory dialysis.

Low transporters have slow solute transport and slow glucose absorption rates, which leads to efficient UF but relatively poor solute removal. In contrast, high transporters have accelerated clearance of small molecules but relatively poor UF because of the rapid absorption of glucose from the dialysate. These patients, who have high peritoneal permeability, consistently demonstrate a high degree of technique failure and an increased mortality, which is independent of their Kt/V, residual renal function, plasma albumin, body size, age, and sex (9). It is possible that chronic fluid overload contributes to cardiovascular morbidity and poor clinical outcome in high transporters.

Regardless of the initial PET results, increased peritoneal membrane permeability to water, glucose, and proteins is a constant feature of peritonitis. Inflammatory cytokines and arachidonic acid metabolites synthesized by macrophages and mesothelial cells are responsible for these changes (10). Repeated episodes of peritonitis often are associated with permanent deterioration of the function of the membrane.

Optimizing Peritoneal Dialysis

The possibilities of PD optimization are presented conceptually in Figure 37.1. This schema is predicated on the notion that blood flow to the peritoneum, the area and permeability of the membrane, the volume and composition of dialysate, and the rate of lymphatic absorption all can be modulated to improve peritoneal mass transport.

Normal peritoneal blood flow, which averages 60 to 100 mL per minute, can be increased by intravenous or intraperitoneal administration of numerous vasodilators, but only local infusion of sodium nitroprusside produces clinically meaningful results. In general, splanchnic vasodilatation augments transport of small, highly diffusible solutes, but only modestly. It is important to note that splanchnic vasodilators tend to increase the vascular exchange surface area as a result of dilatation of the functioning capillaries in combination with the opening up of the reserve capillaries. During this process, the capillary wall thickness decreases and the pores widen, thereby enhancing vascular permeability. Larger solutes are transported relatively faster in these environments (11).

Maintenance of a high chemical gradient between the blood and dialysate in the peritoneal fluid maximizes diffusive transport capability and promotes more efficient clearance of smaller solutes. This goal can be achieved by either

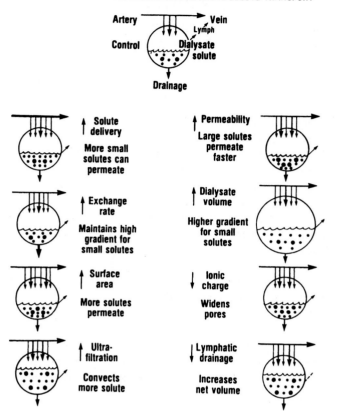

FIGURE 37.1. A schematic representation of solute removal by peritoneal dialysis. The *circles* represent the peritoneum containing small solutes (*dots*) and larger compounds. The *long horizontal arrow* above the *circle* represents peritoneal blood flow. *Vertical arrows* above the *circle* display transfer of small (*thin lines*) and large (*thick lines*) solutes. The *lower arrow* indicates drainage, and the *side arrow* indicates lymphatic absorption. (Reprinted from Gokal R, Nolph KD. *The textbook of peritoneal dialysis*, 1st ed. The Netherlands: Kluwer Academic Publishers, 1994:7, with permission.).

increasing the exchange rate or using a larger volume of dialysate per exchange. It has been our experience that most patients eventually are able to tolerate a dialysate volume of 3 L, although such volume may need to be introduced incrementally.

The rate of UF, or fluid removal, is largely dependent on the osmotic gradient across the peritoneum. Such gradient is provided by the use of dextrose, which can be provided in different concentrations. Commercially available dialysate contains 1.5%, 2.5%, or 4.25% dextrose. When automated cyclers are used, different concentrations of dextrose can be achieved by having the cycler infuse fluid from bags with different concentrations of dextrose. There is intense interest in evaluating non-dextrose substances, which could be used to provide a source for UF, particularly in diabetic patients, for whom the infusion of large dextrose loads represents a challenge to the maintenance of adequate glycemic control. In this regard, the novel osmotic agent icodextrin (a

mixture of glucose polymers with an average molecular weight of 16,200 daltons) has been in clinical use (12). Polypeptides and amino acids, among other substances, have been investigated for their ability to replace dextrose in PD dialysate. Although such investigations continue, their relative expense compared with dextrose may limit their ultimate widespread use.

Improvement in UF rate by definition results in enhanced convective transport. This, in turn, results in the removal of more solute in all molecular range categories. At present, improvement in UF rate is the only mechanism available to clinicians to improve peritoneal clearance meaningfully.

The gross UF rate and solute mass transfer rate are offset by lymphatic absorption. Thus, any factor that serves to diminish peritoneal lymphatic flow would augment PD clearance of water and solutes. No such agent is currently available for clinical use, although it has been suggested that the beneficial effect of phosphotidilcholine in patients with diminished UF is due to reduction in peritoneal lymph flow.

MAJOR COMPLICATIONS OF PERITONEAL DIALYSIS

The two major problems associated with long-term PD are failure to achieve adequate dialysis, either in terms of solute removal or UF, and peritonitis. These problems, as well as patient fatigue associated with the rigorous discipline required to perform PD over a protracted period, account for the vast majority of patients who decide to switch from PD to another form of renal replacement therapy.

Ultrafiltration Failure and Inadequate Dialysis

Ultrafiltration failure is the major impediment to the delivery of satisfactory PD therapy (13). In practical terms, the rapid dissipation of the dialysate/plasma (D/P) glucose gradient (type I UF failure) and reduction in peritoneal membrane surface area (type II UF failure) are the major causes of inadequate UF. Type I UF failure, observed in high transporters by PET, is associated with superior transport rates of small-molecular-weight solutes. It may be seen at the time of initiation of PD therapy and also occurs in patients with acute peritonitis. In contrast, patients with type II failure have a reduction in the effective peritoneal surface membrane area. This may result from adhesion formation after recurrent episodes of peritonitis or after extensive abdominal surgery. Type II failure is associated with diminished transport rates for both water and solutes. These patients will have low transport rates defined by PET testing. The most severe form of type II UF failure occurs in patients with sclerosing, encapsulating peritonitis, a multifactorial condition in which PD can no longer be continued (14).

Ultrafiltration failure also can result from excessive lymphatic absorption. This is not due to the characteristics of the peritoneal membrane and cannot be detected on PET testing. In the absence of a standardized test for the evaluation of lymphatic flow from the peritoneal cavity, at present, such a diagnosis can be made only by exclusion. Similarly, aquaphorin deficiency is another rare condition associated with low UF rates. Because the low sodium levels in PD ultrafiltrate reflect aquaphorin-related water transport across the peritoneum, an inadequate decrease in D/P ratio of sodium after the instillation of hypertonic dialysate supports the diagnosis of this type of UF failure.

Many of the numerous anatomic and physiologic alterations that have been documented in the peritoneum of CAPD patients are believed to be due to the nonphysiologic nature of dextrose-containing dialysate, episodes of acute or chronic peritonitis, and the use of different chemical agents in some groups of patients (14). Notwithstanding the cause of such changes, they are associated with a gradual loss of peritoneal membrane function. Such loss results in poor solute clearances, diminished UF, and augmented protein losses, which in turn are reflected in poor technique, survival, and increased patient mortality.

Because inadequate dialysis is associated with increased patient mortality, clinical guidelines have been developed to ensure that the combination of peritoneal clearance and residual renal function would sufficiently control the biochemical markers of uremia in each patient. Based on these guidelines, PD patients should currently have a weekly KT/V of greater than 2.0 or a minimum of 60 liters of combined creatinine clearance (1). This recommendation of adequate dialysis is the minimum standard to which patients should be subject. It is also important to note that residual renal function may decline over time, and the dialysis prescription may need to be increased to provide more dialysis in the face of the declining contribution from the patient's native renal function.

Peritonitis Associated with Peritoneal Dialysis

Infection, or peritonitis, is a major problem for patients on PD and is the main reason patients switch from PD to hemodialysis. Over the past three decades, technical advances in PD delivery systems, as well as a better understanding of the mechanisms of infection, have led to a progressive reduction in its incidence. Much of the training of patients for PD concerns the ritualization of technique that is designed to reduce the incidence of infection. Whereas most episodes of infection can be treated easily, a small percentage of infections result in catheter loss; in rare circumstances, sequela result in peritoneal membrane changes that preclude further PD.

Patients with PD are subject to infection for a variety of reasons. Obviously, no matter what method of PD they use,

they must manipulate the catheter and open it (potentially to the environment) daily. PD dialysate, with its dextrose content, is a rich culture medium. Moreover, it may have effects that impair host defenses, such as macrophage function or mesothelial cell function. The periodic "washing" of the peritoneal cavity in PD may result in changes in cytokines that are detrimental to host defenses. Finally, the PD catheter represents an indwelling foreign body. Biofilm (see Chapter 42 for detailed discussion of biofilm) has been detected on PD catheters. This may protect organisms from host defense mechanisms and increase susceptibility to infection.

Peritonitis accompanying PD often results from contamination with skin bacteria. *Staphylococcus epidermidis* and *Staphylococcus aureus* account for about half of all cases of peritonitis. In earlier years, *S. epidermidis* was the predominant species, particularly before the advances in PD delivery systems were widely available. With earlier systems, patients often would "touch" contaminate themselves while performing a bag exchange. With the advent of newer systems, *S. aureus* has increased in relative frequency. This is unfortunate because it is a much more difficult form of peritonitis to treat than that resulting from *S. epidermidis*. Infection resulting from vancomycin-resistant enterococci has become an important cause of nosocomial infections and is particularly difficult to eradicate.

Infections from gram-negative organisms are less common but are not infrequent in association with diarrheal syndromes or diverticulitis. Infection with *Pseudomonas* species are particularly problematic because they are difficult to eradicate, often result in loss of the catheter, and may result in peritoneal sclerosis with loss of ability to be on PD.

Other infectious agents, such as fungi or *Mycobacterium*, cause peritonitis in a small minority of patients. Catheter removal is necessary in most patients, although a brief trial of antimicrobial therapy without catheter removal is not unwarranted (see Chapter 38). We have not used intraperitoneal antifungal agents because they are associated with severe discomfort as well as peritoneal sclerosis.

The diagnosis and treatment of PD-associated peritonitis are relatively straightforward (15). Most patients present with a cloudy bag of dialysate and abdominal pain. Fewer than half have a significant temperature elevation, and a surprising number of patients have remarkably few symptoms. We have a rigorous protocol in which patients are instructed at the first sign of cloudy fluid to seek medical attention immediately. We send an aliquot of the fluid for a cell count, Gram stain, and culture. We also examine the exit site of the PD catheter carefully as well as the subcutaneous tunnel in which the catheter traverses the abdominal wall.

Virtually all patients with PD peritonitis will have PD fluid white blood cell count of greater than 100 cells/cc^3. We are usually able to get that result in about 1 hour in our facility. The Gram stain often is nonrevealing, even if subsequently the culture is positive for organisms. We follow recommendations for antibiotic therapy promulgated by the International Society for Peritoneal Dialysis; these recommendations are updated regularly (15). The current recommendation is to use a first-generation cephalosporin (such as cefazolin or cephalothin) as well as ceftazidime for initial therapy of most patients. The use of vancomycin is strongly discouraged in an attempt to reduce the likelihood of developing vancomycin-resistant organisms. Similarly, we have reduced our use of aminoglycoside antibiotics because they may result in a reduction in residual renal function through their nephrotoxic effects.

Therapy for peritonitis includes either systemic or intraperitoneal antibiotics as well as a change in the dialysis prescription. We tend to reduce the exchange volume so as to minimize abdominal distension and discomfort. Although patients with peritonitis need adequate dialysis, we do not want to inhibit host defense mechanisms that may hasten recovery from peritonitis by excessive washing of the peritoneal cavity. Moreover, peritonitis is associated with significant changes in peritoneal membrane permeability that can result in enhanced protein transport and substantial protein losses into the dialysate. We have regularly observed dramatic reductions in the serum albumin concentration during acute peritonitis. Nutritional support, accordingly, is an important adjunctive measure to antibiotic therapy.

Catheter malfunction is also common in peritonitis. Strands of fibrin often can be seen in the dialysate, and it is for this reason that we use heparin in our dialysate during peritonitis. It is not uncommon to encounter a catheter that will not perform normally: Either fluid will not infuse, or fluid will not drain. The evaluation of such catheters is problematic and requires close consultation between the nephrologist and surgeon or interventional radiologist. Other concerns include tunnel infections, which are extremely difficult to treat, as well as refractory peritonitis and relapsing peritonitis. Because dialysis is required to sustain life in PD patients, decisions to remove catheters are complex and always should be made as carefully as possible. If we do have to remove a catheter because of infection, we maintain the patient with hemodialysis for 4 to 6 weeks. We then offer the patient a new catheter and appropriate retraining for PD if that is the patient's desire. In our experience, patients with mild peritonitis that does not require catheter removal do extremely well. Patients with more severe peritonitis that requires catheter removal often choose not to return to PD even after resolution of the peritonitis.

SELECTION OF PATIENTS FOR PERITONEAL DIALYSIS

It has been our practice to select patients who enter our PD program very carefully. PD is self-dialysis, is done at home, and is dependent on a very highly motivated, compulsive patient. Because patient interest and enthusiasm for the method are essential, it is important to have some selection method in place to ensure that appropriate candidates are selected. We prefer to interview patients who meet most or all of the following characteristics: a history of cooperation with therapeutic recommendations; interested in participating extensively in their own care; trainable in the necessary procedures and problem-solving techniques intrinsic to PD; and sufficient support systems in place to assist them as they assume the majority of their dialysis care. We specifically do not encourage patients who have just learned of their ESRD to embark on self-dialysis because they often have intense adjustment problems learning to deal with the effects of ESRD on their lives. Moreover, we usually do not encourage PD for patients who have not been adherent to medical suggestions, who have unstable home environments, or who are of sufficiently large body habitus that adequate dialysis delivery is unlikely. Finally, we typically do not accept patients who choose PD as a way of "escaping" from the lifestyle changes that are necessary to live with ESRD. The ideal patient for PD is one who has considered all options for RRT and has enthusiastically chosen PD as the method most consistent with his or her lifestyle aspirations. Notwithstanding the above caveats, we routinely reevaluate patients in our hemodialysis populations several times each year and routinely offer all patients the opportunity to consider PD as a possible therapeutic option for their ESRD.

Many patients, particularly those who are referred in a timely fashion to a nephrologist, usually are informed of PD as a possible option for ESRD by their nephrologist or a nurse educator. Ideally, patients are informed of options for renal replacement therapy early in the course of their chronic renal failure and can consider the risks and benefits of all forms of therapy before they reach ESRD. Education and options for RRT are part of our ongoing efforts to improve the care given to patients with progressive renal insufficiency.

When a patient with progressive chronic renal disease indicates substantial interest in PD, we arrange for him or her to be enrolled in the pre-PD selection process. The PD training nurse interviews the patient and assesses his or her ability to learn the cognitive and procedural content necessary to perform PD. We also have a renal nutritionist assess the patient's nutritional status because poor nutrition is a powerful contraindication to PD. We then have the PD nurse and the renal social worker visit the patient at home to assess the suitability of the environment as a place that is adequate for PD. A satisfactory home environment includes adequate storage facilities, an area that can be used repetitively to perform exchanges, electricity and running water, and a telephone. We review as much information as we can obtain from the patient in a multidisciplinary effort and then determine whether the patient is an acceptable candidate for our program. In general, we give great weight to the patient's wishes, although we decline to provide PD to the occasional patient for whom, in our judgment, PD seems contraindicated.

In recent years, patients who have been on long-term hemodialysis, in whom a functional angioaccess is no longer available, have been brought to PD programs by their nephrologists. These patients often have had multiple procedures by both angioaccess surgeons as well as interventional radiologists. Typically, all sites for vascular access have been exhausted. These patients, many of whom have had ESRD for many years, sometimes are offered PD as the "only" option for continued survival. It has been our experience that only a minority of these patients will succeed on PD. Malnutrition, propensity to infection, depression and hopelessness, and advanced, progressive vascular disease often are so extensive that long-term survival with any form of RRT is unlikely. We evaluate such patients carefully because PD, which can aggravate malnutrition, make patients more susceptible to peritonitis, and often will deliver inadequate dialysis, can be detrimental to both the quality and quantity of their lives.

Peritoneal dialysis is not suitable for all patients with ESRD. As with most forms of medical therapy, there are some conditions that represent relative or absolute contraindications to PD. Relative contraindications include centripetal obesity, large body habitus (>90 kg), chronic low back disease, severe chronic obstructive pulmonary disease, enterocutaneous ostomies, and a history of extensive intraabdominal surgery. Absolute contraindications include malnutrition (serum albumin concentrations <3.0 mg/dL after nutritional support), extensive uncorrectable abdominal adhesions, intraperitoneal malignancy, massive obesity, crippling digital arthritis, and untreatable intraabdominal infection. Visual impairment is a barrier to PD that often can be overcome with assistance devices and creative training techniques.

Our PD selection committee reviews the history, physical examination, and laboratory data provided by the attending nephrologist, reports of the PD training nurse, renal dietitian, and renal social worker. We give strong consideration to the wishes of the patient (and family, if appropriate). If we believe that PD is appropriate for the patient, we inform the patient that he or she will be accepted into the program. We then work with the patient to set dates for catheter placement and subsequent PD training.

Nephrologists select which method of PD a patient will use by considering a number of different factors. Obviously, the patient's desires are considered, but the provision of adequate dialysis is the essential component of long-term survival with ESRD. Thus, nephrologists are concerned that whichever method is selected, it will provide adequate dialysis. We use the results of PET to assist us as we determine which method of PD to recommend to our patients.

CATHETER INSERTION AND MAINTENANCE

The provision of PD requires that a peritoneal catheter be placed. A PD catheter is a flexible silicone tube that has an open end port as well as numerous side holes. Catheters come in a variety of shapes (curved, straight, swan-necked), and each has enthusiastic supporters. There is little convincing evidence that one catheter is better than another. The catheter should be placed approximately 4 weeks before initiation of dialysis to allow complete healing of the surgical incisions and the exit site as well as complete sealing of the catheter as it enters the peritoneal catheter. It is essential that an operator with knowledge of PD insert the catheter so that it is placed properly. The catheter can be placed either surgically or percutaneously (see Chapters 38 and 39). In certain patients, laparoscopic assistance is useful. The exit site of the catheter should be placed in a site that will not be constantly rubbed or irritated. Thus, it should be placed away from the belt line, and the exit site should be angled downward to prevent pooling of secretions or liquid in the orifice of the exit site. We do not have strong preferences as to the type of catheter, although most nephrologists favor a dual-cuffed catheter. We do use catheters that have a radioopaque stripe in them so they can be visualized on radiograph. Ideally, the catheter tip should be placed in the left lower quadrant. We ask the surgeon to irrigate the catheter in the operating room by infusing several aliquots of fluid in and out of the peritoneal cavity. This serves to clear the tip of the lumen of serous or hemorrhagic fluid and occasionally will identify catheter malfunction (inadequate drainage) so that the catheter can be repositioned. Most operators give one dose of an antibiotic in the operating room. We have tended to use a cephalosporin to minimize the use of vancomycin.

The experience of the operator who places the catheter has been, in our experience, a major determinant in the subsequent success of the catheter. It is our belief that only operators who are interested in placing PD catheters, place many of them, and are willing to follow the patients postoperatively should be encouraged to place catheters. Catheters that are placed in the correct portion of the abdomen, whose exit site is located in an unobtrusive area, and whose exit site is snug seem to have the longest problem-free life. In most programs, more than 85 % of the catheters are still functional 1 year later. About 10% to 15% of catheters must be removed, usually for intractable infection. None of the catheters resists the accumulation of biofilm (see Chapter 42) on their surface. The development of biofilm may predispose to infection as well as loss of the catheter.

The postoperative care of PD catheters varies from program to program. We leave the operative site untouched for about a week. We then do a very careful dressing change, being as careful as possible not to traumatize the exit site with unnecessary movement of the catheter. We prefer to wait at least 14 days after placement of the catheter. If it absolutely must be used earlier, small volumes of fluid should be used to avoid distension of the peritoneal cavity.

Numerous PD regimens are available for the maintenance therapy of ESRD patients, and they can be divided into *manual* and *automated* forms (16). Manual procedures include continuous ambulatory PD (CAPD), which usually consists of three to four daytime exchanges plus a long bedtime dwell, and daytime PD (DPD), which involves four short day exchanges and no night dwell. Automated procedures include continuous cycling PD (CCPD), which provides one to two long day dwells and three to four short nighttime exchanges; nocturnal intermittent PD (NIPD), which consists of multiple short nighttime exchanges without a day dwell; and intermittent PD (IPD), which consists of three to four rapid cycling sessions each week, with dialysis-free periods between the treatments. There is a general consensus that IPD is adequate only in patients with significant residual renal function.

CONCLUSIONS

Peritoneal dialysis remains a viable option for many patients with ESRD. Compared with its rate of use in other countries, it is probably underused in the United States. Although major advances have occurred in our understanding of the function of the peritoneal membrane, mechanisms of its dysfunction, and the pathophysiology and treatment of infection, major obstacles remain to be overcome before the number of patients on PD will increase substantially. We must learn how to overcome the challenging task of providing adequate PD therapy to patients with large body habitus and those with very low or absent residual renal function. This will require better methods of optimizing peritoneal clearances. At present, this can be accomplished only by increasing the number of exchanges, increasing the exchange volume, and enhancing UF (17). Finally, we need to continue to design catheters and dialysate delivery systems that are associated with an even lower incidence of infection. Progress toward these goals will make PD more attractive to the increasing numbers of patients who require RRT for ESRD.

REFERENCES

1. National Kidney Foundation. K/DOQI Clinical Practice Guidelines for Peritoneal Dialysis Adequacy. *Am J Kidney Dis* 2001;37:S65–S136.
2. Krediet RT, Lindholm B, Rippe B. Pathophysiology of peritoneal membrane failure. *Perit Dial Int* 2000;20(suppl4):S22–S42.
3. Hills BA. Role of surfactant in peritoneal dialysis. *Perit Dial Int* 2000;20:503–515.
4. Galdi P, Shostak A, Jaichenko J, et al. Protamine sulfate induces enhanced peritoneal permeability to proteins. *Nephron* 1991;57:45–51.
5. Ronco C. The "nearest capillary" hypothesis: a novel approach to peritoneal transport physiology. *Peri Dial Int* 1996;16:121–125.
6. Chen TW, Khanna R, Moore H, et al. Sieving and reflection coefficients for sodium salts and glucose during peritoneal dialysis. *J Am Soc Nephrol* 1991;2:92–100.
7. Mactier R, Khanna R, Twardowski Z, et al. Contribution of lymphatic absorption to Loss of ultrafiltration and solute clearances in continuous ambulatory peritoneal dialysis. *J Clin Invest* 1987;80:1311–1316.
8. Twardowski ZJ. Clinical value of standardized equilibration tests in CAPD patients. *Blood Purif* 1989;7:95–108.
9. Davies SJ, Phillips L, Russell GI. Peritoneal solute transport predicts survival on CAPD independently of residual renal function. *Nephrol Dial Transplant* 1998;13:962–968.
10. Chaimovitz C. Peritoneal dialysis (nephrology forum). *Kidney Int* 1994;45:1226–1240.
11. Hirszel P, Lameire N, Bogaert M. Pharmacologic alterations of peritoneal transport rates and pharmacokinetics of the peritoneum. In: Gokal R, Nolph KD, eds. *The textbook of peritoneal dialysis.* New York: Kluwer Academic Publishers, 1994:161–132.
12. Davies DS. Kinetics of icodextrin. *Perit Dial Int* 1994;14:S45–S50.
13. Mujais S, Nolph K, Gokal R, et al. Evaluation and management of ultrafiltration problems in peritoneal dialysis. *Perit Dial Int* 2000;20:S5–S21.
14. Dobbie JW. Ultrastructure and pathology in peritoneal dialysis. In: Gokal R, Nolph KD, eds. *The textbook of peritoneal dialysis.* New York: Kluwer Academic Publishers, 1994:17–44.
15. Keane WF, Bailie GR, Boeschoten E, et al. Adult peritoneal dialysis-related peritonitis treatment recommendations: update. *Perit Dial Int* 2000;20:396–412.
16. Twardowski ZJ. Peritoneal dialysis glossary III. *Perit Dial Int* 1990;6:47–49.
17. Krediet RT, Douma CE, van Older RW, et al. Augmenting solute clearance in peritoneal dialysis. *Kidney Int* 1998;54:2218–2225

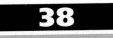

TECHNIQUES OF PERITONEAL CATHETER INSERTION

MICHAEL A. KRAUS

According to data of the 2000 U.S. Renal Data Service (USRDS), as of December 31, 1998, end-stage renal disease (ESRD) affected 346,453 living patients in the United States. Of these, 100,543 had a functioning renal transplant, and 245,910 patients were dependent on dialytic renal replacement therapy (RRT). Peritoneal dialysis was the patients' choice of RRT in 25,273 (10.3%) (1).

Peritoneal dialysis is a relatively simple process with which a patient can perform self-care of RRT at home. The requirements for successful peritoneal dialysis are few: (a) an intact peritoneal cavity; (b) a motivated patient or, in special situations, caregiver; (c) a "clean" environment with the capability of storing supplies; and (d) a functioning peritoneal dialysis catheter. The contraindications to peritoneal dialysis include a lack of any of the preceding requirements and an irreparable or recurrent hernia. Relative contraindications include back pain, which may be worsened by shifting the center of gravity with a full peritoneal cavity; ostomies; recent grafts of an abdominal aortic aneurysm; severe lung disease; or uncontrollable psychiatric illness (2).

Peritoneal dialysis has multiple complications that can lead to significant morbidity and occasionally to mortality. Many causative factors are related directly to the function and placement of the peritoneal dialysis catheter. Catheter implantation–related problems vary but occur in about 1% to 30% of patients (3). Morieras and colleagues reported 137 mechanical complications in 105 catheters over 11 years. Of these events, 61.3 % were catheter related (4). Therefore, the successes of an individual patient's treatment with peritoneal dialysis and the overall quality of the peritoneal dialysis program are dependent on the successful placement and function of peritoneal catheters. Properly implanted catheters will lead to improvement in the infection rates and decreases in the complication rates in a peritoneal dialysis unit.

Surgeons, nephrologists, and interventional radiologists place peritoneal dialysis catheters. Regardless of who places the catheter and the technique used, every physician and care provider involved in the peritoneal dialysis patient's care needs to be aware of the various techniques employed and the complications related to placement of the catheter.

PERITONEAL DIALYSIS CATHETERS

The peritoneal dialysis catheter is essential for successful dialytic therapy. The catheter must allow for the free flow of peritoneal fluid by gravity. Rates of gravity fill and drain must approach up to 3 L in 10 to 15 minutes (300–500 mL per minute) without causing discomfort. Slower rates will lead to unreasonable time to fill or drain the peritoneal cavity and failure of therapy. In addition, fill and dwell flows must be painless. Ideally, the catheter should approach the goal of "stealthness" that is desired in the vascular catheter for access. The catheter should be inert, durable, and free from bacterial growth, which can lead to infectious complications. The peritoneal dialysis catheter also should be designed to limit omental encasement and catheter movement.

Catheters that became available in the year 2001 have varying designs. Catheters are composed of silicone or polyurethane. Catheters are defined based on the design of the extraperitoneal (*subcutaneous*) segment and the design of the intraperitoneal segment. The extraperitoneal segment can be precurved (*arcuate angle*), straight, or preformed into a bucket handle. The precurved design has a hairpin, preformed curve (*arcuate angle*); this design ensures a downward positioning of the exit site. It also has the theoretic advantage of less tension on the extraperitoneal subcutaneous segment, allowing ease in tunneling with less risk of cuff erosion. Those desiring more flexibility in the selection of an exit-site location, not being limited by the precurved design, prefer the straight extraperitoneal segment. In addition, a bucket-handle configuration of the extraperitoneal segment was designed for downward tunneling without tension; the exit-site location with this catheter is the least flexible.

The extraperitoneal segment will have either one or two Dacron cuffs. The single-cuff catheter is used primarily in the pediatric population, in whom patient growth is expected. Most catheters placed in the adult population should have two cuffs. Most studies suggest a decrease in exit-site infections, tunnel infections, and peritonitis with two cuffs (5,6). The proximal (*deep*) cuff is implanted on the preperitoneal surface and the distal (*subcutaneous*) cuff lies in the subcutaneous tunnel. The proximal cuff holds the catheter in place, and fibroblast in-growth reduces entrance site leaks. The distal cuff becomes a barrier to infection and seals the tunnel. Missouri catheters have a unique deep cuff. The Dacron cuff is attached to a Dacron disc at 45-degree angle and then is attached to a Teflon ball. The Teflon ball is implanted intraperitoneally with the disc sewn to the preperitoneal surface.

The intraperitoneal segment of peritoneal dialysis catheters also has multiple designs. The most common two, the *straight* and the *pigtail*, are both hollow tubes with large end holes. The final 10 cm of the catheter contains parallel rows of smaller 1-mm side holes. Most dialysate flow occurs through these side holes. The pigtail design reduces a potentially painful jet-stream effect, which may occur with the straight catheter.

More recently, a T-fluted intraperitoneal design was introduced. The intraperitoneal segment is T-shaped and designed to remain against the anterior peritoneal surface. In addition, the two ends of the "T" are fluted rather than hollow. This design allows more rapid flow and might prevent omental wrap or catheter movement (S. A. Ash, personal communication, 2001.) Other novel designs include the addition of intraperitoneal weights, two Teflon peritoneal discs designed to keep the omentum from attaching (Toronto-Western), and a showerhead design that decreases flow to decrease omental wrap (Lifecath).

Other novel modifications of the arcuate angle coiled catheter include the Moncreif-Popovich catheter; this catheter has a longer distal, subcutaneous, cuff. It is designed for implantation leaving the distal tip subcutaneous at the time of catheter insertion. Four to 6 weeks later, the tip can be externalized, and dialysis can be initiated immediately. It is hoped that implanting the catheter initially will ensure excellent tunnel formation without bacterial colonization (7). Finally, the Missouri swan-neck coiled catheter also is designed with a long subcutaneous tunnel to allow a presternal exit site. This catheter allows patients to bathe safely and may be useful to patients with ostomies (8).

Catheter design does influence implantation technique. Straight and swan-neck catheters with either straight or coiled intraperitoneal segments may be placed by any technique. Missouri, Toronto-Western, and Lifecath catheters must be placed using an open surgical technique with direct visualization of the peritoneal membrane. The T-flute catheter is designed for placement using a peritoneoscope. Catheter selection is usually operator dependent and is based on the method of insertion, ease of insertion, and local expertise.

PREOPERATIVE EXAMINATION

Before placing a peritoneal dialysis catheter, a thorough history and physical examination are mandatory. Most operators use either conscious sedation or general anesthesia. Therefore, the customary preoperative elements of a history and physical examination should be obtained. A history of last oral intake, presence of a designated driver, history of anesthetic reaction (patient and family), complete past medical history, cardiopulmonary history, medication and allergy history, and review of systems, including signs and symptoms of ongoing infection, must be documented. Physical examination should note airway, range of motion of neck, and a thorough cardiopulmonary examination. These elements of history and physical are directed toward standard anesthetic requirements for most procedures using either conscious sedation or general anesthesia.

Certain key elements of the history and physical examination are pertinent to risk stratification and successful placement of peritoneal catheters. A history of prior surgeries is critical. A history of prior hernia repairs may suggest the possibility of a recurrent hernia and leak. Prior abdominal procedures and radiation increase the risk of adhesions and hence perforation. Prior abdominal infections likewise will raise the risk of perforation. Whereas placement of peritoneal catheters is possible in these situations, the patient should be aware of the increased risk of perforation and the increased likelihood of an unacceptable peritoneal cavity (significant adhesions may not allow for free flow of dialysate within the peritoneal cavity). This can lead to compartmentalization of the cavity and may prohibit the ability to perform adequate dialysis as a result of inadequate drainage or inadequate exposure to the complete peritoneal membrane. It is desirable for experienced physicians to place catheters in these patients.

Examination of the abdomen preoperatively is essential. The patient should be examined while both clothed and unclothed as well as standing and supine. Knowledge of the usual location the patient's belt line is necessary. Placement of the exit site should be either below or well above the belt line to prevent irritation that leads to cuff erosion and exit-site infections. Inspection of the abdomen should include evaluation for preexisting umbilical, ventral or inguinal hernias. Larger umbilical and ventral defects should be repaired at time of implantation of the catheter and hence should be done in the operating room by a surgeon. Smaller defects can be followed closely with the patient on peritoneal dialysis; however, the patient should be aware that the hernia may worsen with peritoneal dialysis because of the increased abdominal pressure and might later need to be repaired. This may lead to a disruption of peritoneal dialysis and necessitate a short course of hemodialysis. All known inguinal hernias should be corrected either before or at the same time as catheter placement. Inguinal hernias tend to cause leaks into the scrotum and have an unacceptable risk of incarceration (9).

In obese patients, knowledge of the relationship of the umbilicus to the peritoneal cavity is necessary. In larger patients, the umbilicus could fall below the caudal reflections of the peritoneal cavity; therefore, the umbilicus is a poor landmark to use for entrance site location (see also Chapter 39). Finally, the physician should take note of how the panus moves with positioning. An exit site placed underneath the panus or in the downward reflection is predisposed to infection.

Some physicians prefer to obtain preoperative ultrasound mapping of the epigastric artery within the abdominal rectus sheath. This has the advantage of reducing the likelihood of inadvertent perforation or tear of the artery. No studies have demonstrated the need for this study, and this is not part of the routine preoperative examination.

Preoperative laboratory examinations include platelets, hemoglobin, prothrombin time, and a partial thromboplastin time. Physicians may opt to know recent electrolytes, creatinine, and blood urea nitrogen levels and may perform an electrocardiogram. Chest radiographs may be desirable for general anesthesia or when symptoms of congestive heart failure or pulmonary infection exist.

PATIENT PREPARATION

Patients planning to undergo peritoneal dialysis catheter placement should take nothing orally (NPO) for 6 hours before the procedure. If the procedure is planned as an outpatient procedure, the patient should be told to bring a designated driver. Some centers prefer to have the patient scrub his or her abdomen with an antibiotic soap on the day before and the day of the procedure. Laxatives may be given the day before to decrease the possibility of constipation. Antihypertensives should be taken the day of the procedure, and diabetic medications need to be adjusted for the NPO period.

The patient should be instructed of the risks, benefits, and alternatives to catheter placement. In addition, the risks and benefits of anesthesia are explained. The patient or the patient's guardian should sign an informed consent before the procedure. The risks of peritoneal catheter placement by any technique are bleeding, infection, viscus perforation, and an inability to place a catheter or placement of a nonfunctioning catheter.

The patient is asked to void and defecate before the procedure to decrease risk of bowel or bladder perforation. Some physicians prefer to place a bladder catheter before the procedure, but this is not routine. Dentures and glasses are removed.

The patient should be taken to a procedure suite when possible. Catheters placed by Seldinger technique or with a peritoneoscope can be placed in a patient's room when necessary (i.e., when the patient is an unstable intensive care unit patient). A dedicated sterile procedure room or operating room environment is preferred, however, to minimize perioperative infections and to maximize patient comfort and privacy. Prophylactic antibiotics may be administered. One gram of intravenous cephazolin sodium is adequate. In the cephalosporin-allergic patient, 150 mg of clindamycin or 1 g of vancomycin and an aminoglycoside may be administered. The patient then is positioned supine on the procedure table. When using a peritoneoscope or laparoscope, the table must have the capability to go into Trendelenburg position. The patient's abdomen is scrubbed with povidone–iodine or chlorhexidine scrub and then carefully draped in a standard fashion. If povidone–iodine is used, complete drying is necessary for the full antimicrobial effect.

Conscious sedation is usually adequate to ensure patient comfort and decrease anxiety. Occasionally, general anesthesia is used for patient or surgeon preference. Blood pressure, telemetry, and oxygen concentration are monitored continuously monitored until the patient is discharged. The operator should perform a full scrub and wear standard surgical attire.

CATHETER PLACEMENT TECHNIQUES

There are six technique options for the placement of permanent peritoneal dialysis catheters (Table 38.1). Preferred surgical techniques are placement of catheters via dissection with mini-laparotomy or laparoscopic placement. Nephrologists use a peritoneoscopic placement or a modified Seldinger technique with a guidewire and peel-away sheath. Placement of catheters with a Tenckhoff trocar is also possible but is not performed so frequently (because it results in more pain and morbidity). The percutaneous placement of catheters by interventional radiologists is discussed in Chapter 39. Herein, the techniques of surgical, laparoscopic, Seldinger, and peritoneoscopic placement are presented in detail.

Entrance-site Selection

The knowledge of normal anatomy is essential. Lateral to the midline (umbilicus) and anterior to the peritoneal cav-

TABLE 38.1. TECHNIQUES FOR PERITONEAL DIALYSIS CATHETER PLACEMENT

Surgical
    Dissection with minilaparotomy
    Laparoscopic

Nephrology
    Tenckhoff trocar
    Modified Seldinger with peel-away sheath
    Peritoneoscopy

Interventional Radiology
    Fluoroscopic guided with peel-away sheath

ity are the abdominal rectus muscles. Traversing through the middle of the abdominal rectus sheath are the inferior and superior epigastric arteries. Sites for entrance of the catheter into the peritoneal cavity are defined in relation to the abdominal rectus sheath. *Lateral* refers to an entrance site at the lateral edge of the abdominal rectus sheath. The *paramedian* site is located on the medial aspect of the abdominal rectus sheath and the *midline* approach between the abdominal rectus sheaths (Fig. 38.1). Care must be taken to avoid damage to the arteries. Surgeons prefer to place catheters by either the lateral or paramedian approach. Placements by peritoneoscope or guidewire peel-away approaches are either lateral or midline.

The level of the entrance site should be cephalad to a horizontal line drawn between the anterior superior iliac crests. In a thin person, the entrance site should be between the umbilicus and the level of the anterior iliac crests. In an obese patient, the umbilicus is an unreliable marker and may not even be anterior to the peritoneal cavity. In these patients, the entrance site should be selected 2 to 3 cm cephalad to a line drawn connecting the anterior superior iliac crests.

Lateral and paramedian entrance sites allow the proximal (deep) cuff to be implanted within the abdominal rectus muscle. These approaches carry an increased risk of damag-

ing the epigastric arteries. The midline entrance site is avascular, usually 1 cm below the umbilicus in the thin or normal body habitus. It may need to be above the umbilicus in the morbidly obese patient. This approach virtually eliminates the risk of injuring the epigastric artery, but it does not allow implantation of the proximal cuff into the abdominal rectus muscle. The midline approach has higher leak and hernia rates (10).

Placement of Peritoneal Dialysis Catheters Via Peritoneoscopy

The placement of peritoneal dialysis catheters using the Y-Tec peritoneoscope (Medigroup) was first described by Ash and colleagues in 1983 (11) and has undergone some modifications. The patient is brought to the procedure suite after the history is taken, physical examination is performed, and the preparations are done as described previously. Conscious sedation is used for patient sedation and comfort. General anesthesia is not desirable because the patient will need to tense his or her abdomen to facilitate entry to the peritoneal cavity. After preparation and draping, the patient is asked to tense the abdomen and the lateral aspect of the abdominal rectus muscle is palpated. Then 1% lidocaine is infiltrated locally over the lateral edge of the abdominal rectus muscle 2 to 3 cm cephalad to the line between anterior superior iliac crests. A 1.5- to 2-cm incision is created with a no.11 scalpel blade. Hemostasis is obtained using hemostats or cautery. Using a straight hemostat, blunt dissection is performed to the abdominal rectus sheath. The sheath can be recognized by the striations felt when rubbing the hemostat over the muscle; 1% lidocaine then is infiltrated generously into the abdominal rectus sheath to obtain adequate anesthesia.

At this point, the patient is asked to tense their abdomen and a Verres (insufflation needle) can be introduced into the peritoneal cavity. There is usually a series of two to three "pops" to obtain entry into the peritoneal cavity. There also may be a transient sharp, sudden pain with entry into the peritoneal cavity. The patient is placed into Trendelenburg position, and the abdomen is insufflated with approximately 1 L of filtered air to create a pocket for peritoneoscopy (more may be required for obese patients). The Verres needle then is withdrawn. The patient once again tenses the abdomen, and the Y-Tec trocar and quill assembly guide are introduced into the peritoneal cavity. The trocar is withdrawn, leaving the cannula and quill guide in place. The 2.2-mm peritoneoscope is placed through the cannula, and visualization of the intraperitoneal contents is usually easily possible. If the viscera are not easily seen, the peritoneoscope may be withdrawn slowly at 1-mm increments, watching for a flash of the air pocket. Common reasons for failure to visualize intraperitoneal contents include insufflation of the preperitoneal planes with the Verres needle (usually painful), preperitoneal placement of the peritoneoscope, or

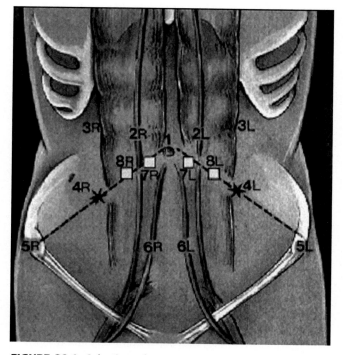

FIGURE 38.1. Selection of entrance site for peritoneal dialysis catheter placement. Landmarks for placement. *5R* and *5L*, anterior superior iliac crests. Entrance site should be a minimum of 2 cm above a line connecting the two. The lateral entrance sites are located at three and four. The paramedian sites are located at *8R* and *8L*. The medial entrance site is either just above or just below the umbilicus (*1*). Note the position of the epigastric arteries (*2R* and *2L*) and the inferior epigastric arteries (*6R* and *6L*). (Illustration courtesy of Medigroup, Inc., North Aurora, IL, U.S.A.)

significant adhesions. Adhesions can be anticipated if the abdomen is observed during insufflation; in the presence of loculated adhesions, air will form an asymmetric bulge on entry into the peritoneal cavity.

The procedure, as originally described by Ash and colleagues, used the Y-Tec trocar (quill catheter guide) for initial peritoneal puncture and insufflation. I prefer to use the Verres needle for insufflation, which decreases the risk of viscus perforation on initial entry into the peritoneal cavity, and prior insufflation makes it technically easier to visualize the intraperitoneal cavity when the Y-Tec trocar and quill assembly guide are introduced into the air pocket.

After visualization of the intraperitoneal contents, limited peritoneoscopy is performed to note the presence of adhesions, the location and size of the omentum, and the size of the bladder. The peritoneoscope, with the cannula and quill guide attached, are advanced to the contralateral anterior peritoneal cavity. In the presence of significant adhesions, any open area of the caudal peritoneal cavity can be used. The peritoneoscope is withdrawn, leaving the cannula and quill guide in place. The cannula is withdrawn from the quill guide, and a straight hemostat is applied to the quill guide, securing it in place. The entrance site then is dilated to the width of the peritoneal dialysis catheter. The catheter is placed over a stylet and into the quill guide. The catheter and stylet are gently advanced to the pouch of Douglas. There should be no pain or resistance as the catheter is advanced. The stylet is withdrawn from the catheter 2 to 3 cm, and the intraperitoneal segment of the catheter is slid over the stylet into the peritoneal cavity. The peritoneal dialysis catheter is advanced until the proximal (deep) cuff is against the abdominal rectus sheath. Using the Y-Tec implanter, or hemostats, the catheter is advanced to seat the cuff within the muscle. After implanting the cuff, visualization of the muscle/cuff should confirm that it is within the abdominal rectus sheath. Then the quill guide can be withdrawn while the catheter and stylet are held in place. The stylet is withdrawn from the catheter, and 60 mL of saline can be infused through the catheter by using a syringe. There should be no resistance to flow. The catheter is aspirated using the syringe; frequently, a mixture of fluid and air will return. Free flow of fluid and air confirms intraperitoneal positioning. Watching fluid movement within the catheter during respiration also confirms intraperitoneal catheter position; the fluid column decreases with inspiration and increases with expiration, corresponding to changes in abdominal pressure.

The intraperitoneal segment of the catheter is now in place. An exit site is selected, paying close attention to belt line and shifts in panus with standing. The exit site always should be directed downward to decrease risk of infection (12); 1% lidocaine is infiltrated locally at the desired exit site. A stab wound is created with a no. 11 scalpel blade, and the tunnel is created. The exit site should be snug around the catheter; no sutures are needed at the exit site; 700 to 1000 mL of either saline or dialysate is infused through the catheter via gravity. After instillation, the entrance site is examined for evidence of leaking. If a leak exists, the deep cuff may be either in the peritoneal cavity or on top of the muscle. It can be adjusted with tension or hemostats to reposition if necessary. After draining by gravity, the entrance site wound is closed with suture, staples, or Durabond. The drain volume should be examined grossly to rule out significant hemoperitoneum, cloudiness, or fecal contamination. The patient is observed for at least 1 hour and then can be discharged to home.

Guidewire–Peel-Away Sheath

Placement of peritoneal dialysis catheters with a guidewire and peel-away sheath is performed using a modified Seldinger approach. The entrance site is usually lateral or midline. The patient is prepared as described for the peritoneoscopy approach. A 1.5- to 2-cm incision is created above the desired entrance site and hemostasis is obtained. Blunt dissection is carried to the abdominal rectus sheath with the lateral approach or to the peritoneum in the midline approach. The peritoneal cavity is cannulated either with an 18-gauge angiocath, Verres needle, or 18-gauge needle. The peritoneal cavity can then be filled with 600 mL of saline or dialysate. If the needle or angiocath is properly placed, the patient should not experience pain or resistance to filling the cavity. It should be noted that some operators opt not to instill fluid or air into the peritoneal cavity.

After the cavity has been entered, a 0.035-inch soft-tipped guidewire is advanced carefully into the peritoneal cavity. The needle or angiocath is removed. A dilator and peel-away sheath are carefully advanced over the wire and toward the dependent peritoneal cavity. There should be no resistance to advancement of the dilator after the peritoneal cavity is entered. The wire is withdrawn, and the dilator is removed, leaving the peel-away sheath in place. A peritoneal catheter with a stiffening stylet in place is advanced through the peel-away sheath (some operators advance the catheter through the peel-away sheath without the use of a stylet). The intraperitoneal segment is advanced over the stylet until the deep cuff is against the rectus muscle or on top the peritoneal cavity. The peel-away sheath then is cracked and removed. If the lateral approach is being used, the deep cuff then can be seated into the abdominal rectus sheath with a hemostat. The stylet is removed, and the catheter is checked for function as noted already (placement via peritoneoscopy). An exit site is selected, and a tunnel is created with one of a number of available devices. The abdomen then can be filled with up to a total of 1 L of fluid and drained as described previously. The entrance site is closed and the patient observed.

Surgical Placement Via Cutdown

Many slight modifications are made in the placement of peritoneal dialysis catheters, depending on the surgeon and his or her training. In general, an overview of this technique involves cutdown to the abdominal rectus muscle, identification of the epigastric artery, and dissection through the abdominal rectus muscle to the peritoneal cavity. Most surgeons prefer either the lateral or the paramedian approach as described herein. Frequently, this procedure is done with the patient under general anesthesia, although conscious sedation can be used. After selection of an appropriate entrance site, as discussed previously, the surgeon makes a 4- to 6-cm incision over the abdominal rectus muscle. Blunt dissection is taken down to the abdominal rectus muscle. The muscle then is dissected carefully free and identified. Attempts are made to localize the epigastric artery. The abdominal rectus muscle is incised horizontally, exposing the peritoneal surface. At this point, many surgeons prefer to place a pursestring suture into the peritoneal wall itself. The peritoneum is lifted up with forceps, and an incision is created that is large enough to allow passage of the continuous ambulatory peritoneal dialysis (CAPD) catheter. The CAPD catheter is placed over a stylet, and the stylet and catheter are advanced into the peritoneal cavity anteriorly to the contralateral gutter. Care is taken to avoid any resistance. If the patient is awake, there should be no pain. The intraperitoneal segment then is slid off the stylet, and the cuff is advanced to the surface of the peritoneal cavity. If a Missouri catheter is being used, the Teflon ball is placed into the peritoneal cavity while the Dacron disc is sewn directly to the anterior portion of the peritoneal surface. After dissection of the abdominal rectus muscle superior or cephalad to the initial incision, the catheter is passed directly through the belly of the abdominal rectus muscle. This buries the cuff directly within the abdominal rectus muscle, forcing the catheter intraperitoneally in a downward direction, hopefully decreasing intraperitoneal malposition. The original dissection of the abdominal rectus muscle then is sewn closed. Once again, care must be taken to avoid damaging the epigastric artery. The catheter is flushed, and the peritoneal cavity is aspirated assuring good flow of the catheter without kinks. A tunnel then is created, either with the hemostats or a tunneling device, and care should be maintained to ensure that the exit site is facing downward. As with the other techniques, the exit site is usually lateral and caudal to the entrance site. The abdomen is filled with 1 to 2 L of saline or dialysate, and the entrance site is observed for evidence of leak. The dialysate is allowed to drain, and the original incision over the entrance site is closed with staples or suture. The drained dialysate is inspected for evidence of significant hemoperitoneum, fecal contaminants, or cloudiness. The patient is observed postoperatively and either maintained in the hospital overnight or discharged after a period of observation.

Laparoscopic Technique

The laparoscopic technique is becoming more popular because of its success in general surgical procedures. It offers the advantage of being able to perform a partial omentectomy or stapling of the omentum when indicated during the initial catheter placement. Placement via laparoscope usually involves use of a 2- to 10-mm laparoscope with an insufflation of CO_2 or nitrous oxide. Smaller scopes are adequate and often preferred. Nitrous oxide allows for pneumoperitoneum without general anesthesia. Various techniques have recently been described (13–18). These involve either a two- or three-puncture approach. This technique differs from peritoneoscopic placement in that the abdominal cavity is entered under direct visualization through the laparoscope. The puncture sites are usually the lateral aspects of both abdominal rectus muscles and the umbilicus. The periumbilicus site is used for insufflation with CO_2 or nitrous oxide and for placement of the laparoscope. One lateral entrance site is used for passage of instruments and the other for the entrance site of the peritoneal dialysis catheter. Using this method, an entrance site can be selected that is free from surrounding adhesions, and the risk of viscus puncture is minimized. The entrance site can be created either with a trocar system, or with dissection. The CAPD catheter again is placed over a stylet through the entrance into the peritoneum and advanced into the lower portion of the peritoneum under direct visualization with the laparoscope. A pursestring can be used at the entrance site at the preference of the surgeon. The laparoscope is withdrawn, and the scope entrance site can be left to close on its own, although some surgeons prefer to close this with suture. The tunnel is created as described already, and completion of the procedure is identical.

COMPARISON OF TECHNIQUES

Multiple reports of experience of catheter placement by the various techniques are in the literature. Complication rates as described by physicians with expertise are minimal. Comparative studies of peritoneoscopic versus surgical placement have been reported. Initially, comparisons for peritoneoscopic placement versus historical surgical controls were reported, for example, by Cruz and Faber (19). These comparisons demonstrated better initial and long-term function of catheters placed via peritoneoscope; however, interpretation of these studies are limited by the use of historical controls and, hence, there may be differences in catheter survival unrelated to placement. Also, there may be bias in patient selection that is not reported. In 1991, Pastan and colleagues (20) reported a comparative study of peritoneoscope versus surgical placement of PD catheters placed during the same period. They found catheter survival to be significantly better in catheters placed via peritoneoscope, although no differences were found in the complication rate. Of note, there was a high rate of leak in both groups, and catheters were used to a great extent without a break-in period. This study is potentially faulted by selection bias because the patients were not randomized, and more obese patients were sent to surgery.

Gadallah and colleagues (21) in 1999 described a prospective, randomized control study comparing surgically placed catheters with peritoneoscopy. Over 3 years, 148 catheters were placed and randomized by month of placement. All catheters were two-cuffed, arcuate-angle, coiled catheters. The catheters were allowed to break in for at least 1 week. Randomization was equivalent in all studied factors, including age, weight, incidence of diabetes, and prior surgery. The rate of early complications, including peritonitis, malfunction, leak, or perforation, was significantly greater in the surgical group: 33.3% versus 13.2%. The difference could be ascribed to the rate of early peritonitis (12.5% in the surgical group compared with 2.6% in the peritoneoscopy group) and leak (11.1% in the surgery group compared with 1.3% in the peritoneoscopy group). The incidence of late complications was statistically equivalent.

Wright and colleagues (22) described a comparison of laparoscopic versus open placement of catheters. In this study of 50 patients, conventional placement was found to be significantly quicker, 14 versus 22 minutes, and there was no difference noted in complication rate, catheter survival, pain score, or length of stay (see also Chapter 39 for comparison of radiologic and surgical techniques).

Hence, all techniques of placement of peritoneal dialysis catheters appear to have acceptable complication rates. Some studies demonstrated an advantage to peritoneoscopic placement, although this may depend heavily on expertise. Theoretically, methods of implantation that allow visualization of the peritoneal contents—laparoscopic and peritoneoscopic—should have a higher success rate, particularly in the complicated patient. The technique used to place catheters is dependent on many factors.

FACTORS THAT INFLUENCE WHO SHOULD PLACE PERITONEAL CATHETERS

Catheter design may directly influence the technique used to place the CAPD catheter. All catheters with the Missouri ball disc system require surgical placement with direct visualization of the peritoneal surface and dissection of the abdominal rectus muscle. Therefore, programs that use these catheters will mandate open placement of all peritoneal dialysis catheters. Similarly, the Toronto-Western Teflon disc catheter and the Lifecath showerhead catheters require direct visualization of the peritoneal surface with a relatively large incision of the peritoneal surface. Therefore, these catheters also mandate open dissection with surgical placement.

Patients who require another surgical intervention at the time of peritoneal dialysis placement, such as the repair of a large hernia, will benefit from surgical placement because this can be done in the same setting as the hernia repair. Patients with known or suspected adhesions can have successful placement of a peritoneal catheter; however, the risk of viscus perforation increases significantly in the presence of adhesions. The presence of significant adhesions leading to loculation of the abdominal cavity may require a minilaparotomy with adhesionolysis. Frequently, this cannot be diagnosed preoperatively.

There is great debate at many hospitals as to who should place peritoneal dialysis catheters. Techniques are described that allow placement by surgeons, nephrologists, or interventional radiologists. There are pros and cons to placement by any of these three specialists; however, certain factors are necessary to promote success of the peritoneal dialysis program at an institution. Catheters should be placed by a physician skilled in the placement technique with knowledge of the function and needs of a peritoneal dialysis catheter. The physician must have knowledge of the anatomy of the abdominal wall as well as the early and late complications of peritoneal dialysis. Physicians who place peritoneal dialysis catheters should have a vested interest in the success of the peritoneal dialysis program and participate in follow-up care. Ideally, all peritoneal dialysis programs should monitor their catheters with respect to complications as well as longevity and patency of peritoneal dialysis catheters, as has been described in the hemodialysis literature. The success of peritoneal dialysis depends greatly on the inserting physician's understanding of the complications noted by the nephrologist and how they relate to placement of peritoneal dialysis catheters.

POSTOPERATIVE MANAGEMENT

After placement of the peritoneal dialysis catheter by any of the preceding techniques, the catheter should be dressed with dry, nonocclusive dressings. The dressing should be large enough to secure the catheter against the abdominal wall to prevent any possibility of trauma to the catheter or tension on the exit site. Most centers favor leaving the dressing untouched for a period of 5 to 7 days postoperatively. Bleeding should be minimal, but, if necessary, the bandage can be reinforced. Some programs favor daily irrigation of the catheter with 100 to 500 mL of saline or dialysate. Other programs favor no irrigation. No data suggest the superiority of one method over another. My personal preference is not to irrigate the catheter; we have had no incidence of nonfunctioning of catheters because of clogging. After 4 to

7 days, the dressing is carefully removed, making sure not to put tension on the exit site; daily dressings can be done subsequently. It is the routine practice of the peritoneal dialysis unit at Indiana University to apply mupirocin cream to the exit site on a daily basis as has been described by Bernardini and colleagues (23). Marked improvements in exit site and tunnel infections have been described. In our institution, *Staphylococcus aureus* infections have reduced from a 55% incidence rate to 10% of all peritonitis and exit-site infections. In addition, overall peritonitis rates have improved from one episode per every 13 months to one episode per every 25 months.

Although CAPD catheters can function immediately after placement, the risk of leak is markedly increased. Pastan and colleagues noted a 25% leak rate in catheters without break-in regardless of placement technique (20). When it is absolutely necessary to institute peritoneal dialysis prior to 2 weeks of healing, low-volume (i.e., 1 L) exchanges and, when possible, supine exchanges or CCPD with dry days should be used to minimize the risk of leak. If a 2-week waiting period is used, we find a less than 1% leak rate, even when dialysis started with standard volumes of dialysis (i.e., 2–2.5 L) per exchange.

COMPLICATIONS OF PERITONEAL DIALYSIS CATHETER PLACEMENT

Complications after placement of a peritoneal dialysis catheter are early (within 30 days) or late (>30 days) after placement (see also Chapter 39). *Early complications* include viscus perforation, bleeding, wound infection, peritonitis, outflow failures, and leaks.

Viscus perforation is the complication of greatest concern. It occurs in 0.5% to 1.5% of all catheter placements, regardless of technique. Perforation can occur during entrance of the peritoneal cavity via needle, trocar, or scalpel or can occur while advancing a catheter and stylet into the lower quadrant of the peritoneal cavity. Significant perforation is suspected with the onset of significant pain, nausea, vomiting, or rapid occurrence of a rigid abdomen. If the perforation is large or includes the colon, peritonitis will ensue shortly. Intravenous antibiotics should be initiated along with careful observation. More than likely, surgical exploration will need to be undertaken with catheter removal and repair of the perforation. Occasionally, a small perforation can occur during peritoneoscopy. It can be diagnosed by direct visualization of the leak during limited peritoneoscopy or suspected by significant and persistent pain on entrance of the peritoneal cavity with the trocar. In this case, the perforation may be small enough to close without surgical intervention. Careful observation with broad-spectrum antibiotics may be reasonable.

Bleeding is rarely a significant complication after any technique. Blood-tinged dialysate that clears with rapid exchange is relatively common, but significant intraperitoneal bleeding should be a very rare complication. Persistent bleeding may occur at the exit site and usually can be stopped with direct pressure or thrombin administration to the exit site. Rarely, a suture will need to be applied around the catheter. If this is done, care must be taken not to puncture the peritoneal dialysis catheter. Severe preperitoneal bleeding during placement of the peritoneal dialysis catheter can be the result of damage to the epigastric artery. Hemostasis will need to be obtained by use of hemostats and surgical repair will likely be necessary.

Wound infection should be relatively uncommon postoperatively. If it is a recurrent theme, evaluation of surgical technique and evaluation for areas of contamination should be undertaken. Usually, antibiotics are sufficient to treat superficial wound infections. Rarely, the entrance-site wound will have to be opened.

Early peritonitis with catheter placement may be a sign of poor surgical technique or poor sterile technique in the procedure suite. If the peritoneal fluid becomes cloudy and associated with pain, and the white blood cell count of the peritoneal fluid is greater than 200 polymorphonuclear leukocytes, bacterial peritonitis is present. Dialysate should be cultured, Gram stain obtained, and appropriate antibiotics administered. Occasionally, the patient develops a cloudy effluent without pain or fever. Cell count of the peritoneal fluid in this case reveals predominant eosinophilia. Eosinophilic peritonitis is a rare cause of nonbacterial peritonitis, the cause of which is unknown. It has been postulated to be secondary to the plastics in the dialysate bags or the composition of the peritoneal dialysis catheter itself. Eosinophilic peritonitis may be persistent but almost always will resolve eventually, and no treatment is generally indicated (24).

Outflow failures may be due to multiple causes, including clots or fibrin within the catheter, kink in the subcutaneous tunnel, constipation, placement of the peritoneal dialysis catheter within the omentum, development of omental wrap, or loculated adhesions within the abdominal cavity. Repair of the problem is dependent on the cause. In the case of fibrin or clots, the catheter may be forcefully irrigated with a 60-mL syringe of saline. Intraperitoneal heparin may be instilled in the dialysate to prevent recurrence. If the subcutaneous tunnel is kinked, incision over the kink and repositioning of the catheter can be performed. Constipation is a common cause of catheter malfunction that usually leads to incomplete drainage of the peritoneal dialysate. Laxatives may be administered overnight, and return of catheter function is noted the following day. Omental wrap or capture of the catheter within adhesions is a significant problem that can be difficult to repair. Manipulation of the catheter as described by Savader and colleagues (25) with a guidewire may

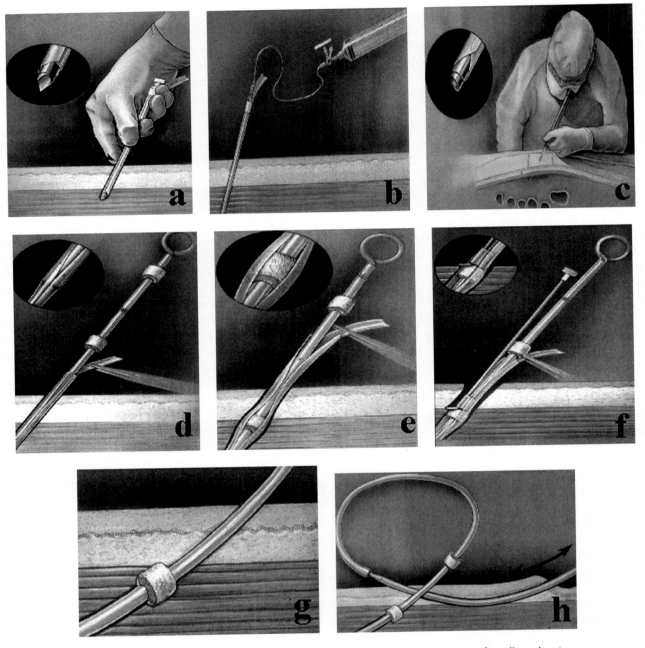

FIGURE 38.2. Placement of peritoneal dialysis catheter via peritoneoscopy. After dissection to the abdominal rectus sheath the Y-Tec trocar and quill guide assembly is introduced into the peritoneal cavity (**A**). The trocar is withdrawn, leaving the cannula and quill guide in place. The patient is placed into the Trendelenburg position and insufflated with 1,000 mL of filtered air (**B**). The peritoneoscope is placed through the cannula, and inspection of the peritoneal contents is performed (**C**). The peritoneoscope and cannula are withdrawn, and the entrance site is dilated (not shown). The catheter is placed over a stylet and passed into the peritoneal cavity through the quill guide (**D**). The catheter is advanced so that the deep cuff is to the rectus sheath (**E**) and then advanced into the rectus muscle using the Implantor (Y-tec, Medigroup) (**F**). In the **inset**, note that the design of the Implantor prevents placement of the cuff through the rectus sheath, preventing placement into the peritoneal cavity. Proper placement of the deep cuff is within the abdominal rectus muscle (**G**). A tunnel is created (**H**), and the entrance site is closed. (Illustration courtesy of Medigroup, Inc., North Aurora, IL, U.S.A.)

be successful (see Chapter 39). It carries little morbidity and may be attempted twice before considering salvage of the catheter with a guidewire a failure. Other techniques for repositioning under fluoroscopy include manipulation of the catheter with Fogarty balloons (26), malleable bars (27), and gastric forceps (28). If omental wrap persists, a minilaparotomy with partial omentectomy can be performed and the catheter repositioned in the lower peritoneal cavity. This also can be performed laparoscopically but requires either partial omentectomy or stapling of the omentum up against the peritoneal surface to prevent recurrence. In the event of severe loculated adhesions, adhesionolysis may be undertaken with success, but it is a significantly larger surgery, and consideration for hemodialysis also may be entertained.

Pain with inflow and occasionally outflow may occur in up to 10% of patients initiating peritoneal dialysis. This may be slightly greater with a straight catheter because of the jet effect of inflow (6). Generally, mild analgesics may be administered, and the pain usually resolves within 2 weeks.

Leak of dialysate from the entrance site to the surrounding tissue can be suspected with drainage of fluid through the exit site or with the appearance of a bulge directly underneath the entrance site incision. This is a very rare complication of properly inserted catheters that have been allowed to heal for 10 to 14 days prior to use. Causes of entrance site leaks are hernia at the entrance site resulting from too large a surgical incision, positioning the deep cuff either on top of the abdominal rectus muscle or intraperitoneally, and trauma (i.e., pulling of the catheter). When leak is suspected or confirmed, catheter rest with a dry abdomen for 2 weeks is a reasonable approach. If the leak is to resolve, it likely will do so within 2 weeks. If not, surgical repair of the entrance site or placement of a new peritoneal catheter will be necessary.

Care must be taken not to confuse large serous drainage from the exit site with a dialysate leak. The glucose of serous drainage should be that of serum. Serous drainage is a common finding, particularly in obese and diabetic patients. Serous drainage usually resolves spontaneously, although occasionally the application of silver nitrate around the exit site to encourage epithelialization is required.

Late complications (>30 days) include exit site infections, peritonitis, tunnel infections, outflow failures, and leaks. *Infections* of the catheter can be related to positioning of the exit site. The incidence of infections attributable to exit-site positioning can be reduced with an adequate physical examination prior to catheter placement. If the exit site is placed at or directly beneath the belt line, significant irritation can occur, which may lead to catheter cuff extrusion and recurrent infections, including exit site, tunnel infections, and peritonitis. Superficial cuffs placed too close to the exit site may be prone to extrusion and infection as well. An upward directed exit site is prone to collecting fluid and dirt leading to an increased incidence of infection (29).

Outflow failure beyond 30 days is likely due to constipation and is relieved with laxatives. Other causes include omental wrap, which can occur at any time and also can lead to movement of the catheter out of the pelvis. Repair is similar to that of early outflow failure.

Leaks and hernias may lead to ultrafiltration failure, doughiness of the abdomen with a "peau de orange" appearance, or scrotal swelling. Leaks can result from ventral or umbilical hernias. A common cause of scrotal swelling and leak is the presence of a patent processus vaginalis that is clinically silent before the start of peritoneal dialysis. Leaks also can occur at the catheter entrance site. Catheter malfunction, leaks, and hernias can be investigated with computed tomography (CT) scan using intraperitoneal contrast (30). Intravenous contrast (100 mL) is placed in a 2-L dialysate bag. The patient is encouraged to ambulate for at least 30 minutes before lying supine for the CT scan. Then the CT scan can more easily visualize the presence of a hernia or leak as well as the cause. CT scan also will determine whether there is a bilateral patent processus vaginalis when only a unilateral leak is suspected (Fig. 38.2–38.4).

CONCLUSION

A successful peritoneal dialysis program is quite dependent on the proper placement of permanent peritoneal dialysis catheters. Knowledge of the techniques and complications of catheter placement is essential for all members of the health care team. All catheters should be monitored for evidence of complications and techniques of placement revisited when appropriate. Catheters can be successfully placed by a variety of techniques as described herein. Catheter placement is driven by results and local expertise.

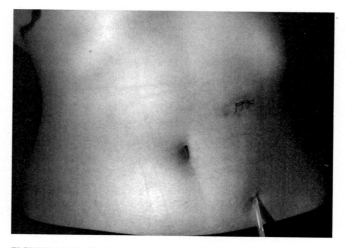

FIGURE 38.3. Photograph of an abdomen 3 days after placement of a peritoneal dialysis via peritoneoscopy. Suture line is above the entrance site. Exit site is in a location to avoid irritation by the belt line.

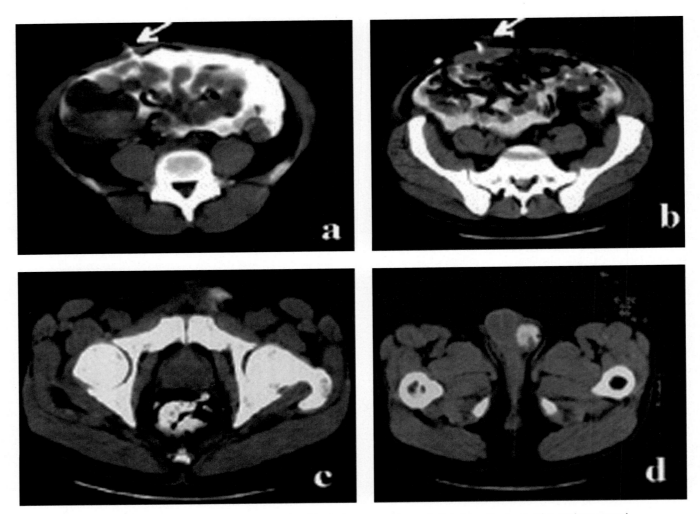

FIGURE 38.4. Computed tomography scans of leaks in two peritoneal dialysis patients. **A:** The patient experienced swelling in the labia and abdominal wall after significant trauma to the catheter. Note the catheter entrance site (*white arrow*). Contrasted fluid was leaking around the catheter to the preperitoneal soft tissue. **B–D:** The patient experienced scrotal swelling after 6 weeks of peritoneal dialysis. **B:** Entrance site (*white arrow*) without evidence of leak. **C,D:** Leak through a patent processus vaginalis into the scrotum.

REFERENCES

1. U.S. Renal Data System (USRDS). *USRDS 2000 annual data report: atlas of end-stage renal disease in the United States.* Bethesda, MD: National Institutes of Health, National Institute of Diabetes and Digestive and Kidney Diseases, 2000.
2. National Kidney Foundation Dialysis Outcomes Quality Initiative (NKF-DOQI). *Clinical practice guidelines for peritoneal dialysis adequacy.* New York: National Kidney Foundation, 1997:80–82.
3. Ash SA. *Clinical dialysis,* 3rd ed. Norwalk, CT: Appleton and Lange, 1995:295–321.
4. Moreiras PM, Cuina L, Goyanes GR, et al. Mechanical complications in chronic peritoneal dialysis. *Clin Nephrol* 1999;52:124–130.
5. Diaz-Buxo JA, Geisenger WT. Single cuff versus double cuff Tenckhoff catheter. *Peritoneal Dialysis Bull* 1984;4:S100–S102.
6. Twardowski ZJ, Khanna R. Peritoneal dialysis access and exit site care. In: *Textbook of peritoneal dialysis,* 1st ed. Dordrecht, The Netherlands: Kluwer Academic Publishers, 1994.
7. Moncreif JW, Popovich RP, Broadrick LJ, et al. Moncreif-Popovich catheter: a new peritoneal access technique for patients on peritoneal dialysis. *ASAIO J* 1993;39:62–65.
8. Twardowski ZJ, Nichols WJ, Nolph KD, et al. Swan neck presternal peritoneal dialysis catheter. *Perit Dial Int* 1993;13(Suppl 2):S130–S132.
9. Morton JH. Abdominal wall hernias. In: *Principles of surgery,* 4th ed. New York: McGraw-Hill, 1986.
10. Helfrich GB, Pechan BW, Alijani MR, et al. Reduced catheter complications with lateral placements. *Perit Dial Bull* 1983;3(Suppl 4):S2–S4.
11. Ash SA, Handt AE, Bloch R. Peritoneoscopic placement of the Tenckhoff dialysis catheter: further clinical experience. *Perit Dial Bull* 1983;3:8–12.
12. Eaton A, Penn A, Bungy M, et al. HD support for a PD program. In: *Aspects of renal care 1,* Eastbourne, U.K.: Balliere Tindall, 1986:87–92.
13. Crabtree JH, Fishman A. Videolaparoscopic implantation of long-term peritoneal dialysis catheters. *Surg Endosc* 2000;13:308–309.

14. Poole GH, Tervit P. Laparoscopic Tenckhoff catheter insertion: a prospective study of a new technique. *Aust N Z J Surg* 2000;70: 371–373.

15. Zadrony D, Draczkowski T, Lichodziejewska-Niemierko M. Two-millimeter minisite mini-laparoscopy for rescue of dysfunctional continuous ambulatory peritoneal dialysis catheters. *Surg Laparosc Endosc* 1999;9:369–371.

16. Crabtree JH, Fishman A, Huen IT. Videolaparoscopic peritoneal dialysis catheter implant and rescue procedures under local anesthesia with nitrous oxide pneumoperitoneum. *Advances in Peritoneal Dialysis* 1998;14:83–86.

17. Lessin MS, Luks FI, Berm AS, et al. Primary laparoscopic placement of peritoneal dialysis catheters in children and young adults. *Surg Endosc* 1999;13:1165–1167.

18. Skipper K, Dickerman R, Dunn E. Laparoscopic placement and revision of peritoneal dialysis catheters. *JSLS* 1999;3:63–65.

19. Cruz C, Faber MD. Peritoneoscopic implantation of catheters for peritoneal dialysis: effect on functional survival and incidence of tunnel infection. *Contrib Nephrol* 1991;89:35–39.

20. Pastan S, Gassensmith C, Manatunga AK, et al. Prospective comparison of peritoneoscopic and surgical implantation of CAPD catheters. *ASAIO Trans* 1991;37:M154–M156.

21. Gadallah MF, Pervez A, el-Shahawy MA, et al. Peritoneoscopic versus surgical placement of peritoneal dialysis catheters: a prospective randomized study on outcome. *Am J Kidney Dis* 1999;33:118–122.

22. Wright MJ, Bel'eed K, Johnson BF, et al. Randomized comparison of laparoscopic and open peritoneal dialysis catheter insertion. *Perit Dial Int* 1999;19:372–375.

23. Bernardini J, Piraino B, Holley J, et al. A randomized trial of *Staphylococcus aureus* prophylaxis in dialysis patients: Mupirocin calcium ointment 2% applied to the exit site versus cyclic oral Rifampin. *Am J Kidney Dis* 1996;27:695–700.

24. Steiner R. Clinical observations on the pathogenesis of peritoneal dialysate eosinophilia. *Perit Dial Bull* 1982;2:118–119.

25. Savader SJ, Lund G, Scheel PJ, et al. Guidewire manipulation of malfunctioning peritoneal dialysis catheters: a critical analysis. *J Vasc Interv Radiol* 1997;8:957–963.

26. Gadallah MF, Arora N, Arumugan R, et al. Role of Fogarty catheter manipulation in management of migrated, nonfunctional peritoneal dialysis catheters. *Am J Kidney Dis* 2000;35: 301–305.

27. Simons ME, Pron G, Voros M, et al. Fluoroscopically-guided manipulation of malfunctioning peritoneal dialysis catheters. *Perit Dial Int* 1999;19:544–549.

28. Ohira N, Yorioka N, Ito T, et al. Correction of CAPD catheter displacement using gastric biopsy forceps: the push-pull method. *Int J Artif Organs* 1999;22:202–204.

29. Twardowski ZJ, Nolph KD, Khanna R, et al. The need for a "swan neck" permanently bent, arcuate peritoneal dialysis catheter. *Perit Dial Bull* 1985;5:219–223.

30. Twardowski ZJ, Tully RJ, Nichols WK, et al. Computerized tomography in the diagnosis of subcutaneous leak sites during continuous ambulatory peritoneal dialysis (CAPD). *Perit Dial Bull* 1984;4:163–166.

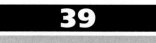

PERCUTANEOUS RADIOLOGIC PLACEMENT AND MANAGEMENT OF PERITONEAL DIALYSIS CATHETERS

TECHNIQUE AND RESULTS

SCOTT SAVADER

The "time line" for the conception and implementation of artificial dialysis methods spanned the greater part of the last century. In 1923, Ganter initially tested peritoneal dialysis (PD) in guinea pigs (1); however, 23 years passed (1946) before Fine and colleagues described their experience in the use of PD for patients with acute renal failure (2). The Brescia–Cimino fistula was not described until an additional 20 years later (1966), whereas catheter-directed hemodialysis (HD) lagged behind by an additional 3 years (1969) (3,4). Thus, PD was the first method of artificial dialysis to be used successfully in a large patient population. In 1978, the U.S. Food and Drug Administration approved the sale of commercially prepared dialysis solutions, thus beginning the modern era of PD.

According to the United States Renal Data System (USRDS) 2000 annual report, 323,160 persons in this country alone were using some form of dialysis as of December 1998. From this group, 25,206 (7.8%) persons were reported to use some form of PD for their primary method of dialysis (5). PD requires a greater degree of motivation than does HD because the patient, by necessity, must assume responsibility for his or her own dialysis care. In return, PD offers its participants freedom from the rigors and restrictions associated with HD and, in many cases, the additional and invaluable benefit of improved overall health. During the last 10 years, the trend has been for fewer patients to use PD and more to use HD. Objective evaluation of this trend is somewhat difficult but could reflect more stringent Dialysis Outcomes Quality Assurance (DOQI) guidelines for dialysis dose imposed on an aging and more obese population. As the age of the dialysis population increases, more patients may opt for care provided at the dialysis center rather than the self-imposed rigors of home PD.

PHYSIOLOGY AND MECHANICS OF PERITONEAL DIALYSIS

Peritoneal dialysis is similar to HD in that there are three components to the system: a blood-filled compartment (the visceral and peritoneal vessels), a compartment for the dialysate (the peritoneal cavity), and a semipermeable membrane to separate the two compartments (the peritoneal membrane). On the other hand, PD is quite unique compared with HD in that no artificial membranes, pumps, or sophisticated machinery are required. A single-lumen catheter, an adequate supply of dialysate, and an intact peritoneal surface constitute the engine necessary for PD; the natural forces of passive diffusion, ultrafiltration, convection, and gravity fuel this dialysis system (6). Diffusion is the primary driving force behind solute transfer during PD, but bulk convective flow also can contribute. *Convection* is the process by which solutes are lost during ultrafiltration, whereas *ultrafiltration* is the movement of water from the blood in the vessels of the peritoneum to the peritoneal cavity as a result of the osmotic gradient set up by the dialysate (6). (See Chapter 37 for a detailed discussion of physiology.)

Advantages

Peritoneal dialysis has physiologic advantages compared with HD in that patients experience a greater "steady state" in terms of their hemodynamics, extracellular fluid volumes, coagulation and nutritional status, and general health.

Disadvantages of Peritoneal Dialysis

Disadvantages associated with PD include time-consuming fluid exchanges, a continued necessity for sterile exchange, protein loss, and an excessive glucose load (6). The efficiency of PD decreases disproportionately as the patient's weight increases because the increase in peritoneal surface area in larger patients cannot keep pace with the relative increase in creatinine and urea production. In addition, PD is not as *mechanically efficient* as HD because the peritoneal surface is thicker and has a relatively small surface area compared with an artificial membrane. Also, the fluid is somewhat stagnant within the peritoneal cavity compared with the rapidly flowing blood passing through an artificial kidney (6). Nevertheless, PD remains an invaluable and relatively inexpensive method for artificial dialysis; it has more widespread use in other countries than in the United States.

CATHETER CHOICE

There are as many PD catheters on the market as there are HD catheters; and, of course, each manufacturer can state why their device is superior to the competitors' device. Basically, PD catheters come straight or pigtailed, single- or double-cuffed, of various lengths, and are 5 to 11 French (*pediatric*) to 11 French to 16 French (*adult*) in size. Polyurethane and silicone are the most commonly used catheter materials. Catheters generally come with a spiraling array of side holes along the functional part of the device. This pattern is designed to minimize malfunction; the catheter is enveloped by constantly moving loops of bowel and omentum. The pigtail design, as is the case for angiography catheters, is to minimize trauma to the surrounding soft tissues. The cuff arrangement is designed both to secure the catheter to the surrounding soft tissues and to provide protection against encroachment of offending organisms from the patient's skin. Length is variable, and obviously one particular length will not necessarily serve the needs of an entire PD population, particularly if pediatric patients are included.

For percutaneous placement in adult patients, I have used a 57-cm-long (catheter tip to beginning of pigtail), pigtail designed, double-cuffed catheter, which accommodates a wide variety of sizes of adults with minor adjustments in catheter placement position. The pigtail would seem to be less traumatic than the straight designs, although literature supporting this statement is difficult to find. The double-cuff design allows the "deep" cuff to be positioned within or on the rectus muscle or rectus sheath, and the "superficial" cuff rests within the subcutaneous tunnel, analogous to the cuff of an HD catheter.

INDICATIONS AND CONTRAINDICATIONS FOR PERITONEAL DIALYSIS CATHETER PLACEMENT

Exclusionary criteria for radiologic placement are similar to those for many interventional procedures and include an uncorrectable bleeding diathesis, a febrile state, and lack of a signed consent form. It also should be kept in mind that patients with end-stage renal disease (ESRD) can have many inherent deficiencies throughout the coagulation system that are not detectable by routine testing of standard coagulation parameters, such as prothrombin time, activated partial thromboplastin time, and platelet count (7). These defects often impact on platelet function and, hence, clot formation. The best defense against this problem is to begin with a "well-dialyzed" patient. Desmopressin (DDAVP), cryoprecipitate, or platelet transfusions may be required to stem postprocedure bleeding, particularly if an artery (i.e., inferior epigastric artery) is transgressed. Percutaneous placement of a PD catheter should be performed on the virgin side of the abdomen, that is, the side without scars or prior surgery, such as an appendectomy, renal transplant, or prior PD catheter. In addition, the comprehensive guidelines for absolute and relative contraindications as set forth by DOQI Clinical Practice Guidelines for PD should be followed (Table 39.1) (8). The nephrologist should screen patients for these criteria before referral (see Chapter 38), but it certainly behooves one to have some concept of these principles to avoid procedures on inappropriate patients.

TECHNIQUE FOR PERCUTANEOUS INSERTION OF A PERITONEAL DIALYSIS CATHETER

Procedures can be performed on an outpatient basis. After obtaining informed consent, prophylactic antibiotic therapy

TABLE 39.1. DOQI GUIDELINES FOR PD CATHETER INSERTION: RELATIVE AND ABSOLUTE CONTRAINDICATIONS

Relative contraindications
  New intraabdominal foreign body (i.e., aortic graft): wait 4 months
  Peritoneal leaks
  Body size limitations
  Intolerance to necessary PD volumes (based on past history)
  Inflammatory or ischemic bowel disease
  Abdominal wall or skin infection
  Morbid obesity
  Severe malnutrition
  Frequent episodes of diverticulitis

Absolute contraindications
  Documented loss of peritoneal function
  Extensive abdominal adhesions
  Physically or mentally incapable patient without appropriate assistant
  Uncorrectable mechanical defect that prevents PD or increases risk of infection (e.g., irreparable hernia, omphalocele, gastroschisis, diaphragmatic hernia, and bladder extrophy)

DOQI, National Kidney Foundation's Dialysis Outcome Quality Initiative; PD, peritoneal dialysis.

consisting of cefazolin (1 g) or ceftriaxone (1 g) is administered intravenously 30 to 60 minutes before the procedure (any broad-spectrum antibiotic can be substituted for these two suggestions). Conscious sedation using midazolam hydrochloride and fentanyl citrate is titrated to the patient's needs under full physiologic monitoring.

The patient's abdomen is prepared and draped. Initial preference is always to place the catheter on the "virgin" side of the abdomen. A starting point for peritoneal access is chosen about 2 to 4 cm superior to and 4 cm lateral to the umbilicus (Fig. 39.1) (9). This region is fully infiltrated both superficially and deep with 1% lidocaine. A 2-cm horizontal incision, approximately the depth of the blade, is made with a no. 11 scalpel. A 15-cm 22-gauge Chiba needle (Cook, Inc., Bloomington, IN, U.S.A.) is advanced from within the incision, along a line parallel to the sagittal plane, at a 45-degree angle to the patient's abdomen, and directed caudally toward the peritoneum. A distinct "loss of resistance" or a "wince" from the patient are both signs that indicate penetration of the peritoneum by the needle. Then 1 to 2 mL of radiographic contrast is injected slowly under fluoroscopic control. If a stain is obtained, the needle is still in the subcutaneous soft tissues and must be advanced until one of the aforementioned signs is realized. If, on the other hand, the contrast flows freely without resistance between loops of bowel, peritoneal access has been achieved and the needle is advanced no farther. The 0.018-inch guidewire from a Micropuncture set (Cook, Inc.) is advanced through the needle and into the peritoneal cavity. The micropuncture sheath then is used to exchange the 0.018-inch guidewire for a 0.035-inch Rosen wire (Cook, Inc.). De

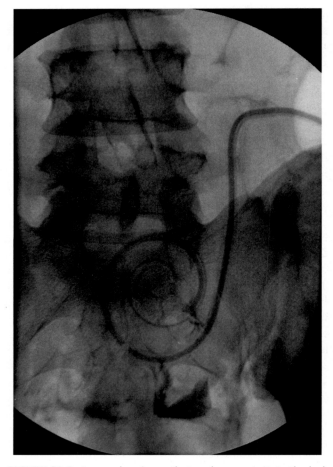

FIGURE 39.2. Image showing catheter placement. Note the lack of any buckling in the catheter. (Reproduced from Savader SJ. Percutaneous radiologic placement of peritoneal dialysis catheters: long-term results. *J Vasc Interv Radiol* 2000;11:965–970, with permission.)

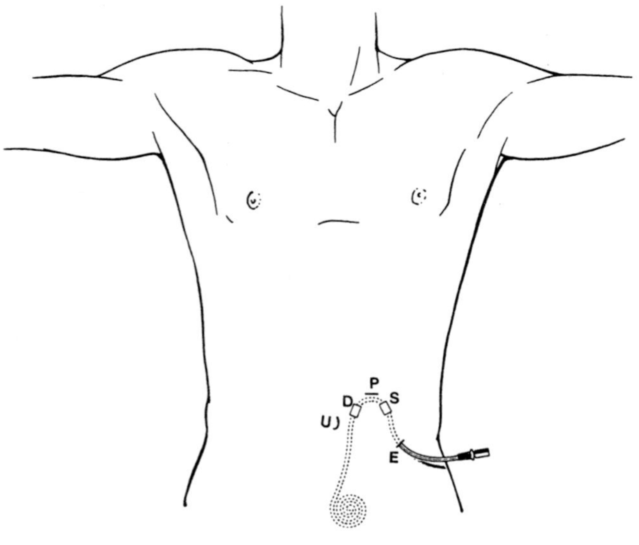

FIGURE 39.1. Diagram showing the relationship between the umbilicus (*U*), primary incision (*P*), deep (*D*) and superficial (*S*) cuffs, and catheter exit site (*E*). (Reproduced from Savader SJ. Percutaneous radiologic placement of peritoneal dialysis catheters: long-term results. *J Vasc Interv Radiol* 2000;11: 965–970, with permission)

pending on the length of the needle tract, particularly in obese patients, the standard 10-cm-long micropuncture sheath may not be long enough to reach from the skin to the peritoneal cavity. For this reason, it is beneficial to have extra-long (20-cm; special order product) micropuncture sheaths available, if possible.

The sheath–dilator assembly from the catheter kit is advanced, without predilatation, over the 0.035-inch guidewire and into the pelvis. The dilator is removed, and the flushed PD catheter is wiped using a wet gauze and is advanced through the sheath into the pelvis (Fig. 39.2). A radiopaque line on many of the catheters allows easy visualization of the orientation of the device. The catheter can be gently rotated if necessary until it is oriented properly, tension free, and the "pig-tailed" peritoneal section is reformed.

Attention then is directed to creation of the subcutaneous tunnel. The tunnel should be oriented at about a 45-degree angle caudal to the peritoneal access site and long enough so that the proximal cuff on the catheter is 4 to 5 cm from the exit site. The tunnel and exit site should be oriented to avoid skin folds, scars, and the belt line (Fig. 39.1).

The soft tissues again are infiltrated generously with 1% lidocaine, and the tunneling device is used in the standard fashion, creating the tunnel from the peritoneal access site to the skin exit site. The peel-away sheath is removed while the catheter is held in place. The catheter is attached to the tunneling device and pulled through the tunnel without reducing the "loop." A 4-0 Vicryl (Ethicon, Johnson and Johnson, Sommerville, NJ, U.S.A.) suture is passed through the Dacron fibers of the deep cuff, and the needle is subsequently passed through the rectus sheath or deep subcutaneous tissues and recovered (Fig. 39.3). The deep cuff of the catheter is gently advanced onto the rectus sheath while applying traction at the exit site to reduce the loop in the catheter. When the loop is reduced, the catheter is checked fluoroscopically for proper placement and orientation. The 4-0 Vicryl suture is then tied, securing the deep cuff. The peritoneal access site is closed at the subcutaneous level with additional 4-0 Vicryl suture and superficially with 2-0 Ethilon (Ethicon, Johnson and Johnson) suture. The catheter is secured at the skin exit site with 2-0 Ethilon suture, and an antimicrobial ointment is applied followed by a sterile dressing.

After completion of the procedure, patients should be recovered for a minimum of 2 hours or until they have meet an institution's requirements for conscious sedation recovery. During this period, patients should be seen by a PD nurse. At this time, the patients can receive "care and handling" instructions for their PD catheter. In addition, while this conversation is proceeding, a liter of dialysate can be passed through the new PD catheter and gravity drained to flush any blood clots from the peritoneum and to ensure that the catheter is functional before the patient is discharged.

Patients should receive information about how to contact the interventional radiologist for concerns or mechanical problems with the catheter. Patients are seen in 10 days, at which time their wounds are checked and sutures removed (if the wound is adequately healed).

Peritoneal dialysis can be initiated at the discretion of the referring nephrologist and typically is based on the patient's immediate need to begin treatment or on the presence or absence of a working HD access site. It is best if use of the PD catheter can be delayed 4 to 6 weeks after the time of placement. This will allow for greater healing of the transabdominal tract and reduce the incidence of dialysate leakage during use of the catheter. If the patient must initiate PD immediately or within the 4- to 6-week window after the procedure is performed, multiple low-volume exchanges should be used rather than the typical four exchanges per day with a 4-hour dwell time. Twelve-hour overnight dwells

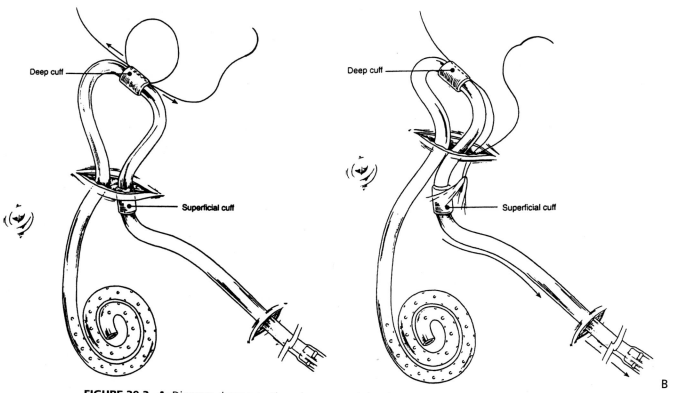

A

B

FIGURE 39.3. A: Diagram demonstrating placement of the absorbable suture into the deep cuff of the peritoneal dialysis catheter. **B**: Securing of the cuff and catheter to the deep tissues of the anterior abdominal wall. The catheter is subsequently pulled in the direction of the arrows and the suture is tied. (Reproduced from Savader SJ. Percutaneous radiologic placement of peritoneal dialysis catheters: long-term results. *J Vasc Interv Radiol* 2000;11:965–970, with permission).

should be avoided until the integrity of the transabdominal tract is confirmed.

COMPLICATIONS (SEE ALSO CHAPTER 38)

Procedure-Related Complications

Procedure-related complications include peritonitis, sepsis, bowel transgressions, abdominal wall hematoma, catheter malfunction, and dialysate leakage.

Postprocedure peritonitis can occur in 4% to 5% of cases and can occur as a result of inadequate patient preparation, contamination of any of the instruments used (or of the catheter itself) during the procedure, or perforation of the colon. If there is any suspicion that the colon has been violated, the procedure should be terminated and the patient admitted for overnight observation. Prophylactic antibiotics should be considered; however, with the emergence of an ever-increasing variety of resistant organisms, the option to begin antibiotics only after an elevated white blood cell count or fever is documented might be considered more prudent. Aggressive intraperitoneal and intravenous antibiotic therapy is a necessity for peritonitis, but catheter salvage may not be possible in most cases (9,10). Sepsis generally necessitates catheter removal. The use of intraperitoneal dialysate or carbon dioxide to help separate the anterior abdominal wall from the viscera, and thus decrease the risk of a bowel perforation during catheter insertion, has been described (11,12). Carbon dioxide could possibly be the better of the two agents because it will collect anteriorly, thus truly separating the anterior abdominal wall from the loops of bowel. Fluids, on the other hand, provide a medium for the bowel loops to float within and may not provide the same degree of separation as with gas. Carbon dioxide might be particularly helpful in patients without a virgin abdomen, but this remains to be demonstrated.

Strict adherence to the operating room principles of sterile technique and limited room access should be observed. The patient should wear a cap and mask and should be shielded from the operating field with a divider and drape. In addition, the catheter should not be allowed to lay on the procedure table unprotected. Rather, it should be placed aside wrapped within a sterile drape or towel until it is ready to be inserted.

Catheter malfunction is uncommon and can occur secondary to excessive intraperitoneal bleeding, with clot formation around or within the catheter, or secondary to a kink in the device. Postplacement flushing of the peritoneum with dialysate will minimize clot-related dysfunction. Whether low-dose thrombolytics can be used safely immediately after the procedure to remedy this problem has yet to be demonstrated. The incidence of catheter kinking should be minimized with fluoroscopic guidance, but if it occurs, it would be addressed in the standard fashion (i.e.,

guidewire or catheter manipulation with replacement over a guidewire, if necessary).

Abdominal wall hematomas occur in 0% to 7% of cases (9,10). They are most likely to occur in those in whom the inferior epigastric artery is transgressed but also can be seen in patients with ESRD-associated bleeding diatheses. Avoidance of this complication necessitates knowledge of anterior abdominal wall anatomy, attention to anatomic landmarks, and some good old-fashioned luck.

The leakage of dialysate from the peritoneal cavity around the catheter can occur in up to 5% to 24% of patients (6,13–17). Placing the catheter 3 months before it is needed most effectively minimizes this complication. Previous investigators have reported placing the catheter up to 12 months before use, tunneling the entire device, and then exposing the hub at the time the catheter is to be used.

Late (Nonprocedure) Complications

Late complications associated with PD catheters are not dependent on the placement technique but rather on the nature of the device itself and the care and handling the catheter receives. This group of complications includes mechanical dysfunction from spontaneous catheter repositioning, adhesions, or omental wrapping; spontaneous catheter or cuff extrusion; and (delayed) peritonitis.

Mechanical dysfunction, collectively occurring at a rate of 9% to 20%, can occur from a number of different causes (8,13,14,18). The PD catheter may spontaneously undergo repositioning from a dependent to a nondependent portion of the abdomen, effectively reducing dialysate return at the end of the dwell. Numerous techniques have been described for catheter repositioning, but returning the catheter tip to a dependent position behind the omentum is all but impossible (19). Adhesions or omental wrappings can trap the catheter within a small volume of peritoneal cavity, resulting in pain during dialysate instillation or an inability to tolerate adequate dialysate volumes to perform effective PD. Fortunately, this can be addressed with a noninvasive procedure termed *guidewire manipulation*. Savader and colleagues demonstrated that 75% of patients can achieve at least one period of long-term catheter patency following this simple and inexpensive procedure, with primary 6- and secondary 12-month patencies of 0.54 (19).

Catheter or cuff extrusion is relatively uncommon but can occur when continuous pressure is applied to the catheter by normal bowel activity. Stitching the deep cuff of the PD catheter to the rectus sheath is not an absolute guarantee against this event. It is suggested, however, that all attempts be made to place the catheter so that the body is straight and not buckled within the peritoneal cavity. This will help to minimize the pressure applied to the catheter by the bowel, which can contribute to extrusion of the device.

Infection related to a PD catheter can occur in 6% to 30% of patients (6,13,14). Late episodes of peritonitis are the most devastating PD catheter–related complication. The mean cumulative risk of developing peritonitis *after* initiation of PD is 60% to 80% during the first 12 months, and recurrent peritonitis is problematic in 20% to 30% of patients (20,21). Peritonitis can result in catheter loss for 9% of patients (13) and has an associated mortality rate of 6% (15). I recently reported a non–procedure-related peritonitis rate of 2.3 infections per 1,000 catheter days with percutaneous radiologic placement of PD catheters, a figure well within that described in current literature for other placement techniques (9,11,15,18,20,21). Our incidence of exit-site infections at 0.52 episodes per 1,000 catheter days was also well within accepted limits (9).

CATHETER PATENCY (SURVIVAL)

The primary goal of catheter placement, for whatever purpose that device might actually serve, is to provide reliable access until the patient's needs no longer require it. Because catheters often can be placed by many different techniques, it is important to compare catheter patency ("survival") to determine whether one technique offers clear advantages over another. An often unfortunate result of this type of data search is the realization not all researchers report survival in the same manner, despite well-defined methods for doing so. Catheter survivals can best be compared when reported using the technique of life-table analysis or the Kaplan–Meier method for survival analysis.

Savader and colleagues, using a Kaplan–Meier survival analysis, reported 6-, 12-, and 24- month probabilities of catheter survival of 0.89 [95% confidence intervals (CI), 0.74 to 1.0], .81 (95% CI, 0.61–1.0), and 0.81 (95% CI, 0.61–1.0), respectively, after percutaneous insertion. The mean and median catheter survivals at the end of the study period were 320 and 289 days, respectively. The range for catheter survival was 33 to 823 days. In another radiologic series, Jacobs and colleagues reported a 20% overall failure rate for 45 PD catheters placed using a strictly percutaneous technique, with 63% still functional at the end of the study period (10). Catheter survival in these radiologic studies would seem to be comparable to that achieved by others reporting surgical and endoscopic placement techniques. Direct comparisons are difficult, however, because most investigators have failed to use a consistent or standardized method to determine catheter survival. Rubin and colleagues reported a 50% loss of catheters at 300 days after surgical placement (18). Cronen and colleagues reported a mean catheter survival of 2.2 months after surgical placement (17). Nissenson and colleagues noted a 12% and 20% replacement rate at 12 and 24 months postplacement, respectively, in a large surgical group (14). Allon and co-workers placed 154 catheters using a percutaneous endoscopic technique with 12- and 24-month catheter survival rates of 65% and 49%, respectively (11). These data suggest that

catheter survival is variable, at best. (See also Chapter 38 for surgery/laparoscopy technique comparisons.)

EVALUATION AND TREATMENT OF THE DYSFUNCTIONAL PERITONEAL DIALYSIS CATHETER

Physicians who place PD catheters are guaranteed to see patients with poor or nonfunctioning catheters. Mechanical catheter malfunction can occur in 6% to 26% of patients with PD catheters, and this can occur by a number of different mechanisms (22–24). PD catheters can undergo spontaneous repositioning into an unfavorable position for efficient dialysis (10%–30%). PD catheters can become loculated within adhesions, omentum, or a fibrinous sheath (15%), thus reducing the surface area available for dialysis and, in fact, rendering PD impossible. In addition, dialysis actually can become quite painful (17%) because of the stretching of adhesions and mesentery. Patients can present with any single complaint or a multiplicity of PD catheter–related problems.

Evaluation of the PD catheter should begin with a problem-focused history. Painful, limited-volume dialysate infusions are symptoms of a "trapped" catheter. A catheter that will instill but not return dialysate indicates that a one-way valve mechanism is occurring, be it a fibrinous sheath or a partial trapping of the catheter by an anatomic structure. Right or left upper-quadrant pain with or without associated ipsilateral shoulder pain often indicates that the catheter has repositioned itself into this location. Mild to moderate pain experienced while the entire prescribed volume of dialysate is instilled, followed by painless return, can indicate that the patient is trying to instill the dialysate too rapidly or that the dialysate being used is too cold. A febrile state, hypotension, continuous abdominal pain, or a tender abdomen on physical examination can be indications of peritonitis. Arrangements should be made for these patients to see their nephrologist immediately, that is, before leaving the hospital.

The next step is radiologic evaluation of the catheter. Some PD catheters are radiolucent, and contrast will have to be injected to visualize them adequately. The catheter should be scanned for any kinks that could impair flow. These are most likely to occur where the catheter traverses the peritoneum and enters the peritoneal cavity. Unfortunately, if this is identified, little can be done from a noninvasive standpoint, and catheter revision most likely will be necessary.

If the patient's primary symptoms are painful dialysate infusion and an inability to instill the required volumes or to recover that volume after PD has been complete, then it is quite possible that a simple procedure will greatly improve or resolve the problem. Many investigators have reported PD catheter "repositioning" (22,25–27). In this simple technique, a device, such as a malleable rod, guidewire, cannula, or tip-deflecting wire, is inserted into the catheter and used to redirect or reposition the catheter's tip into a more favorable position for PD. Results are variable and reportedly range from 33% to 77% (20,23,26,27). As noted for catheter patency data, reporting standards on this subject are not commonly followed up, and it is often difficult to cull out true figures that are helpful or in a form that will allow comparison among various reports.

I have described a variation of this simple technique in which a hydrophilic guidewire is inserted, under sterile conditions, through the PD catheter's lumen and into the peritoneal cavity. The guidewire is advanced until the PD catheter buckles or the patient experiences abdominal pain (the abdominal pain usually can be avoided by simply redirecting the wire into a different region of the abdomen). This process is repeated two to four times. The catheter most likely will return to the same position from which it started. This technique is not terribly effective at actually "repositioning" the catheter back into the pelvis and behind the mesentery, but that is not necessarily the goal.

Let me explain. For the variety of symptoms I have mentioned here as appropriate for treatment in this fashion, the fact that the catheter may not lie in its original position most likely is not the cause for the dysfunction. Mechanical catheter dysfunction most commonly occurs because the functional end of the catheter is "trapped." For example, it may lie within a small peritoneal space defined by adhesions and matted loops of bowel, or omentum may have insinuated itself around the catheter. This would effectively exclude the greater part of the peritoneum from participating in the PD process and preventing recovery of dialysate after the dwell time is completed. In these cases, the necessity is not to get the catheter back into the most dependent part of the pelvis; rather, it is to free the catheter from the surrounding soft tissues.

It has been well documented that guidewire manipulation can rescue a significant number of PD catheters with the above-mentioned problem and that success rates are dependent on the "age" of the PD catheter and the number of manipulations the patient receives. Savader and colleagues defined an early and late catheter failure as one that occurred less than 30 days and more than 30 days after (surgical) placement, respectively (19). Patients with *early* catheter failures and a *single* manipulation (one procedure) achieved a durable (>30 days' patency) success rate of 25%, with a mean patency of 81 days. Patients with a *late* catheter failure and a *single* manipulation achieved a durable success rate of 65% with a mean patency of 159 days. Patients with an *early* catheter failure and *multiple* manipulations (typically two procedures) achieved a durable success rate of 50% with a mean patency of 98 days. Patients with a *late* catheter failure who underwent *multiple* manipulations had durable success rate of 82% with a mean patency of 267 days. A Kaplan–Meier survival analysis from this study yielded primary 3, 6, and 12-month patency rates of 0.61, 0.54, and 0.11, respectively; secondary 3, 6, and 12-month patency rates were 0.75, 0.69, and 0.54, respectively. One of 23 patients (34 manipulations) developed postprocedure peritonitis resulting in catheter loss. These data clearly indicate that catheters that fail "late" and treated with at least two attempts at guidewire manipulation have the greatest chance for return of long-term patency.

SUMMARY

Peritoneal dialysis catheters can be placed efficiently and expediently in an interventional radiology suite without compromising patient care, sterility, pain control, complications, or long-term catheter patency. In addition, interventionists can handle a great number of the mechanical problems that befall these devices using a simple guidewire technique. Although not perfect, guidewire manipulation can result in a very respectable salvage rate for mechanically impaired PD catheters. The cost is minimal, as is the time invested by the patient and interventionist. The complication rate is low and the outcome, particularly in PD catheters that fail late, is almost always positive.

REFERENCES

1. Ganter G. Uber die Beseitigung giftiger Stoffe aus dem Blute durch Dialyse. *Muench Med Wochenschr* 1923;70:1478–1480.
2. Fine J, Frank H, Seligman AM. The treatment of acute renal failure by peritoneal irrigation. *Ann Surg* 1946;124:857–875.
3. Brescia MJ, Cimino JE, Appel K, et al. Chronic hemodialysis using venipuncture and a surgically created arteriovenous fistula. *N Engl J Med* 1966;275:1089–1092.
4. Erben J, Kvasnicka J, Bastecky J, et al. Experience with routine use of subclavian vein cannulation in hemodialysis. *Proc Eur Dial Transplant Assoc* 1969;6:59–64.
5. U.S. Renal Data System (USRDS). *USRDS 1999 annual report.* Section C. Methods of treatment. Ann Arbor, MI: USRDS Coordinating Center, 1999:C2.
6. Baillie GR, Eisele G. Continuous ambulatory peritoneal dialysis: a review of its mechanics, advantages, complications, and areas of controversy. *Ann Pharmacother* 1992;26:1409–1420.
7. Zachee P, Vermylen J., Boogaerts MA. Hematologic aspects of end-stage renal failure. *Ann Hematol* 1994;69:33–40.
8. National Kidney Foundation Dialysis Outcome Quality Initiative (NKF-DOQI). *Clinical Practice guidelines for peritoneal dialysis adequacy.* New York: National Kidney Foundation, 1997: 80–82.
9. Savader SJ. Percutaneous radiologic placement of peritoneal dialysis catheters: long-term results. *J Vasc Interv Radiol* 2000;11: 965–970.
10. Jacobs IG, Gray RR, Elliott DS, et al. Radiologic placement of peritoneal dialysis catheters: preliminary experience. *Radiology* 1992;182:251–255.
11. Allon M, Soucie JM, Macon EJ. Complications with permanent peritoneal dialysis catheters: experience with 154 percutaneously placed catheters. *Nephron* 1988;48:8–11.
12. Rosen DM, Lam AM, Chapman M, et al. Methods of creating

pneumoperitoneum: a review of techniques and complications. *Obstet Gynecol Surv* 1998;53:167–174.

13. Gloor HJ, Nichols WK, Sorkin MI, et al. Peritoneal access and related complications in continuous ambulatory peritoneal dialysis. *Am J Med* 1983;74:593–598.

14. Nissenson AR, Gentile DE, Soderblom RE, et al. Morbidity and mortality of continuous ambulatory peritoneal dialysis: regional experience and long-term prospects. *Am J Kidney Dis* 1986;7: 229–234.

15. Robison RJ, Leapman SB, Wetherington GM, et al. Surgical considerations of continuous ambulatory peritoneal dialysis. *Surgery* 1984;96:723–729.

16. Piraino B, Bernardini J, Sorkin M. The influence of peritoneal catheter exit-site infections on peritonitis, tunnel infections, and catheter loss in patients on continuous ambulatory peritoneal dialysis. *Am J Kidney Dis* 1986;8:436–440.

17. Cronen PW, Moss JP, Simpson T, et al. Tenckhoff catheter placement: surgical aspects. *Am Surg* 1985;51:627–629.

18. Rubin J, Adair CM, Raju S, et al. The Tenckhoff catheter for peritoneal dialysis: an appraisal. *Nephron* 1982;32:370–374.

19. Savader SJ, Lund G, Scheel PJ, et al. Guide wire directed manipulation of malfunctioning peritoneal dialysis catheters: a critical analysis. *J Vasc Interv Radiol* 1997;8:957–963.

20. Linblad AS, Novak JW, Nolph KD, et al. The 1987 USA National CAPD registry report. *Trans Am Soc Artif Intern Organs* 1988;34:150–156.

21. Pollock CA, Ibels LS, Caterson RJ, et al. Continuous ambulatory peritoneal dialysis: eight years experience at a single center. *Medicine* 1989;68:293–308.

22. Moss JS, Minda SA, Newman GE, et al. Malpositioned peritoneal dialysis catheters: a critical reappraisal of correction by stiff-wire manipulation. *Am J Kidney Dis* 1990;15:305–308.

23. Nissenson AR, Gentile DE, Soderblom RE, et al. Medical Review Board, NCC 34, Los Angeles, California. *Am J Kidney Dis* 1986; 8:229–234.

24. Maher ER, Stevens J, Murphy C, et al. Comparison of two methods of Tenckhoff catheter insertion. *Nephron* 1988;48:87–88.

25. Seigel RL, Nosher JL, Gesner LR. Peritoneal dialysis catheters: repositioning with a new fluoroscopic technique. *Radiology* 1994; 199:899–901.

26. Degesys GE, Miller GA, Ford KK, et al. Tenckhoff peritoneal dialysis catheters: the use of fluoroscopy in management. *Radiology* 1985;154:819–820.

27. Jaques P, Richey W, Mandel S. Tenckhoff peritoneal dialysis catheter: cannulography and manipulation. *AJR Am J Roentgenol* 1980;135:83–86.

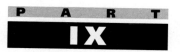

CURRENT INNOVATIVE
CONCEPTS

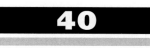

VASCULAR ACCESS CENTERS

AN INNOVATIVE APPROACH FOR VASCULAR ACCESS CARE

W. PERRY ARNOLD
SANFORD D. ALTMAN
GERALD A. BEATHARD

BACKGROUND

Placing and maintaining accesses to the vascular system traditionally have been hospital-based services using both surgical (since 1962) and percutaneous (since 1988) techniques. Initially, surgical thrombectomy, with or without correction of flow-limiting stenoses, was the only option available for clotted grafts and fistulae. Although the surgical approach was technically successful at recanalization, long-term patency was less than desirable. Attempts at percutaneous declotting with prolonged thrombolytic infusion were fraught with complications and yielded poor results (1,2). By the early 1990s, with the advent of high-pressure balloons and pulse spray catheters and the availability of urokinase, percutaneous declotting of failed vascular accesses delivered outcomes similar to or better than conventional surgery (3–5). At the same time, interventional radiologists were becoming increasingly aware of the special needs of dialysis patients, and image-guided catheter placement became more prevalent (6,7). Many studies documented improved catheter placement with lower morbidity and mortality compared with non–image-guided catheter placement in the operating room. The ability to cannulate the internal jugular vein proximally with ultrasound guidance, sparing the subclavian vein from future stenosis and thrombosis, was an added benefit for the dialysis patient. Today many techniques exist, as reviewed in prior chapters, to treat dialysis accesses percutaneously. Do these endovascular procedures need to be performed in a hospital, or can they be performed in an outpatient setting? What are the considerations in developing a freestanding interventional access center? What are the most cost effective and clinically successful techniques to deliver care at a freestanding center? This chapter attempts to answer these questions and will (a) introduce the concept of focused and dedicated access care in a freestanding outpatient facility, (b) discuss startup con-

siderations, (c) set forth facility requirements, and (d) describe techniques to optimize vascular access care.

The Philosophy of Focused Care

A dedicated access care facility focuses on all aspects of hemodialysis vascular access care management including preplacement imaging and evaluation, "best access" creation, regular access monitoring, appropriate elective and acute intervention, and continuous quality improvement. The physician focused on access care understands the importance of vascular access for the dialysis patient; it is the patient's lifeline. The goal of focused care is to create the best access for the individual patient to achieve the longest patency with the fewest interventions. Perhaps the single greatest advantage of providing access care outside the traditional hospital setting is the delivery system created. Consider the following two scenarios.

The Hospital-based Model

When a patient requires dialysis and has a clotted access, there is a scurry of activity at the dialysis center without specific coordination. The dialysis technician or nurse notifies the nephrologist, vascular surgeon, or interventionist involved in the patient's care. Then, through a series of phone calls, arrangements are made to treat the patient in the surgical or interventional suite of a nearby hospital, if room time is available. Unfortunately, a busy hospital often does not treat a clotted access as a true emergency. Instead, the patient often is sent to the emergency department for placement of a temporary catheter, allowing elective access declotting at a later date. Although this serves the needs of the busy hospital, it has a negative impact on the dialysis patient and on the overall cost to the health care system. The central vein used for catheter placement (medically unnecessary in >90%) may be damaged for future appropriate access needs; the patient may miss one or more dialysis treatments; or the patient may be admitted to the hospital for acute dialysis and eventual surgery. Even when the patient is treated appropriately and on the same day, the patient may have to wait many hours because of a fully booked schedule or inpatient emergencies that take precedence in the hospital setting. The patient, the dialysis center, and the referring physician are often frustrated with the less than desirable or timely care delivered, and unnecessary medical costs have been incurred.

The Access Center Model

If a freestanding vascular access center is available, the same thrombosis is dealt with in a much different manner. After discovery of a clotted access, a single telephone call is made by the dialysis center to the access center, followed by a facsimile transmission of patient information. The patient then is scheduled for timely access intervention; 2- to 6-hour turnaround time is not unusual. The patient can undergo dialysis later that day if time is available or early the next day. The access center staff discusses specific patient issues with the dialysis center. These include the results of monthly laboratory tests (potassium, urea reduction ratio, Kt/V, international normalized ratio), post-thrombectomy dialysis plans including day and shift time (because many busy dialysis facilities must assign a station for dialysis at a set time), and patient transportation issues. In more than 90% of the procedures, percutaneous recanalization is successful, and use of the same graft or fistulae for dialysis is continued. In the remainder of cases, when percutaneous intervention is unsuccessful or not appropriate, the patient is discharged from the center with a dialysis catheter along with an organized plan for future coordinated access surgery or intervention. Because ultrasound and fluoroscopic guidance are always available at the access center (unlike some hospital surgery suites), a tunneled catheter access placed in accordance with the National Kidney Foundation's Dialysis Outcomes Quality Initiative (DOQI) guidelines will give the patient the best catheter for high-flow, long-term dialysis. Patient follow-up by the access center is dialysis specific. Issues addressed may include whether or not the flow rates are normal, the kinetics have improved, the patient still has prolonged bleeding post dialysis, and the arm is still swollen.

As in any specialty, focused care leads to improved technical expertise and clinical judgment by the access center team, which, in turn, reduces procedure times and improves outcomes. The sharing of outcome data and anatomic information with referring surgeons and nephrologists improves current and future access care. Patients appreciate such focused care and develop trusting relationships with access center personnel. The access center physician often becomes a patient's first resource when access problems arise.

The History of Focused Care

A focused approach for percutaneous intervention of clotted accesses was first suggested in the late 1980s and early 1990s by interventional radiologists, including the groups Bookstein (4) and Kumpe (5). They were able to demonstrate that through coordinated interventional care, clotted accesses could be successfully treated percutaneously, yielding acceptable patency in a manner less invasive for the patient and at the same time preserving outflow veins for future surgical revision. In the early 1990s, Gerald Beathard, one of the first specialists in interventional nephrology, established an in-hospital interventional nephrology service in Austin, Texas, to deliver hemodialysis access care primarily for outpatients. It was funded and underwritten by the hospital and used a dedicated operating room suite for the delivery of service. Initially, Dr. Beathard percutaneously declotted accesses by pharmacomechanical thrombolysis using pulse spray urokinase. He then developed a technique for mechanical thrombolysis with pulse spray saline, reporting patency rates equal to or better than urokinase thrombolysis and interventions by his surgical counterparts (8). After Turmel-Rodrigues and colleagues showed improved long-term patency of accesses that are carefully monitored and aggressively treated by endovascular techniques (9), the groups of Schwab, Trerotola, Beserab, Strauch and O'Connell, Neyra, and others (10–14) focused attention on techniques to identify access stenoses, which occur in more than 80% of clotted accesses before causing thromboses.

In 1994, Sanford Altman, an interventional radiologist in Miami, Florida, who recognized the importance of regular access monitoring and prethrombotic intervention, developed the first alternative site to hospital-based access care. The fact that many end-stage renal disease (ESRD) patients were reluctant to travel to a hospital for treatment led to the development of a mobile access interventional service. As a major component of this service, Dr. Altman educated nephrologists and dialysis centers on the importance of access monitoring combined with elective intervention. Services eventually were provided in more than 300 dialysis centers in eight states. Dialysis centers were instructed on monitoring techniques to identify access stenosis before thrombosis, including charting dynamic venous pressures, conducting physical examinations of the graft site, noting symptoms such as prolonged bleeding, enlarging aneurysm/pseudoaneurysm and arm swelling, and measuring static venous pressures and flow dilution. Based on abnormal hemodynamic indicators, patients were referred for imaging and intervention. A mobile interventional suite would be sent to the dialysis center, where the referred patients would be evaluated and treated by an interventional radiologist. Dramatic results were obtained, documenting a 1-year secondary patency of 92% and a 60% reduction in access thrombosis without an increase in overall procedures performed per patient-year. Patients with Kt/V less than 1.2

increased from 1.13 before percutaneous transluminal angioplasty (PTA) to 1.4 post-PTA (15). Patient satisfaction and compliance were high, with more than 95% of referred patients appearing for evaluation in the mobile clinic. This was a significant improvement compared with the compliance of patients referred for elective intervention in the hospital setting. Although the clinical results were encouraging, the mobile service was not viable from a business perspective. With improved monitoring and increased elective interventions, procedure needs declined precipitously. The cost of maintaining a fully stocked interventional suite on the road, with a physician and crew, was greater than the revenue generated.

With thousands of patients receiving treatment safely in the mobile setting and even greater numbers of percutaneous procedures being safely performed on an outpatient basis in a hospital setting, it was evident that non–hospital-based freestanding access centers were viable from a patient care perspective. In 1997, the first dedicated freestanding outpatient dialysis vascular access center was opened in Baltimore, Maryland, under the direction of W. Perry Arnold, an interventional radiologist. Working in close cooperation with referring nephrologists and vascular surgeons in the region, Dr. Arnold was able to establish a focused coordinated delivery system meeting, in some instances exceeding, the DOQI guidelines for vascular access placement and maintenance (16). Following these initial successes, freestanding access centers have become a "hot topic" for consideration by dialysis access care providers.

STARTUP CONSIDERATIONS

Feasibility Studies

A physician evaluating the possibility of creating a freestanding vascular access center in his or her community must carefully analyze whether such a center would be a viable business. This can be accomplished by looking at the availability of existing services and potential patient volumes. Among other things, local nephrologists, vascular surgeons, and dialysis center personnel should be queried as to their satisfaction with the quality of available services. To justify the expense of a freestanding facility, there must be a reasonable assumption that the workload will be sufficient for full-time operation. Personnel will not be used for multiple purposes, as in a hospital. If the access center is being developed to support a full-time physician, a minimum referral base of 750 to 1,000 dialysis patients will be needed. On the assumption that the average dialysis patient undergoes 1.2 interventions annually, this would mean approximately 1,000 patient encounters during the first year. The dedicated center must routinely handle seven to eight cases during an average 8-hour workday, about one per hour. In any given location, the optimum patient population will

depend on a number of variables, such as the percentage of fistulae within the population, the degree of surveillance for venous stenosis being practiced, the mortality rate, the transplantation rate, and the chronic catheter use rate. In all events, the patient base will have to expand over time for a center to remain financially viable because improved patient care will reduce the number of procedures required per patient per year. Lower reimbursement rates for prethrombotic interventions will replace higher reimbursements for declotting procedures. Similarly, an expected increase in the creation of native arteriovenous fistulae, as recommended by DOQI and realized outside the United States, also will reduce the total number of access procedures per patient-year.

If the analysis has determined that there is a need for such a center, such efforts have likely identified the best geographic location for the center based on patient demographics, competition, and referral sources. Additional considerations governing the future site of the access center should include proximity to a hospital in case of emergency, traffic patterns, and space availability.

Legal Issues

A law firm should be consulted to answer questions pertaining to state and local requirements for licensing or obtaining a certificate of need and to advise on the legal structure of the entity. Federal and state prohibitions against self-referral, kickbacks, and the corporate practice of medicine will impact on who can own a financial interest in the center, who can provide care in the center, and who can refer patients to the center. A legal opinion should be obtained if the center is to be owned and operated by a multispecialty group practice or by outside investors. If the center is to be owned or operated by a group practice, the lawyer might advise on issues concerning equity participation, performance of procedures, variations in pay, and scope of duties. Are there restrictive covenants in place that may prevent certain physicians from providing care in the center? Limited liability and tax considerations should be addressed. The attorney also may advise on the implications of affiliating the center with a hospital or of directly competing with a hospital. Should this facility operate as an office or a Medicare approved ambulatory surgery center? Certainly, all these issues do not need be resolved before determining the feasibility of opening a freestanding access facility; however, they must be addressed during the startup phase.

Business Plan

As part of the initial planning, the physician should develop a business plan, perhaps with the assistance of an accountant or business advisor. This exercise will help to quantify the philosophical outlook and the scope of services to be provided at the access facility. The business plan should include a mission statement. Ideally, this is a statement that can be placed on the wall for the physicians, staff, and patients to see daily. We hope the center will be a "center of excellence" that is interested primarily in quality care rather than being business driven to maximize profits. That being said, the primary purpose of the business plan is to estimate the financial viability of the center based on a number of assumptions and projections.

Once the scope of service has been determined, the expected revenue per procedure should be ascertained by consulting local billing and collection personnel and the local Medicare carrier. Next, the physician must try to estimate the expected procedure mix. Although this varies from region to region, a good rule of thumb would be to assume that of the total yearly patient encounters, 35% to 40% will be declotting procedures, 35% to 40% will be angiography with or without balloon angioplasty, and 20% to 30% will be dialysis catheter procedures. The number of procedures performed per year will be related to the patient base and affected by the number of grafts, fistulae, and catheters in place. Once this has been determined, the revenue side of the equation is in place.

Both fixed and variable expenses should be estimated. These costs will vary greatly, depending on whether the center will be outfitted as an office or as an ambulatory surgery center; whether the equipment will be new or used, purchased or leased; whether there will be more than one interventional suite; and whether the center will include a vascular laboratory. Real estate costs, staffing requirements, patient transportation needs, billing and collection arrangements, information management systems, and inventory costs also will impact the expense side of the equation. Once the business plan is put together, the physician will be able to determine whether a freestanding vascular access center will be financially viable in his or her community.

If the answer is yes, the next determination is how to fund its development and growth. The initial investment will likely be between $500,000 and $1,000,000. An additional $250,000 to $500,000 may be needed until referrals have stabilized and cash flow is consistent. Experience has shown that this will be likely to occur when 1,000 procedures are being performed per year.

Personnel

The benefits of a freestanding dedicated access center are compromised unless dedicated and skilled personnel staff the facility. Dialysis patients have unique problems that impact considerably on their general management. It is important that personnel at the center understand these patients and their needs. Because ESRD comorbidities will affect the safety and success of the procedures being performed, it is imperative that the staff members know what to do as well as what not to do. Having dedicated, specifically trained persons working as a team provides for the communication

that is essential for optimum vascular access management. To have a full-time physician equivalent, at least two and preferably three interventionists must be available. In addition to the interventionist, three other staff members are needed over the course of each patient encounter. A nurse must be available to premedicate or sedate the patient, if necessary, and to monitor the patient during and after the treatment. If possible, hiring a nurse with previous dialysis center experience is recommended. One radiology technician is needed in the procedure room to handle the fluoroscope and another to assist the physician. All medical personnel must be appropriately licensed. In addition, the center should have adequate clerical personnel to handle scheduling, patient registration, billing, and record keeping. The staff's training, experience, and dedication to service have a great influence on the quality of care delivered.

Operations

The next step is to organize the operating process by developing policies and procedures for all aspects of the practice. These should be memorialized in the form of a written operating manual. The manual should set forth the center's hours of operation and policies with respect to anesthesia, analgesia, and conscious sedation. Job descriptions are mandatory, as are written employment policies. Patient referral and intake forms should be developed as well as the form of report that will be sent to referring physicians and dialysis centers. The manual should reference pertinent local, state, and federal laws such as the Occupational Safety and Health Act (OSHA) guidelines, radiation safety, and licensing requirements. A section should be devoted to the steps to be followed in the case of medical emergencies. Statistically, serious medical complications, including death, will occur, even though center outcomes may be better than those achieved in a hospital setting. One must always be mindful that the dialysis population is at high risk for complications because of their renal failure and comorbidities, such as diabetes and cardiac disease, contributing to a mortality rate of 10% to 20%. Transfer agreements with local hospitals should be documented. Appropriate staff should be advanced cardiac life support (ACLS) certified. A quality assurance program should be implemented for tracking outcomes according to the Society of Cardiovascular and Interventional Radiology (SCVIR) practice standards (17) for dialysis access interventions so that successes, failures, and complications can be appropriately recorded and communicated to the other members of the access care team. The manual also should address patient education and follow-up concerns.

Third-Party Payers

Because the process of negotiating and qualifying for third-party payer contracts may be lengthy, it would be wise to begin well in advance of the center's projected opening date. Consider meeting with payer medical directors or corporate officers to discuss the benefits of focused access care, such as improved outcomes, reduced hospitalizations, and cost savings. Contact the local Medicare carrier and review the International Classification of Diseases (ICD)-9 and Current Procedural Terminology (CPT) codes pertinent to the scope of services to be performed in the center to verify expected reimbursements. If an outside billing service is to be engaged, ask other physicians for references and interview several companies in the area to ascertain their qualifications and experience. Billing for any new service, especially for procedures that traditionally have been either component billed or globally billed in the hospital setting, can be quite complicated. The billing and collection personnel engaged on behalf of the center should have an in-depth understanding of the services performed and the codes to be billed. Payment for procedures will be denied from time to time. To defend the services billed during a review or hearing, operative reports should adequately and consistently reflect all services performed. Billing, collections, accounts receivable, aging, and payment denial reports should be reviewed on a regular basis.

Marketing

A marketing plan should be formulated during the planning stages. The results obtained by other freestanding outpatient vascular access centers may be the best marketing tool. It is imperative to spend time educating local vascular surgeons, nephrologists, dialysis centers, and patients about the benefits of proper access care in a dedicated center. Invite referring physicians to observe a procedure. Treat the nurses at referring dialysis centers to lunch while the access facility's nurses conduct a training seminar. Contact the local chapter of the American Association of Kidney Patients (AAKP) or the local branch of the National Kidney Foundation and offer a lecture for patients. Once the facility is operating, set a date for an "open house" to allow health care providers in the community an opportunity to visit the center. A modest budget for marketing tools such as brochures, business cards, referral pads, or magnets with the center's phone number and address would be well spent.

The Facility

A freestanding dedicated vascular access center should be specifically designed, equipped, supplied and staffed at the level of sophistication required for the limited types of procedures that will be performed. It is possible to do this for a fraction of the cost of the usual hospital angiography suite with no sacrifice in quality. These are the goals of a freestanding access facility: quality patient care and cost savings to the health care system.

Design

Many dialysis patients have some degree of physical disability to be considered when a freestanding facility is planned. Doorways and elevators must accommodate not only wheelchairs but also stretchers and emergency equipment. Maximum barrier protection is essential for vascular access procedures, especially catheter placement. The procedure rooms in a freestanding center should resemble an operating room more than a general angiography suite. Because infection is a major complication of vascular access, a surgical environment is critical. The size of the space required for the construction of a freestanding facility is determined largely by state and federal requirements for medical facilities and certification of an ambulatory surgery center. This usually results in a space comprising more square footage than is practically needed. Patient care areas consisting of at least one procedure room of a 400 square feet minimum and a combination of a patient preparation and recovery area that can accommodate two to three stretchers are essential. Additional needs are for adequate storage, patient reception, clerical staff offices, record storage, dressing rooms, physician offices, and a staff lounge.

A state-of-the-art data management system is necessary to make individualized patient information readily available to the facility staff, referring physicians, and dialysis centers. The system also should be capable of continuously assessing and analyzing quality, costs, and outcomes according to SCVIR guidelines (17).

Equipment

A portable C-arm fluoroscope is the optimum imaging system for dialysis access procedures performed in a freestanding center. The images are excellent, digital subtraction and road mapping are possible, and the price is considerably lower than that of the larger, stationary C-arm found in a hospital angiography suite. The table should be radiolucent so as not to interfere with imaging. It should be movable to allow for ease of setup in the procedure room because access site and procedure type will necessitate different positioning of equipment. The tabletop should be able to move laterally and is extremely valuable if it can float and swivel. Being able to swing the patient in and out of the fluoroscopic field is helpful for economy of time and effort because the operator works and images at the same site. Multidirectional mobile tables are relatively expensive ($25,000–$65,000). An ultrasound device for the placement of central venous catheters is mandatory. This will decrease the time required and enhance the safety of the cannulation of central veins for catheter placement. Monitoring of the patient's electrocardiogram, pulse oximeter, and blood pressure is also required. A full cardiac "crash cart" is also necessary for the infrequent but inevitable patient needing full cardiopulmonary resuscitation.

Supplies

An inventory of catheters, sheaths, wires, and other devices must be stocked; however, because the variety of procedures performed and the number of operators in the dedicated access center are limited, the requisite supply items are relatively minimal compared with a hospital angiography suite. By stocking only supplies that are specifically needed, avoiding duplication and nonessential equipment, considerable savings can be achieved.

Hours of Operation

A successful dedicated facility will have hours of operation that support the dialysis centers. Although some patients can be electively scheduled for evaluation, many require urgent treatment. Because of the need for dialysis, the thrombosed access becomes an emergent problem, especially in the patient with a tendency toward fluid and electrolyte problems. Even though most dialysis units operate three shifts, it is not necessary for the center to offer evening hours. A normal 8-hour day, beginning at 8:00 a.m., will allow the center to receive patients presenting at the early shift and continue to see patients referred from the second shift. Patients from the evening shift can generally be treated the next morning. An evening shift patient with a serious fluid or electrolyte problem will require hospitalization for treatment; fortunately, these will be few. Because dialysis facilities operate on weekends and holidays, a freestanding facility electing to be closed during these periods should arrange for coverage with local hospitals or with other physicians.

Transportation

Transportation is generally not provided as part of the Medicare entitlement program for hemodialysis. Getting to a freestanding center, even if the center is well located, may present problems for some patients, especially for the indigent, elderly, or disabled. For patients to benefit from expedient care, reliable transportation from and to dialysis is needed to maintain the patient's normal schedule. Contracting with a local transport company can ensure that referrals become patients. Although this is an added expense, it is essential to proper patient care.

Techniques

Today's interventional armamentarium is expansive and expensive. Because a hospital-based physician has no incentive to regulate expenses, many interventionists perform procedures unaware of the cost consequences. A hospital may receive payment for certain supplies not reimbursable outside the hospital setting. On the other hand, to remain financially viable, a freestanding center must identify the most cost-efficient means to deliver care and at the same time se-

lect the best procedure for the individual patient. Today there are many devices and techniques available for declotting grafts and fistulae. The goal of every declotting technique is to ensure that the entire clot is removed. If this is accomplished, the technique is successful. Because to date no single technique has proven to yield superior results or to affect outcomes, cost-effectiveness is an important consideration. Current materials and methods used to remove clots may cost $50 to $1,000 or more. Because the reimbursement for declotting in an office or an ambulatory surgery center is fixed regardless of the technique used, the least expensive technique will produce the greatest profitability for the center. That is not to say that more expensive techniques are inappropriate under certain circumstances. The current focus of recanalization procedures has shifted to the more important correction of the underlying cause of thrombosis: stenoses within the access circuit, hypoperfusion causes, coagulopathies, and external mechanical compression.

Aspiration–Extrusion Thrombectomy/Percutaneous Transluminal Angioplasty

W. Perry Arnold developed one of the least expensive access declotting techniques, aspiration–extrusion thrombectomy with PTA (AET/PTA) (18). A modification of aspiration techniques (19,20), AET/PTA can be performed quickly and safely on an outpatient basis. In Dr. Arnold's hands, the mean procedure time is 33 minutes, with an average fluoroscopy time of 8 minutes and an average room time of 1 hour. The procedure requires no thrombolytic drugs or mechanical devices. Major complications are less than 2%. From the standpoint of disposable goods and time needed for completion of a declotting procedure, this has proven to be a time- and cost-efficient procedure. The outcomes exceed the DOQI guidelines of 40% patency at 3 months (16). Dr. Arnold attributes the success of his technique to dilatation of not only the venous anastomosis but also the entire length of the access from the arterial anastomosis to the venous anastomosis during the aspiration and extrusion process. This procedure provides very tight wall contact during PTA of the entire length of the graft to crush mural thrombus and intimal hyperplasia. This loosened tissue then can be removed through the percutaneous entrance sites (aspirated and extruded). Aspiration and extrusion of the thrombus minimize the potential for both arterial and venous emboli by trapping and removing the thrombus from the dialysis circuit.

Dr. Arnold also found that dilating venous outflow stenoses to 8 mm can increase patency safely. In a series of patients presenting with graft thromboses in which the same stenosis in the same access was treated with either a 6-mm or 8-mm balloon at different times of thrombosis, the patency almost doubled when the 8-mm balloon was used (21).

Lyse and Aspirate

Another cost-effective declotting technique, lyse and aspirate, is a modification of the currently popular "lyse and wait" technique (22). Dr. Sanford Altman uses this technique in more than 80% of his recanalization cases. In this technique, 1.5 mg of tissue plasminogen activator (t-PA) in 5 mL of normal saline is used to soften clot but not to reestablish flow. The partially lysed thrombus then is aspirated through two 7-French open-ended sheaths directed toward each other, one positioned in the graft near the arterial anastomosis and the second positioned in the graft near the venous anastomosis. Using a 20-mL syringe, lysed thrombus is aspirated through one sheath with simultaneous injection of saline through the second sheath. This is repeated and reversed until there is no thrombus and only clear saline is aspirated. There appears to be less clot migration into the outflow veins with this technique compared with the traditional lyse and wait technique. Following aspiration, a 7-mm balloon is used to cross the venous anastomosis. Contrast is injected to confirm adequate outflow veins. PTA is performed at the venous anastomosis and venous limb of the graft. The balloon is pulled back to the graft apex, and blood is aspirated from the venous side sheath, confirming a patent venous anastomosis. This sheath then is capped and 1,000 U of heparin is administered. The balloon is reintroduced and advanced across the arterial anastomosis, and arteriography is performed to confirm the size of the inflow artery. Brachial and axillary arteries usually can withstand mild (5–10 atm) inflations with a 7-mm balloon used to dislodge the arterial plug. The inflated balloon then is pulled back toward the apex/midgraft with simultaneous aspiration through the sheath near the arterial anastomosis. In most cases, the platelet plug is aspirated through this sheath. Angiography then is performed from the inflow artery, through the graft, back to the heart. If thrombus is identified, it is aspirated often utilizing a 7-French guiding catheter. The entrance sites are closed with pursestring sutures using 2-0 Prolene. These sutures are removed in 24 hours.

Using this technique, procedure times, technical success, and patency rates [continuous quality improvement (CQI) data] are similar to or better than those reported by others and recommended by DOQI. The cost savings compared with many other techniques is significant.

CONCLUSION

Long-term stability of a dedicated freestanding vascular access center in any community can be achieved only if the center is delivering high-quality patient care. The interventionist focused on dialysis access care should be well versed in all aspects of ESRD and related interventions. Obtain a copy of the DOQI guidelines and refer to them regularly.

Subscribe to radiology, nephrology and surgery journals to stay abreast of the most current access literature. Develop and lead an access management team for your community.

The team should set goals for all aspects of access care, including preplacement evaluation, access creation, access monitoring, and access intervention. The success of this team depends on the level of commitment and frequency of communication among all members. Involvement of vascular surgeons is important because they are responsible for creating the best accesses for patients. It is hoped that DOQI guideline recommendations will be realized and more native arteriovenous fistulae will be created. Nephrologists are responsible for the overall well-being of patients with renal disease and should be encouraged to improve routine access monitoring to allow for timely identification of access stenoses before access thromboses. This will decrease the burden of acute care needs placed on the dialysis center staff when a patient presents with a clotted access. Interventionists are responsible for maintaining access patency by using cost-effective and safe endovascular techniques. Placing and maintaining the access appropriately will reduce the number of hospitalizations and procedures required by the dialysis patient, improving quality of life. Nurses and technologists from the dialysis centers play a vital role in the access team, being most involved in the day-to-day care of dialysis patients. The access center staff is responsible for communicating with referring physicians and dialysis centers to ensure that appropriate referrals are made and that the best care for the patient is delivered. The fact that a procedure can be performed does not necessarily mean that it should be performed. The patient's best interest always should be the team's primary focus. Clinical pathways should be developed by the team to help direct proper access care.

REFERENCES

1. Rodkin RS, Bookstein JJ, Henney DJ, et al. Streptokinase and transluminal angioplasty in the treatment of acutely thrombosed hemodialysis access fistulae. *Radiology* 1983;149:425–428.
2. Graor RA, Risius B, Young JR, et al. Low dose streptokinase for selective thrombolysis: systemic effects and complications. *Radiology* 1984;152:35–39.
3. McNamara TO, Fischer JR. Thrombolysis of peripheral arterial and graft occlusions: improved results with high-dose Urokinase. *AJR Am J Roentgenol* 1985;144:769–775.
4. Bookstein JJ, Fellmeth B, Roberts A, et al. Pulsed-spray pharmacomechanical thrombolysis: preliminary clinical results. *AJR Am J Roentgenol* 1989;152:1097–1100.
5. Kumpe DA, Cohen MA, Durham JD. Treatment of failing and failed hemodialysis access sites: comparison of surgical treatment with thrombolysis/angioplasty. *Semin Vasc Surg* 1992;118–127.
6. Denys BG, Uretsky BF, Reddy PS. Ultrasound-assisted cannulation of the internal jugular vein: a prospective comparison with the external landmark-guided technique. *Circulation* 1993;87:1557–1562.
7. Teichgraber UKM, Benter T, Gebel M, et al. A sonographically

guided technique for central venous access. *AJR Am J Roentgenol* 1997;169:731–733.

8. Beathard GA, Welch BR, Maidment HJ. Mechanical thrombolysis for the treatment of thrombosed hemodialysis access grafts. *Radiology* 1996;200:711–716.

9. Turmel-Rodrigues L, Pengloan J, Blanchier D, et al. Insufficient dialysis shunts: improved long-term patency rates with close hemodynamic monitoring, repeat percutaneous balloon angioplasty, and stent placement. *Radiology* 1993;187:273–278.

10. Schwab SJ, Raymond JR, Saeed M, et al. Prevention of hemodialysis fistula thrombosis: early detection of venous stenosis. *Kidney Int* 1989;36:707–711.

11. Trerotola SO, Scheel PJ, Powe NR, et al. Screening for dialysis access graft malfunction: comparison of physical examination with US. *J Vasc Interv Radiol* 1996;7:15–20.

12. Besarab A, Frinak S, Sherman RA, et al. Simplified measurement of intra-access pressure. *J Am Soc Nephrol* 1998;9:284–289.

13. Strauch BS, O'Connell RS. The role of color Doppler flow imaging in the assessment of the hemodialysis vascular access. *Seminars in Dialysis* 1995;142–146.

14. Neyra NR, Ikizler TA, May RE, et al. Change in access blood flow over time predicts vascular access thrombosis. *Kidney Int* 1998;54:1714–1719.

15. Altman SD, Arthur TS, Altman NR, et al. Maintenance angioplasty of hemodialysis access stenoses in a mobile setting. In: Henry MG, Ferguson RM, eds. *Vascular access for hemodialysis—V.* Chicago: W.L. Gore & Associates and Precept Press, 1997:178.

16. National Kidney Foundation Dialysis Outcomes Quality Initiative (NKF-DOQI). *Clinical practice guidelines for vascular access.* New York: National Kidney Foundation, 1997:58.

17. Aruny JE, Lewis CA, Cardella JF, et al. Quality improvement guidelines for percutaneous management of the thrombosed or dysfunctional dialysis access. *J Vasc Interv Radiol* 1999;10:491–498.

18. Arnold WP. Aspiration and extrusion thrombectomy with percutaneous transluminal angioplasty: technique, efficacy, and patency in hemodialysis access management. *Cardiovasc Interv Radiol* 1999;22(Suppl 2):S120(abst).

19. Turmel-Rodrigues L, Sapoval M, Pengloan J, et al. Manual thromboaspiration and dilation of thrombosed dialysis access: mid-term results of a simple concept. *J Vasc Interv Radiol* 1997;8:813–824.

20. Sharafuddin MJA, Kadir S, Joshi SJ, et al. Percutaneous balloon-assisted aspiration thrombectomy of clotted hemodialysis access grafts. *J Vasc Interv Radiol* 1996;7:177–183.

21. Arnold WP. The effect of venous outflow angioplasty balloon size on primary patency in hemodialysis vascular access graft recanalization. *J Vasc Interv Radiol* 2000;11:182(abst).

22. Cynamon Y, Lakritz PS, Wahl SI, et al. Hemodialysis graft declotting: description of the "lyse and wait" technique. *J Vasc Interv Radiol* 1997;8:825–829.

PHARMACOLOGIC APPROACHES TO PREVENTING HEMODIALYSIS ACCESS FAILURE

JONATHAN HIMMELFARB
MARK D. VANNORSDALL

With the introduction of the external arteriovenous (AV) shunt by Quinton and colleagues in the 1960s, intermittent hemodialysis for the treatment of ESRD became a reality. This early era was characterized by development of the endogenous AV fistula and subsequent development of prosthetic interposition bridge grafts. From the 1960s to the present, there has been a lack of significant technical progress in developing new forms of permanent hemodialysis vascular access. Furthermore, recent data indicate that the cost of monitoring and repairing permanent hemodialysis vascular access in the United States is enormous and continues to increase. Although it is difficult to obtain an accurate estimate of current combined inpatient and outpatient costs for vascular access monitoring and repair, recent estimates suggest that these costs exceed 1 billion dollars per year in the United States alone.

The lack of technical progress in developing new forms of vascular access and the spiraling costs associated with maintaining vascular access have prompted a recent reexamination of the role of pharmacologic approaches to preventing vascular access failure in this patient population. From a pharmacoeconomic perspective, because the costs of maintaining vascular access are so high, any pharmacologic strategies that effectively decrease the development of venous stenosis or thrombosis will have the potential to save thousands of dollars per patient at risk per year. In addition to economic savings, it must be remembered that there are substantial medical and psychological benefits to patients if vascular access failure can be prevented pharmacologically.

VASCULAR ACCESS PHARMACOLOGY

To develop and implement logical pharmacologic strategies for preventing access failure, it is necessary to understand the biology of access failure. A major advance in our understanding of the pathogenesis of vascular access failure oc-

curred with the recognition that most cases are related to the development of pseudointimal or neointimal hyperplasia. This is particularly true for expanded polytetrafluoroethylene (ePTFE) graft failure, the most commonly used permanent vascular access in the United States. Whereas it was recognized that even Scribner shunts could develop intimal hyperplasia (1), most of the time Scribner shunts failed because of a purely thrombotic process (2,3). Similarly, endogenous AV fistulae frequently fail shortly after placement because of a thrombotic process. Even with endogenous AV fistulae, after several months, most failures occur because of the subsequent development of intimal hyperplasia.

The extent to which the development of intimal hyperplasia underlies most cases of ePTFE graft thrombosis became apparent only after the widespread use of angiographic studies that comprehensively evaluate the anatomy associated with graft thrombosis. In earlier surgical series without angiography, an anatomic cause for ePTFE graft thrombosis was demonstrable 40% to 60% at the time of thrombectomy (4,5). In radiologic series, however, ePTFE graft thrombosis occurs in the setting of a stenosis at or distal to the venous anastomosis at least 85% of the time (6). From these observations, the paradigm has developed that thrombosis is the final event but that progressive intimal proliferation is the hidden cause in most cases of graft failure.

The pathophysiology of progressive intimal hyperplasia is complex, and many etiologic factors contribute to its development. It is generally believed that intimal hyperplasia results from an initial vascular injury, which then sets in motion a cascade of biological events (7–9) (Table 41.1). The initial vascular injury may be traumatic and related to the vascular access surgery itself. In the case of prosthetic dialysis grafts, it also has been suggested that repetitive needle cannulation induces injury to the graft (10). Additionally, the constant transmission of arterial pressures to the venous anastomosis, particularly if there is turbulent flow, can lead to progressive injury of the venous wall (11). Compliance

TABLE 41.1. PATHOGENESIS OF INTIMAL HYPERPLASIA

Medial VSMC proliferation
VSMC migration across intima
Intimal VSMC proliferation
Intimal extracellular matrix excretion

VSMC, vascular smooth-muscle cell.

mismatch between the graft and the vein at the anastomosis site contribute to biophysical injury.

A key component of vascular wall injury that contributes to the development of intimal hyperplasia is disruption of endothelial cell integrity and function (7,8). This is particularly important in prosthetic grafts because it has been demonstrated repeatedly that ePTFE grafts fail to endothelialize completely. To date, attempts to improve endothelialization of prosthetic grafts by seeding or sodding endothelial cells in matrix have not been successful (12). Whereas endothelial dysfunction may initiate the process of intimal hyperplasia, the proliferating cell that causes most of the injury is the vascular smooth muscle cell (13,14).

Whereas shear stress, vessel compliance mismatch, and other hemodynamic factors have been suggested as leading to the development of intimal hyperplasia, components of the blood that interact with the vessel wall at a site of injury also may play an important role. Ross and colleagues formulated a "response to injury" hypothesis to explain the development of intimal hyperplasia, which shares common characteristics with the development of atherosclerosis (15). In this hypothesis, platelets play an important role in the response of the vessel wall to injury. Exposure of the subendothelium in injured vascular walls can result in platelet adhesion, with subsequent release of adenosine diphosphate as well as thromboxane A2. A prominent role in this hypothesis also is given to the secretion of platelet-derived growth factor (PDGF) by adherent platelets (15).

The discovery of PDGF in 1974 led to a tremendous expansion in our understanding of how peptide growth factors affect the vascular wall. PDGF is a potent mitogen that causes proliferation and tissue remodeling of the vascular wall (16). Because PDGF has a short half-life in the circulation, it has been thought to act in a paracrine or autocrine fashion near the site of release (17). In addition to being mitogenic for vascular smooth-muscle cells, PDGF has a chemotactic effect that may be particularly important in the migration of vascular smooth-muscle cells during the early phases of intimal hyperplasia formation (16,18).

Initially thought to be a predominantly platelet-derived growth factor, PDGF now is known to be synthesized and secreted by a variety of cell types, including both endothelial cells (19,20) as well as vascular smooth-muscle cells (21). In animal models of arterial vascular injury, the administration of PDGF increases the formation of intimal hyperplasia (21). Alternatively, the use of antibodies to PDGF can reduce intimal hyperplasia formation after vascular injury in animal models (22). It is clear that targeting PDGF-induced development of intimal hyperplasia may be an effective pharmacologic approach to preventing the development of intimal hyperplasia and subsequent vascular access failure in hemodialysis patients.

In addition to PDGF, other growth factors have been established as important in the development of intimal hyperplasia (Fig. 41.1). In particular, basic fibroblast growth factor (bFGF) is known to be an important stimulator of angiogenesis (23). bFGF is released from injured vascular smooth-muscle cells to an extracellular pool, where it can bind to both high- and low-affinity receptors (24). bFGF appears to be critical for stimulating the first wave of vascular smooth-muscle cell replication (7). Infusion of bFGF causes a dramatic increase in vascular smooth-muscle cell replication, and daily infusion of bFGF leads to a striking increase in intimal hyperplastic lesions in animal models (25–27). Thus, bFGF effects on the vessel wall are also a logical target for pharmacologic manipulation to prevent intimal hyperplasia formation. Other growth factors including, insulin growth factor-1 (IGF-1), transforming growth factor beta and epidermal growth factor also may contribute to smooth-muscle migration and proliferation (Fig. 41.1).

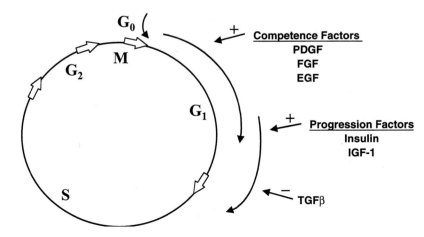

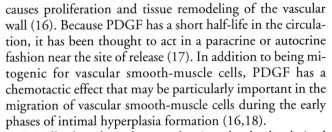

FIGURE 41.1. Peptide growth factors and signal transduction. *EGF,* endothelial growth factor; *FGF,* fibroblast growth factor; *IGF*-1, insulin growth factor-1; *PDGF,* platelet-derived growth factor; TGFβ, transforming growth factor β. *G, M,* and *S* represent cell cycle stages. +, stimulatory; −, inhibitory. (Adapted from Sidawy AN, Mitchell ME, Neville RF. Peptide growth factors and signal transduction. *Semin Vasc Surg* 1998;11:149–155, with permission.)

In addition to the effects of platelet and platelet-derived products on the vascular wall, recent investigators have implicated inflammatory cell pathways in the pathogenesis of both atherosclerosis and intimal hyperplasia (28). In particular, investigators have elucidated pathways by which inflammatory cells, including both neutrophils and monocytes, adhere to injured endothelium (29,30). Injury to endothelium can result in upregulation of a variety of cell adhesion molecules, including intercellular adhesion molecule-1 (ICAM-1) (31,32), endothelial–leukocyte adhesion molecule-1 (ELAM-1) (CD62-e) (33), platelet-activating factor (34), and p-selectin (CD62-p) (35). Leukocyte adherence to injured endothelium results in leukocyte activation, further endothelial cell injury, and the release of chemotactic and mitogenic factors for subsequent smooth-muscle cell proliferation. Products of inflammatory cell activation include oxidants, which may affect the composition of low-density lipoproteins; these altered lipoproteins can be incorporated in monocytes in the subendothelium, leading to the formation of foam cells and the initiation of atherosclerosis (36). Recently, a great deal of interest has been directed toward markers of inflammation that may predict predisposition to atherosclerotic events, including myocardial infarction. Inflammatory and oxidant stress pathways may be particularly relevant in hemodialysis patients as contributors to vascular disease. Of note, a recent study demonstrated that patients on chronic hemodialysis begin to develop venous intimal hyperplasia even before an AV access is created, and that length of time on dialysis correlates with the extent of intimal hyperplasia (37). At present, the extent to which inflammatory cells contribute to the development of hemodialysis access–associated intimal hyperplasia remains uncertain.

Some clues to the pathogenesis of intimal hyperplasia at or distal to the venous anastomosis of small ePTFE grafts in hemodialysis patients come from histologic studies of graft and venous material removed at the time of surgical revision. Studies by Swedberg and colleagues clearly demonstrated the intimal hyperplastic nature of material causing graft and venous stenosis in hemodialysis patients (38). Roy-Chaudhury and colleagues significantly extended these observations by using immunohistologic staining of material obtained both from ePTFE grafts and from the venous anastomosis in hemodialysis patients undergoing graft revision surgery (39). These investigators demonstrated exuberant neovascularization contained within the intima. They further demonstrated extremely high levels of immunohistochemical staining around the areas of neovascularization with antibodies to bFGF and PDGF. Of note, these investigators also developed a pig model of PTFE graft–induced intimal hyperplasia that bears considerable histologic resemblance to the lesions obtained from hemodialysis patients (40). Further investigations of both explanted material obtained from hemodialysis patients with ePTFE-associated intimal hyperplasia as well as animal models are likely to lead to improved understanding of the pathogenesis of intimal hyperplasia in hemodialysis patients.

In summary, a unified theory to explain the pathophysiology of intimal hyperplasia is emerging, although not yet complete. Within the vessel wall, there is normally an intricate balance occurring as a result of communication and interactions between the endothelium and vascular smooth muscle. Disruption of endothelial cell integrity leads to activation and proliferation of vascular smooth-muscle cells. Components of the circulation, including platelets and inflammatory cells, also can contribute to the activation of vascular smooth-muscle cells. These are largely mediated through peptide growth factors, including PDGF and bFGF. From these observations, it can be derived that pharmacologic approaches to preventing this process can occur at several or multiple steps, including the following:

1. Enhancing endothelial cell integrity and function
2. Preventing platelet and inflammatory cell activation when these cells come into contact with an injured vessel wall
3. Preventing PDGF from causing migration and proliferation of smooth-muscle cells

THROMBOSIS

The final common pathway in complete vascular access failure is the development of thrombosis. Several risk factors aside from the development of venous stenosis have been identified for the development of thrombosis in ePTFE grafts. Studies have suggested that age and the presence of diabetes mellitus are risk factors for ePTFE graft thrombosis (41). Whether the use of recombinant human erythropoietin increases the risk for ePTFE graft thrombosis is controversial but is supported by recent data, especially when predialysis hematocrit is normalized (42). Patients with elevated levels of homocysteine, lipoprotein (a), and anticardiolipin antibodies also may be at increased risk for thrombosis attributable to associated hypercoagulability (43–45). It also has been suggested that exposure to topical bovine thrombin perioperatively may lead to antibody formation and subsequent thrombosis (46,47).

The initiating events in thrombosis involve collagen and tissue factor (48). Tissue factor is released from injured cells and expressed on activated endothelial cells, activating the extrinsic pathway of coagulation. Disruption of the endothelium exposes the underlying collagen to platelets, resulting in platelet adhesion and activation. Studies have shown that platelets repetitively bind to ePTFE graft material during the hemodialysis procedure (49). In this fashion, the lack of complete endothelialization of ePTFE graft material contributes to the thrombotic process in addition to intimal hyperplasia development.

The stage is set for the coagulation proteins to assemble into the prothrombinase complex, catalyzing the formation of thrombin, once a platelet plug has formed at the site of injury (48). The formation of thrombin is central to the development of thrombosis. Thrombin cleaves fibrinopeptides from fibrin, leading to cross-linking and subsequent fibrin polymerization strengthening clot formation. Thrombin also is known as a potent agonist for vascular smooth-muscle cells (50,51). Thus, repetitive microthrombosis related to graft cannulation and the development of intimal hyperplasia within and distal to the graft are probably linked.

The many sites of action of the coagulation cascade provide a variety of pharmacologic targets to inhibit vascular access thrombosis. Heparin, first discovered in 1916, consists of mixture of sulfated polysaccharide molecules. Heparin acts to potentiate the antithrombotic effects of antithrombin III by catalytically accelerating the reaction between thrombin and antithrombin III. The use of heparin to prevent extracorporeal thrombosis during the dialysis procedure is of course a common practice.

Oral anticoagulant therapy may be a more practical approach to the long-term prevention of vascular access thrombosis. Warfarin acts by interfering with the synthesis of vitamin K–dependent factors II, VII, IX, X, protein C, and protein S. Warfarin is active in the liver in preventing the gamma-carboxylation of these peptides. The carboxyglutamic acid residues are essential for these peptides binding to phospholipid membranes and are therefore necessary for the formation of the prothrombinase complex on the surface of activated platelets. In particular, crystalline warfarin sodium (Coumadin) is commonly used as an anticoagulant. Although Coumadin is effective at inhibiting the coagulation cascade, there may be a substantial increase in the frequency of bleeding complications with this pharmacologic approach. Although Coumadin is frequently used clin-

ically in an effort to prevent vascular access thrombosis, there have been few clinical trials evaluating its efficacy and safety in preventing either AV fistula or ePTFE graft thrombosis (see later discussion).

Pharmacologic Trials for Prevention of Hemodialysis Vascular Access Failure

Given the magnitude of the problem of hemodialysis access thrombosis, remarkably few controlled trials have examined pharmacologic approaches to preventing access failure (Table 41.2). All the trials conducted to date have small sample sizes, limited statistical power, and short-term observation periods. Most published trials were conducted more than a decade ago, when patient population and techniques of hemodialysis therapy were markedly different.

Scribner Shunt

The major physiologic process associated with external access failure was thrombosis, and intimal hyperplasia clearly played a much smaller role in Scribner shunt thrombosis than is now the case with ePTFE grafts (1–3). Trials of both anticoagulation and antiplatelet therapy have been conducted. Early attempts at pharmacologic prevention of hemodialysis access failure with warfarin anticoagulation were described by the groups of Boyd (2) and Wing (3). Wing and colleagues demonstrated a lower shunt thrombosis rate in the warfarin group compared with controls (1.4 clots per patient-year versus 4.6 clots per patient-year). Trials of antiplatelet therapy were conducted as well. Harter and colleagues found that low-dose (160 mg daily) aspirin versus placebo reduced thrombosis from 72% to 32% (52). Low-dose aspirin may provide a greater protective antiplatelet effect through the inhibition of synthesis of thromboxane than a harmful antiendothelial effect via in-

TABLE 41.2. PHARMACOLOGIC TRIALS TO PREVENT VASCULAR ACCESS FAILURE[a]

Study	Drug	No. of Patients	Follow-up	Results
Shunts				
Kaegi et al., 1974 (53)	Sulfinpyrazone	52	6 mo	76% thrombosis reduction
Harter et al., 1979 (52)	Aspirin	44	5 mo	56% thrombosis reduction
Kobayashi et al., 1980 (54)	Ticlodipine	107	3 mo	21% thrombosis reduction
Radmilovic et al., 1987 (55)	Pentoxifylline	51	5 mo	48% thrombosis reduction
AV fistulae				
Andrassy et al., 1974 (57)	Aspirin	92	4 wk	4% vs 23% thrombosis
Grontoft, 1994	Ticlodipine	36	4 wk	11% vs 47% thrombosis
Grontoft et al. 1998 (60)	Ticlodipine	260	4 wk	12% vs 19% thrombosis
PTFE grafts				
Sreedhara et al., 1994 (62)	Dipyridamole	84	18 mo	Dipyridamole RR 0.35, $p = 0.02$
	Aspirin			ASA RR 1.99, $p = 0.18$

AV, arteriovenous; PTFE, polytetrafluoroethylene; RR, relative risk; ASA, acetyl salicyclic acid.
[a] Confined to studies with ≥20 patients with at least ten patients in each arm.

hibiting vascular synthesis of prostacyclin (52). Similarly, trials of other antiplatelet agents, such as sulfinpyrazone, ticlopidine, and pentoxifylline, also were associated with a reduction in AV shunt thrombosis rates (53–55). The high incidence of thrombotic events observed with external shunts allows a pharmacologic treatment effect to be demonstrated with relatively small sample sizes.

Arteriovenous Fistulae

In 1966, Brescia and colleagues developed the AV fistula as a form of permanent hemodialysis access (56). Early failure of AV fistula frequently results from technical problems related to the small caliber of the vein used for the anastomosis. Based on the results of earlier studies with Scribner shunts, it was logical to attempt to use antiplatelet therapy to prevent early fistula failure from thrombosis. Studies using short-term antiplatelet therapy demonstrate a reduction in early native fistula failure. Aspirin given in a dose of 1 g daily was associated with a 4% thrombosis rate at 2 weeks versus 23% with placebo (57). Ticlopidine given at a dose of 250 mg twice daily was associated with 11% thrombosis at 1 month versus 47% with placebo (58). Similarly, another smaller trial showed a 25% thrombosis rate at 1 month in new AV fistulas treated with ticlopidine versus 50% in the placebo group (59). In the largest prospective trial of ticlopidine to date, Grontoft and colleagues found a trend toward a lower rate of thrombosis in the ticlopidine group (12%) compared with that in the placebo group (19%) (60), although this difference was not significant. In summary, antiplatelet agents, including ticlopidine and low-dose aspirin, may provide a clinically useful reduction in early AV fistula thrombosis, thereby allowing an opportunity for subsequent fistula maturation. No studies reported to date, however, have clearly demonstrated an increase in the development of native AV fistulae suitable for dialysis use as a consequence of pharmacologic therapy. Furthermore, previous studies were conducted in an era in which most AV fistulae created for dialysis were radiocephalic, whereas there is currently an increasing tendency to use both brachiocephalic and brachiobasilic fistulae, which have different flow and patency rates. Thus, a larger-scale trial of antiplatelet agents to support AV fistula maturation by preventing early thrombosis is clearly warranted.

Whereas patency rates of mature AV fistulae are regarded as superior to ePTFE grafts, late thrombosis does occur, often in conjunction with the development of stenotic lesions. To date, no long-term prospective pharmacologic trials have been reported that attempted to prevent late endogenous fistula failure. Warfarin anticoagulation has been associated with lower thrombosis rates in some retrospective trials as has angiotensin converting enzyme inhibition (61). These and other retrospective analyses suggest the need for further prospective study.

Expanded Polytetrafluoroethylene Grafts

Despite the growing use of ePTFE grafts for hemodialysis access, there has been only one prospective, randomized, placebo-controlled study reported of pharmacologic approaches to reducing the rate of ePTFE thrombosis (62). In this study, 84 patients with new ePTFE grafts were randomized to receive dipyridamole 75 mg three times daily, aspirin 325 mg daily, dipyridamole plus aspirin or placebo (62). Patients were followed up for 18 months. In addition, 23 type 2 patients, who began therapy after thrombectomy or revision of a previously placed ePTFE grafts, were randomized to the same drug treatments.

In new ePTFE graft patients, the actuarial cumulative thrombosis rate was 21% in those treated with dipyridamole alone, 25% in patients on dipyridamole plus aspirin, 42% on placebo, and 80% on aspirin alone (Fig. 41.2). The relative risk of thrombosis for patients treated with dipyridamole was 0.35 ($p = 0.02$). In contrast, the relative risk of thrombosis for patients treated with aspirin alone was 1.99 ($p = 0.18$). In patients receiving therapy after a thrombotic event, differences between groups were not statistically significant, possibly reflecting small sample size. Analysis of thrombosis rates in combined patients showed no statistically significant difference between the either dipyridamole group and placebo, possibly reflecting differences between primary and secondary prevention.

The results of this study were somewhat surprising, given that dipyridamole is a relatively weak antiplatelet agent and that aspirin is frequently used in many disorders to prevent thrombotic complications. What is the role by which dipyridamole may inhibit vascular smooth muscle-cell proliferation? Actuarial analysis suggests an increasing reduction of thrombosis by dipyridamole over time with respect to placebo (Fig. 41.2). This may reflect an antiproliferative effect rather than an antiplatelet one. It has been difficult to establish a role for dipyridamole as a platelet inhibitor (63–68); however, experiments using human aortic smooth-muscle cell preparations demonstrate that dipyridamole inhibits PDGF- and bFGF-induced vascular smooth-muscle cell proliferation (69). Several other recent studies also demonstrated that dipyridamole may have a direct effect on vascular smooth-muscle cell proliferation (70–72). This effect does not appear to be cyclic adenosine monophosphate (cAMP) mediated, nor does it appear related to a toxic effect of dipyridamole. These results were obtained with concentrations of dipyridamole comparable to therapeutic plasma concentrations obtained with conventional doses. The direct effect of dipyridamole on PDGF- and bFGF-mediated vascular smooth-muscle cell proliferation is the best explanation for its clinical effect in decreasing ePTFE graft thrombosis in hemodialysis patients.

The seemingly paradoxic effects of aspirin on graft thrombosis in this study may be secondary to dose-related effects on platelet vascular smooth-muscle cell and endothe-

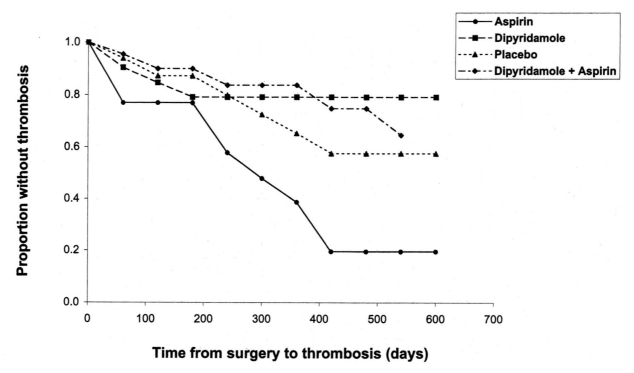

FIGURE 41.2. Antiplatelet therapy and expanded polytetrafluoroethylene graft thrombosis: results of a prospective, randomized, double-blind study. (Adapted from Sreedhara R, Himmelfarb J, Lazarus JM, et al. Antiplatelet therapy in graft thrombosis: results of a prospective, randomized double-blind study. *Kidney Int* 1994;45:1477–1483, with permission.).

lial cell function. Tenfold dose increments in aspirin have antithrombotic, analgesic/antipyretic, and antirheumatic effects, respectively (73). Low-dose aspirin (30–130 mg daily) inhibits platelet function by irreversibly acetylating the cyclooxygenase enzyme, which catalyzes the formation of thromboxane A_2 from arachidonic acid. The antithrombotic effect of low-dose aspirin is as effective as higher doses, supporting the acetylization of cyclooxygenase as the mechanism by which aspirin exerts its antithrombotic effect. Thromboxane A_2 is also a potent vasoconstrictor and smooth-muscle cell agonist; thus, aspirin-mediated thromboxane inhibition would be expected to reduce intimal hyperplasia as well.

Recent evidence also suggests that aspirin (possibly at higher doses) may adversely effect eicosanoid production in smooth-muscle cells, thus promoting intimal hyperplasia (74,75). Prostaglandin E_2 (PGE_2), which can suppress smooth-muscle cell activation and proliferation, is reduced by aspirin at doses greater than 100 mg daily. This inhibition of PGE_2 could increase proliferation of smooth-muscle cells. Additionally, the major lipoxygenase product of arachidonic acid production in vascular smooth-muscle cells is 12-L-hydroxy-5,8,10,14-eicosatetraenoic acid (12-HETE) (76). 12-HETE is an important intracellular messenger and mitogen during the activation of vascular smooth-muscle cells (76–83). Aspirin-induced shunting of arachidonic acid into the lipoxygenase pathways (12-

HETE) and away from the cyclooxygenase pathways (PGE_2) could increase the proliferation of vascular smooth muscle cells.

Eicosapentaenoic Acid (Fish Oil)

Eicosapentaenoic acid (EPA), the active ingredient in fish oil, has also been proposed as a potential agent to reduce ePTFE thrombosis (84). EPA is an inhibitor of both cyclooxygenase and lipoxygenase pathways of arachidonic acid metabolism, in contrast to aspirin, which inhibits only cyclooxygenase. EPA may exert a more beneficial effect on the proliferation of vascular smooth-muscle cells than does aspirin (85). Fish oil modifies lipids and reduces platelet aggregation in hemodialysis patients (86). Additionally, EPA reduces intimal hyperplasia formation in autogenous vein grafts used for arterial bypass in dogs (87–89) and in a rodent model of arterial injury (90). A recent abstract describes a prospective, randomized, controlled trial comprising 34 hemodialysis patients with ePTFE grafts who were given either enriched fish oil (4,000 mg daily) or corn oil. At 1 year, the fish oil group had a higher primary patency rate (77%) compared with the corn oil group (29%). Time to first thrombosis was longer in the fish oil group as well (228 ± 34 days versus 109 ± 40 days). EPA, through either an antiplatelet effect or via inhibition of intimal hyperplasia, may reduce early and long-term graft thrombosis.

Heparinoids

Heparin and heparin-like molecules (*heparinoids*) such as heparin sulfate proteoglycans have been demonstrated to inhibit vascular smooth-muscle cell activity and collagen synthesis *in vitro* and *in vivo* (91–96). Decreased extracellular matrix production and secretion do not appear to be dependent on the anticoagulation properties of heparinoids. Heparinoids may have the benefit of inhibiting proliferation of vascular smooth-muscle cells without the risks of bleeding associated with heparin anticoagulation. Preliminary data indicate that orally active pentosan sulfate decreases both cellular proliferation and matrix syntheses in explants from vascular tissue obtained from the venous end of stenotic AV grafts in hemodialysis patients. To date, no controlled trials have evaluated heparinoids for preventing intimal hyperplasia and subsequent ePTFE graft thrombosis.

Warfarin

The nephrologist is often confronted with the decision of whether to institute warfarin anticoagulation in a patient with graft or fistula thrombosis. No prospective trials have been performed to guide the physician in selecting dialysis patients who might benefit from long-term anticoagulation therapy. It remains controversial whether hemodialysis patients in general, and those with specific laboratory markers of hypercoagulability in particular, are in a hypercoagulable state (97,98). Further, no trials have prospectively or retrospectively evaluated markers of hypercoagulability in graft thrombosis in the absence of radiographically determined stenosis.

Of the common laboratory markers of hypercoagulability, including protein C and S deficiency, factor V Leiden mutation, antithrombin III deficiency, anticardiolipin antibody, antiphospholipid antibody, and lupus anticoagulant, some, but not all, have been studied retrospectively in hemodialysis patients with respect to access thrombosis. Several studies noted an increased incidence of positive anticardiolipin antibody in dialysis patients with PTFE grafts, although in one study, average levels were not increased (43). Retrospective studies have yielded inconsistent results regarding the association between elevated anticardiolipin antibody levels and graft thrombosis. Similarly, other studies have shown an association between antiphospholipid antibody and graft thrombosis, but not anticardiolipin antibody (99). Hyperhomocystinemia, which is highly prevalent in dialysis patients, has been evaluated with respect to hemodialysis graft thrombosis with mixed and inconclusive results (100,101).

Trials of systemic warfarin anticoagulation to prevent fistula or graft thrombosis are limited. The risks associated with long-term anticoagulation of hemodialysis patients is significant, however (102). In a retrospective surgical series, PTFE grafts in patients regarded as hypercoagulable experienced 1.2 thrombotic events per year in those on warfarin therapy versus 4.0 in those not undergoing anticoagulation (103). Stenotic lesions, including central lesions, were not radiographically excluded in most patients in this study. These investigators noted that all thromboses in the warfarin group occurred with international normalized ratios (INR) below 2.7. Maintaining patient INRs between 2.7 and 3.0 was understandably problematic in this series of patients, and a 10% annual incidence of severe bleeding complications was noted, often in association with elevated INR levels.

In the absence of randomized controlled trials, few recommendations regarding warfarin anticoagulation to prevent or reduce graft thrombosis can be made. Long-term warfarin anticoagulation certainly cannot be recommended prophylactically for the vast majority of patients with new grafts or fistulas. Evidence of recurrent graft thrombosis and a negative radiographic workup for stenosis should be sought before considering long-term anticoagulation. Similarly, anticoagulation for patients with abnormal serum coagulation studies in the absence of a clinical thrombotic syndrome cannot now be recommended. Finally, attention needs to be paid to the patient's risk of serious bleeding complications relative to the risk of fistula or graft loss.

Other Agents

Numerous pharmacologic agents have been demonstrated *in vitro* and *in vivo* to reduce or prevent proliferation of vascular smooth-muscle cells and associated intimal hyperplasia. Retrospective human trials have shown potential benefits in reducing ePTFE access thrombosis with varying agents, including angiotensin converting enzyme (ACE) inhibitors, calcium-channel blockers, human menopausal gonadotropin (HMG) Co-A reductase inhibitors, ketanserin, and misoprostol, among others (84,104). ACE inhibitors are of particular interest because of their potential to blockade angiotensin-induced smooth-muscle proliferation.

Radiation Therapy

Although it is not strictly a pharmacologic approach, there is increasing evidence that neointimal formation, particularly after arterial angioplasty or stent placement, can be inhibited by local delivery of ionizing radiation (105–107). Ionizing radiation can be delivered as either external beam irradiation or as brachytherapy using an endovascular approach. Both beta- and gamma-emitting sources have been used for brachytherapy. Endovascular brachytherapy now has been demonstrated in several large clinical trials to be clinically effective in reducing the rate of restenosis after coronary artery angioplasty or stent placement (108,109). Numerous clinical problems, however, remain before endovascular brachytherapy will be clinically widely. These include logistic considerations, concerns with late thrombosis after stent placement, and problems of "candy-wrapper effect," where accelerated intimal hyperplasia may form at the boundaries of the irradiated field.

It should be noted that virtually all the endovascular brachytherapy studies to date have involved the arterial side of the circulation, and much fewer data on the efficacy of brachytherapy for venous intimal hyperplasia exist. A recently presented animal study suggested that external beam radiation is modestly effective in preventing venous intimal hyperplasia distal to an ePTFE graft (110). A single case report documents mild efficacy in treating a proximal venous stenosis in a hemodialysis patient (111). Issues concerning local oncogenesis, the effect of perigraft scarring on hemostasis, and possible late effects on graft thrombosis have not been systematically evaluated in either animal or human models of brachytherapy for venous intimal hyperplasia associated with ePTFE grafts. Thus, considerable work remains before these techniques can be considered for the hemodialysis access population (see Chapter 44).

BIOLOGICAL APPROACHES TO THE PREVENTION OF VASCULAR ACCESS FAILURE

To date, all pharmacologic approaches to the prevention of vascular access failure have relied on the systemic administration of pharmacologic agents. Because the problem of intimal hyperplasia and subsequent thrombosis related to vascular access is in essence a local problem, it is theoretically possible that the local administration of therapy to the site of the access itself may have more biological efficacy with less systemic toxicity. Biologic approaches to modifying ePTFE or other graft biomaterials in an effort to reduce thrombotic potential and to increase endothelialization are logical and have been studied in animal models for more than 15 years (112). To date, no clinical human studies have been performed that use these relatively novel approaches to improving vascular access function for hemodialysis patients.

It is well recognized that one of the problems contributing to the development of both intimal hyperplasia and eventual thrombosis of dialysis access grafts is the lack of complete normal endothelialization that occurs using ePTFE biomaterial. A theoretic solution to this problem would be the establishment of an endothelial cell monolayer on the luminal surface of the graft before implantation, a technique known as *graft seeding* (113). Another technique that has been used experimentally is to apply directly harvested microvascular endothelial cells to the graft without a cell culture step (known as *endothelial sodding*). Studies incorporating both endothelial seeding and endothelial sodding in human studies of arterial bypass grafts have shown modest clinical benefit in some but not all studies (114–118). Endothelial cells seeded onto a graft can survive

for periods *in vivo* but eventually are usually replaced by cells derived from local sources (119,120). Recently, it was suggested that applying shear stress to endothelial cells *ex vivo* prior to implantation on the graft will increase endothelial cell adherence to the graft and improve the extent to which endothelial integrity can be maintained on the graft *in vivo* (121). Clinical results from such an approach are not yet available.

Several groups have proposed that incorporating gene therapy with endothelial cell seeding may be a means to improve vascular access graft outcome (112,122,123). Endothelial cells can be modified genetically either to decrease the likelihood of thrombosis or to decrease the likelihood of the growth of vascular smooth-muscle cells and development of intimal hyperplasia. These approaches to improving graft function are highly promising but are currently in their infancy. A recent study examined the seeding of vascular grafts with endothelial cells genetically modified to secrete large amounts of tissue plasminogen activator (tPA) (124). Grafts secreting large local amounts of tPA should have the benefit of decreased thrombosis from the fibrinolytic actions of this agent. On implementation *in vivo*, endothelial cells transduced with tPA were retained on the graft at a significantly lower rate than nontransduced endothelial cells. This suggests that the proteolytic tPA may have had the adverse effect of degrading matrix proteins required for adherence of the endothelial cells to the graft material. This example serves to illustrate some of the biological complexities likely to become apparent with further efforts to genetically modify graft biomaterials.

A highly promising approach for the future would be to modify graft biomaterials, either directly or via genetic modification of seeded endothelial cells, to inhibit peptide growth factors such as PDGF and bFGF. Local inhibition of PDGF and bFGF should reduce stimulation for vascular smooth-muscle cells to migrate and proliferate, resulting in decreased intimal hyperplasia. One suggested approach to achieve this outcome is to transduce seeded endothelial cells with a nonfunctional bFGF receptor. The use of vascular endothelial growth factor (VEGF) also may increase the endothelialization of new ePTFE grafts.

GENE THERAPY TO PREVENT VASCULAR ACCESS STENOSIS

Because the problem of vascular access stenosis in ePTFE grafts is largely a local problem (located at the graft/vein anastomosis), vectored approaches using gene therapy theoretically could be highly effective for the prevention of local neointimal hyperplasia formation while causing less systemic toxicity than systemic pharmacologic therapy. In experimental models, vectored gene therapy approaches that target inhibition of the cell cycle, overexpression of vascular smooth-muscle cell growth inhibitors, such as nitric oxide synthase, and inhibition of transcription factors have been highly successful (125–129). Gene therapy for the treatment of human diseases is in its infancy, however, with concerns about safety and immunogenicity, especially with viral vectors for gene delivery. Of note, a gene therapy strategy using an E2F transcription factor decoy oligodeoxynucleotide delivered directly by pressure (without a viral vector) into vein grafts has been demonstrated in a human trial to have efficacy (130). In the future, we are likely to see numerous approaches to vectored gene therapy to prevent venous neointimal hyperplasia associated with ePTFE grafts in both animal studies and human trials.

NATIONAL INSTITUTES OF HEALTH–SPONSORED HEMODIALYSIS VASCULAR ACCESS CLINICAL TRIALS

With the growing perception of the clinical importance and expense of hemodialysis vascular access failure, the National Institutes of Health (NIH) developed a dialysis access consortium. The stated goal of this consortium is to conduct multicenter, randomized, placebo-controlled clinical trials of drug therapies to reduce the failure rate of both AV grafts and fistulas in hemodialysis patients. Currently, clinical trials are being designed in an attempt to reduce both ePTFE graft and native AV fistula access failure. The results of these multicenter, large-scale, clinical trials may have a substantial impact on pharmacologic approaches to preventing hemodialysis vascular access failure.

SUMMARY

The morbidity and cost associated with vascular access failure continues to plague the treatment of ESRD with chronic hemodialysis therapy. Biological processes that lead to vascular access failure are beginning to be well understood; these include the development of intimal hyperplasia with consequent venous stenosis followed by eventual thrombosis. In addition, a subset of patients with thrombosis in the absence of stenosis is in the process of being characterized. Pharmacologic approaches to preventing intimal hyperplasia and thrombosis are logical and, if successful, likely to be cost effective.

Studies to date have demonstrated that antiplatelet therapy can reduce early AV fistula failure. These agents are recommended for the first 4 to 6 weeks after fistula creation. To date, a single controlled trial has demonstrated the benefit of dipyridamole in reducing ePTFE graft thrombosis. Further research is needed before these and other potential agents can be recommended with confidence for large groups of patients. Additionally, research is needed in the group of patients at high risk for restenosis and thrombosis

after angioplasty and thrombectomy. Risk factors for thrombosis in the absence of stenosis and indications for warfarin anticoagulation need to be better characterized. Newer biologic approaches to modulating the propensity for both intimal hyperplasia formation and thrombosis are now being intensively investigated, with further data likely to become available in the near future.

REFERENCES

1. Glasham RW, Walker F. A histologic examination of Quinton Scribner shunts. *Br J Surg* 1968;55:189–192.
2. Boyd SJ, Dennis MB, Nogami RT, et al. Prophylactic coumadin and AV cannula function. *J Appl Physiol* 1974;37: 6–7.
3. Wing AJ, Curtis JR, DeWardener HE. Reduction of clotting of Scribner shunts by long-term anticoagulation. *BMJ* 1967;3: 143–145.
4. Munda R, First MR, Alexander JW, et al. Polytetrafluoroethylene graft survival in hemodialysis. *JAMA* 1983;249:219–222.
5. Palder SB, Kirkman RL, Whittemore AD, et al. Vascular access from hemodialysis: patency rates and results of revision. *Ann Surg* 1985;202:235–239.
6. Kanterman RY, Vesely TM, Pilgram TK, et al. Dialysis access grafts: anatomic location of venous stenosis and results of angioplasty. *Radiology* 1995;195:135–139.
7. Kraiss LW, Clowes AW. Response of the arterial wall to injury and intimal hyperplasia. In: Sidawy AN, Sumpio BE, DePalma RG, eds. *The basic science of vascular disease.* Armonk, NY: Futura Publishing Company, 1997:289–317.
8. Neville RF, Sidawy AN. Myointimal hyperplasia: basic science and clinical considerations. *Semin Vasc Surg* 1998;11:142–148.
9. Andrade EA. Blood-materials interactions: 20 years of frustration. *Trans Am Soc Artif Intern Organs* 1981;27:659.
10. Delorme JM, Guidoin R, Canizales S, et al. Vascular access for hemodialysis: Pathologic features of surgically excised ePTFE grafts. *J Vasc Surg* 1992;6:517–524.
11. Zarins CK, Zatina MA, Giddens DP, et al. Shear stress regulation of artery lumen diameter in experimental atherogenesis. *J Vasc Surg* 1987;5:413–420.
12. Quinones-Baldrich WJ. Myointimal hyperplasia: a lesion. In: *Anonymous pharmacological suppression of intimal hyperplasia.* Georgetown, TX: R.G. Landes Company, 1993:1–10.
13. Clowes AW, Clowes MM, Fingerle J, et al. Regulation of smooth muscle cell growth in injured artery. *J Cardiovasc Pharmacol* 1987;14:S12–S15.
14. Cox JL, Chaisson DA, Gotlieb AI. Stranger in a strange land: the pathogenesis of saphenous vein graft stenosis with emphasis on structural and functional differences between veins and arteries. *Prog Cardiovasc Dis* 1991;34:45–68.
15. Ross R. Atherosclerosis: a defense mechanism gone awry. *Am J Pathol* 1993;143:987–1002.
16. Grotendorst GR, Chang T, Seppa HEJ, et al. Platelet-derived growth factor is a chemoattractant for vascular smooth muscle cells. *J Cell Physiol* 1982;113:261–266.
17. Raines EW, Bowen-Pope DF, Ross R. Platelet-derived growth factor. In: Sporn MB, Roberts AB, eds. *Peptide growth factors and their receptors.* Heidelberg, Germany: Springer-Verlag, 1990:173–262.
18. Jawein A, Bowen-Pope DF, Lindner V, et al. Platelet-derived growth factor promotes smooth muscle migration and intimal thickening in a rat model of balloon angioplasty. *J Clin Invest* 1992;89:507–511.

19. Fox PL, DiCorleto PE. Regulation of production of a platelet-derived growth factor-like protein by cultured bovine aortic endothelial cells. *J Cell Physiol* 1984;121:298–308.

20. DiCorleto PE, Bowen-Pope DF. Cultured endothelial cells produce a platelet-derived growth factor-like protein. *Proc Natl Acad Sci USA* 1983;80:1919–1923.

21. Libby P, Warner SJ, Salomon RN, et al. Production of platelet-derived growth factor-like mitogen by smooth-muscle cells from human atheroma. *N Engl J Med* 1988;318:1493–1498.

22. Ferns GAA, Raines EW, Sprugel KH, et al. Inhibition of neointimal smooth muscle cell accumulation after angioplasty by an antibody to PDGF. *Science* 1991;253:1129–1132.

23. Folkman J, Klagsbrun M. Angiogenic factors. *Science* 1987;235:442–447.

24. Gospodarowicz D, Ferrara N, Schweigerer L, et al. Structural characterization and biological functions of fibroblast growth factor. *Endocr Rev* 1987;8:95–114.

25. Lindner V, Lappi DA, Baird A, et al. Role of basic fibroblast growth factor in vascular lesion formation. *Circ Res* 1991;68:106–113.

26. Lindner V, Reidy MA. Proliferation of smooth muscle cells after vascular injury in inhibited by an antibody against basic fibroblast growth factor. *Proc Natl Acad Sci USA* 1991;88:3739–3743.

27. Olsen NE, Chao S, Lindner V, et al. Intimal smooth muscle cell proliferation after balloon catheter injury: the role of basic fibroblast growth factor. *Am J Pathol* 1992;140:1017–1023.

28. Quinones-Baldrich WJ. The role of anti-inflammatory agents in the control of intimal hyperplasia. In: Quinones-Baldrich WJ, ed. *Pharmacological suppression of intimal hyperplasia.* Georgetown, TX: RG Landes, 1993:22–32.

29. Harlan JM. Leukocyte-endothelial interactions. *Blood* 1985;65:513–525.

30. Butcher EC. Cellular and molecular mechanisms that direct leukocyte traffic. *Am J Pathol* 1990;136:3–11.

31. Luscinskas FW, Cybulsky MI, Keily JM, et al. Cytokine-activated human endothelial monolayers support enhanced neutrophil transmigration via a mechanism involving both endothelial-leukocyte adhesion molecule-1 and intercellular adhesion molecule-1. *J Immunol* 1995;146:1617–1625.

32. Smith CW, Marlin SD, Rothlein R, et al. Cooperative interactions of LFA-1 and Mac-1 with intercellular adhesion molecule-1 in facilitating adherence and transendothelial migration of human neutrophils *in vitro. J Clin Invest* 1989;83:2008–2017.

33. Bevilacqua MP, Pober JS, Mendrick DL, et al. Identification of an inducible endothelial-leukocyte adhesion molecule. *Proc Natl Acad Sci USA* 1987;84:9238–9242.

34. Zimmerman GA, McIntyre TM, Mehra M, et al. Endothelial cell-associated platelet-activating factor: a novel mechanism for signalling intercellular adhesion. *J Cell Biol* 1990;110:529–540.

35. McEver RP, Beckstead JH, Moore SL, et al. GMP-140, a platelet alpha-granule membrane protein, is also synthesized by vascular endothelial cells and is localized in Weibel-Palade bodies. *J Clin Invest* 1989;84:92–99.

36. Steinberg D, Parthasarathy S, Carew TE, et al. Beyond cholesterol: Modifications of low-density lipoprotein that increase its atherogenicity. *N Engl J Med* 1989;320:915–924.

37. Feinfeld DA, Batista R, Mir R, et al. Changes in venous histology in chronic hemodialysis patients. *Am J Kidney Dis* 1999;34:702–705.

38. Swedberg SH, Brown BG, Sigley R, et al. Intimal fibromuscular hyperplasia at the venous anastomosis of PTFE grafts in hemodialysis patients. *Circulation* 1989;80:1726–1736.

39. Roy-Chaudhury P, Whiting J, Miller M, et al. Venous neointimal hyperplasia in PTFE dialysis grafts: a role for cytokines, M?, and angiogenesis. *J Am Soc Nephrol* 1998;9:181A(abst).

40. Roy-Chaudhury P, Heffelfinger SC, Miller M, et al. Venous stenosis in PTFE dialysis grafts: development of a pig model of AV graft stenosis. *J Am Soc Nephrol* 1998;9:181A(abst).

41. Windus DW, Jendrisak MD, Delmez JA. Prosthetic fistula survival and complications in hemodialysis patients: effects of diabetes and age. *Am J Kidney Dis* 1992;92:448–452.

42. Churchill DN, Muirhead N, Goldstein M, et al. Probability of thrombosis of vascular access among hemodialysis patients treated with recombinant human erythropoietin. *J Am Soc Nephrol* 1994;4:1809–1813.

43. Prakash R, Miller C, Suki WN. Anticardiolipin antibody in patients on maintenance hemodialysis and its association with recurrent arteriovenous graft thrombosis. *Am J Kidney Dis* 1995;26:347–352.

44. Goldwasser P, Avram MM, Collier JT, et al. Correlates of vascular access occlusion in hemodialysis. *Am J Kidney Dis* 1994;24:785–794.

45. Hernandez E, Praga M, Alamo C, et al. Lipoprotein(s) and vascular access survival in patients on chronic hemodialysis. *Nephron* 1996;72:145–149.

46. Sands JJ, Nudo SA, Ashford RG, et al. Antibodies to topical bovine thrombin correlate with access thrombosis. *Am J Kidney Dis* 2000;35:796–801.

47. Ortel TL, Mercer MC, Thames EH, et al. Immunologic impact and clinical outcomes after surgical exposure to bovine thrombin. *Ann Surg* 2000;233:88–96.

48. Furie B, Furie BC. Molecular and cellular biology of blood coagulation. *N Engl J Med* 1992;326:800–806.

49. Windus DW, Santoro S, Royal HD. The effects of hemodialysis on platelet deposition in prosthetic graft fistulas. *Am J Kidney Dis* 1995;26:614–621.

50. Huang CL, Ives HE. Growth inhibition by protein kinase C late in mitogenesis. *Nature* 1987;329:849–850.

51. Berk BC, Taubman MB, Griendling KK, et al. Thrombin-stimulated events in cultured vascular smooth muscle cells. *Biochem J* 1991;274:799–805.

52. Harter HR, Burch JW, Majerus PW, et al. Prevention of thrombosis in patients on hemodialysis by low dose aspirin. *N Engl J Med* 1979;301:577–579.

53. Kaegi A, Pineo GF, Shimizu A, et al. Arteriovenous shunt thrombosis. *N Engl J Med* 1974;290:304–306.

54. Kobayashi K, Maeda K, Koshikawa S, et al. Antithrombotic therapy with ticlopidine in chronic renal failure patients on chronic maintenance hemodialysis: a multicenter collaborative double-blind study. *Thromb Res* 1980;20:255–261.

55. Radmilovic A, Boric Z, et al. Shunt thrombosis prevention in hemodialysis patients: a double blind randomized study: pentoxifylline vs. placebo. *Antilogy* 1987;38:449–506.

56. Brescia MJ, Cimino JE, Appel K, et al. Chronic hemodialysis using venipuncture and a surgically recreated arteriovenous fistula. *N Engl J Med* 1966;275:1089–1092.

57. Andrassy K, Malluche H, Bornefeld H, et al. Prevention of p.o. clotting of av. cimino fistulae with acetysalicyl acid: results of a prospective double-blind study. *Klin Wochenschr* 1974;52:348–349.

58. Grontoft KC, Mulec H, Gutierrez A, et al. Thromboprophylactic effect of ticlopidine in arteriovenous fistulas for hemodialysis. *Scand J Urol Nephrol* 1985;19:55–57.

59. Fiskestrand CE, Thompson LW, et al. Double-blind randomized controlled trial of the effect of ticlopidine in arteriovenous fistulas for hemodialysis. *Artif Organs* 1985;9:61–63.

60. Grontoft KC, Larsson R, et al. Effects of ticlopidine in AV-fistula surgery in uremia. *Scand J Urol Nephrol* 1998;32:267–283.

61. Sone M, Moriyama T. Angiotensin II inhibition prevents the occlusion of arterio-venous fistula in hemodialysis patients: a case control study. *J Am Soc Nephrol* 2000;11:197A.

62. Sreedhara R, Himmelfarb J, Lazarus JM, et al. Antiplatelet therapy in graft thrombosis: results of a prospective, randomized double-blind study. *Kidney Int* 1994;45:1477–1483.

63. Rajah SM, Crow MJ, Penny AF, et al. The effect of dipyridamole on platelet function: correlation with blood levels in man. *J Clin Pharmacol* 1977;4:129–133.

64. Emmons PR, Harrison MJG, Honour AJ, et al. Effect of dipyridamole on human platelet behaviours. *Lancet* 1965;2:603–606.

65. Saniabadi AR, Lowe GDO, Barbenel JC, et al. A comparison of spontaneous platelet aggregation in whole blood with platelet rich plasma: Additional evidence for the role of ADP. *Thromb Haemost* 1984;51:115–118.

66. Eliasson R, Bygdeman S. Effect of dipyridamole and two pyrimido-pyrimidine derivatives on the kinetics of human platelet aggregation and on platelet adhesiveness. *Scand J Clin Lab Invest* 1969;24:145–151.

67. Kon ND, Hansen KJ, Martin MB, et al. Inhibition of platelet deposition on polytetrafluoroethylene grafts by antiplatelet agents. *Surgery* 1984;96:870–873.

68. Golden MA, Tina Au YP, Kenagy RD, et al. Growth factor gene expression by intimal cells in healing polytetrafluoroethylene grafts. *J Vasc Surg* 1990;11:580–585.

69. Himmelfarb J, Couper L. Dipyridamole inhibits PDGF- and bFGF-induced vascular smooth muscle cell proliferation. *Kidney Int* 1997;52:1671–1677.

70. Singh JP, Rothfuss KF, Wiernick TR, et al. Dipyridamole directly inhibits vascular smooth muscle cell proliferation *in vitro* and *in vivo*: implications in the treatment of restenosis after angioplasty. *J Am Coll Cardiol* 1974;23:665–671.

71. Ingerman-Wojenski CM, Silver MJ. Model system interaction of platelets with damaged arterial wall. II. Inhibition of smooth muscle cell proliferation by dipyridamole and AH-P719. *Exp Mol Pathol* 1988;48:116–134.

72. Grunwald J, Haudenschild CC. The influence of antiplatelet drugs on injury-stimulated migration of cultured smooth muscle cells. *Artery* 1985;12:324–336.

73. Roth GR, Calverley DC. Aspirin, platelets, and thrombosis: theory and practice. *Blood* 1994;83:885–898.

74. Brinkman HJ, van Buul Wortelboer MF, van Mourik JA. Involvement of cyclooxygenase and lipoxygenase-mediated conversion of arachidonic acid in controlling human vascular smooth muscle cell proliferation. *Thromb Haemost* 1990;63: 291–297.

75. Loesberg C, Van Wijk R, Zandbergen J, et al. Cell cycle-dependent inhibition of human vascular smooth muscle cell proliferation by prostaglandin E1. *Exp Cell Res* 1985;160:117–125.

76. Nakao J, Koshihara Y, Ito H, et al. Enhancement of endogenous production of 12-L-hydroxy-5,8,10,14-eiosatetraenoic acid in aortic smooth muscle cells by platelet-derived growth factor. *Life Sci* 1985;37:1435–1442.

77. Nakao J, Ito H, Chang WC, et al. Aortic smooth muscle cell migration caused by platelet derived growth factor is mediated by lipoxygenase product(s) of arachidonic acid. *Biochem Biophys Res Commun* 1983;112:866–871.

78. Nakao J, Ooyama T, Ito H, et al. Comparative effects of lipoxygenase products of arachidonic acid on rat smooth muscle cell migration. *Atherosclerosis* 1982;44:339–342.

79. Nakao J, Ito H, Ooyama T, et al. Calcium dependence of aortic smooth muscle migration induced by 12-L-hydroxy-5,8,10,14-eicosatetraenoic acid: effect of A23187, nicardopine and trifluoperazine. *Atherosclerosis* 1983;46:309–319.

80. Nakao J, Ito H, Kanayasu T, et al. Stimulatory effect of insulin on aortic smooth muscle cell migration induced by 12-L-hydroxy-5,8,10,14-eicosatetraenoic acid and its modulation by elevated extracellular glucose levels. *Diabetes* 1985;34:185–191.

81. Nakao J, Ito H, Koshihara Y, et al. Age related increase in migration of aortic smooth muscle cells induced by 12-L-hydroxy-5,8,10,14-eicosatetraenoic acid. *Atherosclerosis* 1984;51:179–187.

82. Saito F, Hori MD, Ideguchi Y, et al. 12-Lipoxygenase products modulate calcium signals in vascular smooth muscle cells. *Hypertension* 1992;20:138–143.

83. Natarajan R, Gu JL, Rossi J, et al. Elevated glucose and angiotensin II increase 12-lipoxygenase activity and expression in porcine aortic smooth muscle cells. *Proc Natl Acad Sci USA* 1993;90:4947–4951.

84. Diskin CJ, Stokes TJ, Pennell AT. Pharmacologic intervention to prevent hemodialysis access thrombosis. *Nephron* 1993;64: 1–26.

85. Heller A, Koch T, Schmeck J, et al. Lipid mediators in inflammatory disorders. *Drugs* 1998;55:487–496.

86. Rylance PB, Gordge MP, Saynor R, et al. Fish oil modifies lipids and reduces platelet aggregability in hemodialysis patients. *Nephron* 1986;43:196–202.

87. Landymore RW, MacAulay MA, Cooper JH, et al. Effects of cod liver oil on intimal hyperplasia in vein grafts used for arterial bypass. *Can J Surg* 1986;29:129–131.

88. Landymore RW, Kinley CE, Cooper JH, et al. Cod liver oil for prevention of intimal hyperplasia of autogenous vein grafts used for arterial bypass. *Thorac Cardiovasc Surg* 1985;59:351–357.

89. Cahill PD, Saris GE, Cooper AD, et al. Inhibition of vein graft intimal thickening by eicosapentaenoic acid: reduced thromboxane production without change in lipoprotein levels or low density lipoprotein density. *J Vasc Surg* 1988;7:108–118.

90. Schmitz PG, Tyler LD. Fish oil inhibits intimal hyperplasia in a rodent model of injury. *J Am Soc Nephrol* 2000;11:196A.

91. Hoover RL, Rosenberg R, Haering W, et al. Inhibition of rat arterial smooth muscle cell proliferation by heparin. II. *In vitro* studies. *Circ Res* 1980;47:578–583.

92. Clowes AW, Karnovsky MJ. Suppression by heparin of smooth muscle cell proliferation in injured arteries. *Nature* 1977;265: 625–626.

93. Castellot JJ, Addonizio ML, Rosenberg R, et al. Cultured endothelial cells produce a heparin-like inhibitor of smooth muscle cell growth. *J Cell Biol* 1981;90:372–379.

94. Fritze LMS, Reilly CF, Rosenberg RD. An antiproliferative heparin sulfate species produced by post-confluent smooth muscle cells. *J Cell Biol* 1985;100:1041–1049.

95. Elliot S, Striker LJ, Stetler-Stevenson WG, et al. Pentosan polysulfate decreases proliferation and net extracellular matrix production in mouse mesangial cells. *J Am Soc Nephrol* 1999;10: 62–68.

96. Koyama N, Kinsella MG, Wight TN, et al. Heparin sulfate proteoglycans mediate a potent inhibitory signal for migration of vascular smooth muscle cells. *Circ Res* 1998;83:305–313.

97. Sitter T, Schiffl H. Anticardiolipin antibodies in patients on regular hemodialysis: an epiphenomenon. *Nephron* 1993;64:655–656.

98. Ishii Y, Yano S. Evaluation of blood coagulation fibrinolysis system in patients receiving chronic hemodialysis. *Nephron* 1996; 73:407–412.

99. Brunet P, Aillaud MF, et al. Antiphospholipids in hemodialysis patients: relationship between lupus anticoagulant and thrombosis. *Kidney Int* 1995;48:794–800.

100. Manns BJ, Burgess ED, et al. Hyperhomocystinemia, anticardiolipin antibody status, and risk for vascular access thrombosis in hemodialysis patients. *Kidney Int* 1999;55:315–320.

101. Shemin D, Lapane KL, Bausserman L, et al. Plasma total homocysteine and hemodialysis access thrombosis: a prospective study. *J Am Soc Nephrol* 1999;10:1095–1099.

102. Biggers JA, Remmers AR, et al. The risk of anticoagulation in hemodialysis patients. *Nephron* 1977;18:109–113.

103. LeSar CJ, Merrick HW, et al. Thrombotic complications resulting from hypercoagulable states in chronic hemodialysis vascular access. *J Am Coll Surg* 1999;189:73–81.

104. Petrik PV, Law MM, Moore WS, et al. Dexamethasone and enalapril suppress intimal hyperplasia individually but have no synergistic effect. *Ann Vasc Surg* 1998;12:216–220.

105. Fareh J, Martel R, Kermani P, et al. Cellular effects of beta-particle delivery on vascular smooth muscle cells and endothelical cells: a dose-response study. *Circulation* 1999:99:1477–1484.

106. Diamond DA, Vesely TM. The role of radiation therapy in the management of vascular restenosis. Part II. Radiation techniques and results. *J Vasc Interv Radiol* 1998;9:389–400.

107. Tierstein PS, Massullo V, Jani S, et al. Three-year clinical and angiographic follow-up after intracoronary radiation: results of a randomized clinical trial. *Circulation* 2000;101:360–365.

108. Verin V, Popowski Y, De Bruyne B, et al., and the Dose Finding Group. Endoluminal beta-radiation therapy for the prevention of coronary restenosis after balloon angioplasty. *N Engl J Med* 2001;344:243–249.

109. Leon MB, Teirstein PS, Moses JW, et al. Localized intracoronary gamma-radiation therapy to inhibit the recurrence of restenosis after stenting. *N Engl J Med* 2001;344:250–256.

110. Kelly BS, Heffelfinger SC, Narayana A, et al. External beam radiation (EBR) reduces venous neointimal hyperplasia (VNH) in PTFE dialysis grafts. *J Am Soc Nephrol* 2000;11:187A(abst).

111. Basile DP. Prevention of restenosis of central venous stricture after percutaneous transluminal angioplasty and endovascular stenting by brachytherapy. *Kidney Int* 1999;55:742–743.

112. Clowes AW. Improving the interface between biomaterials and the blood: the gene therapy approach. *Circulation* 1996;93:1319–1320.

113. Schneider PA, Hanson SR, Price TM, et al. Durability of confluent endothelial cell monolayers on small-caliber vascular prostheses *in vitro*. *Surgery* 1988;103:456–462.

114. Yue X, van der Lei B, Schakenraad JM, et al. Smooth muscle cell seeding in biodegradable grafts in rats: a new method to enhance the process of arterial wall generation. *Surgery* 1988;103:206–212.

115. Ortenwall P, Wadenvik H, Kutti J, et al. Endothelial cell seeding reduces thrombogenicity of Dacron grafts in humans. *J Vasc Surg* 1990;11:403–410.

116. Herring M, Smith J, Dalsing M, et al. Endothelial seeding of polytetrafluoroethylene femoral popliteal bypasses: the failure of low-density seeding to improve patency. *J Vasc Surg* 1994;20:650–655.

117. Zilla P, Deutch M, Meinhart J, et al. Clinical *in vitro* endothelialization of femoropopliteal bypass grafts: an actuarial follow-up over three years. *J Vasc Surg* 1994;19:540–548.

118. Fasol R, Zilla P, Deutch M, et al. Human endothelial cell seeding: evaluation of its effectiveness by platelet parameters after one year. *J Vasc Surg* 1989;9:432–436.

119. Miyata T, Conte MS, Trudell LA, et al. Delayed exposure to pulsatile shear stress improves retention of human saphenous vein endothelial cells on seeded ePTFE grafts. *J Surg Res* 1991;50:485–493.

120. Rosenman JE, Kempszinski RF, Pearce WH, et al. Kinetics of endothelial cell seeding. *J Vasc Surg* 1985;2:778–784.

121. Dardick A, Liu A, Ballermann BJ. Chronic *in vitro* shear stress stimulates endothelial cell retention on prosthetic vascular grafts and reduces subsequent in vivo neointimal thickness. *J Vasc Surg* 1999;29:157–167.

122. Newman KD, Nguyen N, Dichek DA. Quantification of vascular graft seeding by use of computer-assisted image analysis and genetically modified endothelial cells. *J Vasc Surg* 1991;14:140–146.

123. Sackman JE, Freeman MB, Petersen MG, et al. Synthetic vascular grafts seeded with genetically modified endothelium in the dog: evaluation of the effect of seeding technique and retroviral vector on cell persistence *in vivo*. *Cell Transplant* 1995;4:219–235.

124. Dunn PF, Newman KD, Jones M, et al. Seeding of vascular grafts with genetically modified endothelial cells: secretion of recombinant TPA results in decreased seeded cell retention *in vitro* and *in vivo*. *Circulation* 1996;93:1439–1446.

125. Svensson EC, Schwartz LB. Gene therapy for vascular disease. *Curr Opin Cardiol* 1998;13:369–374.

126. Walsh K, Perlman H. Molecular strategies to inhibit restenosis: modulation of the vascular myocyte phenotype. *Semin Interv Cardiol* 1996;1:173–179.

127. Clowes AW. Vascular gene therapy in the 21st century. *Thromb Haemost* 1997;78:605–610.

128. Morishita R, Nakagami H, Taniyama Y, et al. Oligonucleotide-based gene therapy for cardiovascular disease. *Clin Chem Lab Med* 1998;36:529–534.

129. Ohno T, Gordon D, San H, et al. Gene therapy for vascular smooth muscle cell proliferation after arterial injury. *Science* 1994;265:781–784.

130. Mann MJ, Whittemore AD, Donaldson MC, et al. *Ex vivo* gene therapy of human vascular bypass grafts with E2F decoy: the PREVENT single-centre, randomised, controlled trial. *Lancet* 1999;354:1493–1498.

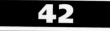

PHYSICAL AND BIOLOGIC CONSIDERATIONS FOR HEMODIALYSIS CATHETERS (BIOFILM, LOCKS, AND PORTS)

THOMAS M. VESELY

Central venous catheters are a suboptimal method of providing vascular access for hemodialysis. The common occurrence of catheter-related complications has limited their acceptance as a desirable method of vascular access. Catheter-related infections are one of the most serious complications encountered in this patient population. Infectious complications include exit site or tunnel infections, bacteremia and sepsis, and metastatic seeding of blood-borne bacteria, which can lead to endocarditis or discitis. Catheters can incite central venous stenosis and thrombosis, a significant problem that limits the availability of future vascular access sites. (See Chapter 25.) Catheter-related thrombosis and fibrin sheath formation are discussed in Chapter 36. Finally, many catheters are unable to achieve or sustain adequate blood flow rates for hemodialysis. Failure to provide the necessary blood flow rates can limit the efficiency of dialysis and lead to inadequate treatment or prolonged hemodialysis treatment times.

Despite these numerous problems, central venous catheters continue to have an important role in the management of vascular access for hemodialysis patients. Our continued reliance on catheters is based on several useful attributes (1). Catheters can be inserted easily and quickly into most patients, and they can be used for hemodialysis immediately after placement. Patients prefer that needle punctures not be required with catheter access and that once hemodialysis is completed there is no need to hold needle sticks for approximately 10 minutes to achieve thrombostasis.

The most common indication for a hemodialysis catheter is the need for a temporary vascular access in patients who are awaiting the maturation of an arteriovenous fistula or synthetic graft. In the past decade, however, there has been an increasing reliance on catheters as a permanent method of vascular access for hemodialysis. The reasons for using a catheter as a permanent vascular access include (a) exhaus-

tion of peripheral vascular access sites in chronic hemodialysis patients, (b) an inability to find suitable vessels for a fistula or graft in elderly or diabetic patients, and (c) patients with cardiovascular compromise who cannot support or tolerate a fistula or graft.

Because of our continuing reliance on hemodialysis catheters, extensive efforts have been made to reduce the incidence of catheter-related complications and improve catheter performance. Substantial research has been directed toward understanding the complex biological processes that are responsible for catheter-related infections. Recent advances in catheter construction have focused on the development of new materials that may prevent or inhibit these infections (see Chapter 35). In addition, technological efforts have been directed toward creating new catheter designs that can provide higher and more reliable flow rates during hemodialysis.

The first section of this chapter reviews the pathogenesis of catheter infections and several of the methods that have been used to prevent their occurrence. This is followed by a description of catheter materials, design, and performance. This material serves as a foundation for a description of new concepts in hemodialysis catheters, including hemodialysis ports and catheter-locking solutions.

CATHETER INFECTION

The pathogenesis of catheter-related infections is complex, multifactorial, and continues to be a topic of intense research. Catheter infections are the result of a sequence of events that begins with contamination of the catheter surfaces, followed by bacterial colonization and the subsequent development of a biofilm layer.

The initiating event can be caused by bacterial skin flora that gain access to the external surface of the catheter at the time of insertion or by bacteria that migrate from the skin surface onto the catheter once it is in position. Alternatively, the internal surfaces of a catheter can become contaminated with bacteria by frequent manipulation of the catheter hub or by hematogenous spread from another source. The duration of catheter placement is thought to be an important determinant of the source of infection (2). Colonization of the external surfaces by skin flora is the most common source of infection during the first 10 days after catheter placement. Colonization of the internal (luminal) surfaces of the catheter, likely due to contamination of the hub, predominates after 30 days of catheter placement.

Bacterial attachment to the catheter surface is the first and most important step in the pathogenesis of infection. To become adherent to the catheter, the invading bacteria must overcome a variety of physical forces, including gravitational forces, shear forces, electrostatic forces, and surface tension, which act to prevent bacterial attachment (3). Characteristics of the catheter surface, such as the type of material, surface smoothness, and hydrophilicity, can affect the bacterial attachment process. Exposure of the catheter to the subcutaneous tissues can change these surface characteristics. This process, known as *surface conditioning*, has been demonstrated to occur with silicone catheters and can alter the ability of bacteria to attach to the external surfaces (3,4). Certain blood proteins, such as albumin, fibrinogen, and fibronectin, can deposit on the catheter surface and serve as ligands for bacterial attachment (5). Contact-activated platelets also may have a role in bacterial attachment to intravascular surfaces.

Following successful attachment to the catheter surface, the bacteria multiply and begin to form undifferentiated microcolonies. An extracellular signaling process initiates the maturation of these bacterial colonies and triggers the cells to secrete an amorphous polysaccharide matrix termed the *glycocalix*. The maturation and growth of the bacterial colonies, combined with the continued secretion of the glycocalix, create a confluence of microorganisms embedded within an extracellular matrix. When combined with host substances, such as blood proteins and platelets, this complex microenvironment is called a *biofilm*.

A biofilm is defined as a complex structure of bacterial cells enclosed in a self-produced glycocalix that allows survival in a hostile environment (6). Biofilms are ubiquitous throughout our environment and commonly are found on persistently wet surfaces. The development of biofilm within humans, such as on the surface of an implanted medical device, is responsible for a significant number of chronic bacterial infections.

The bacterial community within a biofilm comprises two forms: sessile bacteria that remain embedded within the glycocalix and planktonic bacteria that are released into the bloodstream and colonize other areas throughout the body. Sessile bacteria that are located within the glycocalix are protected from the host's immune responses and are less sus-

ceptible to antibiotics. Many antimicrobial agents are unable to penetrate into the glycocalix or are inactivated in the outer layers of the biofilm. In addition, some of the sessile bacteria within the biofilm are in a slow-growing or nongrowing state and are less susceptible to antimicrobial agents.

The periodic multiplication and release of the planktonic forms of bacteria are thought to be responsible for the sudden onset of symptoms associated with a catheter-related infection. These planktonic bacteria shed from the protective biofilm can be killed, however, using antimicrobial therapy. It is for this reason that antibiotic treatment may alleviate the acute symptoms of a catheter-related infection but cannot eradicate the sessile bacteria located deep within the biofilm (6).

Colonization and formation of a biofilm layer on the surfaces of a hemodialysis catheter may not necessarily lead to a catheter-related infection. Raad and colleagues used electron microscopy to quantify the amount of biofilm on the surfaces of infected and noninfected silicone catheters (2). The extent of biofilm on catheters that were removed for infection did not differ from the amount of biofilm found on noninfected catheters. The multiplication and release of planktonic bacteria from the biofilm are believed to correlate with a clinical infection. The regulatory mechanisms responsible for the release of planktonic bacteria from the biofilm are not well known.

CATHETER DESIGN AND CONSTRUCTION

Numerous strategies have been developed to prevent or inhibit the cascade of biological events that lead to a catheter-related infection. A variety of approaches have been used to prevent bacterial contamination of the catheter at the time of insertion. These include the use of different cutaneous disinfectants, intravenous antibiotics, fastidious catheter-site care, and different types of catheter dressings. Catheters can be cuffed, tunneled, or buried in a subcutaneous pocket (*ports*) to decrease the migration of skin bacteria onto the catheter. Most recently, the physical nature of the catheter material has been modified by the addition of antimicrobial, antibiotic, or antithrombotic coatings. Several of these catheter modifications are discussed in more detail herein.

Catheter Materials

The ideal material for the construction of long-term hemodialysis catheters should have several characteristics, including structural integrity, long-term biostability, low bacterial adhesion, low thrombogenicity, and resistance to kinking. This section focuses on the materials that are used in the construction of the current generation of long-term hemodialysis catheters.

For the past decade, silicone has been the primary material used for the construction of many types of central venous access devices, including peripherally inserted central catheters, ports, and tunneled central venous catheters. Silicone is classified as a thermoset elastomer, a group of polymers that are known for their thermal, chemical, and enzymatic stability (7). Silicone is advantageous as a material for catheter construction because of this biostability and also because it is a soft material with excellent kink resistance; however, silicone catheters are not very stiff and often require an introducer sheath for insertion. Some silicone materials have a high coefficient of friction that imparts a tacky feel to the catheter surface. This can create resistance between the external surface of the catheter and the inner surface of an introducer sheath during the insertion procedure. Silicone has limited tensile strength, and catheters constructed of this material can be damaged if mishandled.

Polyurethanes are classified within a broad group of polymers called *thermoplastics*. This group of materials also includes polyvinyl chloride, polyethylene, polyamides, and polyesters. Polyurethanes are becoming increasingly popular for use in medical devices because of the ability to adjust specific characteristics of the material during the manufacturing process. Polyurethane has three to ten times the tensile strength of silicone. This valuable characteristic has been used to improve the performance of hemodialysis catheters. Polyurethane catheters can be designed to have very thin walls and will maintain excellent structural integrity. Decreasing the thickness of the catheter walls will lead to an increase in the inner luminal dimensions while maintaining the same outer diameter. Larger inner luminal dimensions should increase catheter flow rates. Some polyurethanes are designed to be slightly stiff under room temperature conditions, which allows easier insertion, but they soften after exposure to the increased temperature and moisture within the central veins.

Silicone catheters have an increased risk of infection compared with polyurethane, polyvinyl chloride, or Teflon catheters (4). The reason for this increased risk of infection is likely multifactorial. Hydrophobic material such as silicone tends to attract bacteria more than hydrophilic materials. Scanning electron microscopy has revealed that silicone catheters have a rougher surface compared with polyurethane catheters; this may play a role in bacterial adherence (8). Silicone also causes activation of the complement system, which has been suggested to increase the risk of infection (9).

New technologies have been developed to modify the surfaces of silicone and polyurethane catheters to decrease the thrombogenicity of the material and prevent bacterial adherence. The addition of a heparin coating decreases the deposition of plasma proteins and platelets onto the catheter surface. By decreasing the number of bacterial attachment sites, the heparin coating may interfere with bacterial colonization and subsequent biofilm formation. Appelgren and colleagues used a heparin coating with long-term (>4 months) stability on vascular catheters and demonstrated a reduction in catheter-related infections compared with noncoated catheters (10).

A wide variety of antimicrobial substances have been applied to the surfaces of vascular catheters to prevent infection. Most investigational trials have used nontunneled catheters with antimicrobial coatings. These catheters, which were used for short-term (<10 days) implantation, had mixed results (11–16). Some of the antimicrobial coatings decreased the incidence of infection, but this benefit was short-lived. The chemical coating leached into the blood or surrounding tissues, which decreased the local concentration of the agent, and thereby diminished its effectiveness. New methods to create long-term bonding of antimicrobial agents to catheter surfaces are under development and may prove beneficial for use in long-term hemodialysis catheters. The widespread use of antibiotic-coated catheters is an important public health concern, however, because of the potential for developing antibiotic resistant strains of bacteria. Several guidelines for the future development of antimicrobial-coated catheters have been proposed to address this important issue (17,18).

Ion implantation and ion beam–assisted deposition can be used to alter the physical and chemical structure of the outer surface of catheter materials. These ion beam processes affect only the extreme outer layer (1 μm) of the material; therefore, the structural integrity of the catheter is not affected. These ion-beam processes can be used to alter surface characteristics that affect biocompatibility. Increasing the critical surface tension of catheter materials can increase their ability to resist the deposition of plasma proteins. This can create a less thrombogenic surface that is more resistant to infection (19). In addition, an ion-beam process can be used to deposit extremely thin layers of coatings onto the surface of catheters. Thin layers of silver have been applied to catheters to create an infection-resistant and thrombus-resistant outer surface (20,21).

Catheter Design

The dual-lumen configuration is the most common design used for the current generation of tunneled, long-term hemodialysis catheters. Dual-lumen catheters have either a circular or oval external shape. All these catheters have a central internal septum that creates two "D"-shaped internal lumina. The Ash split catheter (Medcomp, Harleysville, PA, U.S.A.) is a variant design of the dual-lumen configuration. After the Ash split catheter is tunneled through the subcutaneous tissue, the distal 5 to 7 cm of the central septum is manually separated ("split") immediately before insertion. This separation of the distal tips is thought to improve blood flow and decrease recirculation.

An alternative design, the Tesio twin catheters (Medcomp), consists of two separate single-lumen silicone catheters that are inserted in parallel subcutaneous tunnels for long-term vascular access. The Schon catheter (Angio-Dynamics, Queensbury, NY, U.S.A.) is a variant of the single lumen design. The Schon catheter consists of two separate single-lumen catheters that are permanently joined at one point along the length of the catheters. When buried within the subcutaneous tissue, this junction point effectively prevents accidental dislodgment. The Schon catheter requires two separate subcutaneous tunnels but only one vascular entry site.

Theoretic evaluation of these two different catheter designs suggests that the use of two single-lumen catheters (i.e., Tesio) should provide higher and more reliable blood flows compared with a dual-lumen catheter (22,23). The combined internal luminal dimension of two separate single-lumen catheters is larger than the internal lumina of one dual-lumen catheter. The detrimental aspect of this greater luminal capacity is that it is achieved using two large-diameter catheters. From a different perspective, the incorporation of an internal septum has a negative effect on catheter performance. Using a derivation of Poiseuille's law to estimate the effect of a noncircular cross-section on catheter performance suggests that the central septum creates a sevenfold increase in resistance to flow compared with a circular tube of equal diameter.

The arterial and venous end holes, located at the distal tip of the catheter, are staggered (1–3 cm) to minimize mixing (*recirculation*) of the blood during hemodialysis. The average recirculation for a well-positioned catheter, with the tips positioned in the upper right atrium, should be less than 5% (23).

Several of the long-term hemodialysis catheters are designed with multiple side holes or perforations along their distal end. These holes function to decrease intraluminal pressure and thereby facilitate blood flow (22). The lumina of catheters constructed of soft material can partially or temporarily collapse when subjected to the high negative pressures (300–350 mm Hg) used to achieve maximal flow rates during hemodialysis. The addition of side holes may prevent this collapse when these high negative pressures are imposed. (24). These side holes also may be beneficial in preventing the formation of a confluent fibrin sheath along the distal aspect of the catheter.

The *sine qua non* of most long-term hemodialysis catheters is the cuff attached to the external surface. This cuff promotes tissue ingrowth, thereby anchoring the catheter to the subcutaneous tissue in the tunnel. The cuff is also thought to be a barrier to infection, but this function has not been demonstrated for long-term hemodialysis catheters. Antimicrobial impregnated cuffs have shown variable results in their ability to decrease the rate of catheter colonization and infection (25). Unfortunately, the use of antimicrobial impregnated cuffs also can decrease the ingrowth of fibroblasts and predispose the cuff to dislodgement (26). The Schon catheter is currently the only long-term hemodialysis catheter that does not have an external cuff.

Catheter-related Hemodynamics

Blood flow through a hemodialysis catheter is related to the pressures applied by the hemodialysis machine and the resistance created within the catheter lumina. Poiseuille's law mathematically describes the specific parameters that determine this relationship (Fig. 42.1). Blood flow increases by the fourth power of the radius of the inner lumen. Because of this exponential influence, the dimension of the internal lumen is the most critical determinant of blood flow. Slight increases in the radius of the internal lumen will dramatically increase the blood flow. For this reason, the type of material used for catheter construction can affect catheter performance. Silicone catheters will have reduced blood flow compared with a polyurethane catheter of equal outer diameter. As previously described, the greater tensile strength of polyurethane allows catheters to be constructed with thinner walls, thereby providing a larger inner luminal diameter.

The currently available long-term dual-lumen catheters range from 12 to 16 French (4–5 mm) in diameter. The Vaxcel catheter (Boston Scientific, Natick, MA, U.S.A.) has a 16-French shaft near the external hubs that tapers to 14 French at the distal tip. The single-lumen Tesio catheters are available in 10 French and 12 French. Using Poiseuille's law, if the wall thickness of a catheter remains constant, increasing the outer diameter from 10 French to 12 French will double the rate of blood flow through the catheter. Further increasing the outer diameter of the catheter to 15 French will provide a five times greater flow rate compared with a 10-French catheter. Figure 42.2 depicts the proportional relationships between a 15-French catheter and the internal luminal diameters of several central venous segments.

As also described by Poiseuille's law, increasing the catheter length will directly increase the resistance to blood flow. Longer catheters will have decreased performance compared with shorter versions with equal luminal dimensions. Long (36–55 cm) hemodialysis catheters are available

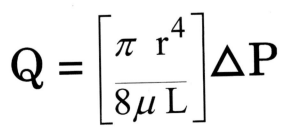

$$Q = \left[\frac{\pi \, r^4}{8 \mu \, L} \right] \Delta P$$

FIGURE 42.1. Poiseuille's law. Catheter blood flow (*Q*) is proportional to the radius (*r*) of the inner lumen and the pressure difference (*ΔP*) but inversely proportional to the viscosity (*μ*) and the length (*L*).

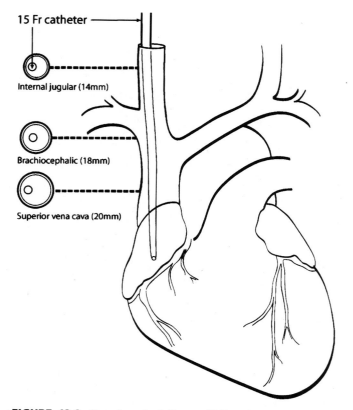

15 Fr catheter

Internal jugular (14mm)

Brachiocephalic (18mm)

Superior vena cava (20mm)

FIGURE 42.2. Drawing depicting a 15-French catheter positioned within the right central veins. The cross-sectional images along the left side of the drawing depict the proportional relationship of the 15-French catheter to the luminal diameters of the venous segments.

and are used primarily for alternative vascular access sites, such as through femoral, translumbar, or transhepatic routes.

The viscosity (μ) of blood is another determinant of blood flow through a hemodialysis catheter. Because of hemoconcentration, the viscosity of blood increases during a hemodialysis treatment (27). According to Poiseuille's law, if viscosity is increased by 20%, the blood flow will decrease by 16.67%. The viscosity of blood is related to the hematocrit level. In the hematocrit range of 25% to 60%, a 10% increase in hematocrit will increase the blood viscosity by about 20% (28). Using a 15-cm-long, 11-French-diameter catheter in a patient with a hematocrit of 25%, a prepump pressure of 80 mm Hg is required to achieve a blood flow rate of 300 mL per minute. If the patient's hematocrit is increased to 40%, the viscosity of the blood increases, and a prepump pressure of 260 mm Hg is needed to obtain the same flow rate.

Catheter Performance

High-efficiency hemodialyzers require a vascular access that can sustain blood flows of at least 350 mL per minute, preferably 400 mL per minute, to achieve maximum efficiency (23). Grafts and arteriovenous fistulae typically pro-

vide blood flows greater than 400 mL per minute. Whereas manufacturers often claim that hemodialysis catheters can consistently sustain blood flows of 400 mL per minute or greater, this level of performance is seldom achieved in a diverse patient population. More commonly, the average blood flow through a long-term hemodialysis catheter ranges from 300 to 350 mL per minute (29–31).

Several clinical studies have reported the performance capabilities for several long-term catheters. The blood flows achieved using Tesio twin catheters range from 300 to 400 mL per minute (23,31,32). Perini and colleagues reported that the blood flows obtained using Tesio catheters increased from 286 mL per minute at the time of insertion to 306 mL per minute after 6 months of placement. The blood flows reported for the Ash split catheter range from 295 to 422 mL per minute (31,33). Reported flows for the Perm-Cath (Kendall, Mansfield, MA, U.S.A.) range from 280 to 380 mL per minute (23,31).

One of the most important factors to ensure a well-functioning hemodialysis catheter is correct positioning of the catheter tip. (See Chapters 32, 33, and 36 for optimal catheter tip position regarding catheter function.) The historical concern regarding the placement of catheter tips in the right atrium is related to the potential for vascular injury. Years ago, some vascular catheters were constructed of stiff materials that could be injurious; however, the current generation of long-term hemodialysis catheters is constructed of soft materials that can be positioned safely within the upper right atrium. Numerous studies have demonstrated that the tip of a hemodialysis catheter should be positioned within the superior aspect of the right atrium or at the cava–atrial junction (34–36). McCarthy and colleagues found that catheters positioned in the right atrium had a longer duration of function (116 days) than catheters with tips in the superior vena cava (100 days) or in the brachiocephalic vein (12 days) (37).

HEMODIALYSIS PORTS

Vascular catheters with external components are susceptible to infection by migration of bacterial skin flora along the subcutaneous tunnel or by contamination of the hubs. Removal of these external components may eliminate these mechanisms of infection. Vascular access ports are devices that are implanted into the subcutaneous tissue ("port pocket") and have no external components. A vascular catheter is inserted into a central vein and then subcutaneously tunneled to connect with the port device. Access to the port is obtained by the use of special needles. Vascular access ports are commonly used for chemotherapy and are reported to have lower infection rates than traditional catheter designs (38,39).

Traditional vascular catheters often place limitations on the patient's lifestyle and may alter the patient's body image.

Implantable ports require minimal maintenance and no changes in the activities of daily living.

The design and construction of subcutaneous ports for hemodialysis require advanced technology that is not found in conventional ports used for chemotherapy. Hemodialysis ports must be able to endure frequent punctures with large-caliber needles, and they must be capable of providing sustained high blood flow rates during hemodialysis.

This section describes two recently developed hemodialysis port systems. Each of these port systems has a unique and technologically sophisticated percutaneous access mechanism that is capable of enduring multiple, large-bore needle punctures. Both of these port systems use two separate single-lumen catheters for aspiration and return of blood from the hemodialysis machine. As we have previously learned, this design is advantageous for achieving high blood flows.

Subcutaneous ports should be implanted into an anatomic region that provides stabilization of the device and does not interfere with patient motion. The port should be implanted at the correct depth (10–15 mm) within the subcutaneous tissue. Insufficient tissue coverage of the port can cause tissue necrosis, and excessive depth can lead to difficult needle cannulation.

Although the initial costs of hemodialysis ports are high, nearly ten times the cost of a conventional catheter, these devices may prove to be more economical if catheter-related complications can be reduced. Continued clinical study of these devices is needed before we will be able to more thoroughly assess their benefits.

Lifesite Hemodialysis Access System

The LifeSite hemodialysis access system (Vasca, Inc., Tewksbury, MA, U.S.A.) consists of a subcutaneous port, or valve, attached to a single-lumen catheter (Fig. 42.3). Two separate ports and catheters are necessary for each patient, one for aspirating and the other for returning blood from the hemodialysis machine. The two ports typically are implanted side by side in the right anterior chest wall inferior

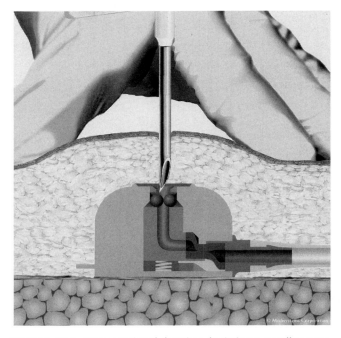

FIGURE 42.4. Cross-sectional drawing depicting a needle entering the LifeSite hemodialysis port.

to the clavicle. The catheters are separately tunneled to the vascular entry site, most commonly the right internal jugular vein.

The LifeSite port, which measures 17 mm in height and 32 mm in diameter, has a titanium alloy outer housing and an internal valve mechanism constructed of silicone and stainless steel. A 12-French (4-mm) silicone catheter is attached to the base of each port during the implantation procedure. The luminal diameter of the catheter is 2.46 mm, and the distal tip has one large end hole and six side holes. Each catheter initially measures 65 cm in length but is cut to the appropriate length at the time of implantation.

To gain access to the LifeSite port, a 14-gauge needle is inserted into the valve entry site with a twisting motion until it locks in position. Insertion of the 14-gauge needle opens an internal pinch clamp, allowing blood flow through the port and catheter (Fig. 42.4). When the needle is withdrawn, the pinch clamp closes and seals the valve. The access needle is intentionally inserted into the exact same skin site for each cannulation, which leads to the development of a fibrous tract between the LifeSite valve entrance and the overlying skin entry site. This is referred to as the *buttonhole technique*. Over time, needle cannulation of the port valve becomes easier and can be performed using blunt needles without causing pain to the patient.

The LifeSite port is designed to allow irrigation of the valve mechanism and surrounding port pocket with an antimicrobial solution. A 25-gauge needle is inserted into port and used to instill 1 mL of a 70% isopropyl alcohol solution. This volume of irrigant fluid overfills the valve mechanism and allows seepage of the antimicrobial solution into the

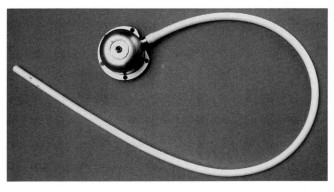

FIGURE 42.3. The LifeSite hemodialysis port with attached 12-French catheter.

port pocket and along the buttonhole tract. The 25-gauge needle will not open the internal pinch clamp and thus prevents irrigant fluid from entering the catheter or vascular system. The manufacturer recommends irrigating the Life-Site port with 70% isopropyl alcohol before and after each cannulation. At the end of each hemodialysis treatment, before removing the 14-gauge access needle, the lumen of each catheter is filled with a standard heparin lock solution.

The performance and durability of the LifeSite hemodialysis access system have been compared with those of Tesio catheters (40). An average blood flow of 359 mL per minute was achieved using the LifeSite port compared with 332 mL per minute using the Tesio catheters. During the 6-month follow-up period, the device-related infection rate in the LifeSite group (1.3 per 1,000 patient-days) was less than the Tesio group (3.3 per 1,000 patient-days).

Dialock Hemodialysis Access Device

The Dialock (Biolink Corp., Middleboro, MA, U.S.A.) hemodialysis access device is an implantable, subcutaneous port that has two separate needle accessible passages, each of which leads to a single lumen vascular catheter (Fig. 42.5). A single Dialock device provides vascular access for both aspiration and return of blood from the hemodialysis machine.

The Dialock device is constructed of titanium and measures about 50 mm × 30 mm × 20 mm. The needle entry area has a trough-like design to aid the user in accessing the two needle passageways. To minimize blood flow turbulence through the device, the Dialock was designed to provide straight-line alignment of the access needle and the vascular catheter. Insertion of the proprietary 15-gauge needle opens a septum-valve mechanism to provide access to the channel connecting to the vascular catheter. The septum-valve mechanism closes when the needle is withdrawn to prevent backflow of blood through the port.

Two 11-French vascular catheters are attached to the Dialock device during the implantation procedure. The catheter is constructed of very thin-walled silicone tubing, providing an inner luminal diameter of 2.5 mm. A thin reinforcing wire extends circumferentially along the length of the catheter. Each catheter has a single notched end hole. The catheter is initially 40 cm long and is cut to the appropriate length during the insertion procedure. After attaching the two catheters to the Dialock device, they are secured by the use of a locking tool and the insertion a locking pin.

The Dialock device is accessed using a proprietary cannula (needle) set. The 15-gauge cannula has an internal stylet that is used to access the port and open the septum-valve mechanism. After "docking" the cannula within the port, the stylet is removed. The 15-gauge cannula is attached to silicone rubber tubing fitted with a standard Luer-lock connector to provide linkage between the patient and the hemodialysis machine. After completion of dialysis, a catheter-locking solution (see later) flush solution, including taurolidine, has been used to prevent infectious complications.

Two clinical trials of the Dialock hemodialysis access device have been described. Levin and colleagues reported av-

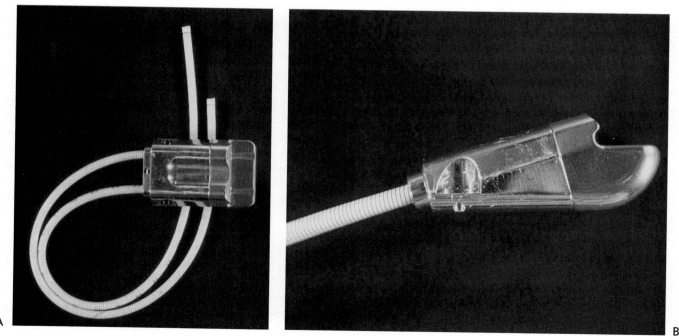

FIGURE 42.5. A: The Dialock hemodialysis port with attached 11-French catheters. **B:** Lateral view of the Dialock device.

erage blood flows of 326 mL per minute in a small group of ten patients who received the Dialock device (41). They reported their infection rate as 2.3 episodes of bacteremia per 1,000 patient-days, and none of the devices were removed because of infection. In another small group of ten patients, Canaud and colleagues reported a mean blood flow of 307 mL per minute using the Dialock device (42). Three episodes of bacteremia occurred in two of these study patients, but no infections occurred related to the Dialock device.

CATHETER-LOCKING SOLUTIONS

Hemodialysis catheters are commonly filled, or locked, with concentrated heparin solution after every use. The volume of heparin instilled should correspond precisely to the volume of the catheter lumen. Typically, 1 to 2 mL of concentrated heparin (5,000 IU per milliliter) or nearly 10,000 U of heparin is instilled into each lumen. To prevent the undesirable effects of systemic heparinization, this solution must be withdrawn from the catheter before use.

Despite its beneficial antithrombotic effects, the use of concentrated heparin as a catheter-locking solution can have significant hazards. Inadvertent spillage of concentrated heparin from the catheter into the systemic circulation can lead to a variety of hemorrhagic complications, the most common of which is bleeding around the catheter exit site. Heparin-induced thrombocytopenia occurs in 1% to 3% of patients exposed to unfractionated heparin and can increase greatly the likelihood of vascular thrombotic events (see Chapter 9). The use of heparin as a catheter-locking solution also can interfere with laboratory studies performed on blood that has been withdrawn through the catheter.

Non–heparin catheter locking solutions have been used to avoid the potential problems associated with heparin. Compared with heparin, trisodium citrate and polygeline are equally effective as a catheter-locking solution (43). Citrate is an alternative anticoagulant that is commonly used during hemodialysis for patients who are allergic to heparin. Citrate acts as an anticoagulant by decreasing the level of ionized calcium in blood. Citrate (citric acid) also has some antimicrobial activity, particularly at high concentrations and low pH. Several investigators have reported the successful use of citrate as a hemodialysis catheter lock solution (43,44). On April 17, 2000, the United States Food and Drug Administration issued a warning regarding the use of concentrated (46.7%) citrate solution (TriCitrasol, Medcomp, Harleysville, PA, U.S.A.) because of serious complications that occurred after inadvertent systemic administration. The product has subsequently been withdrawn in the United States. Further investigation of the use of less concentrated citrate locking solutions is continuing.

In addition to antithrombotic activity, it would be advantageous for a catheter-locking solution to possess antibacterial activity. This could inhibit or prevent colonization of the internal luminal surfaces and reduce catheter-related infections. Vercaigne and colleagues evaluated the biochemical stability of combining an antibiotic, such as vancomycin, ceftazidime, or gentamicin with heparin (45). Although some of the antibiotic was absorbed onto the surface of the hemodialysis catheter, thereby reducing the concentration of "free" antibiotic, the remaining antibiotic concentration within the catheter was sufficient to decrease the incidence of infection.

Bastani and colleagues demonstrated that systemically administered antibiotics do not diffuse or otherwise penetrate into a catheter to provide effective intraluminal concentrations of the drug (46). Despite appropriate serum concentrations of vancomycin, the level of antibiotic measured within the catheter hub was too low to be clinically effective. Adequate concentrations of the antibiotic were achieved in only the distal 4 cm of the catheter. Their recommendation was to use both systemic antibiotic therapy plus an antibiotic lock solution.

Capdevial and colleagues evaluated the use of antibiotics given both systemically and as a catheter-locking solution to treat patients with catheter-related sepsis (47). Intravenous antibiotics were administered through the hemodialysis catheter as a 4-hour continuous infusion, half the dose through each lumen. The catheter lock solution (100 μg/mL of antibiotic in 5% heparin) containing either vancomycin or ciprofloxacin was instilled in each catheter lumen between hemodialysis treatments. The catheter-related sepsis resolved in all patients using this therapy. The follow-up quantitative blood cultures were negative, and none of the catheters was removed.

Although effective, the widespread use of conventional antibiotics within a catheter-locking solution may contribute to the emergence or spread of antibiotic-resistant bacterial infections. It would be preferable to use a nonantibiotic agent that has effective antimicrobial activity. Taurolidine, a chemical used for the treatment of bacterial peritonitis, possesses these attributes. It is a nonantibiotic agent that has a broad spectrum of antibacterial and antifungal activity. Taurolidine reduces or prevents the adherence of bacterial or fungal cells to epithelium by altering cell-wall structures and destroying fimbria and flagellae (48). The use of taurolidine as a component in a catheter-locking solution may inhibit bacteria from adhering to, and colonizing, the surfaces of a hemodialysis catheter. Studies have reported a decreased incidence of catheter-related infections when 2% taurolidine was added to the infusion for total parental nutrition. The development of antimicrobial resistance to or other adverse effects from taurolidine has not been reported. Other potential locking solutions needing study include the tissue plasminogen activators, which may prevent biofilm formation and therefore decrease infection risk and prevent clotting.

REFERENCES

1. Schwab SJ, Beathard G. The hemodialysis catheter conundrum: hate living with them, but can't live without them. *Kidney Int* 1991;56:1–17.
2. Raad I, Costerton W, Sabharwal U, et al. Ultrastructural analysis of indwelling vascular catheters: a quantitative relationship between luminal colonization and duration of placement. *J Infect Dis* 1993;168:400–407.
3. Lewis WJ, Sherertz RJ. Microbial interactions with catheter material. *Nutrition* 1997;13:5S–9S.
4. Sherertz RJ, Carruth WA, Marosok RD, et al. Contribution of vascular catheter material to the pathogenesis of infection: the enhanced risk of silicone in vivo. *J Biomed Mater Res* 1995;29:635–645.
5. An YH, Friedman RJ. Concise review of mechanisms of bacterial adhesion to biomaterial surfaces. *J Biomed Mater Res* 1998;43:338–348.
6. Costerton JW, Stewart PS, Greenberg EP. Bacterial biofilms: a common cause of persistent infections. *Science* 1999;284:1318–1322.
7. Tingey KG. Desirable properties for vascular catheter materials: a review of silicone and polyurethane materials in IV catheters. *JVAD* 2000;5:14–16.
8. Linder LE, Curelaru I, Gustavsson B, et al. Material thrombogenicity in central venous catheterization: a comparison between soft, antebrachial catheters of silicone elastomer and polyurethane. *JPEN Parenter Enteral Nutr* 1984;8:399–406.
9. Marosok R, Washburn R, Indorf A, et al. Contribution of vascular catheter material to the pathogenesis of infection: depletion of complement by silicone elastomer in vitro. *J Biomed Mater Res* 1996;30:245–250.
10. Appelgren P, Ransjo U, Bindslev L, et al. Does surface heparinisation reduce bacterial colonisation of central venous catheters? *Lancet* 1995;345:130.
11. Kamal GD, Pfaller MA, Rempe LE, et al. Reduced intravascular catheter infection by antibiotic bonding. *JAMA* 1991;265:2364–2368.
12. Maki DG, Stolz SM, Wheeler S, et al. Prevention of central venous catheter-related bloodstream infection by use of antiseptic-impregnated catheter. *Ann Intern Med* 1997;127:257–266.
13. Raad I, Darouiche R, Dupuis J, et al. Central venous catheters coated with minocycline and rifampin for the prevention of catheter-related colonization and bloodstream infections. *Ann Intern Med* 1997;127:267–274.
14. Trerotola SO, Johnson MS, Shah H, et al. Tunneled hemodialysis catheters: use of a silver-coated catheter for prevention of infection-a randomized study. *Radiology* 1998;207:491–496.
15. Darouiche RO, Raad II, Heard SO, et al. A comparison of two antimicrobial-impregnated central venous catheters. *N Engl J Med* 1999;340:1–8.
16. Veenstra DL, Saint S, Saha S, et al. Efficacy of antiseptic-impregnated central venous catheters in preventing catheter-related bloodstream infection. *JAMA* 1999;281:261–267.
17. Raad II. Vascular catheters impregnated with antimicrobial agents: present knowledge and future direction. *Infect Control Hosp Epidemiol* 1997;18:227–229.
18. Spencer RC. Novel methods for the prevention of infection of intravascular devices. *J Hops Infect* 1999;43(Suppl):S127–S135.
19. Sioshansi P. New processes for surface treatment of catheters. *Artif Organs* 1994;18:266–271.
20. Bambauer R, Mestres P, Schiel R, et al. Surface-treated catheters with ion beam-based process evaluation in rats. *Artif Organs* 1997;21:1039–1041.
21. Bambauer R, Mestres P, Pirrung KJ, et al. Scanning electron microscopic investigation of catheters of blood access. *Artif Organs* 1994;18:272–275.
22. Hoenich NA, Donnelly PK. Technology and clinical application of large-bore and implantable catheters. *Artif Organs* 1994;18:276–282.
23. Atherikul K, Schwab SJ, Conlon PJ. Adequacy of haemodialysis with cuffed central-vein catheters. *Nephrol Dial Transplant* 1998;13:745–749.
24. Vanholder R, Ringoir S. Vascular access for hemodialysis. *Artif Organs* 1994;18:263–265.
25. Maki DG, Cobb L, Garman JK, et al. An attachable silver-impregnated cuff for prevention of infection with central venous catheters: a prospective randomized multicenter trial. *Am J Med* 1988;85:307–314.
26. Hemmerlein JB, Trerotola SO, Kraus MA, et al. In vitro cytotoxicity of silver-impregnated collagen cuffs designed to decrease infection in tunneled catheters. *Radiology* 1997;204:363–367.
27. Wink J, Vaziri ND, Barker S, et al. The effect of hemodialysis on whole blood, plasma and erythrocyte viscosity. *Int J Artif Organs* 1988;11:340–342.
28. Cinar Y, Demir G, Pac M, et al. Effect of hematocrit on blood pressure via hyperviscosity. *Am J Hypertens* 1999;12:739–743.
29. Hassell DD, Vesely TM, Pilgram TK, Audrain JL. Initial performance of Tesio hemodialysis catheters. *J Vasc Interv Radiol* 1999;10:553–558.
30. Perini S, LaBerge JM, Pearl JM, Santiestiban HL, et al. Tesio catheter: radiologically guided placement, mechanical performance, and adequacy of delivered dialysis. *Radiology* 2000;215:129–137.
31. Mankus RA, Ash SR, Sutton JM. Comparison of blood flow rates and hydraulic resistance between the Mahurkar catheter, the Tesio twin catheter, and the Ash split cath. *ASAIO J* 1998;44:M532–M534.
32. Leblanc M, Bosc JY, Vaussenat F, et al. Effective blood flow and recirculation rates in internal jugular vein twin catheters: measurement by ultrasound velocity dilution. *Am J Kidney Dis* 1998;31:87–92.
33. Trerotola SO, Shah H, Johnson M, et al. Randomized comparison of high-flow versus conventional hemodialysis catheters. *J Vasc Interv Radiol* 1999;10:1032–1038.
34. Nazarian GK, Bjarnason H, Dietz CA, et al. Changes in tunneled catheter tip position when a patient is upright. *J Vasc Interv Radiol* 1997;8:437–441.
35. Forauer AR, Alonzo M. Change in peripherally inserted central catheter tip position with abduction and adduction of the upper extremity. *J Vasc Interv Radiol* 2000;11:1315–1318.
36. Kowalski CM, Kaufman JA, Rivitz SM, Geller SC, Waltman AC. Migration of central venous catheters: implications for initial catheter tip positioning. *J Vasc Interv Radiol* 1997;8:443–447.
37. McCarthy M, Sadler D, Sirkis H, et al. Central venous catheters for hemodialysis: effect of catheter tip position on duration of function. *AJR Am J Roentgenol* 1999;172:7(abst).
38. Groeger JS, Lucas AB, Thaler HT, et al. Infectious morbidity associated with long-term use of venous access devices in patients with cancer. *Ann Intern Med* 1993;119:1168–1174.
39. Struk DW, Bennett JD, Kozak RI. Insertion of subcutaneous central venous infusion ports by interventional radiologists. *Can Assoc Radiol J* 1995;46:32–36.
40. Moran J. Use of the LifeSite hemodialysis access system reduces risk of vascular access infections. *Am J Kidney Dis* 2001;37: A25(abst).
41. Levin NW, Yang PM, Hatch DA, et al. Initial results of a new access device for hemodialysis. *Kidney Int* 1998;54:1739–1745.
42. Canaud B, My C, Morena M, et al. Dialock: a new vascular access device for extracorporeal renal replacement therapy. Preliminary clinical results. *Nephrol Dial Transplant* 1999;14:692–698.

43. Buturovic J, Ponikvar R, Kandus A, et al. Filling hemodialysis catheters in the interdialytic period: heparin versus citrate versus polygeline: a prospective randomized study. *Artif Organs* 1998; 22:945–947.

44. Bayes B, Bonal J, Romero R. Sodium citrate for filling haemodialysis catheters. *Nephrol Dial Transplant* 1999;14:2532–2533.

45. Vercaigne LM, Sitar DS, Penner SB, et al. Antibiotic-heparin lock: in vitro antibiotic stability combined with heparin in a central venous catheter. *Pharmacotherapy* 2000;20:394–399.

46. Bastani B, Minton J, Islam S. Insufficient penetration of systemic vancomycin into the PermCath lumen. *Nephrol Dial Transplant* 2000;15:1035–1037.

47. Capdevila JA, Segarra A, Planes AM, et al. Successful treatment of haemodialysis catheter-related sepsis without catheter removal. *Nephrol Dial Transplant* 1993;8:231–234.

48. Jurewitsch B, Lee T, Park J, et al. Taurolidine 2% as an antimicrobial lock solution for prevention of recurrent catheter-related bloodstream infections. *J Parenter Enter Nutr* 1998;22: 242–244.

ENDOLUMINAL GRAFTS

DIERK VORWERK
RICHARD J. GRAY
MARTIN R. CRAIN

Several types of endoluminal graft are now either commercially available or under clinical investigation. These devices initially were used in the treatment of atherosclerotic aneurysms, pseudoaneurysms, arterial ruptures, and peripheral occlusive disease. More recently, they have been applied to dialysis patients.

The use of endoluminal grafts in hemodialysis fistulas and grafts may be beneficial under particular circumstances. These include angioplasty-related venous ruptures and pseudoaneurysms. Endoluminal grafts also have a potential benefit in the treatment of recurrent stenotic lesions, a frequent problem following interventions. Another potential application is inhibition of the aggressive neointimal growth that occurs within stents wherever they have been placed in the venous segments of a dialysis communication. This is especially important for central veins, which after a failed angioplasty have no other treatment alternative than a stent (see Chapter 25). Bare stents maintain luminal patency by preventing elastic recoil; it is intuitive that covering the stent with a low porosity material may improve patency by inhibiting intimal hyperplasia from accumulating in the stent. If endoluminal grafts can prevent elastic recoil without inciting an intimal hyperplastic reaction, they could significantly improve patency relative to standard balloon angioplasty and even become the first-line therapy for *de novo* venous stenosis.

This chapter discusses the current status and future directions of endoluminal grafts in patients with hemodialysis access needs. The roles of device design, the biologic response to graft material, the clinical and experimental experience to date, and potential new directions for percutaneous conduits are explored.

DESIGN AND CHARACTERISTICS OF ENDOLUMINAL GRAFTS

An increasing array of endoluminal grafts is being developed, but only a few have reached a state of being ready for clinical application. Differences are related to their construction principle, the graft material, the type of stent that is used, and the alloy used for the stent. Other differences include the method of delivery to the treatment site and local fixation. The major design principles are outlined subsequently herein.

Stented Graft Versus Covered Stent

In some devices, the body of the endoluminal graft consists of the pure graft material with only its ends connected to stents, which allow local fixation within the vascular lumen. Here the stent serves only to anchor the graft material within the vessel lumen. These *stented grafts* do not have a stent reinforcement along the longitudinal axis. The potential benefits of this design include the flexibility to handle vessel tortuosity and minimization of stent interactions with the vessel wall. Nonreinforced endoluminal grafts may not resist external forces well, however, and therefore are susceptible to kinking if placed in tortuous or stenotic vessels. The Ancure device (Guidant Corporation, Indianapolis, IN, U.S.A.), which is approved in the United States for abdominal aortic aneurysms, is constructed in this fashion.

Covered stents (grafted stents) are completely reinforced by a stent body that is covered by graft material on the inside, outside, or both. Some peripheral arterial devices, such as the Hemobahn (W. L. Gore Inc., Flagstaff, AZ, U.S.A.), the Jomed balloon-expandable stent graft (Jomed Inc., Munich, Germany), and the Passager peripheral graft (Boston Scientific, Nattick, MA, U.S.A.) as well as some tracheoesophageal devices, such as the Wallgraft (Boston Scientific), are based on that principle. In fact, most endoluminal grafts currently available or under development have a reinforcing stent skeleton throughout their length.

Graft Material Composition

Several different polymeric graft coverings are used in endoluminal grafts. The coatings used for endoluminal grafts are generally approved materials, which have been previously used over the years in vascular surgery. This is advantageous because, unless modified, they do not require additional testing for biocompatibility. The most common ones are polyethylene terephthalate (PET, Dacron), which is well known from conventional surgery for aortic repair (1), and polytetrafluoroethylene (PTFE, Teflon), preferentially used for dialysis grafts and infrainguinal arterial bypasses. Other materials, such as polyurethane–polycarbonate, have been developed specifically for stent–graft applications but are not currently approved for vascular use in the United States. The thickness, macroscopic structure, and chemical structure of each of these coverings are responsible for thrombogenicity, biologic tissue response, and resistance against biodegradation. The thickness and macroscopic structure of the covering also affect the diameter and rigidity of any introduction apparatus, which influence the ability to deliver the product safely to the intended intravascular site.

The *PET fabric* is a woven or knitted textile made from PET fibers that have been converted into yarns. Of the two PET textiles, woven PET is the most commonly used fabric for endoluminal grafts because it can be manufactured in thicknesses of 0.1mm or less (2), ultimately facilitating a lower-profile (smaller-diameter) introduction system than knitted PET would afford. Woven PET is more rigid than knitted PET, but it is much thinner. In conventional surgery, PET is most commonly used as graft material for arteries larger than 10 mm in diameter where late failure is due mainly to dilatation, suture-line failure, structural defects, and infection. Experimentally, PET creates a comparably aggressive neointimal and foreign-body inflammatory reaction relative to noncovered stents (3). PET is also more thrombogenic than PTFE. (See "Intravascular Tissue Interactions" to follow) Therefore, PTFE is a preferred graft material for arteries <6 mm, where thrombosis and neointimal reobstruction are more prevalent causes of graft failure.

Biodegradation and retention of tensile strength over time of thin-walled implants remain unknown. PET has been used as a coating for the Wallstent, a stent made from a complex metal alloy known as Elgiloy, to produce the Wallgraft (Boston Scientific), which is approved for tracheoesophageal stenoses and under investigation for several arterial applications. Use of the Wallgraft for dialysis applications is off-label in the United States. PET also covers the nitinol Passager stents (Boston Scientific), which are under investigation for arterial aneurysms, and the nitinol Cragg stent (Cragg Endopro, Mintec, Inc., Tucson, AZ, U.S.A.) widely studied for peripheral arterial and dialysis access applications.

Discovered in 1938 (1), *PTFE* is a fully fluorinated carbon-based polymer. Its molecular weight is between 20 and 120 million. It has a high thermal and mechanical resistance and is chemically stable. Vascular grafts are made from PTFE resins extruded into tubes that are expanded and heated to create soft and microporous tube grafts. PTFE in vascular grafts is therefore known as *expanded* polytetrafluoroethylene, or ePTFE. A large proportion of air after expansion accounts for the ePTFE being white.

Healing patterns of ePTFE depend on its porosity. Grafts with larger pores show quicker healing than do those with small pores, due to capillary ingrowth. If wrapped by an external reinforcement, as most Gore ePTFE materials (W. L. Gore Inc.) are, healing patterns change (1). If not wrapped by an external reinforcement layer, ePTFE is safely dilatable by use of a balloon to at least four times its original size. The porosity of ePTFE actually decreases after radial expansion, but ePTFE does not lose a significant amount of tensile strength (4). This expansile ability, which characterizes the unwrapped Impra (Impra Inc., Tempe, AZ, U.S.A.) ePTFE grafts, originally made this a preferred material for most of the early homemade peripheral grafts that used balloon-expandable Palmaz stents as a carrier for the graft material (5,6). When used in these homemade small-caliber endoluminal grafts as well as some aortic grafts, the ePTFE material has been predilated up to 25 mm in diameter, after which it is wrapped around a stent for insertion into the delivery system (5,7). Peripheral grafts that use ePTFE as a coating include the Hemobahn device (W.L. Gore Inc.) and the Jomed balloon-expandable stent graft (Jomed Inc.).

INTRAVASCULAR TISSUE INTERACTIONS

Much more is understood regarding the biological response to the presence of vascular grafts in arteries than in veins. A brief overview is provided here; the interested reader is referred to comprehensive reviews (1,8).

The primary responses of the human host to the connection of grafts to, or placement within, blood vessels include an inflammatory response, rheologic and thrombogenic factor response, and the development of intimal and medial cellular hyperplastic growth (8). These responses are interrelated in that inflammatory, foreign-body, and cytokine responses can hasten the development of intimal hyperplasia. The biochemical nature and (especially) the porosity of graft material play a significant role in the incorporation of grafts within the subcutaneous tissue, which in turn determines resistance to infection and the degree of cellular ingrowth and pseudointimal thickness. The anatomy and flow physiology of vascular anastomoses also add to the interplay of all the factors involved. In arterial applications, shear stresses predominate in determining the degree of the healing response that is intimal hyperplasia. What is specific to the hemoaccess circuit is the unremitting nature of intimal hyperplasia. In arteries, intimal hyperplasia is stimulated by the injury of an angioplasty but abates and even regresses after 12 to 24 months, whereas it is progressive and unrelenting in the venous outflow of arteriovenous (AV) fistulae and grafts. Thus, the dominant factors that ultimately limit the use of stents or grafts in the venous outflow of AV circuits are the high-volume, turbulent flow state and the unique responses of vein and perivascular tissues to that state (9).

The application of endovascular grafts within vessels has produced mixed results regarding the biologic response and clinical outcome. In the arterial environment, the news is somewhat encouraging. It has been shown in humans that intimal hyperplasia is pronounced only at attachment areas and that the excluded intima and media (i.e., outside the intravascular graft wall) do not appreciably participate in the intimal hyperplastic response (10). The grafts also undergo virtually no incorporation (*scarring*) within the excluded arterial segments. On the other hand, in animal experiments in arteries, endovascular grafts covered by PET or polyurethane–polycarbonate create a more pronounced neointimal coverage than bare stents (3). There are some experimental data showing that ePTFE creates less neointimal growth than PET and is similar to bare stents in animals (11). This may be due to the lower porosity of PTFE relative to PET.

The response within human veins has been less optimistic. Sapoval and colleagues (12) (see "Covered Stents" to follow) found that the neointimal hyperplastic response continued within all the endoluminal grafts placed within veins in their series and inferred that the cellular growth had occurred through the wall of the endoluminal graft. The graft material used was PET. Whether or not the neointimal hyperplasia in vein segments can be modified by different graft characteristics remains to be seen.

CLINICAL EXPERIENCE WITH ENDOLUMINAL GRAFTS FOR DIALYSIS ACCESS

Covered Stents

An example is shown in Figure 43.1. The published clinical experience in dialysis accesses is limited (Table 43.1). The largest series to date was published by Farber and colleagues (13), who used 22 PET-covered Cragg Endopro devices (Fig. 43.2) in 20 patients. Indications for placement included the standard indications for stent deployment using a bare stent (angioplasty failure, early recurrence, and angioplasty-induced rupture) as well as three pseudoaneurysms. They placed the devices in central veins and in upper-arm veins; ten were placed across the venous anastomosis of a dialysis graft. They achieved a primary stent patency of 57% at 6 months and 29% at 12 months. Secondary stent patency was 83% at 6 months and 64% at 12 months.

Sapoval and colleagues (12) used the same type of PET-covered stent in 14 patients for the treatment of various angioplasty failure problems, including venous rupture, recur-

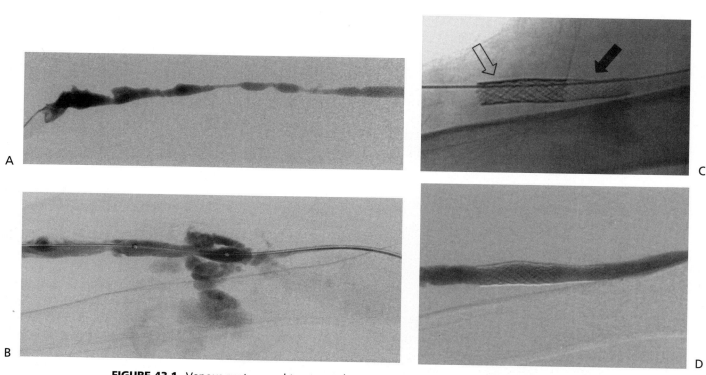

FIGURE 43.1. Venous rupture and treatment by a covered stent. **A:** Multiple stenoses in a right upper-arm brachiocephalic autologous fistula. **B:** After balloon angioplasty, rupture of the cephalic vein occurred that could not be closed by prolonged angioplasty over 20 minutes. **C:** Implantation of a balloon-expandable expanded polytetrafluoroethylene (ePTFE)-covered stent (*transparent arrow*) that followed implantation of a self-expandable Wallstent (*black arrow*), which had failed to seal the rupture. **D:** After placing the endoluminal graft, immediate closure of the rupture was achieved.

TABLE 43.1. COVERED STENTS (CRAGG ENDOPRO)[a]

	Salvage	6 Month Primary Patency	6 Month Secondary Patency
Sapoval et al. (12)	92% (13/14)	28.5%	67.8%
Farber et al. (13)	85% (17/20)	57%[b]	83%[b]
Hausegger et al. (14)	100% (3/3)	—	—

[a] See text for indications.
[b] Stent patencies.

rent stenosis, residual stenosis after angioplasty, and one pseudoaneurysm. At 6 months, the primary circuit patency was 28.5%, and secondary circuit patency was 67.8%. They concluded that the device was helpful after venous rupture from angioplasty but did not prevent neointimal hyperplasia from accumulating within the stent. After noting the poor 6-month primary patency and several local inflammatory reactions around the device, this group abandoned the use of this device for the dialysis access application.

Hausegger and colleagues (14) used again the same type of PET-covered stent in three cases with venous aneurysms at the venous anastomosis of three implant grafts. Although all the aneurysms were primarily excluded, recurrence of the aneurysm occurred in two and the graft thrombosed in one. These researchers gave up the use of these devices for this indication.

Current Status for Covered Stents in Dialysis Access

There is no evidence to date that covered stents will improve patency. On the contrary, the few clinical data available show a patency that is similar to bare stents.

The preceding studies (12–14) suggest that the use of covered stents to seal venous rupture caused by an angioplasty balloon does work acutely. In most venous ruptures, however, a prolonged balloon dilatation over 10 to 15 min-

utes is sufficient. If balloon tamponade fails, placement of a noncovered stent usually seals the leak (15–17). A covered stent becomes necessary only in very rare instances.

For graft pseudoaneurysms and venous aneurysms, the use of covered stents may be technically possible, but surgical resection with interposition or jump grafting is an established procedure that may be more cost-effective. More importantly, surgery avoids the long-term implantation of a device, which is theoretically prone to infection or deformation, especially if placed in a region that will be repeatedly punctured with dialysis needles, the most common site for graft-related pseudoaneurysms.

After placement of a covered stent, all collateral veins at the deployment site are closed, unlike bare stents, which usually do not impede inflow through collaterals. Thus, flow of important tributary veins, for example, internal and external jugular, contralateral innominate or cephalic entering into the placement area may be compromised.

Endoluminal graft technology is considerably more expensive than bare stents. To be cost-effective, the complication-free patency benefit for a covered stent must match the increased cost of the device. For example, the PET-covered Wallgraft (Boston Scientific) is 2.5 times more expensive than a Wallstent (Boston Scientific). To be cost-effective relative to a Wallstent, a Wallgraft would need a 2.5 times longer intervention-free patency than the Wallstent allows while maintaining the same complication rate.

In conventional surgery, ePTFE is the preferred material for 6- to 10-mm grafts. Because it causes relatively little neointimal hyperplasia, it seems more suitable than others as a covering for peripheral endoluminal grafts in low-caliber arteries, such as the femoral arteries. Because many dialysis access–related venous stenoses occur in 6- to 10-mm veins, ePTFE may be suitable for these lesions. Impra currently has an ePTFE-covered, self-expanding, nitinol-based stent under investigation for dialysis graft-related stenoses. This endoluminal graft comes in tubular and flared varieties; the flared device will conform to a size increase at the treatment site, typical at the venous anastomosis, and theoretically promote laminar flow (decreased turbulence) within the stent (Fig. 43.3A). Vascular Architects, Inc. (San Jose, CA, U.S.A.) has an ePTFE partially covered, self-expanding nitinol-based stent graft (aSpire) that is also under investigation for dialysis graft-related stenoses as well as peripheral applications (Fig. 43.3B). The incomplete covering of the venous wall afforded by the spiral design of this device theoretically allows more normal physiology than a complete covering.

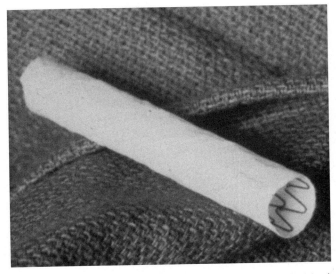

FIGURE 43.2. Polyethylene terephthalate (PET)-covered nitinol Cragg Endopro device. (Courtesy of Luc Turmel-Rodrigues.)

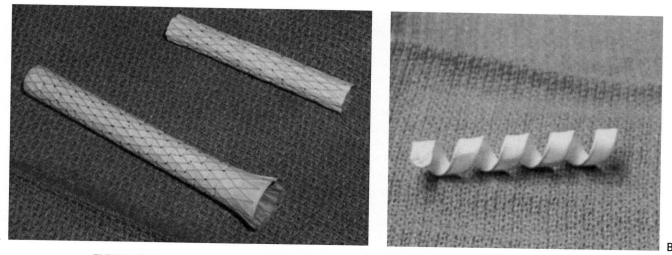

FIGURE 43.3. A: Expanded polytetrafluoroethylene (ePTFE)-covered stent by Impra with tubular and flared designs (see text). **B**: The ePTFE partially covered stent (aSpire) by Vascular Architechs, Inc.

This may decrease mural ischemia and thereby decrease the inflammatory response in the adventitia and the tendency for intimal hyperplasia to accumulate.

Stent–Graft Arteriovenous Fistulae: A Hybrid Endovascular Concept for Graft Creation

Attempts have been made to use endovascular methods to extend vascular grafts to remote, less accessible vessels in situations in which disease or lack of suitable vessel size precludes a more conventional vascular operation. In general, the concept involves handling one end of a prosthetic conduit with conventional surgical anastomotic technique. This will allow the next segment of graft to reside in a subcutaneous tunnel. Then the other end of the graft is introduced into the vessel lumen using an endovascular technique so that its terminal segment can reach a remote intravascular position where the vessel is not diseased and is perhaps larger in caliber. This technique was first described for arterial application by Marin and colleagues (18), who used the endovascular segment of a hybrid graft proximally to bypass atherosclerotic iliac arteries. Then they brought the extravascular graft segment out of the femoral arteriotomy and down to a surgical anastomosis with the profunda or superficial femoral arteries to bypass common femoral disease. The technical aspects of the procedure included suturing the leading edge of a PTFE graft to the midpoint of a Palmaz stent, dilating the entire graft within the artery after securing the stent proximally, and ligating the common femoral artery inferior to the arteriotomy to prevent hematoma formation from back-bleeding. When given the opportunity to explant the graft in several of their patients, Marin and colleagues (19) found that the intimal hyperplastic response was greatest within the bare stent and that there was no intimal hyperplastic response in regions of arterial wall plaque external to the graft.

Essentially the same concept has been applied to create a hemodialysis access circuit, albeit by reversing the segments such that the stent-supported segment is introduced through a venotomy (16-French peel-away sheath) to reach the larger central veins and thus represents the outflow segment. Masuda and colleagues (20) devised an otherwise standard upper-arm curved ePTFE graft, but the venous end was anchored intraluminally in the axillary vein by a Palmaz stent. In this case, the extravascular segment in the subcutaneous tissue was available for hemodialysis needle punctures (Fig. 43.4). Masuda and colleagues (20) created these grafts in eight patients in whom no other dialysis access could be placed in the affected extremity because of insufficient vein

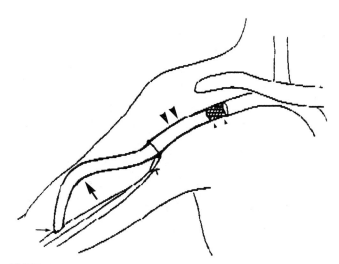

FIGURE 43.4. Diagrammatic depiction of dialysis graft anastomosed to the brachial artery (*tiny arrow*) with central endoluminal extension (*large arrowheads*) anchored by a stent (*tiny arrowheads*) in the axillary vein. Subcutaneous extraluminal segment of graft (*large arrow*) can be punctured for dialysis. (Adapted from Masuda EM, Kistner RL, Eklof B, et al. Stent-graft arteriovenous fistula: an endovascular technique in hemodialysis access. *J Endovasc Surg* 1998;5:18–23, with permission.)

size. Two early failures occurred, one due to stent compression and the other due to ischemic steal phenomenon requiring graft ligation. In the limited follow-up available, three of the remaining six remained patent for longer than 1 year. Venograms of each of the three showed no stenosis at the stent–vein interface or outflow vein. Not surprisingly, some degree of intimal hyperplasia was detected at the stent site when one of the grafts was explanted at 20 months.

This type of stent-modified hemodialysis graft holds promise as a technique for extension of limb vascular access in patients who have exhausted other options for a particular extremity. By extending the graft to larger, less accessible outflow veins, vein segments that are thrombosed or diminutive may be effectively bypassed. It is not certain, however, whether graft secured or supported by stents inside larger veins will be subject to any lesser rate of intimal–medial hyperplasia, which limits surgical anastomoses to smaller arm veins. As with covered stents, covering of valuable venous branches is also a potential drawback, although the veins being bypassed often are already diseased in the population under consideration.

A greater potential limitation of hybrid grafts is graft infection. Explantation of infected grafts from subcutaneous tissue can be a formidable task, and there would be concern about the feasibility and risk involved with removing graft from less accessible central veins, such as in the chest. As opposed to arterial endografts, which may be easily removed by virtue of the limited incorporation in the endovascular position, it is uncertain whether an endovenous graft, even if infected, could be extracted from the venotomy site. Indeed, our experience with this type of hybrid graft implanted in a canine model was that grafts in place for 6 to 12 weeks could not be extracted from the vein without causing disruption of major veins remote from the incision site (21) (Fig. 43.5). Again, whether an infected graft could be more easily extracted has not been determined.

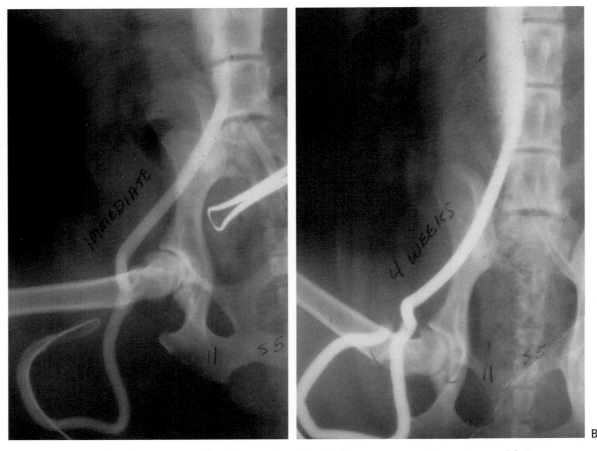

FIGURE 43.5. Hemoaccess graft with stented endoluminal venous segment in a canine model. **A:** Intraoperative angiogram after creation of a graft with 6-mm unsupported subcutaneous segment and a long endovenous extension supported by a 10-mm-diameter Wallstent. Catheter for contrast injection is in the arterial limb laterally, and the venous limb extends to the confluence of the iliac veins. Note the stent support of this graft with Wallstent. Also note a similar graft has been placed on the left (unopacified). **B:** Angiogram of hybrid graft system at 4 weeks. Both unsupported subcutaneous segment and stent-supported endovenous segment are widely patent. Again, note contralateral left iliac stent.

Percutaneous Insertion of Hemodialysis Grafts and Stent Grafts

The concept of a hemoaccess conduit placed completely percutaneously has been tested in a very limited fashion by Trerotola and colleagues (22). In an animal model, silicone-covered Wallstents were introduced by entirely percutaneous means into the femoral arteries and veins to create a subcutaneous circuit for hemoaccess punctures. Because of the lack of a more secure "anastomosis," early dislodgement from the vessels occurred. Although not clinically applicable in its current state, the work points out a promising direction for future research. The technologic development of a percutaneous anastomosis method will open up many exciting clinical and research opportunities.

CONCLUSION

The use of endoluminal grafts in hemodialysis fistulae and grafts thus far has produced marginal results. In cases of venous anastomotic ruptures, venous aneurysms, and pseudoaneurysms, recurrences have led some researchers to conclude that endoluminal grafts require further refinement before they can be accepted for these indications. Furthermore, the success with prolonged balloon dilatation and uncovered stent placement is adequate in many instances.

Greater potential impact of endoluminal grafts exists for treatment of recurrent stenotic lesions through the inhibition of aggressive neointimal growth. The clinical experience with current endoluminal devices, however, has shown that neointimal hyperplasia is not prevented from accumulating within the grafted segment. In addition, the relatively poor 6-month primary patency and several local inflammatory reactions around devices led some groups to abandon the use of endoluminal grafts in their current form for this application. Currently, routine use of endovascular grafts in this patient population cannot be recommended.

A better understanding of the host responses to the placement of grafts within hemoaccess circuits and veins will allow a more targeted and sophisticated development of devices for application in vessels with relatively unique flow physiology. Modification of graft characteristics and modulation of the host's inflammatory and biophysiologic responses need to be pursued to limit or eliminate the development of the aggressive neointimal and medial hyperplastic growth that has hampered the clinical application of endografts to date.

More novel applications, such as a partially or completely percutaneously created AV hemoaccess circuit, remain an intriguing possibility that requires more laboratory and clinical investigation. The limited survival and frequent need for interventional and surgical maintenance of hemodialysis fistulae and grafts will continue to drive product and idea development for this beleaguered patient population. Endoluminal grafts may play a significant role in the improvement of these patients' lives.

REFERENCES

1. Kowligi R, Edwin T, Banas C, et al. Vascular grafts: materials, methods and clinical application. In: Wise D, Trantolo D, Altobelli D, et al., eds. *Encyclopedic handbook of biomaterials and bioengineering.* Part B: Applications, vol 2. New York, NY: Marcel Dekker, 1995:979–996.
2. Blum U, Voshage G, Lammer J, et al. Endoluminal stent-grafts for infrarenal abdominal aortic aneurysms. *N Engl J Med* 1997; 336:13–20.
3. Schürmann K, Vorwerk D, Uppenkamp R, et al. Iliac arteries: plain and heparin-coated Dacron-covered stents compared with noncovered metal stents: an experimental study. *Radiology* 1997; 203:55–64.
4. Palmaz F, Sprague E, Palmaz JC. Physical properties of polytetrafluoroethylene bypass material after balloon dilatation. *J Vasc Interv Radiol* 1996;7:657–663.
5. Richter G, Palmaz J, Allenberg J, et al. Die transluminale Stentprothese beim Bauchaortenaneurysma. *Radiologe* 1994;34;511–518.
6. Vorwerk D, Günther RW, Marschall H, et al. Adaptierbarer Sanduhrstent zur Reduktion des Shuntflusses nach TIPS—Anlage. *Fortschr Röntgenstr* 1995;162:436–438.
7. Murphy K, Richter G, Henry M, et al. Aortoiliac aneurysms: management with endovascular stent-graft placement. *Radiology* 1996;198:473–480.
8. Back MR, White RA. The biologic response of prosthetic dialysis grafts. In: Wilson SE, ed. *Vascular access: principles and practice,* 3rd ed. St. Louis: Mosby, 1996:137–149.
9. Fillinger MF, Reinitz ER, Schwartz RA, et al. Graft geometry and venous intimal-medial hyperplasia in arteriovenous loop grafts. *J Vasc Surg* 1990;11:556–566.
10. Marin ML, Veith FJ, Cynamon J, et al. Human transluminally placed endovascular stented grafts: preliminary histopathologic analysis of healing grafts in aortoiliac and femoral artery occlusive disease. *J Vasc Surg* 1995;21:595–603.
11. Cejna M, Xu Z, Schoder M, et al. Evaluation of different types of covered stents in the sheep model. *Eur Radiol* 1999;9:90(abst).
12. Sapoval M, Turmel Rodrigues L, Raynaud A, et al. Cragg covered stents in hemodialysis access: initial and midterm results. *J Vasc Interv Radiol* 1996;7:335–342.
13. Farber A, Barbey M, Grunert J, et al. Access related venous stenoses and occlusions: treatment with percutaneous transluminal angioplasty and Dacron-covered stents. *Cardiovasc Interv Radiol* 1999;22:214–218.
14. Hausegger K, Tiessenhausen K, Klimpfinger M, et al. Aneurysms of hemodialysis access grafts: treatment with covered stents: a report of three cases. *Cardiovasc Interv Radiol* 1998;21:334–337.
15. Rundback JH, Leonardo RF, Poplausky MR, et al. Venous rupture complicating hemodialysis access angioplasty: percutaneous treatment and outcomes in seven patients. *AJR Am J Roentgengol* 1998;171:1081–1084.
16. Welber A, Schur I, Sofocleous CT, et al. Endovascular stent placement for angioplasty-induced rupture related to the treatment of hemodialysis grafts. *J Vasc Interv Radiol* 1999;10:547–551.
17. Funaki B, Szymski GX, Leef JA, et al. Wallstent deployment to

salvage dialysis graft thrombolysis complicated by venous rupture: early and intermediate results. *AJR Am J Roentgenol* 1997; 169:1435–1437.

18. Marin ML, Veith FJ, Sanchez LA, et al. Endovascular repair of aortoiliac occlusive disease. *World J Surg* 1996;20:679–686.

19. Marin ML, Veith FJ, Cynamon J, et al. Human transluminally placed endovascular stented grafts: preliminary histopathologic analysis of healing grafts in aortoiliac and femoral artery occlusive disease. *J Vasc Surg* 1995;21:595–603.

20. Masuda EM, Kistner RL, Eklof B, et al. Stent-graft arteriovenous fistula: an endovascular technique in hemodialysis access. *J Endovasc Surg* 1998;5:18–23.

21. Crain MR, Mewissen MW, Seibold C, et al. Novel arteriovenous access graft with stented endovenous extension: initial study in a canine model. *J Vasc Interv Radiol* 1998;9(S):197(abst).

22. Trerotola SO, Johnson WM, Winkler, et al. Percutaneous creation of arteriovenous hemodialysis grafts: work in progress. *J Vasc Interv Radiol* 1995;6:675–681.

VASCULAR BRACHYTHERAPY

RON WAKSMAN
RICHARD J. GRAY

With the growing popularity of peripheral vascular medicine, identifying a reliable treatment to the plaguing recurrence of restenosis will increase and augment the benefits of vascular intervention. Investigators have shown that the endovascular delivery of radiation therapy is one such treatment. Combating restenosis in the peripheral vascular system is contingent on understanding the processes, mechanisms, and potential targets affected by using brachytherapy. The successful outcome of clinical trials in coronary arteries facilitated recognition of vascular brachytherapy as a standard of care for the treatment of in-stent restenosis. Expansion of the indications to *de novo* lesions identified the potential and limitations of the technology (late thrombosis and edge effect). Simultaneously, investigators embarked on a series of studies using vascular brachytherapy as adjunct therapy for intervention in peripheral arteries. The outcome of these trials will determine the future role of vascular brachytherapy as a tool for prevention of restenosis in the peripheral vascular system.

As the manifestation of coronary atherosclerosis and peripheral artery disease is primarily evident in older patient populations, and with the generation of baby boomers nearing their 60s, the full impact of peripheral and coronary atherosclerosis in the United States is upon us. Whereas coronary vascular procedures increase at a rate of 8% per year, there is greater growth in the frequency of peripheral procedures, estimated at 19% per year. Despite new advances such as stents, atherectomy devices, thrombectomy and endoluminal grafts, the restenosis rate after peripheral artery intervention continues to compromise the overall success of these procedures. Restenosis and the need for repeat revascularization remain the main limitations of intervention in peripheral arteries.

Vascular brachytherapy is a promising technology with the potential to reduce restenosis rates. Nearly 5,000 patients enrolled in clinical trials helped to evaluate the effectiveness and safety of this technology. Five-year follow-up of clinical and angiographic data collected on patients treated with intracoronary radiation for the prevention of restenosis was released recently. These studies demonstrate different levels of efficacy and raise further questions regarding proper dosimetry, the incidence of edge effect, the late thrombosis phenomenon, and late restenosis. Whereas most vascular brachytherapy trials have focused on the use of radiation therapy for the prevention of coronary in-stent restenosis, more data are needed to determine the effectiveness of beta and gamma sources and the use of centering delivery systems.

Currently, the clinical experience with vascular brachytherapy for the peripheral system is limited, and planned trials are designed to evaluate the restenosis rates of several vascular sites with the use of endovascular radiation therapy following vascular intervention (e.g., balloon angioplasty, stent placement, atherectomy, or laser ablative techniques). Target sites for such preventive therapy have been identified as superficial femoral artery (SFA) lesions, renal artery stenosis, patients undergoing hemodialysis with the arteriovenous (AV) graft stenosis, a subclavian or brachiocephalic vein, and following transjugular intrahepatic portosystemic shunt (TIPS) procedures for patients with portal hypertension.

MECHANISMS OF RESTENOSIS

The use of percutaneous transluminal angioplasty (PTA) has considerably improved the revascularization rates of many patients. Unfortunately, the long-term efficacy of PTA is limited by its 6- to 12-month high rate of restenosis (1). Restenosis following PTA occurs in response to the healing process associated with overinflation of the balloon during angioplasty and subsequent overstretching of the vessel. The main mechanisms of restenosis are acute recoil, intimal hyperplasia, and late vascular constriction (*negative remodeling*) (2–5).

In the peripheral system, restenosis following PTA is seen mainly in small and medium peripheral arteries, such as the femoral and renal arteries. Although not as common, and found to have less of an effect on patency, lower rates of restenosis following intervention also have been reported in larger arteries, such as the aortoiliac and carotid arteries (6–12). Other sites affected by restenosis include bypass graft anastomosis, AV dialysis grafts, and following placement of TIPS (13). Factors that effect long-term vessel patency following PTA include the length of the lesion, the degree of the stenosis, the plaque burden, vessel size, and proximal and distal flow. For peripheral short focal lesions, short-term (6-month) patency rates as high as 75% have been reported. In contrast, more complex and longer areas of stenosis, those with poor distal runoff, and those performed for limb salvage may have a 6-month patency as low as 25% and a 5-year patency of only 16% (14).

Many attempts have been made to reduce restenosis by adding adjunct pharmacologic therapy to PTA or by the use of mechanical devices, including atherectomy, laser angioplasty, and intravascular stenting. It appears that instrumentation of these vessels, by balloon or device, is responsible for inducing restenosis because none of these alternative approaches significantly retards the neointimal hyperplasia or improves and preserves long-term vascular patency (15–18). Indeed, the hyperplastic response post revascularization remains an outstanding issue for all vascular interventional modalities.

Intraluminal delivery of radiation following vascular intervention is viewed as a viable solution to inhibit restenosis (19–29). Exposing the vessels to low-dose radiation following angioplasty modifies wound healing by inhibiting the excessive neointima formation. Intravascular radiation in the peripheral system, however, requires special considerations when selecting the isotope and the delivery system to deliver the radiation to the target site.

RADIATION PHYSICS AND DOSIMETRIC CONSIDERATIONS

Different isotopes on various platforms and systems have been developed for the use of endovascular brachytherapy. The main platforms for radiation delivery are catheter-based systems and radioactive stents. Catheter-based systems contain a solid form, such as line source wires, radioactive seeds, and radioactive balloons, or nonsolid sources, such as radioactive gas- and liquid-filled balloons.

Several different gamma and beta isotopes are available, and selecting the most appropriate one depends on the anatomy of the vessel, the properties of the treated lesion, and proper identification of the target tissue needing treatment. Anatomically important parameters that also need consideration include the diameter and the curvature of the vessel, the eccentricity of the plaque, the lesion length, the composition of the plaque, the amount of calcium, and the presence or absence of a stent in the treated segment. These factors influence which source to use, as different sources have varying properties that warrant using one over another.

Requirements for choosing the ideal radiation system for vascular brachytherapy should include dose distribution of a few millimeters from the source with a minimal dose gradient, low-dose levels to surrounding tissues, and a dwell time less than 15 minutes. Other considerations for source selection include source energy, half-life for multiple applications, available activity, penetration, dose distribution, radiation exposure to the patient and the operator, shielding requirement, availability, and cost.

To determine an accurate dosimetry, it is essential to identify the target tissue, the right dose, and the treatment margins. It has been argued that the adventitia is the target, but when considering the success of previous trials, it is difficult to deny the fact that the high-dose exposure to the vessel wall and residual plaque may be essential to obtain efficacy (30,31). The doses prescribed today in clinical studies are empirical; they are based on doses used in animal studies and the limited experience gained from treating other benign diseases. Because a wide range of doses demonstrated effectiveness in preclinical studies, a therapeutic window must exist that allows some flexibility in selecting the isotope for this application.

Understanding Gamma Radiation

Gamma rays are photons originating from the center of the nucleus; they differ from x-rays, which originate from the orbital outside of the nucleus. Gamma rays have deep penetrating energies between 20 keV to 20 MeV, which require an excess of shielding, as compared with beta and x-ray emitters. The only gamma ray isotope currently in use is iridium-192 (Ir-192). There are isotopes that emit both gamma and x-rays, such as iodine-125 (I-125) and palladium-103 (Pd-103). These isotopes have lower energies, however, and require higher activity levels to deliver a prescribed dose in the acceptable dwell time (<15 minutes). Using these isotopes for vascular brachytherapy is difficult, as they are either not available in high activity levels or too expensive for this application. The dosimetry of Ir-192 is well understood and is associated with an acceptable dose gradient, as Ir-192 has a lesser fall-off in dose than beta emitters. Ir-192 is available in activities of up to 10 Ci, but, due to high penetration, patients need to be transferred to a shielded radiation oncology room because the average shielding of a catheterization laboratory will not be enough to handle more than 500 mCi source in activity. Focal stenosis in smaller-diameter arteries can be treated with lower activities of Ir-192 in the catheterization laboratory and will require an average of 20 minutes of dwell time for doses above 15 Gy when prescribed at 2 mm radial distance from the source.

Understanding Beta Radiation

Beta rays are high-energy electrons emitted by nuclei and contain too many or too few neutrons. These negatively charged particles have a wide variety of energies, including transition energies, particularly between parent–daughter cells, and they have a diverse range of half-lives, from several minutes (Cu-62) up to 30 years (Sr/Y90). Beta emitters are associated with a higher gradient to the near wall, as they lose their energy rapidly to surrounding tissue and their range is within 1 cm of tissue. Vascular brachytherapy using beta emitters appears promising; safety levels are high when radiation exposure to nontargeted areas is low. To use beta emitters for the peripheral application, they must be in proximity with the vessel wall and should be used with as high an activity level as possible.

RADIATION SYSTEMS FOR THE PERIPHERAL VASCULAR SYSTEM

Several radiation systems for peripheral endovascular brachytherapy have been suggested and are currently under development. These systems are as follows:

External Radiation

External-beam radiation is a viable option for the treatment of peripheral vessels. It allows for a homogeneous dose distribution with the possibility of fractionation. To date, an attempt to treat SFA lesions and AV dialysis grafts with external radiation was reported without success to reduce the restenosis rate. Using sterotactic techniques to localize the radiation to the target area may improve the results of this approach.

Radioactive Stents

Radioactive stents are attractive devices because they require minimum shielding and are easy to use. The dosimetry of radioactive stents is even more complicated and depends on the geometry of the stent, which varies across stent designs. Current tested radioactive stents lack dose homogeneity across the entire length of the stent, which could affect the biological response to radiation, especially at the stent edges. The lack of even dose distribution also might result in an improper delivery to specific injured sites, causing additional growth. This problem, known as *edge effect*, and identified as the major limitation of radioactive stents in coronary trials, may result from a stimulatory response from the vessel. Low-activity radioactive stents may be associated with an ineffective low-dose rate. Whereas radioactive stents with high activities may deliver toxic doses to the stented area that delay reendothelialization, higher radiation doses might promote stent thrombosis and tissue necrosis to the area surrounding the stent. New studies are under way that will evaluate whether higher activities will minimize the edge-effect phenomenon. Other approaches used to improve the results with radioactive stents include changes to the geometry of the stent and altering the isotope or the activity level at the stent's edges. A new approach with the use of radioactive nitinol self-expanding stents, which use gamma emitters, is currently under investigation as a potential therapy for primary SFA lesions.

Catheter-based Systems

Several catheter-based systems are available for the peripheral vascular system; however, the only system used in clinical trials is the MicroSelectron-HDR (Nucletron-Odelft, Veenendaal, The Netherlands). The system uses a high-dose-rate afterloader that consists of a computerized system, which delivers a 3-mm stepping 10 Ci in activity of 192-iridium source into a centered closed-end lumen segmented balloon radiation catheter. There are many advantages to using a remote afterloading system for vascular brachytherapy. Namely, the remote afterloading system drives the radiation source quickly to the treatment site, avoiding radiation exposure to untreated arteries. In addition, radiation exposure to the clinical personnel is eliminated by remotely programming the automatic advancement of the radiation source from a shielded safe to the treatment site. The radiation dose can be controlled and shaped using the computerized afterloader device to adjust accurately the source position and treatment time. By using an afterloader, it continually monitors the radiation dose and automatically retracts the source into the shielded safe after treatment. Treatment time is automatically adapted for the radioactive decay of the source, and the afterloader can handle a very high activity source (10 Ci), resulting in shorter dwell times. The afterloader used in the MicroSelectron-HDR system is pictured in Figure 44.1.

The Peripheral Brachytherapy Centering Catheter (the PARIS catheter) (Guidant, Santa Clara, CA, U.S.A.) is currently being used in the multicenter Peripheral Artery Radiation Investigational Study (PARIS). This catheter is a double-lumen catheter with multiple centering balloons near its distal tip. One lumen is used for inflation of the centering balloon, and the second lumen is used for the guidewire and the closed-end lumen sheath, which, once the catheter is in position, is introduced following removal of the guidewire. The inflated balloons engage the walls of the vessel and allow centering. The shaft diameter is a 7-French closed-end lumen catheter (Fig. 44.2) and comes with balloons 4 to 8 mm in diameter and 10 to 20 cm long and enables the catheter to be in the center of the lumen of large peripheral vessels during inflation. Other designs of catheters, such as the helical balloon, overcome the centering problem and provide flow and perfusion during centering.

Another catheter-based system, available for use in the catheterization laboratory, includes the use of an Ir-192 radioactive wire delivered either manually or automatically into a closed-end lumen catheter. The activity of the source is limited to 500 mCi, and the system is practical to use only for short lesions in small vessels (diameters <4.0 mm) that require a dwell time of at least 20 minutes. Similar to this gamma system, the eventual use of a catheter-based system using high-activity beta sources also may be an option for intermediate-sized vessels.

Hot Balloons

The angioplasty balloon is another platform that can be used to deliver radiation for the peripheral system. These balloons can be filled with either a liquid isotope, such as Re-188 or Re-186, or radioactive xenon-133 gas. The advantage of using these systems is the uniform dosimetry and proximity of the beta emitter to the vessel wall. Special care, however, is required when using the liquid-filled balloon to prevent spilling of the isotope outside the balloon. The radioactive balloon catheter (Radiance Medical Systems, Inc., Irvine, CA, U.S.A.) is particularly attractive for peripheral applications because it is associated with the apposition of a solid beta P-32 source attached to the inner balloon surface.

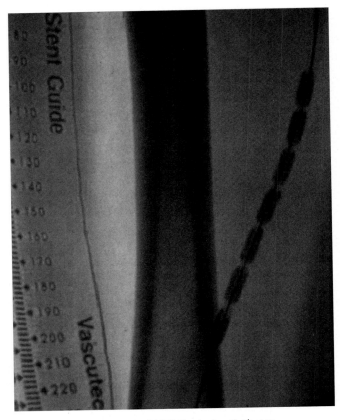

FIGURE 44.2. PARIS Centering Catheter.

With inflation of the balloon, the source is attached to the lumen surface. The system is limited to lesions smaller than 33 mm long with one step, but it can accommodate longer lesions with manual stepping. To date, there are no clinical data to support the use of this technology in peripheral arteries.

An alternative and attractive approach could be the use of low x-ray energy delivered intraluminally via catheter. The emitter would be between 5 to 7 mm long and 1.25 to 2.0 mm in diameter. It could be administered distally to the lesion and pulled back to cover the entire lesion length. If effective, it would alleviate the need for the use of radioisotopes in the catheterization laboratory. Miniaturizing the emitter is a technical challenge, and there are no preclinical data yet to support this theory.

CLINICAL TRIALS

Performed in the peripheral arteries, the first application of vascular brachytherapy for the prevention of restenosis was initiated by Liermann and colleagues in Frankfurt, Germany. Known as the *Frankfurt Experience*, the first pilot study of endovascular radiation was conducted in 30 patients with in-stent restenosis in their saphenous femoral arteries (32). The patients underwent atherectomy and PTA, followed by endovascular radiation using the MicroSelec-

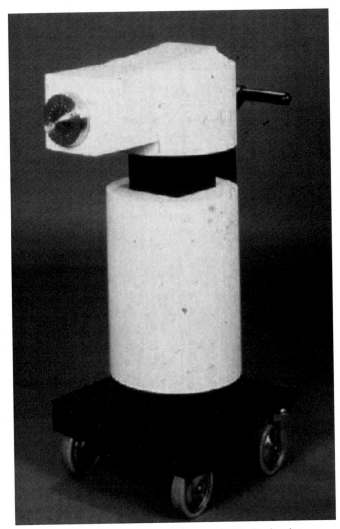

FIGURE 44.1. The MicroSelectron-HDR afterloader.

tron-HDR afterloader and a noncentering catheter. The gamma source Ir-192 was used to deliver a dose of 12 Gy, 3 mm into the vessel wall. The actual dose, however, varied from 8 to 28 Gy. No adverse effects from the radiation treatment were reported with up to 7 years of follow-up. The 5-year patency rate of the target vessel was 82%, with only 3 of 28 (11%) stenoses within the treated segment reported. Late total occlusion developed in 2 of 28 patients (7%) after 16 and 37 months, respectively.

The Emory Experience

A subsequent pilot study was conducted at Emory University in 1994, which examined the effects of endovascular radiation in the superficial femoral arteries of four patients following PTA and stenting. Of the four patients, one with a Palmaz stent needed subsequent surgery 1 year after radiation therapy because of a crushed stent. The histology of the irradiated stent segment in this patient demonstrated minimal intimal hyperplasia surrounding the stent struts, thus indicating the inhibitory effect of radiation therapy in stented SFAs (33).

The Vienna Experience

The effectiveness of the MicroSelectron-HDR system was tested in a randomized, placebo-controlled trial in Vienna in which 113 patients (63 men, 50 women; mean age 71 years) with *de novo* or recurrent femoropopliteal lesions were included. This study compared the restenosis rate after PTA plus BT (brachytherapy)(57 patients, PTA+BT group) with PTA (56 patients, PTA group) without stent implantation. The mean treated length was 16.7 cm (PTA+BT group) versus 14.8 cm (PTA group). For patients randomized to PTA plus BT, a dose of 12 Gy was applied by an Ir-192 source 3 mm from the source axis. Follow-up examinations included measurement of the ankle-brachial index, color-flow duplex sonography, and angiography. The primary endpoint of the study was patency after 6 months. The overall recurrence rate after 6 months was 15 of 53 (28.3%) in the PTA+BT group versus 29 of 54 (53.7%) in the PTA group (chi^2 test, $p<0.05$). The cumulative patency rates at 12 months of follow-up were 63.6% in the PTA+BT group and 35.3% in the PTA group (log-rank test, $p<0.005$) (34). The group from Vienna continued to investigate a series of patients with higher-dose 18 Gy to improve the outcome of the radiation group.

In another series of studies, the effectiveness of radiation as adjunct therapy with primary stenting of the SFA was evaluated in 33 patients. In this series, the recurrence rate at 6 months was 10 of 33 (30%), but this was attributed to a high rate of late thrombosis, nearly 10%, whereas only 4 of 33 (12%) had in-stent restenosis. Late thrombosis was reduced significantly once prolonged antiplatelet therapy was administered, as shown in Vienna 5, in which 90 patients randomly received stent plus radiation treatment versus stent alone for the treatment of SFA lesions.

The PARIS Trial

The PARIS study was the first FDA approved, multicenter, randomized, double-blind control study involving 300 patients following PTA to SFA stenosis using gamma radiation 192-Ir source. Utilizing the MicroSelectron-HDR afterloader, the treatment dose is 14 Gy, delivered via a centered, segmented end-lumen balloon catheter. The primary objectives of this study are to determine angiographic evidence of patency and a reduction of greater than 30% of the treated lesions' restenosis rate at 6 months. A secondary endpoint is to determine the clinical patency at 6 and 12 months by treadmill exercise and by the ankle–brachial index (ABI). The clinical endpoints are improvements in treadmill exercise time of longer than 90 seconds, improvement of ABI 0.10 compared with pre-PTA values, and an absence of repeat interventions to the treated vessel. This study was designed based on recently published recommendations and general principles of the evaluation of new interventional devices and technologies (35,36). Ultimately, the data from this study should determine whether endovascular radiation therapy has a role in the prevention of restenosis in patients following PTA for SFA lesions.

In the feasibility phase of PARIS, 40 patients with claudication were enrolled. The mean lesion length was 9.9 $\pm$ 3.0 cm, with a mean reference vessel diameter of 5.4 $\pm$ 0.5 mm. Following successful PTA, a segmented balloon-centering catheter was positioned to cover the PTA site (37). The patients were transported to the radiation oncology suite and treated with radiation using a high-dose rate MicroSelectron-HDR afterloader. The isotope used for this study was Ir-192 (maximum of 10 Ci in activity), and the prescribed dose was 14 Gy to 2 mm into the vessel wall. ABI and maximum walking time were evaluated with a repeat angiogram at 6 months. Radiation was delivered successfully in all but two patients because of technical difficulties. There were no procedural, in hospital, or 30-day complications in any of the treated patients. Maximum walking time on treadmill was increased from 3.56 $\pm$ 2.7 minutes at baseline to 4.53 $\pm$ 2.7 minutes at 3 months ($p = 0.01$); ABI also improved from 0.7 + 0.2 to 1.0 + 0.2. Among the first 20 patients who returned for 5-month angiographic follow-up, one patient required revascularization of the treated site. There has been no evidence of arterial aneurysms or perforations. The 6-month angiographic follow-up was completed on 30 patients; 13.3% had evidence of clinical restenosis. The feasibility study of PARIS demonstrated that the delivery of a high-dose rate gamma radiation via a centering catheter is feasible and safe following PTA to SFA lesions. Completion of the randomization phase for this study, scheduled for the end of 2001, should report its results sometime in 2002.

Arteriovenous Dialysis Studies

Although experience with brachytherapy for inhibiting intimal hyperplasia after angioplasty of arterial stenoses has been promising, the etiology, pathophysiology, and anatomy for the dialysis venous access are considerably different (38). First, the stimulus for intimal hyperplasia in arteries is the injury of angioplasty. In contrast, the abnormal hemodynamics of the permanent dialysis access provides a continuous, chronic proliferative stimulus for intimal hyperplasia. Second, in contrast to an artery, which generally is treated once or twice, restenosis due to intimal hyperplasia inevitably will require multiple treatments, and the cumulative lifetime radiation tolerance of the veins and perivenous tissues will become an issue. Third, unlike arteries, the thicknesses of the venous wall layers are not definable by endoluminal ultrasound, which leaves the thickness of the target tissue and the optimal dose penetration uncertain. Fourth, targeting a certain layer of the wall to receive a predetermined dose will be difficult at some anatomic locations

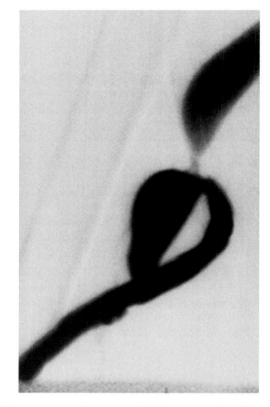

FIGURE 44.4. Arteriovenous dialysis graft-related eccentric stenosis in the vein adjacent to the venous anastomosis.

(i.e., the typical increase in the lumen diameter across the autologous arteriovenous fistula or AV graft venous anastomosis) (Figs. 44.3 and 44.4). Fifth, the composition of venous stenoses varies depending on the location; central catheter-related lesions and intragraft stenoses have a significant fibrous component, whereas venous anastomotic lesions are predominantly intimal hyperplasia (39). Further, the composition of an individual venous stenosis is not uniform, as evidenced by the typical focal bands of resistance to balloon dilatation within longer lesions (Fig. 44.5). Sixth, the intimal hyperplasia seen in AV dialysis stenoses is predominantly extracellular matrix, less cellular than intimal hyperplasia at other locations (see Chapter 8). Seventh, many failing AV grafts have more than one lesion that will require treatment. Eighth, the effect of graft material on the dose distribution is unknown, a potentially major factor given the high frequency of stenoses that bridge or are adjacent to the venous anastomosis (40) (Figs. 44.3 and 44.4). Finally, delivery of a uniform prescribed dose to the target layer will be challenged by the eccentric morphology of many lesions (Fig. 44.4) and by adjacent lesions with different characteristics or that bridge veins of different caliber (Fig. 44.6).

A pilot study was initiated at Emory University in 1994 to determine whether intravascular low-dose radiation retards neointimal hyperplasia in patients for whom PTA failed at the distal venous anastomosis of AV dialysis grafts

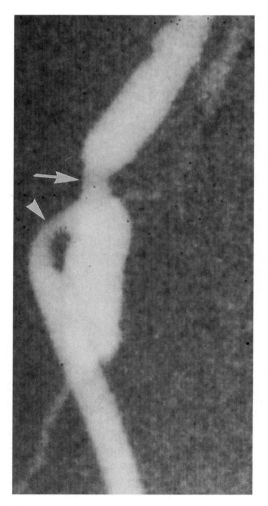

FIGURE 44.3. Typical venous anastomosis with stenosis (*arrowhead*) within the graft that extends across the anastomosis into the vein (*arrow*). Note the difference in lumen diameter between the graft and the vein, also seen in Figure 44.4.

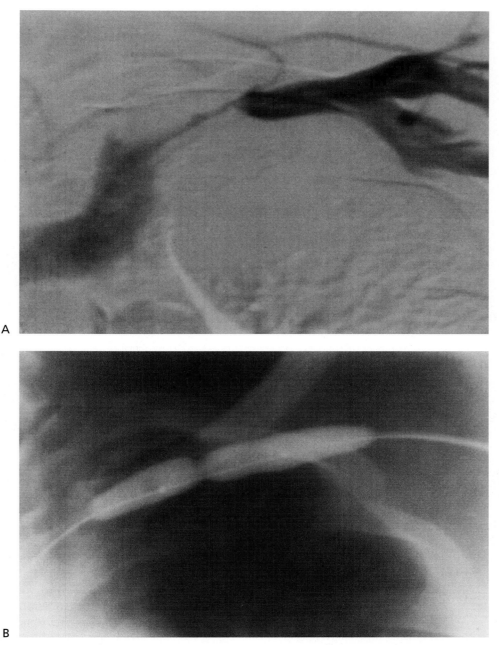

FIGURE 44.5. A: Subclavian stenosis. **B**: Typical focal waist on dilated balloon in the subclavian vein (same patient as A). (From Gray RJ. Central venous stenosis in hemodialysis patients. In: *SCVIR Syllabus: Venous Interventions*. Fairfax, VA: Society of Cardiovascular and Interventional Radiology, 1995:123–135, with permission.)

(33). Patients for whom prior PTAs to their AV graft failed and who had less than 50% luminal stenosis were enrolled in the study and underwent balloon dilatation at the narrowed segment. Following PTA, a sheath was placed across the lesion, and a closed-end lumen 5-French noncentered radiation delivery catheter was positioned at the angioplasty site. The catheter position was verified by radioopaque marker bands on a dummy source wire that was placed into the catheter. The sheath and the catheter were fixed to the skin, and the patients were transported to the radiation on-cology suite. The patients were treated with a high-activity Ir-192 source delivered to the treatment site by a MicroSe-lectron-HDR afterloader. The treatment dose was 14 Gy delivered to a depth of 2 mm into the arterial wall. After the radiation treatment, the sheath and the catheter were re-trieved, and the patients were sent home on the same day. Bimonthly clinical follow-up, including color-flow Doppler evaluation, was performed, and most patients underwent angiographic follow-up at 6 months. Eleven patients with 18 lesions were treated. A 40% patency rate at 44 weeks was

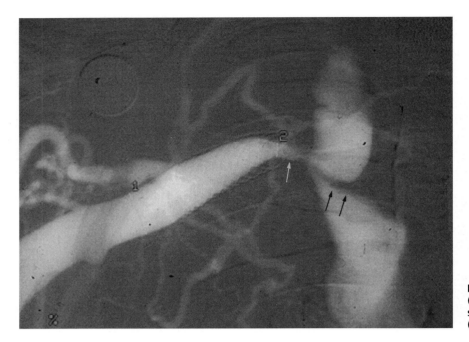

FIGURE 44.6. Concentric subclavian stenosis (*white arrow*) partially within indwelling stent and a tandem weblike eccentric stenosis (*black arrows*) in the larger innominate vein.

reported. Although the procedure was successful in all patients, the long-term results of this study were similar to the practice reported so far by stand-alone PTA without radiation. In summary, this study demonstrated only the feasibility and safety of intravascular radiation therapy post PTA using the MicroSelectron-HDR afterloader for patients with AV dialysis graft stenosis.

This feasibility study had several limitations: The study population was small and heterogeneous; many patients had several PTA failures prior to the procedure, and there was heterogenicity on the type of the treated grafted shunts. Several patients in this study had thrombotic events within 3 months following the procedure and underwent thrombectomy or lytic therapy. Although the prescribed dose was 14 Gy, the actual calculated dose given to the patients ranged from 7 to 90 Gy. This occurred because a centering catheter was not used in a large conduit. The effectiveness of intravascular radiation therapy in the AV dialysis grafts, however, is unclear. Using a centered catheter to deliver radiation to large vessels is essential to control the uniformity of the dose given to the vessel wall in such large conduits; however, the distended balloon may render the endoluminal surface ischemic, thus increasing radioresistance. The vessel wall may be moved away from the source, and higher doses will be delivered to the intima than to the deeper layers, particularly if beta sources are used (38). Larger randomized studies are required to determine the value of this new technology for patients with AV dialysis graft failure.

External beam radiation therapy has several advantages compared with endoluminal catheter-delivered therapy. It requires no special equipment, is less expensive, is noninvasive, and is available virtually everywhere. Therefore, it can be ad-

ministered without significantly altering the daily routines of the interventional suite or the radiation therapy department. Further, the dosimetry for external beam therapy is well established. It can be delivered with uniform, precise, fractionated doses to a defined target volume; hence, some of the problems of dose-nonhomogeneity that endoluminal sources carry (e.g., eccentric lesions, change in lumen caliber at lesion sites, uncertain target layer thickness) are avoided. Further, the superficial location of the typical dialysis autologous fistula or AV graft is ideal for external beam. Parikh and Nori reported a pilot study that used external radiation for AV dialysis (38). In this study, dialysis patients with stenosis at AV graft were subjected to balloon angioplasty and external radiation doses of 12 and 18 Gy in a fractionated method (two fractions for each dose). At 6 months, the TLR was 40%, but by 18 months all grafts failed and required intervention.

Cohen and colleagues (41) reported on the efficacy of low-dose, external beam irradiation in 31 patients with a heterogeneous group of 41 lesions (28 peripheral, 13 central) in their dialysis shunts. The patients were randomized to PTA with or without stent placement alone versus PTA with or without stent placement followed by external radiation prescribing 14 Gy in two 7 Gy fractions, one immediately after PTA and the second at 48 hours. The restenosis rate at 6 months was 45% in the irradiated group and 67% in the control group; however, the difference in restenosis did not reach statistical significance.

Because stents can maintain luminal patency by preventing elastic recoil, one logical strategy to improve patency after endovascular therapy is to inhibit in-stent restenosis by radiating the stent immediately following deployment. Trerotola and colleagues (42) reported a study in canines in which five dogs underwent implantation of bilateral polytetrafluoroethylene (PTFE) grafts with Wallstents (BSCI) deployed at the venous anastomosis. One side was endoluminally radiated with a 12 Gy gamma source using Ir-192. The other side was not radiated. Monthly follow-up angiographies over 10 months, or until thrombosis, demonstrated a lower degree of stenosis and smaller volume of intimal hyperplasia on the radiated sides of all animals. Late total occlusion at 11 months was seen in one case. Although Cohen's group (41) included stented lesions in their clinical study, no human experience specifically examining the results of stent deployment followed by radiation has been presented.

New studies for this application are currently under way using low-dose external radiation to reduce restenosis of vascular access for AV grafts in hemodialysis patients. Other studies using a centering device to deliver an accurate homogeneous dose of radiation following PTA are currently under design.

More recently, a new study was initiated utilizing endovascular radiation therapy for the prevention of restenosis following TIPS for patients with portal hypertension. Overall, the restenosis rate attributable to intimal hyperplasia of TIPS at 6 months has been reported as high as 70%. Complete thrombosis as early as 2 weeks after the procedure also has been reported (43). Over the long term, brachytherapy may be the best means of preventing occlusion for these patients.

Other potential targets for vascular brachytherapy include renal arteries and subclavian vein stenosis.

LIMITATIONS TO BRACHYTHERAPY

Although clinical trials using vascular brachytherapy for both coronary and peripheral applications have demonstrated positive results in reducing restenosis rates, these trials also identified two major complications related to the technology: late thrombosis and edge stenosis effects seen at the edges of radiation treatment segments. Late thrombosis is probably due to the delay in healing associated with radiation. It has been estimated that late thrombosis can be remedied through the prolonged administration of antiplatelet therapy following intervention.

Identified as a major limitation to radioactive stents and explained earlier ("Radiation Systems for the Peripheral Vascular System: Radioactive Stents"), the edge-effect phenomenon is not exclusive to stented lesions. The incidence of edge effect also has been known to occur with catheter-based systems that use both beta and gamma emitters, especially when the treated area is not covered with wide enough margins. The main explanation for the incidence of edge effect is a combination of low doses at the edges of the radiation source and injury created by the device for intervention, which is not covered by the radiation source. It is hypothesized that wider radiation margins of radiation treatment to the intervening segment may eliminate or significantly reduce the edge effect seen so far in all radiation trials.

CONCLUSION

Despite new technologies and devices, restenosis remains the major limitation of intervention in the peripheral vascular system, including AV dialysis. The results from preliminary studies demonstrate that radiation has the potential to alter the rate of restenosis following intervention. With the progression of these studies and their promising results, the use of vascular brachytherapy will dramatically change the practice of peripheral intervention, resulting in an improved long-term patency for our patients.

REFERENCES

1. Tripuraneni P. Catheter-based radiotherapy for peripheral vascular restenosis. *Vascular Radiotherapy Monitor* 1999;1:70–77.
2. Haude M, Erbel R, Issa H, et al. Quantitative analysis of elastic recoil after balloon angioplasty and after intracoronary implantation of balloon-expandable Palmaz-Schatz stents. *J Am Coll Cardiol* 1993;21:26–34.
3. Consigny PM, Bilder GE. Expression and release of smooth muscle cell mitogens in arterial wall after balloon angioplasty. *J Vasc Med Biol* 1993;4:1–8.
4. Mintz GS, Popma JJ, Pichard AD, et al. Arterial remodeling after coronary angioplasty: a serial intravascular ultrasound study. *Circulation* 1996;94:35–43.
5. Isner JM. Vascular remodeling. Honey, I think I shrunk the artery. *Circulation* 1994;89:2937–2941.
6. Murray RR Jr, Hewews RC, White RI Jr, et al. Long-segment femoro-popliteal stenoses: is angioplasty a boon or a bust? *Radiology* 1987;162:473–476.
7. Johnston KW. Femoral and popliteal arteries: re-analyzes of results of balloon angioplasty. *Radiology* 1992;183:767–771.
8. Vroegindeweij D, Kemper FJ, Teilbeek AV, et al. Recurrence of stenosis following balloon angioplasty and Simpson atherectomy of the femoropoplilteal segment: a randomized comparative 1 year follow-up study using color flow duplex. *Eur J Vasc Surg* 1992;6:164–171.
9. Rees CR, Palmaz JC, Becker GJ, et al. Palmaz stent in atherosclerotic stenosis involving the ostia of the renal arteries: preliminary report of a multicenter study. *Radiology* 1991;181:507–514.
10. Hunink MFM, Magruder CD, Meyerovitz MF, et al. Risks and benefits of femoropopliteal percutaneous balloon angioplasty. *J Vasc Surg* 1993;17:183–194.
11. White GF, Liew SC, Waugh RC, et al. Early outcome of intermediate follow-up of vascular stents in the femoral and popliteal arteries without long term anticoagulation. *J Vasc Surg* 1995;21:279–281.
12. Kotb MM, Kadir S, Bennett JD, et al. Aortoiliac angioplasty: is there a need for other types of percutaneous intervention. *JVIR* 1992;3:67–71.
13. Dolmath BL, Gray RJ, Horton KM, Rundback JH, Kline ME. Treatment of anastomotic bypass graft stenosis with directional atherectomy: short term and intermediate-term results. *J Vasc International Radiology* 1995;6:105–113.
14. Johnston KW. Femoral and popliteal arteries: reanalysis of results of angioplasty. *Radiology* 1987;162:473–476.

15. KA Robinson. Arterial biologic response to ionizing radiation. In: Waksman R, Bonan R, eds. *Vascular brachytherapy: state of the art.* London: Remedica Publishing, 1999;15–24.

16. Hillegass WB, Ohman EM, Califf RM. Restenosis: the clinical issues. In: Topol EJ, ed. *Textbook of interventional cardiology,* 2nd ed. vol 1. Philadelphia: WB Saunders, 1994;415–435.

17. Pickering JG, Weir L, Jekanowski J, et al. Proliferative activity in peripheral and coronary atherosclerotic plaques among patients undergoing percutaneous revascularization. *J Clin Invest* 1993; 91:1469–1480.

18. Strandness DE, Barnes RW, Katzen B, et al. Indiscriminate use of laser angioplasty. *Radiology* 1989;172:945–946.

19. Waksman R, Robinson KA, Crocker IR, et al. Long term efficacy and safety of endovascular low dose irradiation in a swine model of restenosis after angioplasty. *Circulation* 1995;91:1533–1539.

20. Weidermann JG, Marboe C, Amols H, et al. Intracoronary irradiation markedly reduces restenosis after balloon angioplasty in a porcine model. *J Am Coll Cardiol* 1994;23:1491–1498.

21. Weiderman JG, Marboe C, Amols H, et al. Intracoronary irradiation markedly reduces neointimal proliferation after balloon angioplasty in swine: persistent benefit at 6-month follow-up. *J Am Coll Cardiol* 1995;25:1456–1461.

22. Mazur W, Ali MN, Dabhagi SF, et al. High dose rate intracoronary radiation suppresses neointimal proliferation in the stented and balloon model of porcine restenosis. *Int J Radiat Oncol Biol Phys* 1996;36:777–788.

23. Borok TL, Bray M, Sinclair I, et al. Role of ionizing irradiation for keloids. *Int J Radiat Oncol Biol Phys* 1988;15:865–870.

24. Van den Brenk HAS, Minty CCJ. Radiation in the management of keloids and hypertorphic scar. *Br J Surg* 1959/1960;47:595–605.

25. Nickson JJ, Lawrence W, Rachwalsky I, et al. Roentgen rays and wound healing: fractionated irradiation: experimental study. *Surgery* 1953;34:859–862.

26. Insalsingh CHA. An experience ein treating 501 patients with keloids. *Johns Hopkins Med J* 1974;134:284–290.

27. Grillo HC, Potsaid MS. Studies in wound healing. *Ann Surg* 1961;154:741.

28. MacLennon I, Keys HM, Evarts CM, Rubgin P. Usefulness of post-operative hip irradiation in the prevention of heterotrophic bone formation in a high risk group of patients. *Int J Radia Oncol Biol Phys* 1984;10:49–53.

29. Van den Brenk HAS. Results of prophylactice post-operative irradiation in 1300 cases of pterygium. *AJR* 1968;103:723.

30. Mintz GS, Pichard AD, Kent KM, et al. Endovascular stents reduce restenosis by eliminating geometric arterial remodeling: a serial intravascular ultrasound study. *J Am Coll Cardiol* 1995;35A:701–705.

31. Waksman R, Rodriquez JC, Robinson KA, et al. Effect of intravascular irradiation on cell proliferation, apoptosis and vascular remodeling after balloon overstretch injury of porcine coronary arteries. *Circulation* 1996;96:1944–1952.

32. Liermann DD, Bottcher HD, Kollath J, et al. Prophylactic endovascular radiotherapy to prevent intimal hyperplasia after stent implantation in femoropopliteal arteries. *Cardiovasc Intervent Radiol* 1994;17:12–16.

33. Waksman R, Crocker IA, Kikeri D, et al. Long term results of endovascular radiation therapy for prevention of restenosis in the peripheral vascular system. *Circulation* 1996;94I-300:1745.

34. Minar E, Pokrajac B, Maca T, et al. Endovascular brachytherapy for prophylaxis of restenosis after femoropopliteal angioplasty: results of a prospective randomized study. *Circulation* 2000;102:2694–2699.

35. Sacks D, Marinelli DL, Martin LG, et al. General principles for evaluation of new interventional technologies and devices: Technology Assessment Committee. *J Vasc Interv Radiol* 1997;8:133–136.

36. Sacks D, Marinelli DL, Martin LG, et al. Reporting standards for clinical evaluation of new peripheral arterial revascularization devices: Technology Assessment Committee. *J Vasc Interv Radiol* 1997;8:137–149.

37. Waksman R, Laird JR, Jurkovitz CT, et al. Intravascular radiation therapy after balloon angioplasty of narrowed femoropopliteal arteries to prevent restenosis: results of the PARIS Feasibility Clinical Trial. *J Vasc Interv Radiol* 2001;12: 915–921.

38. Parikh S, Nori D. Radiation therapy to prevent stenosis of peripheral vascular accesses. *Semin Radiat Oncol* 1999;9:144–154.

39. Gray RJ, Dolmatch BL, Buick MK. Directional atherectomy treatment for hemodialysis access: early results. *J Vasc Interv Radiol* 1992;3:497–503.

40. Kanterman RY, Vesely TM, Pilgram TK, et al. Dialysis access grafts: anatomic location of venous stenosis and results of angioplasty. *Radiology* 1995;195:135–139.

41. Cohen GS, Freeman H, Ringold MA, et al. External beam irradiation as an adjunctive treatment in failing dialysis shunts. *J Vasc Interv Radiol* 2000;11:321–326

42. Trerotola SO, Carmody TJ, Timmerman RD. Brachytherapy for the prevention of stenosis in a canine hemodialysis graft model: preliminary observations. *Radiology* 1999;212:748–754.

43. Raat H, Stockx L, Ranschaert E, et al. Percutaneous hydrodynamic Thrombectomy of acute thrombosis in transjugular intrahepatic portosystemic shunt (TIPS): a feasibility study in five patients *Cardiovasc Intervent Radiol* 1997;20:180–183.

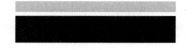

SUBJECT INDEX

SUBJECT INDEX

Page numbers ending in "f" refer to figures. Page numbers ending in "t" refer to tables.